Spine Technology Handbook

Spine Technology Handbook

Dr. Steven M. Kurtz

Dr. Avram Allan Edidin

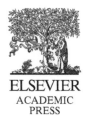

ELSEVIER
ACADEMIC
PRESS

AMSTERDAM • BOSTON • HEIDELBERG • LONDON
NEW YORK • OXFORD • PARIS • SAN DIEGO
SAN FRANCISCO • SINGAPORE • SYDNEY • TOKYO

Academic Press is an imprint of Elsevier
30 Corporate Drive, Suite 400, Burlington, MA 01803, USA
525 B Street, Suite 1900, San Diego, California 92101-4495, USA
84 Theobald's Road, London WC1X 8RR, UK

This book is printed on acid-free paper. ♾

Library of Congress Cataloging-in-Publication Data
Application Submitted

British Library Cataloguing-in-Publication Data
A catalogue record for this book is available from the British Library.

ISBN 13: 978-0-12-369390-7
ISBN 10: 0-12-369390-X

For information on all Academic Press publications
visit our Web site at www.books.elsevier.com

Printed and bound by CPI Group (UK) Ltd, Croydon, CR0 4YY

Transferred to Digital Print 2011

"To myself I am only a child playing on the beach, while vast oceans of truth lie undiscovered before me."

Sir Isaac Newton

Editors' Dedications:

To Katie, Peter, Michael, Sophia, and Andrew Kurtz for their patience during the time I worked on this little project.

To my wife, Cathleen, and my daughter, Alex, for their love and support as this challenge moved from conceptual kernel to finished work. And, to my parents, Profs. Michael and Ruth Edidin, for instilling in me a love of inquiry and science from an early age.

Contents

Contributors

Steven M. Kurtz
Exponent, Inc.
Drexel University
Philadelphia, PA

Avram Allan Edidin
Drexel University
Philadelphia, PA

Stanley A. Brown
Research Biomaterials Engineer
Office of Science and Engineering
  laboratories
Center for Devices and Radiological
  Health
U.S. Food and Drug Administration

Heather Anne L. Guerin
Department of Mechanical
  Engineering and Applied
  Mechanics
Department of Orthopaedic Surgery
University of Pennsylvania
  Philadelphia, PA

Dawn M. Elliott
McKay Orthopaedic Research
  Laboratory
University of Pennsylvania
  Philadelphia, PA

Tony M. Keaveny
Orthopaedic Biomechanics
  Laboratory, Department of
  Mechanical Engineering
Department of Bioengineering
The University of California,
  Berkeley, CA

Jenni M. Buckley
Orthopaedic Biomechanics
  Laboratory, Department of
  Mechanical Engineering
The University of California,
  Berkeley, CA

Peter A. Cripton
Shannon G. Reed
Amy Saari
Division of Orthopaedic Engineering
  Research
Departments of Mechanical
  Engineering and Orthopaedics
University of British Columbia
Vancouver, B.C.

Vijay K. Goel
Koichi Sairyo
Sri Lakshmi Vishnubhotla
Ashok Biyani
Nabil Ebraheim
Spine Research Center, Department
  of Bioengineering, University of
  Toledo, and Department of
  Orthopedic
Surgery, Medical University of Ohio,
  Toledo, Ohio

Marta L. Villarraga
Exponent, Inc.
Drexel University
Philadelphia, PA

Bill McKay
Steve Peckham
Jeff Scifert
Medtronic Sofamor Danek
Memphis, TN

Michele S. Marcolongo
Marco Cannella
Department of Materials Science and
    Engineering
Drexel University Philadelphia, PA

Christopher J. Massey
Department of Mechanical
    Engineering and Mechanics
Drexel University Philadelphia, PA

Karen Talmadge
Executive Vice President, Co-
    Founder and Chief Science Officer
Kyphon Inc., Sunnyvale, CA

Jove Graham
Mechanical Engineer, Office of
    Science and Engineering
    Laboratories, Center for Devices
    and Radiological Health, Food and
    Drug Administration

Chris Espinosa
Exponent, Inc.
Menlo Park, CA

Anton Bowden
Exponent, Inc.
Drexel University
Philadelphia, PA

Janice M. Hogan
Hogan & Hartson, LLP
Philadelphia, PA

Jordana Schmier
Michael Halpern
Exponent, Inc.
Alexandria, VA

Preface

This book is geared toward bioengineers inclined to the historical and contemporary study of spine implant technology. Of great value to the practicing clinician, the book is authored by spine implant experts and allied professionals, and is also of interest to the general bioengineering audience. To focus on current spine technologies we have intentionally restricted the scope of the book to topics that have some track record in the peer-reviewed literature. Newer technologies in this rapidly evolving field, such as facet replacement and dynamic posterior instrumentation, are still under development and thus outside the scope of our review. Nonetheless, we have strived to make the book a valuable reference for bioengineers working on the newest technologies.

Our strategy when developing the scope for this book was first to cover bioengineering fundamentals, followed by detailed review of current spine implant technologies, including key activities required to bring new devices to market. To achieve both the desired breadth and necessary depth in each of the selected topics, we have recruited leading experts in the field. We thus wish to profoundly thank the authors who took time away from their research, teaching, and professional duties to contribute to this book.

—*Steven Michael Kurtz, Ph.D.*
Avram Allan Edidin, Ph.D.
January 2006

Chapter 1

The Basic Tools and Terminology of Spine Treatment

S. M. Kurtz[1,2] and A. A. Edidin
(1) Exponent, Inc., Philadelphia, PA
(2) Drexel University, Philadelphia, PA

1.1 Introduction

Technology-based therapies form the foundation of modern spinal disorder treatments. Such therapies may be pharmaceutical, biological, or mechanical, but they are all primarily focused on relieving chronic, intractable back pain. While specific modalities are effective to a degree, the aggregate spine disease treatment remains problematic in that there are few clear technological solutions that can completely alleviate chronic back pain, especially when due to advanced disc degeneration. In the late stages of spine degenerative disease, implant technology has shown potential to relieve some, but not all, back pain.

Early intervention with new spine implant technologies has the potential to mitigate and possibly forestall the painful cascade of degenerative changes that occur with age. One must therefore approach spine implants today with the understanding that the new implant technologies have not reached full maturity. As such, the field of spine implant technology geared toward earlier intervention in the degenerative disc cascade is effectively a new field that is evolving rapidly around the world.

The primary standard treatment for intractable back pain unresponsive to nonsurgical treatment is decompression and fusion, which consists of immobilizing the spine using bone graft, metal plates or rods, and screws. Because fusion is irreversible and stops all motion at the implanted level, it can be perceived as an end-stage procedure, naturally opening the door to many earlier-stage motion-preserving technologies for treating the diseased spine. Motion-preservation technologies cover a wide range of techniques, including nucleus repair, total disc replacement, and vertebral fracture repair. Novel motion-preserving technologies, many of which are still under design, will require innovative implants and instruments for deployment in the body.

Although treating chronic, intractable back pain is the underlying motivation for creating and developing new spine implants, the origins and causes of such pain are complex, involving organic disease, as well as psychological and societal factors. Because of the psychosocial aspect of back pain, simply treating the organic disease does not necessarily imply that a patient's pain symptoms will be totally alleviated. The magnitude of the psychosocial aspect of back pain distinguishes spine surgical intervention markedly from other elective procedures, such as hip or knee replacement.

The typical candidate for total joint replacement is elderly, greater than 65 years in age, and has retired from his or her professional activities [NIH 1994; NIH 2003]. Therefore, at least in North America, the hip or knee replacement patient typically has a remaining life expectancy of one or two decades. Joint replacements are, by and large, successful and durable procedures [NIH 1994; NIH 2003]. In the elderly patient population, for example, hip and knee replacement survival rates typically exceed 90% after 10 years [NIH 1994; NIH 2003].

Candidates for spine surgery are typically middle aged (i.e., less than 65 years) and still working. The national demographics for patients in the United States receiving a fusion at any level of the spine are summarized in Figure 1.1. These patients have many remaining decades of life expectancy, placing extraordinary design requirements on a load-bearing implant design, as it must remain *in vivo* for a long period of time. Chronic back pain can be severe and debilitating, and patients may be effectively incapacitated by the time they are ready to consider spine surgery as a viable option. During a recent clinical trial for total disc replacement, for example, 29 out of 39 (74%) surgical candidates were already taking narcotic medication for pain management [Zigler 2004].

Treatment of patients is the provenance of physicians, whereas the creation of tools and instruments is the traditional purview of engineers. When the tools and instruments are intended to modify or enhance parts of the human body, they are designed by bioengineers. The fields of medicine and bioengineering are intertwined and mutually interdependent. For this reason, bioengineering should not be considered subordinate to medicine, or vice versa. The fields mutually enhance and reinforce. Even the most perfectly conceived implant solution could have disastrous results if it is implanted for the wrong reason, in the wrong patient, or in the wrong location.

Spine implant technology provides a unique and important motivation for studying bioengineering. Beginning in the 1970s and 1980s, bioengineering played a fundamental role in the development of orthopedic hip and knee implants, to great clinical and commercial success. By the late 1990s, orthopedic bioengineering reached a period of stable, predictable growth (Figure 1.2).

Demographics for U.S. Patients Receiving Spine Fusions

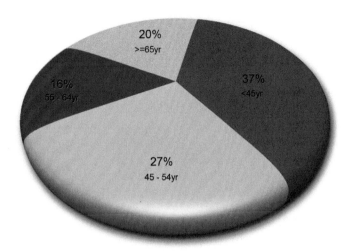

Fig. 1.1.

Patient demographics (gender, age) for fusion procedures in the United States (2003). *(Data source: National Hospital Discharge Survey. Courtesy of Kevin Ong, Exponent, Inc.)*

On the other hand, the expansion of spine implant technologies has been comparatively explosive, with the global market for spine implants growing at an expected rate exceeding 20% per year at the start of the twenty-first century (Figure 1.2). Between 1990 and 2003, the total number of primary cervical and lumbar fusion procedures in the United States alone grew from 121,400 to 281,300, representing an increase of 170% (Figure 1.3). For motion-preserving alternatives to fusion, researchers have predicted the creation of a new $2 billion market by 2010 [Singh 2004]. There is, and will continue to be, a strong demand for bioengineering talent among the producers of spine implant technology.

The thrust of this book is to provide a foundation of concepts, principles, and data crucial to bioengineers for the design, development, and clinical deployment of new spine implant technologies. The bioengineer is responsible for materials selection, component design, and testing of promising new implants. Once a promising device is developed, its release is subject to the stipulations of multiple regulatory agencies. In addition, an important consideration is the payer. In the United States this is usually private insurance or a federal program, such as Medicare or Medicaid. As a result, the successful introduction of a new spine implant technology in the clinic depends on the complex interplay among engineering, design, materials science, regulation, and health care economics. This book reviews these topics to provide a broad perspective to the engineer considering a career in spine implant development. In this chapter, we review the basic terminology and anatomy underlying the structure and function of the spine.

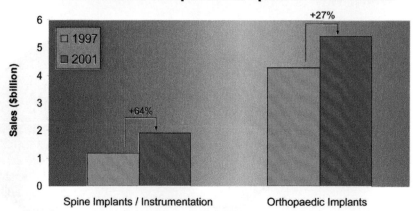

Fig. 1.2.

Growth of the global market for spine implant technology relative to other segments of the ortho-pedic market. *(Data source: 1999–2000 Medical & Healthcare Marketplace Guide, edited by R. C. Smith, M. A. Geier, J. Reno, and J. Sarasohn-Kahn. New York: IDD Enterprises, L.P., 1998. Courtesy of Christo-pher Espinosa, Exponent, Inc.)*

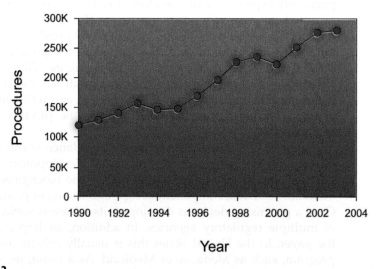

Fig. 1.3.

Primary cervical and lumbar fusion procedures in the United States (1990 to 2003). *(Data source: National Hospital Discharge Survey. Courtesy of Kevin Ong, Exponent, Inc.)*

1.2 Which Way Is Up?

Physicians visualize and operate in terms of both global and anatomical reference frames. To design implants and communicate with surgeons, it is most efficient to adopt a clinical vocabulary not only for anatomical locations but also for anatomic directions. Anatomic reference directions are illustrated in Figure 1.4.

Consider a right-handed coordinate frame, which is centered in a standing person's center of gravity (located near the center of the pelvis). In anatomic coordinates, the vertical direction is *superior*; the downward direction is *inferior*. *Anterior* refers to the front of the human body, whereas *posterior* points toward the back. The person's left and right should be self-explanatory, but both are considered *lateral* to the body. In anatomic terms, the *medial* direction is toward the middle of the body.

People do not spend all of the their time standing, so a more specific vocabulary in local anatomic coordinates is needed. With respect to limbs, for

Anatomic Reference Directions

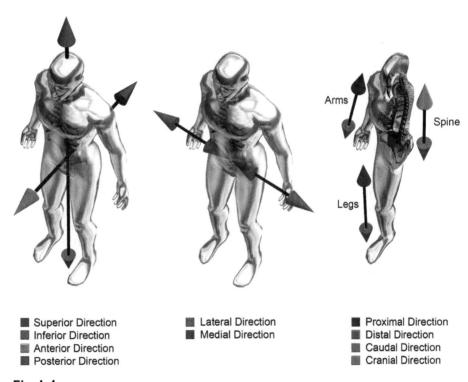

■ Superior Direction
■ Inferior Direction
■ Anterior Direction
■ Posterior Direction

■ Lateral Direction
■ Medial Direction

■ Proximal Direction
■ Distal Direction
■ Caudal Direction
■ Cranial Direction

Fig. 1.4.

Anatomic reference directions. *(Courtesy of Christopher Espinosa, Exponent, Inc.)*

Motions of the Spine

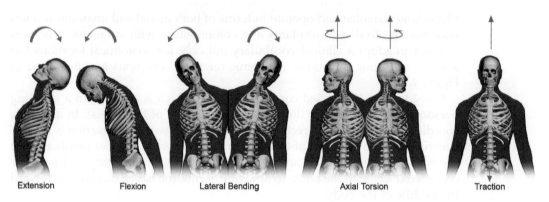

Extension   Flexion   Lateral Bending   Axial Torsion   Traction

Fig. 1.5.
Anatomic terms used to describe the motions of the spine. *(Courtesy of Christopher Espinosa, Exponent, Inc.)*

instance, *proximal* refers to the region closest to the body, whereas *distal* is the furthest away. In the spine, *caudal* means in the direction "toward the tail," and *cranial*, or cephalad, means "toward the cranium, or head."

Finally, additional anatomic terms are used to describe the kinematic motions of the spine. These include *flexion* (bending anteriorly), *extension* (bending posteriorly), *lateral bending*, and *axial torsion* (Figure 1.5). Application of axial displacement to the spine is termed *distraction* instead of tension.

1.3 The Spine

The spine is a complex structure with hard and soft tissue constituents. The bones of the spine, the *vertebrae*, are the hard elements of the structure. They also protect the vulnerable spinal cord and emanating nerves. The structure and function of the vertebrae vary somewhat along the length of the spine. In general, however, each vertebral body consists of an anterior portion that is optimized for sustaining compressive loads and posterior elements that are optimized for protection of the spinal cord while facilitating motion by providing anchorage for muscle attachments.

Between the vertebral bodies, the *intervertebral discs* form a viscoelastic cushion to distribute and attenuate forces with concomitant flexibility. The aggregate spinal column is tied together by ligaments and actuated by muscles. These soft tissues are the subject of Chapter 3, whereas the vertebrae are detailed in Chapter 4.

The spine is divided into *cervical*, *thoracic*, *lumbar*, and *sacral* regions. The seven *cervical vertebrae* of the neck provide maximum flexibility and range of

Regions of the Spine

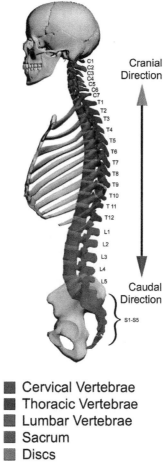

- ▣ Cervical Vertebrae
- ▣ Thoracic Vertebrae
- ▣ Lumbar Vertebrae
- ▣ Sacrum
- ▣ Discs

Fig. 1.6.

Cervical, thoracic, lumbar, and sacral regions of the spine. *(Courtesy of Christopher Espinosa, Exponent, Inc.)*

motion for the head. These vertebrae are designated C1 through C7 in the cranial-to-caudal direction (Figure 1.6). The underside of the cranium, where it attaches to the spine, is designated C0. The discs are identified based on their adjacent vertebral bodies (e.g., C1-C2 for the disc between C1 and C2).

The 12 *thoracic vertebrae* (T1 through T12) support the ribs and the organs that hang from them (Figure 1.6). In the thoracic region, the vertebral bodies are optimized for a combination of structural support and flexibility.

Caudal to the thoracic region, the five *lumbar vertebrae* (L1 through L5) are subjected to the highest forces and moments of the spine (Figure 1.6).

Consequently, they are largest and strongest of the vertebral bodies. These bones are optimized for structural support as opposed to flexibility.

The *sacrum* attaches the spine (at L5-S1) to the illiac bones of the pelvis (at the sacroilliac joint) (Figure 1.6). The coccyx is located inferior to the sacrum, at the most caudal region of the spine. The bones of the coccyx are thought to be the vestiges of a tail, and hence its reference as the "tail bone."

1.4 Overview of the Handbook

This book is intended to serve as a primary text for an undergraduate bioengineering course focused on the spine. The book is divided into three principal sections: Part I covers the fundamentals of spine bioengineering, Part II reviews the historical and current applications of spine technology, and Part III outlines the principal steps of developing a new spine implant technology. Part II is sufficiently detailed so as to serve as the basis for a graduate course in spine implants. Parts II and III, in particular, are also intended as references for engineers and scientists working with spine implants.

The fundamentals section of the text, Part I, presupposes two years of engineering fundamentals. The first six chapters cover, from an introductory perspective: synthetic biomaterials (Chapter 2), the soft and hard tissues of the spine (Chapters 3 and 4), and spine biomechanics (Chapter 5). The properties and geometry of these structures vary considerably from person to person and are further altered by trauma and disease (Chapter 6).

Part II of the text covers spine implant technologies that are well established or currently in the advanced stages of clinical trials. The historical development of spine fusion technology, and current implant concepts, are reviewed in Chapters 7 and 8, respectively. Chapter 9 is devoted to biologic technologies for spine repair. Chapters 10 and 11 describe two different modalities of current motion-preserving technologies intended to treat early and late intervertebral disc degeneration, respectively: disc repair and total disc replacement. Chapter 12 summarizes percutaneous vertebral fracture repair technologies, including vertebroplasty and kyphoplasty.

Part III of the text provides guidance on the process of assessment and commercialization of new spine implant technologies. Some of the unique aspects of spine implant testing are summarized in Chapter 13. Chapter 14 describes the application of finite element methods to spine implants. Chapter 15 reviews the regulatory process for obtaining approval of spine implants in the United States, and Chapter 16 provides an introduction to economic (cost/benefit) assessment of spine implants.

Understanding the properties and limitations of synthetic as well as natural biomaterials is crucial for bioengineers who intend to design future generations of spine implants. Therefore, the second chapter reviews the properties of polymers, metals, and ceramics from which today's spine implants are currently fabricated.

1.5 Acknowledgments

The authors are grateful to Christopher Espinosa and Dr. Kevin Ong of Exponent, Inc., for providing the illustrations for this chapter.

1.6 References

NIH (1994). *NIH Consensus Statement: Total Hip Replacement.* National Institutes of Health Technology Assessment Conference. *http://consensus.nih.gov/1994/1994HipReplacement098html.htm.*

NIH (2003). *NIH Consensus Statement: Total Knee Replacement.* National Institutes of Health Technology Assessment Conference. *http://consensus.nih.gov/2003/2003TotalKneeReplacement117html.htm.*

Singh, K., A. R. Vaccaro, and T. J. Albert (2004). "Assessing the Potential Impact of Total Disc Arthroplasty on Surgeon Practice Patterns in North America," *Spine J.* 4:195S–201S.

Zigler, J. E. (2004). "Lumbar Spine Arthroplasty Using the ProDisc II," *Spine J.* 4:260S–7S.

1.5 Acknowledgments

The authors are grateful to Christopher Espinosa and Dr. Kevin Ong of Exponent, Inc. for providing the illustrations for this chapter.

1.6 References

NIH (1994). NIH Consensus Statement: Total Hip Replacement, National Institutes of Health Technology Assessment Conference. http://consensus.nih.gov/1994/1994HipReplacement098html.htm

NIH (2003). NIH Consensus Statement: Total Knee Replacement, National Institutes of Health Technology Assessment Conference. http://consensus.nih.gov/2003/2003TotalKneeReplacement117html.htm

Singh, K., K. Vaccaro, and F.J. Albert (2006), "Assessing the Potential Impact of Total Disc Arthroplasty on Surgeon Practice Patterns in North America," Spine J. 6:199–205.

Zigler, J. (2004). "Lumbar Spine Arthroplasty Using the ProDisc II," Spine J. 4:260S–7S.

Chapter 2

Synthetic Biomaterials for Spinal Applications

S. A. Brown
Food and Drug Administration

2.1 Introduction

The goal of this chapter is to provide introductory material in the rapidly growing area of biomaterials used in the spine. A spinal device may be composed of one or many materials. It is therefore important to understand the nature of each material in the device, in that if one material is inappropriate the entire device may fail either from adverse biological reactions or material failure. The interaction between a medical device and the host tissues involves a number of material properties. The physical presence of a device alters that local tissue site. Corrosion, degradation, or wear can produce by-products that stimulate an adverse reaction. Therefore, selection of materials must be made with an understanding of these complex interactions. As will be discussed in later chapters, the response of tissues to biomaterials is a function of the mechanical properties of the materials and the tissues to which they are attached. Therefore, discussion of properties of materials in this chapter is often relative to the properties of bone.

The chemical and physical properties of the synthetic materials discussed, as well as the methods for determining these properties, are described by international standards. There are a significant number of organizations developing standards. The primary references used in this chapter are those developed by the American Society for Testing and Materials International (ASTM International), which are published annually. An alphanumeric nomenclature is used for designation of ASTM standards, where the letter indicates the type of standard and the number is assigned sequentially as developed. Those developed by committee F04 on Medical and Surgical Materials and Devices have designations beginning with the letter F and are published in Volume 13.01. A somewhat parallel set of standards has been published by the International Standards Organization (ISO).

2.2 Mechanical Properties and Mechanical Testing

2.2.1 Tensile Testing

Some basic terminology regarding the mechanical properties of materials is necessary for a discussion of materials and their interactions with biological tissues. The most common way to determine mechanical properties is to pull a specimen apart and measure the force and deformation. Standardized test protocols have been developed by ASTM International for a variety of materials, such as E8 for metals or D412 for rubber and plastic materials [ASTM 2006a; ASTM 2006b]. Tensile testing is done with a "dog bone" shaped specimen, the large ends of which are held in some sort of a grip for the narrow midsection to serve as the test section. The midportion is marked as the "gage length," where deformation is measured. A mechanical test machine will use rotating screws or hydraulics to stretch the specimen. Force is measured in Newtons (N), and how much the specimen stretches (deformation) is measured in millimeters. Because specimens of different dimensions can be tested, one must normalize the measurements to be independent of size. Stress σ (N/m^2 or Pascals) is calculated as force divided by the original cross-sectional area, whereas strain ε (%) is calculated as change in length divided by the original length. From these data, stress/strain curves such as those shown in Figure 2.1 are generated. Each of these is discussed in more detail in the respective material sections.

There are a number of material properties that can be determined from these measurements. The "brittle" curve shows a linear relationship between stress and strain and is typical for brittle materials such as ceramics. The slope of this linear region (stress/strain) determines the stiffness of the material and is called the elastic (E) or Young's modulus. The "ductile" curve also has a linear region, but also contains a shoulder (typical of a metallic material). This straight region is known as the elastic portion of the curve. If a small stress is applied to the specimen it will deform elastically, like a rubber band, and will return to its original length when the stress is removed. The shoulder is indicative of the beginning of permanent (plastic) deformation, as will be described subsequently. The onset of permanent deformation—or yield strength (YS)—of the material, is defined as the stress at which the offset is equal to a specified value. For metals, yield is typically defined as 0.2%, whereas a 2% offset is often used for plastics. Figure 2.1 shows a line running parallel to the curve, intersecting at the YS. If the specimen was loaded up to the YS and then unloaded, the stress/strain recording would follow this parallel line, returning to the 0.2% offset or permanent deformation. If a metal is loaded again, the recording will follow this parallel line starting at the offset yield, reaching the upper curve, and continuing to show a gradual increase in stress with increasing strain. This

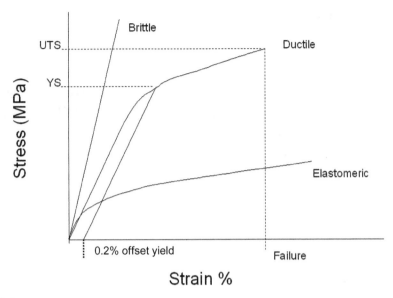

Fig. 2.1.

Typical stress/strain curve for a brittle, a ductile, and a plastic (elastomeric) material.

is known as the plastic region of the curve. Eventually, the ductile metal breaks at the ultimate tensile strength (UTS), and the percent elongation to failure can be determined. Plastic and elastomeric materials deform extensively, like the curve labeled elastomeric.

The area under these curves is force times distance, has units of energy, and is called toughness. The brittle material will absorb much less energy prior to failure than the ductile material. Hit a piece of glass with a hammer and it will shatter; hit a piece of metal and it will bend or deform. The amount of energy absorbed (or toughness) of the plastic/elastomeric material depends on how much it elongates prior to failure.

The properties of a number of common materials are shown in Table 2.1. In general, metals are strong and tough, whereas ceramics are more rigid or stiffer but brittle. Polymers have a lower modulus and are thus softer, and are weaker than metals and ceramics, but often have much higher elongations to failure. Polymer composites are stronger and stiffer, but less ductile. Bone is a composite of brittle ceramic crystallites of hydroxyapatite and tough collagen fibers. Metals are typically ten times stiffer than bone, whereas polymers are much less stiff than bone.

2.2.2 Other Types of Mechanical Testing

Materials are also tested according to other standards, by crushing them in compression or in flexion. The terminology is essentially the same; only the mathematics are different. Compression testing is done by placing a specimen

Table 2.1.

Mechanical properties of some materials. Literature values or minimum values from standards. Strength is measured in tension, except where "fl" indicates the material is testing in flexion.

	Yield (MPa)	UTS (MPa)	Elong. (%)	Modulus (GPa)
Stainless steel alloys				
F138 annealed	170	480	40	200
F138 cold worked	690	860	12	200
F138 wire	—	1,035	15	200
F1586 N strengthened, hard	1,000	1,100	10	193
F2229 low nickel, cold worked	1,241	1,379	12	200
Cobalt alloys				
F75, cast	450	655	8	200
F1537 annealed CoCrMo	517	897	20	240
F1537 hot-worked CoCrMo	700	1,000	12	240
F1537 warm-worked CoCrMo	827	1,192	12	240
Titanium alloys				
F67-1 CPTi	170	240	24	103
F67-4 CPTi	483	550	15	104
F136 Ti 6Al, 4V ELI	795	860	10	114
F1472 Ti 6Al 4V	869	924	8	114
F1295 Ti 6Al, 7Nb	800	900	10	114
F1713 Ti 13Nb, 13Zr	725	860	8	79
F1813, 12Mo, 6 Zr, 2 Fe	897	931	12	80
Ceramics				
F 603 alumina	—	fl 400	0.1	380
F2393 zirconia, (Mg PSZ)		fl 600		180
F1873 zirconia, yttria (Y-TZP)		fl 800		200
LTI pyrolytic carbon		275–500	1.6–2.1	17–28
LTI pyrolytic carbon + 5–12% Si		550–620	2.0	28–31
PAN AS4 fiber	—	3,980	1.65	240

Table 2.1. *Continued*

	Yield (MPa)	UTS (MPa)	Elong. (%)	Modulus (GPa)
Polymers				
PEEK		93	50	3.6
PMMA cast		45–75	1.3	2–3
Acetal (POM)		65	40	3.1
UHMWPE		30	200	0.5
Silicone rubber		7	800	0.03
Composites				
PEEK 61% C fiber, long		2,130	1.4	125
PEEK 61% C fiber, +– 45		300	17.2	47
PEEK 30% C fiber, chopped		208	1.3	17
Biologic tissues				
Hydroxyapatite (HA) mineral		100	0.001	114–130
Bone (cortical)		80–150	1.5	18–20
Collagen		50		1.2

between two flat plates. When a specimen is tested in compression, it generally becomes larger in diameter (cross section) and is compressed. This can produce an artifact due to the movement between the specimen and the plates. There will also be a point after which the increase in load is no longer related to the strength of the specimen. Compression testing is often done with soft polymers, or those difficult to fabricate in tensile specimens. Compressive strength is also an important parameter for devices subjected to in service compressive stresses, such as PMMA bone cement.

Flexural testing is done with specimens—typically flat, rectangular bars suspended between two vertical uprights. A bending force is applied in the middle of the span either at a single contact in the middle of the span or with a pair of contacts centered over the middle. With three-point bending, the stress is maximal under the contact. Four-point bending applies a uniform stress between the loading contacts. In either case, flexural testing applies a tensile stress to the underside of the specimen, whereas the upper surface is in compression.

Fracture toughness is another material property that can be determined by a number of standard methods in tension or bending. Typically the specimen is notched. The rate of crack propagation is measured and the energy absorbed to failure is determined. Fracture toughness testing produces numerical data that are related to the more empirical toughness values one could estimate by integrating the area under a stress/strain curve.

Although not directly available from a stress/strain curve, the strength of a material can be related to its hardness. Stronger materials are typically harder. Hardness is tested by measuring the indentation caused by a sharp object dropped on the material's surface with a known force. Hardness is perhaps the most important property when considering a material's wear resistance.

An additional property, which is not depicted in Figure 2.1, is the fatigue strength or endurance limit of a material. If the material as tested in Figure 2.1 has been loaded to the YS and unloaded, it has been permanently deformed. If this is repeated several times, like bending a paper clip back and forth, eventually it will break. If, however, the metal is loaded only within the elastic region, and then unloaded, it is not deformed or broken. If it is loaded again and unloaded, it still will not break. For some metals, there is a stress level below which the part can theoretically be loaded and unloaded an infinite number of times without failure. In reality, a fatigue limit is defined at a specified number of cycles, such as 10^6 or 10^7. Clearly, fatigue strength is a critical property in the design of load-bearing devices such as total hips, which are loaded on average a million times a year, or heart valves that are loaded 40 million times a year.

Relative motion between parts can cause mechanical damage and release of small particles due to wear. There are several mechanisms that are applicable to biomedical applications. The surface of an implanted material is not perfectly smooth on a microscopic scale, but rather has small protrusions or asperities on the surface. Contact is not across the entire surface but is localized to the asperities. Thus, a relatively low contact pressure for the entire surface can actually result in very high local pressures on the asperities. Such localized contact pressures can result in fusion or adhesion between asperities of two surfaces. Subsequent movement tears the asperities off and produces damage due to adhesive wear. These asperities then break off as particulate debris.

When one surface is much harder than the other, abrasive wear may occur where the harder plows into the softer. This is especially likely in three-body wear that occurs when small particles get trapped between the wear surfaces. This is analogous to sandpaper, made with hard abrasive particles. Three-body wear of the metal component in metal-polymer joints can lead to a confounding situation of polymer wear. The hard particles plow into the polymer and cause wear, but they also scratch the metal surface. Because the metals are ductile, scratching will create a trough, with metal pushed up on each side of the trough, like a plow through dirt. These ridges on each side of the scratches probably contribute to a major portion of the subsequent abrasive wear of the polymeric component. In contrast, ceramic materials are not ductile. They may get scratched, resulting in troughs, but they will not plastically deform to form ridges. This may be one reason for the much lower wear rates observed with ceramic-polymer total joints as compared to metal-polymer combinations.

Wear can occur due to fatigue in situations of point loading or with large sliding distances of a smaller component over a larger surface. Consider sliding your fingertip back and forth across the palm of your hand. The fingertip is constantly loaded, but the palm tissue is loaded and then unloaded as the finger passes by. This is analogous to the loading of a tibial component in a total knee replacement. Now think of sticking your finger down in a bowl of Jell-O. Pushing down and up pushes Jell-O aside, back and forth. There is a shear stress under your finger due to the compressive force of pushing. The same is true for the tissue in your palm or the polymeric bearing of the total knee. Repeated loading and unloading causes cyclic shear stress under the contact point. Eventually this may lead to the formation of fatigue cracks parallel to the joint surface. These flake off and produce particulate debris due to fatigue wear.

2.3 Metals and Metal Alloys

2.3.1 Basics of Metallurgy

Metals are composed of atoms held together by metallic bonds, with each atom surrounded by a "cloud" of valence electrons with high mobility. This mobility gives metals good conductivity of electricity and heat. The concept of a phase is important to understanding alloys. A phase is a singular form (composition or structure) of a material. Ice, water, and steam are three phases of H_2O. When molten metals solidify they undergo a phase transformation from liquid to solid. During solidification, atoms take on an orderly array known as a crystal structure, much like salt crystals that form as salty water evaporates or rock candy forms on a string. For example, atoms may arrange themselves with atoms at eight corners of a cube—with one in the middle called body-centered cubic (BCC), or arranged on the faces of the cube called face-centered cubic (FCC). Some metals (such as iron, cobalt, and titanium) will undergo allotropic transformations (changes in crystal structure with changes in temperature). Molten iron solidifies first as BCC, transforms to FCC, and then back to BCC at room temperature. Some phase transformations involve dimensional changes due to the density or packing factor (FCC to BCC results in an increase in volume).

As molten metal solidifies in a mold, solidification will typically begin on the surface of the mold. At each site, atoms will be laid down on the solid in an orderly crystallographic manner. Solidification will continue until two growth areas meet and form a boundary. Each of these growth sites is called a crystal or grain, whereas each boundary is a crystal or grain boundary.

Metallic alloys are mixtures of several elements in a solid solution. For elements of similar atomic charge, diameter, and crystal structure there is no limit to the solubility of one element in another and thus they solidify as a single phase. For example, titanium and zirconium are fully soluble in each other.

Small differences in the diameter of the two (or more) elements in a single-phase alloy or two-phase alloy provide strengthening. The presence of large atoms in a metal of smaller atoms will produce a localized strain in the crystal lattice which will be under localized compression. Similarly, a few small atoms in the interstices between larger atoms will create local stress fields. These localized strains increase the strength of the metal by a mechanism known as solid solution strengthening.

Elements with markedly different properties or crystal structures will have limited solubility. For example, carbon is much smaller than iron. In small quantities, carbon is soluble in iron, but at higher concentrations it will precipitate out as a second phase (such as graphite) or form a carbide. A number of alloy systems utilize the precipitation of second phases as a strengthening mechanism known as precipitation hardening.

Metals deform by stepwise movement of point or line defects known as dislocations. When a metal solidifies, there are few dislocations. If the metal is then mechanically worked (as in pounding or bending), the dislocation density greatly increases. This is the mechanism of plastic deformation of metals. The increased number of dislocations, each with its localized stress field, makes it more difficult to do more plastic deformation. This explains why, as is shown in Figure 2.1, the 0.2% offset reloading curve goes to a higher value prior to experiencing further plastic deformation. With plastic deformation, the metal gets stronger and harder by the mechanism of cold working (or work hardening). If the deformation results in too many dislocations in a particular location, they will coalesce into a crack and the metal will begin to break. By keeping the grain size small, few dislocations can accumulate within a grain, and thus the metal can deform more before it begins to break.

After extensive cold working, the alloy can be heated to anneal or stress relieve it. This results in the formation of new crystals with few dislocations. Controlling the temperature and time can result in a soft, fine-grained metal that can be subsequently cold worked. This is the process used to produce small pieces of metal from a large ingot. Metal can be rolled to form a heavily cold worked but thinner plate. Before it breaks, the metal is annealed to stress relieve it. It is then rolled again. Similarly, bars and wires are formed by repeated drawing and annealing. The effects of cold work can be seen in Table 2.1 for F138 stainless steel in the annealed condition, cold worked, or highly drawn wire [ASTM 2006e]. Similarly, cast F75 is typically large grained [ASTM 2006c]. Minor compositional differences make the alloy a fine-grained heavily cold worked F1537 [ASTM 2006j].

2.3.2 Metallic Corrosion

Corrosion resistance is one of the most important properties of metals used for implants. There are a number of mechanisms by which metals can corrode. Those of most significance to implant applications in aqueous saline solutions are galvanic (or mixed metal) corrosion, crevice corrosion, and fretting corrosion.

Galvanic (or mixed metal) corrosion results when two dissimilar metals in electrical contact are immersed in an electrolyte. The direction of the reaction can be determined by examining the electromotive force (EMF) series. There are four essential components that must exist for a galvanic reaction to occur: an anode where the metal oxidizes ($M \rightarrow M^+ + e^-$), a cathode where the electron is consumed by a reduction reaction ($4e^- + O_2 + 2H_2O \rightarrow 4OH^-$), an electrolyte as a source of reduction species, and an external circuit to conduct the electrons. Iron is more electronegative than copper and when they are connected and immersed in a saltwater bath iron will be anodic and corrode. The *in vivo* environment contains electrolytes, but a patient with two metallic implants made of different alloys is not subject to mixed metal corrosion if the devices are not in contact with each other (i.e., there is no electrical connection).

Galvanic cells occur not only with different alloys but with differences within an alloy. Carbides, grain boundaries, and different phases within an alloy also present differences in EMF and thus the possibility for localized galvanic cells. Cold working also increases the free energy of metal and thus its susceptibility to corrosion.

Crevice corrosion can occur in a confined space exposed to a chloride solution. The space can be in the form of a gasket-type connection between a metal and a nonmetal or two pieces of metal bolted or clamped together. Crevice corrosion involves a number of steps, which may take six months to two years to develop. Initially there is uniform corrosion (oxidation and reduction) on the free surfaces and within the crevice. Restriction of oxygen diffusion due to the confines of the crevice results in oxygen depletion and thus only metal oxidation with release of M^+ in the crevice and flow of e^- to the free surfaces outside the crevice. This electron flow is balanced by an influx of chloride ion Cl^- into the crevice. Metal chlorides hydrolyze in water and dissociate into an insoluble metal hydroxide and a free acid ($M^+Cl^- + H_2O \rightarrow MOH + H^+Cl^-$). This results in an ever-increasing acid concentration in the crevice, drop in pH, and a self-accelerating reaction.

The surgical alloys in use today all owe their corrosion resistance to the formation of stable, passive oxide films. Titanium forms a tenacious oxide, which prevents further corrosion. Stainless steels and cobalt alloys form chromium oxide films. If the film is damaged, as with scratching, the oxide film reforms or repassivates, resulting in restoration of the passive condition.

Fretting corrosion involves continuous disruption of the film due to relative micro-motion between parts. This results in continuous exposure of the underlying metal and results in a continuous corrosion and repassivation. This has been observed in the contact areas between plates and screws used for fracture fixation, as well as in the tapered junctions of modular total joint prostheses.

2.3.3 Stainless Steels

All of these concepts are utilized in designing the alloy systems used for medical devices. Consider stainless steel as an example of how an alloy "can be designed." Steel is an alloy of iron, carbon, and other elements. Carbon will also influence the crystal structure of iron. At room temperature, iron has a BCC crystal structure and is known as α ferrite. With heating, it undergoes a phase transformation to FCC and is known as γ austenite. With further heating, it goes back to BCC (δ ferrite) before it melts. The spaces, or interstices, between atoms are larger in FCC than BCC. Therefore, the smaller carbon atoms fit better in the FCC and thus have a higher solubility in FCC. This has several implications.

To be self-passivating, stainless steels must contain at least 12% chromium. However, carbon has a strong affinity for chromium, and chromium carbides form with the average stoichiometry of $Cr_{23}C_6$. The formation of a carbide results from the migration of chromium atoms from the bulk stainless steel alloy into the carbide. The result is that the carbide has a high chromium content, whereas the alloy surrounding the carbide is depleted in chromium. If the chromium content is depleted and drops below 12% Cr, there is insufficient Cr for effective repassivation and the stainless steel becomes susceptible to corrosion. As a safety factor, surgical stainless contains 17 to 19% chromium and the carbon content in surgical alloys is kept low, at <0.03%.

Nickel is added to the chromium-iron-carbon steel to solve this apparent dilemma. Nickel is FCC; its addition will stabilize the FCC form of iron and keep the carbon in solution. Stainless steel knives, forks, and spoons are typically "18-8" (18% chromium and 8% nickel). "Surgical" stainless steel according to ASTM F138 (as shown in Table 2.2) contains 17 to 19% chromium and 13 to 15.5% nickel (2 to 3% molybdenum are added for improved corrosion resistance and the carbon is low, at <0.03%) [ASTM 2006e]. The result is a nice, homogeneous, single-phase corrosion resistant stainless steel alloy. Although stainless steel has good corrosion resistance, the options for strengthening mechanisms have been limited to only cold working. As is shown in Table 2.1, the mechanical properties of ASTM F138 surgical stainless steel in the annealed condition can be greatly increased by cold working, and are even higher for heavily drawn wire [ASTM 2006e]. While yield and ultimate strength increase, the ductility (elongation) goes down. Cold working makes stainless steel stronger but more brittle.

Stainless steel per ASTM F138 is often also called 316LVM (using the American iron and steel industry nomenclature), with LVM meaning "low vacuum melted" [ASTM 2006e]. This is the most common of the stainless steels used for implants. Two other alloy types have been developed in recent years, as shown in Tables 2.1 and 2.2. One is nitrogen strengthened, such as F1586 [ASTM 2006k]. The addition of 0.25 to 0.5% nitrogen provides interstitial solid solution strengthening, and stabilizes the FCC austenitic phase. The other alloy is F2229, a low nickel alloy developed because of concerns of allergic reactions to nickel (discussed later) [ASTM 2006o]. In this alloy manganese is used rather than nickel to stabilize the austenitic phase.

2.3.4 Cobalt Chromium Alloys

There is a wide class of cobalt alloys, which was initially developed for high-temperature use in jet engines. Those used in surgical applications are alloys

Table 2.2.
Weight percent chemical composition of some stainless steel, cobalt-chromium, and titanium alloys.

	Cr	Ni	Mo	Mn	C	Other	Balance
F138	17–19	13–15	2–3	<2	<0.03		Fe
F1586	19.5–22	9–11	2–3	2–4.5	<0.08	N 0.25–0.5,	Fe
						Nb 0.25–.28	
F2229	19–23	<0.05	0.5–1.5	21–24	<0.08	N 0.85–1.1	Fe
F75	27–30	<1.0	5–7	<1	<0.25	Fe <0.75	Co
F1537-1	26–30	<1.0	5–7	<1.0	<0.14	<1.5 Fe	Co
F1537-2	26–30	<1.0	5–7	<1.0	0.15–0.35	<1.5 Fe	Co

	Al	V	Zr	Nb	Fe	N	C	H	O	Bal.
F67-1					<0.2	<0.03	<0.1	<0.015	<0.18	Ti
F67-4					<0.5	<0.05	<0.1	<0.015	<0.40	Ti
F136	5.5–6.5	3.5–4.5			<0.25	<0.05	<0.08	<0.012	<0.13	Ti
F1472	5.5–6.75	3.5–4.5			<0.30	<0.05	<0.08	<0.015	<0.20	Ti
F1295	5.5–6.5			6.5–7.5	<0.25	<0.05	<0.08	<0.009	<0.2	Ti
F1713			12.5–14	12.5–14	<0.25	<0.05	<0.08	<0.012	<0.15	Ti
F1813		Mo 10–13	5–7		1.5–2.5	<0.05	<0.05	<0.02	0.08–0.28	Ti

of cobalt, chromium, molybdenum, and carbon. The inherent corrosion resistance of cobalt is such that it was once referred to as stellite, the star among the alloys. Like iron, cobalt undergoes phase transformations with cooling. The metallurgy is more complex than that of stainless steels, but suffice it to say that precipitation of chromium carbides is desirable for precipitation strengthening and enhanced wear resistance, without adverse effects on corrosion resistance. The original use of the alloy was for castings per F75 [ASTM 2006c]. The castings were multiphase with large carbides. The hard carbides gave these castings excellent wear resistance. This alloy work hardens rapidly and is difficult to machine. However, recent advances have developed fine-grained forged and wrought versions. The principles of cold working discussed in reference to stainless steels apply to F1537, as shown in Table 2.1 [ASTM 2006j]. Parts to be made of cobalt alloy that require significant machining, such as bearing surfaces of spinal disc prostheses, will probably be made from F1537. These are fine-grained alloys with very small carbides for wear resistance.

2.3.5 Titanium Alloys

Titanium is a lightweight metal that forms a stable titanium oxide film for high-temperature applications in the aerospace industry. The combination of the oxide's corrosion resistance and the low elastic modulus, which is closer to bone than that of the others discussed, has led to extensive use in orthopedics. However, in some joint replacement applications titanium implants have demonstrated poor wear resistance. It undergoes a phase transformation at 882°C from α HCP at lower temperatures to β BCC at higher. The α phase has good strength and toughness, whereas the β phase has better formability characteristics. There is a wide range of alloys in use, with typical properties and chemical composition listed in Tables 2.1 and 2.2.

Commercially pure (CPTi) F67 is all alpha titanium with interstitial strengthening from oxygen and nitrogen. There are four grades used as implants, with the extremes (grades 1 and 4) of low and high strengthening in the tables. For many years the standard titanium alloy used was, and still is, F136 titanium, 6% aluminum, 4% vanadium [ASTM 2006d]. This is a two-phase alloy with aluminum as the alpha stabilizer and vanadium as a beta stabilizer. This is the extra low interstitial (ELI) version of the alloy, which was developed for jet aircraft applications due to its low notch sensitivity. A non-ELI version of Ti 6,4 is also utilized for medical applications (F1472), which has higher tensile yield and strength (as shown in Table 2.1) [ASTM 2006i]. The properties of the two-phase Ti 6,4 alloys in the wrought and forged conditions have been utilized for the stems of total joint prostheses, with the application of a CPTi coating to facilitate bone attachment or ingrowth. An early method utilized sintering of CPTi beads onto Ti 6,4 stems. However, the sintering temperatures were greater than the beta transition at 882°C, which led to deleterious effects on the mechanical properties of the stems. As a result, bone attachment coatings are applied as diffusion bonded beads or wire meshes, or powder is thermally sprayed onto the surfaces.

Concerns about possible toxic effects of vanadium led to the development of F1295, in which niobium is used as the beta stabilizer [ASTM 2006h]. In an effort to develop alloys with the lower modulus of the beta phase, several all-beta alloys (such as F1713 and F1813) have been developed [ASTM 2006l; ASTM 2006m]. These are relatively new alloys and have not had wide use to date.

2.4 Ceramics

Unlike metals, in which atoms are loosely bound and able to move, ceramics are composed of atoms that are ionocovalently bound into compound forms. This atomic immobility means that ceramics do not conduct heat or electricity. Two very obvious properties that are different from metals are those of melting point and brittleness. Ceramics have very high melting points (generally above 1,000°C) and are brittle, as shown in Table 2.1.

Unlike metals, ceramics have directional bonds that prevent shifting one position at a time by the movement of dislocations. Thus, they are brittle; they do not bend, they crack. If a metal is hit, it will absorb the energy by bending or deforming. A ceramic that is hit will convert the strain energy to surface free energy (i.e., it will form a crack). Ceramics are typically strong and hard, which gives them excellent wear resistance. One method of toughening ceramics is to engineer the grains and grain boundaries, so that the crack tends to go through the boundary and is deflected by the grain. Zirconia ceramics are toughened by a phase transformation. Zirconia is stabilized in the tetragonal phase with compounds such as yttria and magnesia. Under conditions of stress, such as at a crack tip, zirconia will undergo a phase transform to monoclinic. Monoclinic is less dense (i.e., needs more volume), and thus creates a localized compression field at the tip. This localized increase in volume is induced by stress and crack propagation is prevented.

Many of the more common ceramics are metal oxides such as alumina (sapphire, Al_2O_3) and silica (SiO_2). Ceramics also include many non-oxide compounds such as carbides and nitrides, which may be used for hard surface coatings on metal drill bits and bearing surfaces. The gold color of titanium drill bits is probably a titanium nitride coating on a standard tool steel. In some ceramics, many different elements form a single compound such as the mineral phase of bone $Ca_{10}(PO_4)_6(OH)_2$ (hydroxyapatite).

Ceramic parts start out as a powder, which has been specially processed to be of high purity for most biomedical applications. The batched powder is then processed and formed into a shape that is similar to the final part. This unfired green body is then raised to a temperature where the powder coalesces into a single structure in a process called sintering. In sintering, the powder coalesces into a hard material in which the particles have fused together to form grains. In some cases the sintered part is then subjected to hot isostatic pressure (HIP) to reduce porosity and increase mechanical properties. The parts are then machined into their final shape by grinding and polishing methods.

The formation of carbon materials is quite different. Many are formed by pyrolysis or burning of an organic material. Graphite is made by putting coke in a furnace and subjecting it to very high temperatures for several days to burn off all the non-carbon elements. It is too soft for most biomedical applications, so it is coated. One method produces low-temperature isotropic (LTI) pyrolytic carbon. Preformed graphitic bodies are placed in a column through which methane or propane is pumped, to levitate the discs in a "fluidized bed." An alloy of carbon and silicon can be made using methyltrichlorosilane (CH_3SiCl_3). The column is heated to 1,500°C to pyrolyze the gas. The result is the formation of small crystallites of carbon deposited on the graphite discs. The 1,500°C is considered low temperature. The crystallites are random in orientation and thus the coating has isotropic properties, and hence the name LTI carbon. This produces a very strong and hard coating, as shown in Table 2.1.

Carbon fibers can be made from polymeric fibers such as polyacrylonitrile PAN. Fibers are subjected to a multistage process of heating to burn off the non-carbon atoms and create long chains of the hexagonal crystalline carbon structure. Temperatures in the final stages are 1,500 to 2,000°C, depending on the process. The result is very high strength fibers, as shown in Table 2.1.

The spinal applications of ceramics continue to grow. Their corrosion resistance and good wear properties and electrical insulation offer major advantages, whereas their brittleness with catastrophic failure is a disadvantage. New ceramics are currently being investigated that incorporate careful engineering and design.

2.5 Polymers

As the name implies, polymers are made up of many "mers" or basic building blocks. They are formed in long, sometimes branching, chains—with a backbone of carbon or silicon atoms held together with covalent bonds. Perhaps the simplest and most common polymer is polyethylene, which is made from many ethylene molecules. It consists of a long chain of carbon atoms as the backbone with two hydrogen atoms per carbon and as end caps. The number of mers (n) will determine many of the properties of the polymer formed. Low molecular forms of polyethylene are used for such things as soda pop bottles, whereas ultrahigh molecular weight polyethylene (UHMWPE) is used for the bottom of snow skis and the plastic bearing component of total joint replacements. In some cases, the polymer may not be linear but may have side branches. Low-density polyethylene may have a branched structure with side chains of PE coming off at a number of the hydrogen atoms.

In other polymers, one of the hydrogens is replaced with one or more ligands. For example, replacing one hydrogen with a chlorine atom produces poly vinyl chloride (PVC). Replacing all four with fluorine atoms results in poly tetra fluoroethylene (PTFE) or Teflon. Linear polymers can also be made with other elements in the backbone. For example, a common engineering polymer that goes by the name of polyoxymethylene (POM), or acetal or Delrin, is actually a polymer of formaldehyde. It has a backbone of carbon and oxygen atoms, with two hydrogen atoms per carbon. It is often used for making the fixtures used in testing spinal devices.

Polymers can be classified as thermoplastic or thermosetting. A thermoplastic polymer has a linear or branched structure. As a solid it is like a bowl of spaghetti because the chains can slide over one other. With heating, the chains can slide more easily; the polymer melts or flows. Thus, thermoplastic polymers can be heated, melted, molded, and recycled. Differences in properties can be achieved with the addition of different ligands. PVC is more rigid than PE because the chlorine atoms are larger and tend to prevent the sliding of one molecule over another. Polymethylmethacrylate (PMMA), as shown in Table 2.1, is stronger, stiffer, and much more brittle than UHMWPE. In this case, two of the four hydrogen atoms are replaced: one with a methyl group (CH_3) and the other with an acrylic group ($COOCH_3$). These large side groups make sliding much more difficult, and hence the increase in strength and modulus.

They also make it difficult for the molecules to orientate in an orderly, crystalline pattern. As a result of this amorphous structure, PMMA (Plexiglas or Lucite) is optically transparent.

In contrast, a thermosetting polymer is composed of chains that are cross-linked. They do not melt with heating, but degrade. The term *thermoset* implies that there is a chemical reaction, often involving heat, which results in setting in a 3D cross-linked structure. A common example is "5-minute epoxy": when the two parts are mixed, the catalyst causes setting and cross linking of the epoxy. Once set, it cannot be heated and reused. The amount of cross linking affects the mechanical properties. The process of vulcanization, which was developed by Goodyear, used sulfur to form a bridge between chains of natural rubber, and created a 3D structure. Few cross links are used in rubber gloves. Adding more sulfur and cross linking produces a car tire. Even more cross links are added to make the hard casing of a car battery.

One very important consideration for biomedical applications is the nature of polymerization. PE polymers are formed by addition reactions. Heat and a catalyst are used to add ethylene mers to the string. In contrast, nylon is formed by a condensation reaction in which two different molecules are combined and then strung together as a chain. Combining the two molecules releases a by-product, in this case water, which does not have any adverse biological effects. By comparison, the polymerization of silicone adhesive "bathtub caulk" releases acetic acid and the area smells like vinegar. Other condensation reactions release by-products with potentially adverse biological effects. The issue is not only what is released during polymerization but what may be trapped in the material that may slowly leach out over time and expose the patient to potential toxic components.

Mixing two-part polymer systems does not necessarily imply a thermosetting reaction. Bone cement is a two-part system used for fixing total joint replacements. The powder is ground-up polymer (PMMA) with a chemical initiator benzoyl peroxide (BP). The liquid is the monomer (MMA) with an activator. Mixing them softens the powder, resulting in activation of the BP. The BP then causes the polymerization of the monomer, resulting in solidification of the powder-liquid in 5 to 10 minutes. There is no cross linking, so the solid can be heated and molded after solidification.

Another term used to describe the mechanical properties of polymers is *elastomeric*. These can be either thermoplastic or thermosetting. This implies that the polymer will return to its original shape after deformation, like a rubber band. Molecules with zigzag backbone structures can straighten out with stress, and then spring back. Cross-linked thermosets can stretch the bonds and straighten out the structure, and then spring back. Note in Table 2.1 the very high elongation (% deformation) for silicone elastomer.

Many devices are made of plastic. A plastic is a polymer with any number of additives. Colorants are added to make them look nice. Antioxidants may be added to increase stability. Plasticizers may be added to increase softness. These are low molecular weight substances that act as a lubricant so the molecules can slide over each other, much like butter or tomato sauce in a bowl of spaghetti. An early problem with PVC blood bags was the addition of a plasticizer that tended to leak or leach out of the plastic and had toxic effects in the recipients of the blood.

2.5.1 Polymer Degradation

Degradation of polymeric materials can result in alterations in the properties of the material as well as release of degradation products that may cause adverse biological responses in the surrounding tissues. There are a number of ways polymers can degrade, but the mechanisms are beyond the scope of this text. However, discussion of what changes can occur can provide insight into the biological performance of polymers.

Chemical degradation starts with breaking the long polymer chain into smaller fragments, or chain scission. There are a number of mechanisms by which this can happen, such as hydrolysis, where H_2O splits to H^+ and OH^- attacks a bond. This can split the chain and the H^+ and OH^- can attach to the ends of the fragments forming end caps. Some enzymes and ionizing radiation are also capable of attacking polymers. Once split, the smaller fragments may react as free radicals to form end caps, react with other chains to form side branches, or react with other chains to form cross links. Thus, the polymer may get reduced in molecular weight, increasing its solubility and potential for further breakdown, or it may get harder and more brittle due to cross linking. Radiation cross linking of UHMWPE has recently been utilized to make a material with greatly increased wear resistance.

Properties of polymers may degrade over time by physical interaction with the environment. Low molecular weight substances, especially lipids, may adsorb into the material and cause discoloration. These low molecular weight substances may act as plasticizers and soften the material, or get trapped in the matrix of macromolecules and make the material more brittle. Such adsorption may be accelerated by mechanical forces such as cyclic loading or flexing. These mechanical forces can cause a sort of pumping action, with space between molecules opening and closing with each cycle and thus entrapping the low molecular weight substances entering the spaces. Similarly, low molecular weight substances added to the material during manufacture, such as plasticizers, may diffuse out over time. This can result in changes in the mechanical or other physical properties of the device. Such leaching may also stimulate an adverse biological reaction.

2.6 Composites

Composite materials are produced by mixing or joining two or more materials to give a combination of properties of the individual components. Typically, the property of each material is not changed, but rather contributes to the property of the composite. Composites can be placed (based on the shapes of the parts) in three categories: particulate (concrete), fiber (fiber glass), and laminar (plywood). Many properties can be determined by the rule of mixtures, which states that the property of the mixture is equal to the sum of the volume fractions of each constituent times that property for that constituent. For example, density of a polymer-fiber composite is equal to the sum of the fraction of polymer matrix times its density plus the fraction of fiber times its density.

As an example consider composites of carbon fiber in a polyetheretherketone (PEEK) matrix. The tensile strength for PEEK is 93 MPa and its modulus is 3.6 GPa (Table 2.1). For carbon fibers made of polyacrylonitrile (PAN), the values are 3,980 and 240, respectively. A composite made by adding 30% chopped fiber to PEEK has increased the strength (208) and modulus (17). However, the ductility is reduced from 50 to only 1.3%. Long fiber composites produce even higher strength and modulus. A composite made from sheets of 61% carbon fibers and tested in a direction longitudinal to the fibers has a strength of 2,130 and modulus of 125. By using a 45/45 cross ply, the properties drop to 300 and 47, but there is a substantial increase in elongation. Thus, a wide range of mechanical properties can be produced by adjusting the nature and amount of the fibers.

Many biological materials are also composites. Bone, for example, is a composite of mineral hydroxylapatite (HA) and collagen fibers. As shown in Table 2.1, HA is strong, rigid, and brittle. Collagen has a much lower modulus, and though the data are difficult to pinpoint it has much more elongation than HA. The composite bone is a strong and more flexible material.

Because bone growth and structure are responsive to stress, the use of some rigid metallic devices has been associated with alterations in bone healing and structure. Composite technology has been used to tailor materials to match bone. The 30% chopped carbon PEEK has a modulus close to that of bone and has been considered for use as a moderately flexible device to hold a fracture together during healing. The long fiber composites are stiffer than bone, but not as stiff as stainless steel or cobalt alloys. Thus, they have been considered for high strength devices for joint replacement. The nature and amount of the composite constituents can be adjusted to produce the optimum properties.

2.7 Biological Effects

Implantation of a spinal device involves a number of surgical steps initiated with incision of the skin. There are a series of biological responses that are the body's normal defense mechanisms against injury and infection. Understanding the normal reactions and the cells involved is critical to understanding cellular reactions that indicate an adverse reaction to an implant.

2.7.1 Inflammation and Wound Healing

Inflammation is the first response of any vascularized tissue (tissue with blood vessels) to tissue damage. Most of the response is due to changes in those blood vessels. These responses are rapid and are normal. Only when the response becomes prolonged is there a problem. To understand the cellular events, consider the tissue around a splinter. The presence of red blood cells and fluid can be observed early. Vascular damage also triggers the two branches of the blood coagulation system. The first involves activation of platelets, small cells in the blood, which stick to exposed surfaces (or foreign objects) and form a plug. The other involves a series of proteolytic reactions, starting with the activation of a protein circulating in the blood by exposure to damaged vascular tissue or a foreign object. This sequence results in the final pathway of conversion of fibrinogen to fibrin clot.

During the first 24 hours after injury there is an influx of white blood cells. The predominant type of leukocyte is the neutrophil, usually referred to as PMN (polymorphonuclear leukocyte) or poly. This cell has a protective mechanism and its function is phagocytosis, to engulf and destroy foreign material or cellular debris. The second group of white blood cells is the monocyte, which accounts for up to 10% of the white blood cells and is about 10 μm in size. This cell is also a phagocytic cell and has the capability of engulfing and destroying foreign substances. When a monocyte leaves the blood and goes into the tissue, it changes its appearance and differentiates into a macrophage (histiocyte). The macrophage is a large cell (up to about 20 μm in size) and is actively phagocytic. This early pattern is referred to as acute inflammation. If the source of the injury is removed (e.g., the splinter is removed), the response resolves and the tissue will heal. Small vessels begin to grow into the wound. Tissue cells called fibroblasts come in and start to synthesize collagen to close the wound.

If the source of injury is not removed and the response continues it is referred to as chronic inflammation. The biological response is to "invade and destroy, or wall off." If the splinter is relatively clean, the biological response will be to wall it off with a capsule of fibrous tissue, resulting in eventual extrusion of the splinter by skin exfoliation. However, if the splinter or other objects produce fragments or particulates the macrophages may be overwhelmed in their attempt to phagocytize material and coalesce with other cells to form multinucleated giant cells. There is often evidence of foreign material, or wear debris, associated within these cells. The presence of the foreign body giant cell indicates that the phagocytic system is incapable of ridding the body of the foreign matter and tissue destruction often occurs with loss of normal tissue or significant bone resorption, depending on the site of inflammation.

2.7.2 Cellular Responses to Implants

When a biomaterial is inserted into the body the two features described previously are involved: inflammation and healing. If the material is removed quickly, wound healing proceeds normally. However, if the material remains in the body the response is for the fibroblasts in the healing response to lay down layers of a fibrous capsule around the material to "wall it off" from the rest of the body. It is generally believed that the thinner the fibrous capsule the more acceptable the material is to the host (i.e., it is biocompatible). If the material is not biocompatible, or when the irritation is continuous (as with the production of wear debris) the response will continue as a chronic inflammation and progress to giant cells and granulomas.

Formation of a fibrous capsule tends not to occur with porous or textured materials. If the interstices are large enough, local vascularized tissue will grow into the pores rather than form the capsule. Long-term percutaneous catheters have been coated with velour to facilitate ingrowth and anchorage. As we will see, spinal implants may have porous coatings for anchorage by bone ingrowth.

2.7.3 Infection and Immune Responses

Implants do not cause infections, microbes do. However, it is well recognized that the presence of a foreign body greatly increases the infection risk and markedly decreases the number of bacteria required to cause an infection from 10^6 to 10^2. Not only is there an increased risk of infection but the infection will be difficult to cure. Once again, remember your splinter. If the splinter site became infected, the only way to cure the infection is to remove the splinter. Unfortunately, the same is true for implanted devices. The only way to cure the infection is to remove the device. The consequences of this depend on the need for the device. Removal of sutures may cause little impairment to healing, whereas removal of an artificial vertebral disk will be disabling.

The immune system is an important protective system, and it reacts specifically and with memory. This is why vaccinations are important for common diseases such as polio and measles. Lymphocytes are the key element of the immune system in the circulation. There are a number of types of lymphocytes, but those key for biomaterials purposes are the B-cell and the T-cell. When B-cells recognize an antigen to which they are programmed, they produce antibody-producing cells called plasma cells. The T-cells are associated with cytotoxic responses. Although the immune system is an important defense mechanism, sometimes it can cause harm to the host and these reactions are called allergy, or autoimmunity, when the immune system attacks the host tissue as with rheumatoid arthritis.

Allergic responses occur to foreign substances through a variety of mechanisms. One type of allergy is called atopic or type I. The most common example of this is hay fever, which is the result of the formation of specific types of antibodies to ragweed pollen. The current concern in this area is with latex materials, such as surgical gloves, which contain a protein that may cause this type of allergy.

A second type of reaction is T-cell mediated and is called contact dermatitis (type IV). A common example of this is skin reaction from contact with poison ivy. Some of the metals such as nickel, cobalt, and chromium can cause allergy when contacted as metal protein complexes. Allergic reactions to metallic devices can occur, but unless there is corrosion and release of metal ions there will not be allergic responses.

2.7.4 Biological Effects of Corrosion Products and Wear Debris

The distribution and elimination of the metal ions from corrosion must be considered in determining the effect on the host. Many of the elements used in metal alloys are essential trace elements for human metabolism. Nickel, chromium, cobalt, and iron are all necessary for metabolic processes and there are normal mechanisms for maintaining proper concentrations. Thus, only in extreme excess will they impact on the host. Some, such as nickel and cobalt ions, are rapidly excreted in the kidney, whereas others (such as chromium with a valence of 6^+) are stored in the tissues. Thus, the toxicity issues include tissue accumulation as well as total concentration from the material.

Wear may result in the production of small pieces (particles) that can stimulate a biological reaction. Polys and macrophages will attempt to engulf and degrade these foreign particles. If the debris production rate is not too high, there will be no additional response. However, if the cells cannot clear the debris chronic inflammation will result with foreign body giant cells, granulomas, and the release of various soluble mediators. Our understanding of cellular responses to debris in the micrometer range is well advanced. However, refinement of techniques for tissue harvesting and electron microscopic examination have demonstrated debris in the nanometer size range. The response to nanoparticles is still under investigation. The generation of wear particles is a critical issue in evaluation of spinal disk replacements. Of particular concern is the possibility of debris, especially nanoparticles, getting into the spinal fluid and affecting the cord or other neural tissues.

In general, metallic particles will undergo corrosion in the acid environment of the phagocytic cells and be released and eliminated as ions. The ceramics are less prone to corrosion or dissolution, and thus the degradation of any particles from wear may be slow. The polymers are usually very resistant to further degradation. They tend to be the major cause of prolonged cellular response with tissue and organ damage (such as loss of bone) from extensive, yet ineffective, phagocytosis. Not only do the frustrated phagocytes send out signals (cytokines) to recruit more cells but die in their effort to destroy particles, thus releasing all of their intercellular enzymes, acids, and superoxides produced.

2.8 Biocompatibility Testing

Biocompatibility has been defined as the ability of a material to perform with an appropriate host response in a specific application. Will this material stimulate the appropriate biological response for the intended use? The material to be tested must be in the identical form to that when used (i.e., it must be sterilized in the appropriate manner and any surface or bulk modifications completed). The tests may be done *in vitro* using tissue or cell cultures or may involve injection of substances or implantation into the animal.

Biocompatibility evaluation is desired on all new materials or old materials used in new applications. The tests chosen should be carefully considered and matched to the ultimate use of the device. An important first step in biocompatibility evaluation is to conduct a risk assessment through a literature search on the toxicology and biocompatibility of the components, by-products, and degradation products of the material. A risk assessment taking into account the amount of each substance compared to its toxicity level may indicate the material will fail and need not be tested and not used, or that the material is safe in this application and does not need to be tested or requires only minimal testing. Biocompatibility testing is an inexact science and some materials pass the testing but ultimately do not perform as expected in human patients. Despite the limitations, biocompatibility evaluation remains a necessary screening test before a device can be approved.

In some tests the material will be used directly. In other tests the material will be extracted in a liquid and the extract tested. The extract used will vary depending on the test methods to be used or on the nature of the material. The tests are designed to test for cytotoxicity (damage to cells), stimulation of the immune response, irritation to tissues, provocation of chronic inflammation, effects on blood and blood components, and effects on genetic factors including mutations and tumor formation. The selection of tests to be done and the methods used are the subject of much investigation and deliberation. In general, guidelines for the selection of tests and the methods for performing these tests are described in ASTM F748 and ISO standard 10993 [ASTM 2006g]. Regulatory agencies, such as the Food and Drug Administration (FDA) in the United States, will give the developer and manufacturer of devices guidelines about what testing is advisable.

2.9 Summary and Conclusions

With this information as a background, we can now proceed with designing and testing spinal devices, based on material properties and clinical applications. For example, stainless steel has been the traditional material of choice of plates and screws (and rods and hooks) for spinal fusion. Why? Because it is the easiest of the alloys to machine, and can be used in different work hardened conditions with minimal galvanic corrosion problems. Thus, a plate or rod might be manufactured in the annealed condition, with a cold work reserve to permit the surgeon to bend the device to fit the anatomy of the patient. The screws and hooks would be more heavily cold worked for increased strength. If the surgeon is concerned about osteoporotic bone and stress shielding, he or she might prefer to use titanium 6Al 4V with its lower elastic modulus. Similarly, titanium, PEEK, and carbon-fiber-reinforced PEEK are used for spinal cages because they have the low modulus needed to facilitate bone regeneration and fusion. On the other hand, vertebral disk prostheses with articulating bearing surfaces need to be highly wear resistant. Here the materials of choice might be UHMWPE, cobalt chromium alloy, or alumina.

As new materials and applications are developed the mechanical properties and biological effects will have to be evaluated using the methods described.

The following chapters develop the concepts necessary to understand the critical and unique aspects of the various devices used in the spine. It is the understanding of material properties, device design and testing, and the clinical application that is necessary for a clinical success.

2.10 References

ASTM (2006a). "D412, Standard Test Methods for Vulcanized Rubber and Thermoplastic Elastomers—Tension," in *ASTM Standards* (vol. 09.01). Conshohocken, PA: ASTM International.

ASTM (2006b). "E8M, Standard Test Methods for Tension Testing of Metallic Materials," in *ASTM Standards* (vol. 03.01). Conshohocken, PA: ASTM International.

ASTM (2006c). "F75, Standard Specification for Cobalt-28 Chromium-6 Molybdenum Casting Alloy and Cast Products for Surgical Implants (UNS R30075)," in *ASTM Standards* (vol. 13.01). Conshohocken, PA: ASTM International.

ASTM (2006d). "F136, Standard Specification for Wrought Titanium-6 Aluminum-4 Vanadium ELI (Extra Low Interstitial) Alloy for Surgical Implant Applications (R56401)," in *ASTM Standards* (vol. 13.01). Conshohocken, PA: ASTM International.

ASTM (2006e). "F138, Standard Specification for Wrought 18 Chromium-14 Nickel-2.5 Molybdenum Stainless Steel Bar and Wire for Surgical Implants (UNS S31673)," in *ASTM Standards* (vol. 13.01). Conshohocken, PA: ASTM International.

ASTM (2006f). "F603, Standard Specification for High-Purity Dense Aluminum Oxide for Medical Applications," in *ASTM Standards* (vol. 13.01). Conshohocken, PA: ASTM International.

ASTM (2006g). "F748, Standard Practice for Selecting Generic Biological Test Methods for Materials and Devices," in *ASTM Standards* (vol. 13.01). Conshohocken, PA: ASTM International.

ASTM (2006h). "F1295, Standard Specification for Wrought Titanium-6 Aluminum-7 Niobium Alloy for Surgical Implant Applications (UNS R56700)," in *ASTM Standards* (vol. 13.01). Conshohocken, PA: ASTM International.

ASTM (2006i). "F1472, Standard Specification for Wrought Titanium-6 Aluminum-4 Vanadium Alloy for Surgical Implant Applications (UNS R56400)," in *ASTM Standards* (vol. 13.01). Conshohocken, PA: ASTM International.

ASTM (2006j). "F1537, Standard Specification for Wrought Cobalt-28 Chromium-6 Molybdenum Alloys for Surgical Implants (UNS R31537, UNS R31538, and UNS R311539)," in *ASTM Standards* (vol. 13.01). Conshohocken, PA: ASTM International.

ASTM (2006k). "F1586, Standard Specification for Wrought Nitrogen Strengthened 21 Chromium-10 Nickel-3 Manganese-2.5 Molybdenum Stainless Steel Alloy Bar for Surgical Implants (UNS S31675)," in *ASTM Standards* (vol. 13.01). Conshohocken, PA: ASTM International.

ASTM (2006l). "F1713, Standard Specification for Wrought Titanium-13 Niobium-13 Zirconium Alloy for Surgical Implant Applications (UNS R58130)," in *ASTM Standards* (vol. 13.01). Conshohocken, PA: ASTM International.

ASTM (2006m). "F1813, Standard Specification for Wrought Titanium-12 Molybdenum-6 Zirconium-2 Iron Alloy for Surgical Implants (UNS R58120)," in *ASTM Standards* (vol. 13.01). Conshohocken, PA: ASTM International.

ASTM (2006n). "F1873, Standard Specification for High-Purity Dense Yttria Tetragonal Zirconium Oxide Polycrystal (Y-TZP) for Surgical Implant Applications," in *ASTM Standards* (vol. 13.01). Conshohocken, PA: ASTM International.

ASTM (2006o). "F2229, Standard Specification for Wrought, Nitrogen Strengthened 23 Manganese-21 Chromium-1 Molybdenum Low-Nickel Stainless Steel Alloy Bar and Wire for Surgical Implants (UNS S29108)," in *ASTM Standards* (vol. 13.01). Conshohocken, PA: ASTM International.

ASTM (2006p). "F2393, Standard Specification for High-Purity Dense Magnesia Partially Stabilized Zirconia (Mg-PSZ) for Surgical Implant Applications," in *ASTM Standards* (vol. 13.01). Conshohocken, PA: ASTM International.

Ratner, B. D., A. S. Hoffman, F. J. Schoen, and J. E. Lemons (eds.) (2004). *Biomaterials Science*. San Diego: Academic Press.

www.Matweb.com. Good source for material properties.

Chapter 3

Structure and Properties of Soft Tissues in the Spine

Heather Anne L. Guerin, Ph.D.[1] *and*
Dawn M. Elliott, Ph.D.[2]
(1) Department of Mechanical Engineering and Applied
Mechanics (2) Department of Orthopaedic Surgery
McKay Orthopaedic Research Laboratory,
University of Pennsylvania, Philadelphia, PA

3.1 Introduction

The soft tissues of the spine include the intervertebral discs (situated between each of the rigid vertebrae of the spine), the ligaments (which connect the vertebrae at various points), and the spinal cord. The entire spinal column provides structural support for the trunk of the body and protects the spinal cord. The intervertebral discs and spinal ligaments impart flexibility and mobility to the spine, allowing motions of the body such as twisting and bending forward, backward, and side to side. To provide support, the intervertebral discs and ligaments must be stiff enough to maintain stability under large spinal loads. To provide flexibility, the soft tissues of the spine must be soft enough to allow motion in many directions, which can subject these tissues to loading in bending, torsion, tension, compression, and shear. The spinal cord does not support mechanical loads, but must be flexible enough to deform along with the spine during motion without damage. The spinal cord provides motor control and sensory perception to the rest of the body. In this chapter we outline the structure, composition, and mechanical function of each of the soft tissues of the spine: the intervertebral discs, the ligaments, and the spinal cord.

3.2 Intervertebral Discs

The intervertebral discs are soft tissue structures situated between each of the 24 cervical, thoracic, and lumbar vertebrae of the spine. Each intervertebral disc comprises a symphysis, or fibrocartilaginous joint, that connects successive vertebrae. The intervertebral discs are the largest avascular structures in the body (blood vessels reach only the outer areas of the intervertebral disc). Additionally, the intervertebral discs are largely aneural (with nerve endings reaching only the periphery of the tissue), and the intervertebral discs are only sparsely populated with cells. Poor blood supply and low cellularity may contribute to nutritional and degenerative problems in the intervertebral disc. The intervertebral discs vary in size and shape with spinal level. A small, round cross-sectional shape in the cervical spine progresses to a larger, more kidney-like cross-sectional shape in the lumbar spine to accommodate the mechanical requirements at different levels of the spine.

Whereas the size and shape of the intervertebral discs vary with spinal level, the general structure and composition of the intervertebral discs are constant along the length of the spine. The intervertebral discs—like other connective tissues in the body such as ligament, cartilage, and tendon—consist of collagen fibers embedded in a highly hydrated extracellular matrix. Although the material composition of the intervertebral discs is similar to other connective soft tissues, the intervertebral discs have a unique structure that confers multidirectional flexibility and large load-bearing capacity. The structure of each intervertebral disc has three main components: the *annulus fibrosus* (a fibrous ring which surrounds the *nucleus pulposus*); the gelatinous, hydratéd center of the intervertebral disc; and the end plates, which are situated above and below each intervertebral disc, adjacent to the vertebrae (Figure 3.1).

The interaction between the intervertebral disc components is similar to a thick-walled pressure vessel, and allows the intervertebral discs to act as shock absorbers, absorbing and transmitting the loads experienced by the spine. Daily activities such as walking, running, driving, or lifting expose the intervertebral discs to repetitive compressive forces. However, it is not unusual for the intervertebral disc to be loaded in complex combinations of torsion, tension, shear, compression, and bending. External loading may also be exerted upon the intervertebral discs by gravity, abdominal and back muscles, and intra-abdominal pressure [Adams et al. 2002; Stokes and Iatridis 2004].

3.2.1 Nucleus Pulposus

The nucleus pulposus is a translucent, gelatinous, semi-solid structure. It consists of a loose meshwork of randomly distributed collagen fibrils in a hydrated extrafibrillar matrix. In healthy nondegenerated nucleus pulposus tissue, collagens account for approximately 20% of the dry weight of the nucleus pulposus, proteoglycans comprise about 30 to 50% of the dry weight, and the remainder is comprised of noncollagenous proteins. Water constitutes about 70 to 80% of total nucleus pulposus weight [Buckwalter 1996; Eyre 1979].

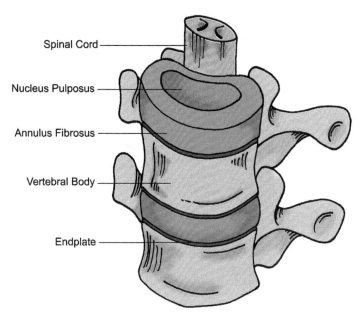

Fig. 3.1.
Spinal motion segment with intervertebral discs and spinal cord.

Collagens are helically organized proteins bundled into fibers that confer mechanical strength to tissues. Type II collagen makes up about 80% of the total collagen content in the nucleus pulposus [Buckwalter 1995; Eyre 1979]. This type of collagen is found in other compressive load-bearing tissues of the body like cartilage. Collagen types V, VI, IX, and XII make up the remainder of the collagen content in the nucleus pulposus. These collagens are thought to interact with other collagen fibrils, to surround nucleus pulposus cells, or to help form networks within tissues, although their exact contribution to nucleus pulposus mechanical function is unclear [Roughley 2004].

Aside from water, proteoglycans are the most abundant material in the nucleus pulposus, and play an important role in the function of this tissue. The major proteoglycan in the intervertebral disc is aggrecan. Aggrecan has a brush-like structure made up of many glycosaminoglycan molecules attached to a core protein (Figure 3.2). Aggrecan is so named because many aggrecan molecules aggregate via link proteins along a long hyaluronan molecule, forming a proteoglycan macromolecule. The glycosaminoglycans contain fixed negative charges. These negative charges attract positively charged ions to the nucleus pulposus in order to achieve electroneutrality within the tissue. When electroneutrality is achieved, the ion concentration in the nucleus pulposus is then higher than the surrounding tissue. This causes osmotic pressure within the nucleus pulposus, as water is attracted into the tissue to balance the ion density in the nucleus pulposus with the surrounding annulus fibrosus and end plates. Thus, the nucleus pulposus has a high water content, which is responsible for the largely fluid-like behavior of the tissue.

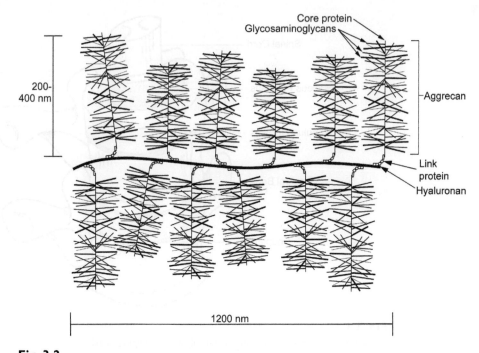

Fig. 3.2.
A proteoglycan macromolecule of aggrecan molecules. Each brush-like aggrecan molecule is made up of glycosaminoglycans bound to a protein core.

The nucleus pulposus tissue is pressurized within the intervertebral disc. The water within the nucleus pulposus, the osmotic imbalance in ion concentrations described previously, and repulsion of the negative charges on the glycosaminoglycan molecules all contribute pressure to the nucleus pulposus. This pressure is constrained by the type II collagen fiber mesh within the nucleus pulposus (which traps the large proteoglycan molecules) and by the surrounding annulus fibrosus and end plates (which confine the entire nucleus pulposus). The total pressure within the nucleus pulposus is called the swelling pressure. The swelling pressure of healthy nucleus pulposus tissue is 0.1 to 0.2 MPa in a recumbent position and may reach as high as 1 to 3 MPa when standing or lifting [Nachemson and Morris 1964; Wilke et al. 1999]. Similarly high pressures have been measured in cadaveric motion segments under externally applied loads [McNally and Adams 1992]. Released from its constraints, excised nucleus pulposus tissue will absorb water, even from the air, and swell to 200% of its original volume.

Nucleus pulposus pressurization enables the tissue to absorb and transmit the compressive loads of the spine. When the intervertebral disc is loaded in compression, the pressure within the nucleus pulposus increases. Over time, water flows out of the nucleus pulposus to reequilibrate this pressure. When the load is removed, water and ions flow back into the nucleus pulposus to equilibrate the pressure within the intervertebral disc. This cycle of fluid flow in and out of the intervertebral disc is also diurnal. Because the intervertebral disc is loaded in compression for about 16 hours a day, a large amount of fluid (up to 20% of total intervertebral disc volume) is expressed. Overnight during rest, the intervertebral disc is rehydrated and repressurized. Intervertebral disc pressure increases overnight by 0.1 to 0.24 MPa, which is between 20 and 50% of the total pressure in the intervertebral disc during relaxed standing [Wilke et al. 1999].

The random organization of nucleus pulposus tissue contributes to isotropic mechanical properties (i.e., mechanical properties are the same in all directions). The compressive modulus of the nucleus pulposus is approximately 1 MPa [Johannessen and Elliott 2005], and the shear modulus has been measured at 6 kPa [Iatridis et al. 1997]. These mechanical properties and the swelling pressures mentioned previously suggest that the nucleus pulposus of the healthy intervertebral disc is largely fluid-like and loads are supported primarily via pressurization.

The cell density in the nucleus pulposus is very low compared to other tissues. Whereas other relatively acellular tissues such as cartilage have cell densities of 14×10^6 cells/cm^3, nucleus pulposus cell density is nearly an order of magnitude lower at 4×10^6 cells/cm^3 [Oegema 1993]. In very early life, the cells in the nucleus pulposus are derived from fetal notochordal cells. These cells completely disappear by early adulthood and are replaced by a lesser number of round cells that resemble the chondrocytes found in tissues subjected to compressive loading, such as articular cartilage [Coventry et al. 1945a]. These cells predominantly produce type II collagen and aggrecan.

3.2.2 Annulus Fibrosus

The annulus fibrosus is a ring of highly organized fibrocartilage that surrounds the nucleus pulposus. It consists of concentric layers of collagen fibers embedded in a proteoglycan matrix, with the fibers of each layer oriented at alternating angles (Figure 3.3). The fibers make an angle of ±28 to 43 degrees with respect to the transverse axis [Cassidy, Hiltner, and Baer 1989; Guerin and Elliott 2005b; Hickey and Hukins 1980; Marchand and Ahmed 1990]. The concentric layers of the annulus fibrosus are not continuous; rather, they are interwoven and incomplete around the circumference of the intervertebral disc. There are between 15 and 40 layers through the thickness of the annulus fibrosus. The anterior annulus fibrosus has more layers than the posterior [Marchand and Ahmed 1990]. The collagen fibers are anchored into the adjacent vertebral bones at the outer periphery of the annulus fibrosus, and into the cartilage end plates in the central intervertebral disc.

The alternating angled, layered structure of the annulus fibrosus is ideal for withstanding large and complex loads in multiple directions, and is extremely important to the overall mechanical function of the intervertabral disc. Under compressive loading of the intervertebral disc, the inner annulus fibrosus is exposed to axial compressive stresses, and outward nucleus pulposus bulging causes radial compressive and circumferential tensile stresses in the outer

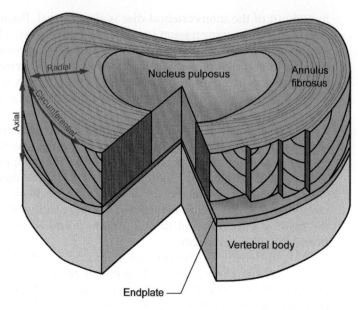

Fig. 3.3.

Annulus fibrosus layered structure (adapted from Iatridis et al. 1998). Each concentric layer of the annulus has collagen fibers oriented at alternating angles to provide for load-bearing in many directions.

annulus fibrosus (Figure 3.4). In bending or torsion, the fibers of the annulus fibrosus may be loaded directly in tension at some point around the circumference of the tissue (Figure 3.4). The intervertebral disc may undergo any combination of these loading scenarios during the motions of normal daily life.

The angled fiber orientation of the annulus fibrosus contributes to anisotropic mechanical properties (i.e., mechanical properties vary with circumferential, radial, and axial orientation), as shown in Figure 3.3. Tensile circumferential modulus is 10 to 20 times greater than in the axial direction, and an order of magnitude greater than in the radial direction (Table 3.1). Additionally, it has been shown that the fibers of the annulus fibrosus reorient during circumferential tensile loading, which may significantly increase mechanical properties in that direction [Guerin and Elliott 2005b]. Anisotropic mechanical properties accommodate the complex loading conditions the annulus fibrosus undergoes. For instance, tensile loading occurs primarily in the circumferential direction. Therefore, the tensile properties are greatest in that direction. Unlike tensile mechanical properties, the compressive mechanical properties are not highly anisotropic, suggesting that they are not strongly inflenced by collagen fiber direction. Like the nucleus pulposus, water content may contribute to the compressive mechanical properties in the annulus fibrosus. The compressive modulus of the annulus fibrosus is 0.6 MPa [Iatridis et al. 1998].

The mechanical properties of the annulus fibrosus also vary spatially. For instance, in the circumferential direction the anterior annulus fibrosus is

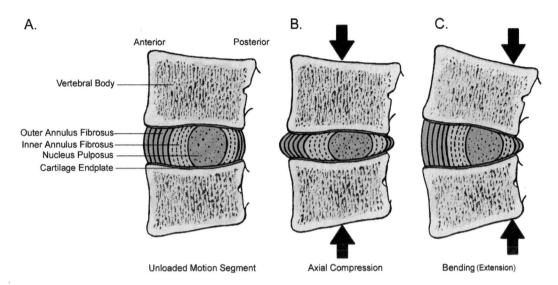

Fig. 3.4.

Motion segment loading scenarios (adapted from Buckwalter et al. 2000a). (A) An uncompressed motion segment. (B) Under axial compression, the nucleus pulposus bulges and transmits tensile loads to the annulus fibrosus. (C) Under bending loads, the nucleus pulposus bulges, and the annulus is loaded in compression and tension in different areas depending on the direction of bending.

stiffer than the posterior. Spatial differences in circumferential moduli are as large as an order of magnitude (Table 3.1). However, little spatial variation in mechanical properties is seen in the radial or axial directions. This may be because collagen fibers do not significantly contribute to mechanical properties in those orientations. Annulus fibrosus structural differences may be responsible for the relative mechanical inferiority of some areas of the intervertebral disc. For instance, the posterolateral region is characterized by incomplete layers, increased fiber-interlacing angles, and loose interconnections of fibers [Marchand and Ahmed 1990]. These regional variations in composition and tensile properties of the posterolateral annulus fibrosus may represent potential areas for compromise of structural integrity, and may contribute to the initiation and propagation of posterior annular tears, fissures, and herniations [Osti et al. 1992].

Also important to the specialized function of the annulus fibrosus are its nonlinear and viscoelastic material properties. Loaded excised tissue samples show a nonlinear stress/strain curve. This curve is characterized by a "toe"–region where low stresses are observed at low strains followed by a high stress and high strain "linear"–region, and then failure of the tissue (Figure 3.5). In the circumferential direction, toe-region modulus is approximately 2 to 5 MPa, whereas the linear-region modulus is approximately 20 MPa [Elliott and Setton 2001; Guerin and Elliott 2005b]. This tenfold increase in modulus with increasing applied strain demonstrates very large nonlinearity. The nonlinearity of annulus fibrosus tissue is similar to the material behavior of other soft

Table 3.1.

Linear region moduli of nondegenerated and degenerated annulus fibrosus tissue. 1. (Acaroglu et al. 1995). 2. (Ebara et al. 1996). 3. (Elliott and Setton 2001). 4. (Fujita et al. 1997). 5. (Guerin and Elliott 2005b).

	Circumferential		Axial		Radial	
	Nondegenerated	Degenerated	Nondegenerated	Degenerated	Nondegenerated	Degenerated
Anterior						
Inner	5.6–10[1-3]	5.0[1]	1.0[3]	N/A	N/A	N/A
Outer	17–29[1-3,5]	22–29[1,5]	0.8[3]	N/A	0.4–0.5[3,4]	0.4[4]
Posterior						
Inner	2.0–6.0[1,2]	4.0[1]	N/A	N/A	0.5[4]	N/A
Outer	13–19[1,2]	8.0[1]	N/A	N/A	N/A	N/A

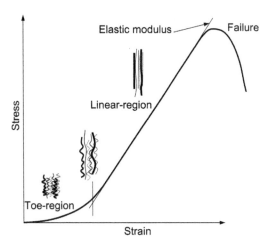

Fig. 3.5.

Nonlinear stress/strain curve. Collagen fibers remain crimped in the nonlinear toe region, but progressively straighten with applied load so that the elasticity of the straightened collagen fibers contributes to the elastic modulus in the linear region.

collagenous tissues such as articular cartilage, tendon, and ligaments. It is thought that uncrimping of collagen fibers contributes to nonlinearity [Kastelic et al. 1980]. Collagen fibers that are initially wavy become uncrimped as load is applied, progressively contributing to the overall stiffness of the tissue. Interactions between the fibers and the proteoglycan matrix as well as collagen fiber cross linking may also contribute to tissue nonlinearity [Guerin and Elliott 2005a]. The transition between the toe and linear regions of the stress/strain curve occurs at approximately 6% strain in annulus fibrosus tissue [Guerin and Elliott 2005b].

Annulus fibrosus viscoelasticity results in time-dependent material behaviors such as stress relaxation or creep. Stress relaxation occurs when the tissue is extended to a given strain and that displacement is held constant for a period of time. The initial stress on the tissue decreases with time, and the tissue relaxes to an equilibrium stress (Figure 3.6a). Creep occurs when the tissue is loaded to a given stress, and strain increases over time to an equilibrium level (Figure 3.6b). Once the load is released, the strain decreases (recovery). Fluid flow through the permeable matrix and frictional interactions between collagen fibers and the proteoglycan matrix may contribute to viscoelasticity in the annulus fibrosus [Woo, Johnson, and Smith 1993; Yin and Elliott 2004].

Biochemical composition also contributes to inhomogeneous and anisotropic mechanical properties. There are significant spatial variations of water, collagen, and proteoglycan content from outer to inner annulus fibrosus and from anterior to posterior annulus fibrosus [Eyre and Muir 1976; Pearce 1993]. The outer annulus fibrosus is dense and fibrous, with clearly defined layers of highly organized fibers. Collagen makes up 60 to 70% of the dry weight of the outer annulus fibrosus, whereas proteoglycans comprise only 10% of the dry

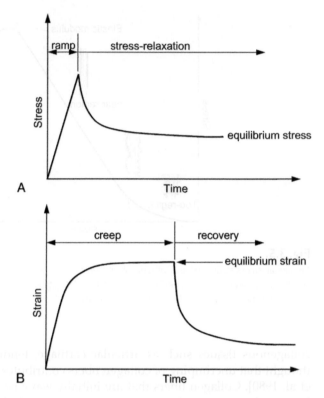

Fig. 3.6.
The viscoelastic mechanical behaviors of stress relaxation (A) and creep (B). Stress relaxation causes load to decrease to equilibrium if displacement is held constant. Under constant load, tissue will creep to an equilibrium strain.

weight of the outer annulus fibrosus, and the remainder is comprised of non-collagenous proteins. The major collagens in the annulus fibrosus are types I and II collagen, with each comprising about 50% of total collagen content in the entire annulus fibrosus in very young humans. However, collagen types and amounts vary with radial position in the annulus fibrosus. The ratio of type I to type II collagen is very high in the outer annulus fibrosus [Buckwalter 1995; Eyre 1979]. Type I collagen allows for tensile load bearing in the outer annulus fibrosus. Moving radially inward through the intervertebral disc, the ratio of type I to type II collagen diminishes, so that type II collagen predominates in the inner annulus fibrosus. Inner annulus fibrosus biochemical composition changes to reflect a lower concentration of collagen altogether (23 to 30% of dry weight), a greater percentage of proteoglycans, and greater hydration [Eyre 1979]. Additionally, the layered structure becomes less distinct and fiber organization diminishes toward the inner annulus fibrosus [Coventry, Ghormley, and Kernohan 1945b]. These changes in composition and structure may accommodate the largely compressive loading patterns in the inner annulus fibrosus.

The cells of the annulus fibrosus vary from inner to outer sites. The inner annulus fibrosus is populated with cells similar to nucleus pulposus cells. These cells are round and chondrocyte-like. Outer annulus fibrosus cells are more fibrocyte-like and elongated, with their major axes aligned along the collagen fiber direction [Setton and Chen 2004]. These cells produce predominantly type I and type II collagen. Like the nucleus pulposus, cell density in the annulus fibrosus is 9×10^6 cells/cm^3, which is very low compared to other tissues.

3.2.3 End Plates

The cartilaginous end plates form a border between the vertebral bodies and the intervertebral disc. The deep calcified layer of the end plates is closest to vertebral bone. This layer is covered by a layer of hyaline cartilage. Hyaline cartilage is comprised of type II collagen, proteoglycans, and water [Buckwalter et al. 2000a]. The uniform layer between the intervertebral disc and vertebral bodies created by this tissue helps to evenly distribute loads across the intervertebral disc [Buckwalter et al. 2000a].

The end plates are the primary path for fluid flow to and from the intervertebral disc. This flow is facilitated through marrow contact channels, which connect the vertebral bone to the mid-layers of the end plate, but do not completely penetrate through the end plates to the intervertebral disc. Fluid flow through the end plates enables rehydration of the intervertebral disc after daily loading and promoting the transport of larger proteins [Ayotte, Ito, and Tepic 2001]. The marrow contact channels also house capillaries for nutrient supply to the intervertebral disc. Capillary density is greatest in the center of the intervertebral disc and decreases toward the outer annulus fibrosus [Urban, Smith, and Fairbank 2004]. Nutrition of the intervertebral disc is provided by diffusion of small molecules such as glucose and oxygen through the end plates [Urban et al. 1982].

Like the other components of the intervertebral disc, the structure and mechanical properties of the end plates vary spatially, though these characteristics have not been widely studied. The end plates are thickest at the periphery of the intervertebral disc, and become thinner moving inward radially, with an average thickness of approximately 0.6 mm [Edwards et al. 2001; Roberts, Menage, and Urban 1989]. Collagen content is greatest at the periphery of the end plate, whereas proteoglycan and water content is greatest at the center [Roberts, Menage, and Urban 1989]. Indentation testing of lumbar vertebral end plates has shown that the failure load of the end plates is between 60 and 180 N, and the stiffness of the end plates is between 80 and 175 N/mm. The highest failure load and stiffness are at the periphery of the intervertebral disc, and the anterior end plates are stronger and stiffer than the posterior [Grant, Oxland, and Dvorak 2001]. These differences may be the result of underlying bone structure and mechanical properties, or may be the result of the progression of fetal development of the spine. For very high axial loads, the end plate may be the intervertebral disc structure that fails first. End plate failure may occur due to bulging of the nucleus pulposus that increases pressure on the end plates and forces the end plates into the vertebral body [Brinckmann et al. 1983].

3.3 Intervertebral Disc Aging and Degeneration

The intervertebral discs, especially the discs of the lumbar spine, undergo dramatic changes in structure, composition, and mechanical function with age. Aging of the intervertebral discs is universal. The intervertebral discs are also susceptible to degenerative disc disease. The effects of normal aging and of degenerative disc disease are very similar and difficult to differentiate. The onset and progression of degenerative disc disease may be influenced by genetics or environmental influences such as working conditions or lifestyle [Battie, Videman, and Parent 2004; Osti and Cullum 1994]. It is thought that individuals whose work involves heavy physical activity or long periods of driving suffer intervertebral disc degeneration or low back pain at higher rates than normal [Osti and Cullum 1994]. However, scientific evidence to support this is inconclusive [Battie, Videman, and Parent 2004], partly because other factors such as socioeconomic status are difficult to separate from employment status. Smoking and obesity are also thought to contribute to intervertebral disc degeneration [Battie et al. 1991].

The nutritional, biochemical, compositional, structural, and mechanical milestones of aging and degeneration are well marked. Overall, the degenerative changes in the intervertebral disc result in a loss of demarcation between the nucleus pulposus and annulus fibrosus, loss of disc height, a decrease in height as the intervertebral disc loses its ability to rehydrate after loading, and altered loading on the intervertebral disc and surrounding tissues. The factors responsible for the initiation of the degenerative process and the specific sequence of events in the process are not known. Degeneration may be related to low back pain, although the connections are not confirmed and the source of low back pain is not known. Low back pain is among the top ten reasons for doctor visits in the United States, with direct costs reaching $25 billion [Frymoyer and Cats-Baril 1991]. Currently, there is no treatment that restores mobility or function to the degenerated intervertebral disc. Therefore, understanding intervertebral disc degeneration may be an important step toward developing successful therapies for low back pain.

3.3.1 Nucleus Pulposus

It is thought that the aging and degenerative processes first affect the nucleus pulposus. Beginning early in life, the large aggregating proteoglycans in the healthy nucleus pulposus break down, so that large aggregating proteoglycans comprise as little as 10% of the total proteoglycan content by adulthood [Johnstone and Bayliss 1995]. Degraded proteoglycan components remain in the nucleus pulposus, which may affect the ability to attract and bind water. Water, which makes up nearly 90% of the weight of nucleus pulposus tissue in childhood, begins to decrease in the nucleus pulposus early in life, until it comprises 70% or less of total nucleus pulposus weight in the elderly [Antoniou et al. 1996; Eyre 1979].

Proteinases, cell metabolism, and nutrition may all play a role in initiating the breakdown of proteoglycans in the nucleus pulposus. In the healthy intervertebral disc, there is a balance (or homeostasis) between proteoglycan synthesis and degradation, and also between inflow of nutrients and outflow of waste products. Degenerated nucleus pulposus tissue has increased levels of matrix metalloproteinases (MMPs), which are enzymes that degrade proteins such as proteoglycans and collagen. In healthy tissues, the production of MMPs by nucleus pulposus cells is regulated by a complex cascade of mechanical and biochemical factors. However, regulation of this cascade with age or degeneration may be disturbed [Goupille et al. 1998]. To compound the problem of proteoglycan degradation, nucleus pulposus cells are unable to synthesize proteoglycans at the rate they are destroyed. Cell production of proteoglycans and collagen may also be affected by decreases in intervertebral disc nutrition that occur with degeneration. Lack of nutrition and buildup of waste products or degraded proteoglycans in the nucleus pulposus adversely affect the cellular environment, causing a reduction in cellular synthesis of proteoglycans and collagen, or even cell death.

Collagen composition and overall structure of the nucleus pulposus also change in the degenerated intervertebral disc. The total amount of type II collagen in the nucleus pulposus decreases, and type I collagen increases [Antoniou et al. 1996; Nerlich, Schleicher, and Boos 1997]. Collagen fibers become denatured. The gelatinous, translucent nucleus pulposus becomes firmer, and progressively white, then yellow or brownish due to oxidation resulting from poor nutrition and accumulation of waste products (Figure 3.7). Noncollagenous proteins and dense granular tissue increase with age and degeneration [Buckwalter 1995]. The nucleus pulposus becomes less like a liquid and more like a solid [Iatridis et al. 1996], taking on more solid-like material properties. Shear modulus increases by up to 80% [Iatridis et al. 1997] and the swelling pressure of degenerated nucleus pulposus tissue decreases dramatically, from 1 to 2 MPa to 0.03 MPa or less (Johannessen and Elliott 2005; Nachemson and Morris 1964; Wilke et al. 1999). Compression stiffness decreases from 1.0 MPa to 0.4 MPa [Johannessen and Elliott 2005]. Changes to the mechanical and biochemical environment of nucleus pulposus cells may further alter cellular synthesis of nucleus pulposus components.

The initiation of nucleus pulposus changes is not possible to pinpoint. Rather, aging and degeneration are inter-related: biochemical changes cause cellular changes that result in mechanical changes, which in turn cause more biochemical and cellular changes. The changes observed in the degenerating nucleus pulposus and their biomechanical consequences may be key factors in further progression of degeneration in the entire intervertebral disc.

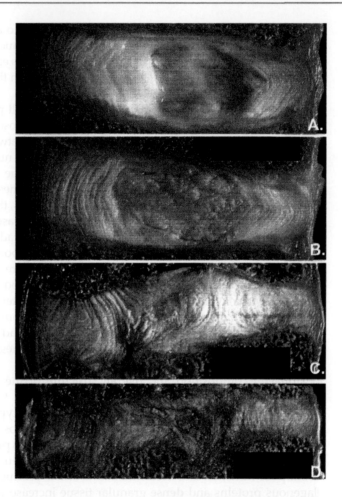

Fig. 3.7.
Progression of intervertebral disc degeneration adapted from Addms, 2002. (A) Nondegenerated, healthy intervertebral disc with distinction between nucleus pulposus and annulus fibrosus, hydrated, shiny, white gelatinous nucleus pulposus and distinct annulus fibrosus layers. (B) Moderately degenerated intervertebral disc, with fibrous nucleus pulposus and yellowing of the nucleus pulposus and annulus fibrosus. (C) Severe degeneration, with loss of distinction between nucleus pulposus and annulus fibrosus, severe fibrosus of nucleus pulposus. (D) Extreme degeneration, with loss of disc height, clefts in the nucleus pulposus, and inward bulging of the annulus fibrosus.

3.3.2 Annulus Fibrosus

The structure, composition, and function of the annulus fibrosus are affected by degeneration. It is thought that these changes may, in part, result from the degenerative changes initiated in the nucleus pulposus. Loss of water in the nucleus pulposus prevents that tissue from pressurizing, and it is thus less able to absorb and transmit the compressive loads of the spine. These compressive loads are directly transferred to the annulus fibrosus. Without nucleus pulposus pressurization, the layers of the inner annulus fibrosus may bulge inward in compression, rather than outward in tension [Meakin, Redpath, and Hukins 2001; Seroussi et al. 1989], and the entire intervertebral disc motion segment may become hypermobile [Johannessen et al. 2005]. Degeneration-induced alterations in mechanical loading in the annulus fibrosus include increased shear stresses and stress concentrations. This may lead to cracks, tears, or fissures in the tissue or delamination of the layers of the annulus [Iatridis and Gwynn 2004] (Figure 3.7).

With aging and degeneration, annulus fibrosus layers become disorganized and less distinct. The number of layers through the radial thickness of the tissue decreases, and the layers become thicker [Marchand and Ahmed 1990]. These structural changes affect the mechanical properties of the annulus fibrosus. Although the circumferential linear-region modulus does not significantly change with degeneration (Table 3.1), the circumferential toe-region modulus in the outer anterior region increases from 2.5 to 5.7 MPa with degeneration, likely because changes in water content affect the nonlinear and viscoelastic behaviors of the tissue [Guerin and Elliott 2005b]. Additionally, the Poisson's ratio decreases by about 50% with degeneration [Acaroglu et al. 1995; Elliott and Setton 2001; Guerin and Elliott 2005b]. Shear modulus increases [Iatridis et al. 1999] and failure strain decreases in degenerated annulus fibrosus tissue [Acaroglu et al. 1995]. These mechanical property changes alter the loading patterns on surrounding tissues including the vertebrae, muscles, and ligaments.

Biochemical and cellular changes in the degenerated annulus fibrosus may be an adaptation to the altered mechanical environment. In degenerated intervertebral discs, type I collagen content decreases from 50 to 40% of total collagen content, and type II collagen content increases from 50 to 60% of total collagen content in the annulus [Eyre 1979], perhaps to better withstand compressive loads. The ratio of type I to type II collagen from outer to inner annulus fibrosus also changes, so that type II collagen increases specifically in the outer annulus fibrosus, and type I collagen increases in the inner annulus fibrosus [Eyre 1979]. Collagen in the annulus fibrosus of degenerated intervertebral discs becomes cross-linked and denatured, and collagen protein modifications and oxidation causes the characteristic discoloration of degenerated annulus fibrosus tissue (Figure 3.7) [Hormel and Eyre 1991].

Altered tissue mechanics may also cause cell death or altered cell synthesis. Like the cells of the nucleus pulposus, annulus fibrosus cells are subject to density and nutritional limitations. Low cell density, cell nutrition, and the buildup of waste products affect the synthesis of collagen and proteoglycans. Matrix metalloproteinases degrade the proteoglycans and collagens of the annulus fibrosus with age and degeneration. As in the nucleus pulposus, cell synthesis of these proteins cannot meet the rate of destruction.

3.3.3 End Plates

Degeneration impacts the cartilagenous end plates of the intervertebral disc. The cartilage of the end plates thins, becomes calcified, and the blood supply to the end plates becomes diminished [Bernick and Cailliet 1982]. These factors, coupled with occlusion of the marrow contact channels with age [Benneker et al. 2005], prevent important nutrients such as glucose and oxygen from entering the intervertebral disc and prevent waste products such as lactic acid from leaving the intervertebral disc [Boos et al. 2002; Urban, Smith, and Fairbank 2004]. End plate changes with degeneration thus may affect the biochemical environment of the entire intervertebral disc, impacting cell metabolism in the nucleus pulposus and annulus fibrosus. However, the specific mechanisms by which end plate calcification and degeneration contribute to disc degeneration are not known.

The mechanical response of the end plate to the changes induced by aging and degeneration has not yet been fully quantified. Increased degeneration is associated with decreased failure properties in the bony end plate, but stiffness is not affected [Grant, Oxland, and Dvorak 2001]. Degenerative changes in the intervertebral disc cause load transfer from the nucleus pulposus to the annulus fibrosus. Therefore, the periphery of the end plates is loaded more in degeneration, possibly contributing to degenerative changes in the end plate [Kurowski and Kubo 1986]. When the periphery of the end plate is loaded in degenerated intervertebral discs, end plate failure typically occurs by fracture at the periphery [Perey 1957].

3.3.4 Intervertebral Disc Degeneration: Relationship to Low Back Pain and Treatments

There are many mechanisms for low back pain that may originate from the intervertebral disc. Loss of disc height and structure may result in pain in the intervertebral disc itself because of increased enervation in degenerated intervertebral discs. Loss of disc height may also contribute to altered loading on the vertebral bodies and facet joints of the spine, resulting in pain and possibly arthritis in the facet joints. Additionally, surrounding muscles of the spine may (voluntarily or involuntarily) increase activation to counteract or restrict painful motion [Stokes and Iatridis 2004]. Bulging of the intervertebral disc can result in nerve root impingement, causing pain in areas of the body enervated by the impinged nerve. Degenerated intervertebral discs may release mediators that sensitize nerve endings [Buckwalter et al. 2000b]. Other painful intervertebral disc-related conditions include spinal stenosis, a narrowing of the vertebral foramen due to thickening of the ligaments, bones, and facet joints adjacent to the space [Spivak 1998]. In herniation, nucleus pulposus material protrudes through weakened areas of the annulus fibrosus. End plate degeneration (or osteophytes, which are bony protrusions on the rims of the vertebral bodies) may also be a source of pain. However, it is not known precisely how any of these conditions, including intervertebral disc degeneration itself, generate low back pain.

Intervertebral disc degeneration is commonly diagnosed using noninvasive imaging methods such as X-ray, magnetic resonance imaging (MRI), or discography. Although only bone is visible on an X-ray image, intervertebral disc degeneration may be identified using this method by observation of narrowing of the disc space between vertebrae. MRI imaging shows both bone and soft tissue. Intervertebral disc degeneration may be identified on MRI by a visible loss of disc height, bulging of the intervertebral disc into the spinal cord, osteophytes, loss of signal intensity in the nucleus pulposus indicating decreased water content, and irregularly shaped end plates [Beattie and Meyers 1998]. However, degeneration of intervertebral discs evidenced by MRI does not always correlate with low back pain. Conversely, patients who experience low back pain may not necessarily show signs of intervertebral disc degeneration on MRI [Haughton 2004]. Discography is used to identify intervertebral discs that are a possible source of pain. A contrast agent is injected into a specific intervertebral disc under fluoroscopic guidance to determine if that disc elicits the same pain response in the patient.

Current treatment options for low back pain are limited, and each has significant drawbacks. Conservative treatments include rest, physical therapy, activity modification, or injections into the epidural space to relieve low back pain. Other treatments include discectomy (removal of all or part of the nucleus pulposus to depressurize the intervertebral disc) or intradiscal electrothermal therapy (a less invasive means of removing tissue using heat or radiofrequency probes). Fusion remains the surgical standard for treatment of low back pain resulting from intervertebral disc degeneration. In this treatment, the intervertebral disc is removed, and grafts and/or hardware implants are inserted in its place to fuse adjacent vertebrae. This treatment removes the degenerated intervertebral disc (the possible source of pain) and restores disc height, but does not always eliminate pain. Range of motion is limited by fusion and mechanics are significantly altered in the vertebrae and intervertebral discs adjacent to fusion, contributing to degeneration of adjacent motion segments [Park et al. 2004].

Intervertebral disc arthroplasty is a promising treatment for low back pain that seeks to retain range of motion, avoid adjacent segment degeneration, and restore disc height and spinal mechanics [Anderson and Rouleau 2004]. However, as this treatment option is new, long-term studies must still be conducted to confirm that these goals are met. Nucleus pulposus replacements are also being developed to restore mechanical function in early stages of intervertebral disc degeneration. Interventional treatment options such as gene therapy or administration of growth factors are also being developed to prevent the progression of degeneration [Masuda, Oegema, and An 2004; Shimer et al. 2004]. Current and future low back pain treatments are more thoroughly discussed in Chapters 1, 7, and 10.

3.4 Ligaments

The ligaments of the spine tether the vertebrae together, providing support to the entire spinal column. They constrain motions of the spine to prevent overextension and injury. Ligaments are comprised primarily of type I collagen fibers embedded in a hydrated extracellular matrix. The structure and composition of the spinal ligaments enable the mechanical function of these tissues.

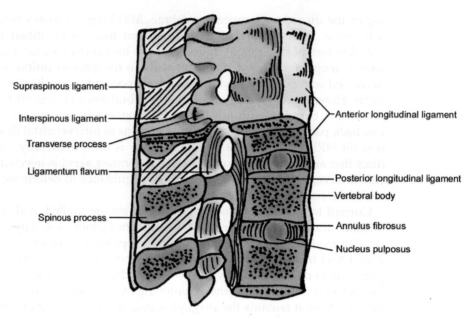

Supraspinous ligament

Interspinous ligament

Transverse process

Ligamentum flavum

Spinous process

Anterior longitudinal ligament

Posterior longitudinal ligament

Vertebral body

Annulus fibrosus

Nucleus pulposus

Fig. 3.8.

Spinal ligaments. Anterior and posterior longitudinal ligaments run the length of the spinal column outside the vertebral bodies. Ligamentum flavum and interspinous ligament join adjacent vertebrae, and supraspinous ligament connects spinous processes.

The main ligaments of the spine are the anterior and posterior longitudinal ligaments (Figure 3.8). Each is continuous along the front (anterior) or back (posterior) of the spinal column, providing strong support for the spinal column from the neck to the sacrum. The anterior longitudinal ligament is the stronger and wider of the two ligaments. Failure of this ligament occurs between 330 and 435 N [Neumann et al. 1992]. The anterior longitudinal ligament is attached to the vertebrae and intervertebral discs at each level. At these insertion points, the fibers of the ligaments interweave with either bone tissue or the fibers of the annulus fibrosus to provide a strong connection. The anterior longitudinal ligament is stretched in tension as the back is extended (i.e., bending backward). The restoring force of this tissue, conferred by its elasticity in the direction of the spine, opposes extension and protects the spine against hyperextension. The posterior longitudinal ligament is smaller and is only attached to the intervertebral discs. It is stretched in flexion, and thus resists hyperflexion (i.e., bending forward too far). By restricting the range of motion of the spine, the anterior and posterior longitudinal ligaments (along with the facet joints and facet joint capsules) help to protect the intervertebral discs from damage due to excessive motions of the intervertebral sympheses.

The anterior and posterior ligaments are comprised of highly organized type I collagen fibers embedded in an extracellular matrix of proteoglycans. Type I collagen, which absorbs and transmits tensile loads, makes up 70% of the dry weight of these ligaments [Woo et al. 2000]. The collagen fibers of the anterior and posterior ligaments are oriented parallel to the length of the spine. This transversely isotropic structure gives these ligaments the greatest elasticity and strength along the fiber direction. Perpendicular to the fiber direction, mechanical properties such as modulus and failure stress are orders of magnitude lower because there is no fiber reinforcement in that direction [Lynch et al. 2003; Quapp and Weiss 1998]. Like the annulus fibrosus, ligaments exhibit nonlinear stress/strain behavior and viscoelastic behaviors such as creep and stress relaxation (Figure 3.6).

The proteoglycans of ligament are different than those of the nucleus pulposus, as they are smaller and nonaggregating, and include decorin and biglycan. Proteoglycans make up less than 1% of the dry weight of the tissue [Frank et al. 1988]. However, the proteoglycans of ligament do attract and bind water to the tissue, so that water makes up 60 to 70% of the total weight of the tissue [Frank et al. 1988].

Other smaller ligaments connect each of the vertebrae together individually. The ligamenta flava connect to the posterior lamina of adjacent vertebrae (Figure 3.8). Like the posterior longitudinal ligament, the ligamenta flava are stretched during flexion of the spine. However, because they are further from the axis of rotation of the motion segment (which is positioned in the intervertebral disc) the ligamenta flava are actually stretched more than the posterior longitudinal ligament for the same amount of flexion [Hukins and Meakin 2000]. This causes higher strains in the ligamenta flava. The collagen fibers of the ligamenta flava are initially disorganized, rather than uniaxially oriented, but become aligned at high strains. This allows the ligamenta flava to withstand these high strains without failure [Hukins and Meakin 2000].

The interspinous ligaments are situated between the spinous processes of adjacent vertebrae (Figure 3.8), and are comprised of collagen fibers oriented in a fan-like arrangement. In this orientation, the fibers are not stretched in flexion or extension. The function of these ligaments is not known, but it may be to transfer stress from the surrounding musculature [Hukins and Meakin 2000]. The supraspinous ligament is a long ligament that extends from the top of the spine to between the third and fifth lumbar vertebra (Figure 3.8). It has little tensile strength. It is thought that the purpose of this ligament is not necessarily to provide mechanical function but to provide cushioning for the spine [Hukins and Meakin 2000].

The ligaments of the spine are affected by age, although to a lesser degree than the intervertebral disc. In young people, the anterior longitudinal ligament is most likely to fail at the mid-substance. In older people, failure is at the bone insertion site [Neumann et al. 1994]. Injury or degeneration of the spinal ligaments may alter the mechanical environment of the spine, particularly in the intervertebral disc, and may predispose the disc to degeneration.

3.5 Spinal Cord

Unlike the other soft tissue structures of the spine, the function of the spinal cord is not mechanical. Rather, the spinal cord is the conduction pathway for

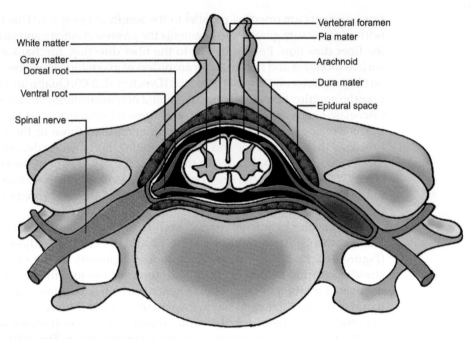

White matter
Gray matter
Dorsal root
Ventral root
Spinal nerve

Vertebral foramen
Pia mater
Arachnoid
Dura mater
Epidural space

Fig. 3.9.

Cross section of spinal cord. White and gray matters compose the spinal cord, which is protected by the *dura mater*, *arachnoid mater*, and *pia mater*. Spinal nerves extend from spinal cord in pairs, and are made up of a dorsal and a ventral root.

nerve impulses between the brain and the rest of the body. The spinal cord is about 1 centimeter wide and resides in the space of the vertebral foramen (Figure 3.9). At each vertebral level, a pair of spinal nerves branches off of the spinal cord and exits from the vertebral foramen to enervate the body.

The spinal cord itself ends at the first lumbar vertebra. It terminates in a cone-shaped structure called the *conus medullaris*. From the *conus medullaris* arise the spinal nerves that enervate the lower regions of the body. These nerves resemble a horse's tail extending from the *conus medullaris*, and are thus called the *cauda equina*. The nerves of the *cauda equina* enervate the lower regions of the body. They travel through the vertebral foramen and exit the spinal column in pairs, like the nerves of the spinal cord.

Each spinal nerve has two origins, or roots, at the spinal cord: one dorsal and one ventral (Figure 3.9). These roots join outside the vertebral body into one spinal nerve. The ventral (efferent) root is made up of motor fibers, and carries outputs from the brain to the muscles. The dorsal (afferent) root is comprised of sensory fibers that carry sensory inputs to the brain. The pair of spinal nerves that exit from each vertebral level enervates the same parts of the body in every person. The specific muscles enervated by a spinal nerve are called myotomes, and the areas of skin are called dermatomes. For instance, the motor nerves that exit at C7 straighten the elbow, and the sensory fibers enervate the tops of the forearms.

The spinal cord itself is divided into gray matter and white matter (Figure 3.9). The gray matter is in the interior part of the spinal cord, and is made up of the nerve cell bodies. The white matter surrounds the gray matter, and is made up of the axons that extend from the nerve cells. The axon is the part of the nerve cell that transmits signals to the nucleus of the nerve cell, and ultimately to the brain. The axons of the white matter are surrounded by a specialized cell (Schwann cell) that forms a protective lipid and protein sheath, called myelin. Myelination also affects the velocity of the conduction signals in the axon.

Mechanically, the spinal cord is a nonlinear, viscoelastic material [Bilston and Thibault 1996]. It is a very soft tissue with low modulus so that it may easily deform under typical spinal motion without suffering high loads. The white and gray matters of the spinal cord have different mechanical properties, with the gray matter the more relatively rigid and brittle of the two [Ichihara et al. 2003]. The tensile modulus of the gray matter (64 to 112 kPa) is nearly twice that of the white matter (30 to 65 kPa). However, the gray matter fails at lower strains. This difference in mechanical properties may cause high shear stresses between the two structures under load, and contribute to injury or degeneration of the spinal cord [Ichihara et al. 2003].

The spinal cord is fragile, and the nerves that make up the spinal cord cannot regenerate once they are destroyed by injury. Therefore, there are several protective mechanisms for this tissue. First, the spinal cord and nerves of the *cauda equina* are housed in the foraminal space of each vertebra along the spinal column, so that the entire spinal cord is surrounded by rigid bone (Figure 3.9). Second, within the vertebral foramen there are three protective layers of soft tissue surrounding the length of the spinal cord (Figure 3.9). The outermost layer, the *dura mater*, surrounds both the brain and the spinal cord, and is the strongest and thickest of the three layers. It is comprised of longitudinally oriented collagen fibers in an extracellular matrix. With aligned collagen fibers conferring the greatest tensile strength in the longitudinal direction, the *dura mater* provides protection for the spinal cord during flexion or extension of the spine [Runza et al. 1999]. Inside the *dura mater* is the *arachnoid mater*, a thin, web-like layer of tissue. Inside the sub-arachnoid space is the cerebrospinal fluid, which cushions the spinal cord. Last, the spinal cord is most closely surrounded by the very thin *pia mater*. The *pia mater* is extremely elastic, with a tensile modulus of 2.3 MPa, and provides constraint for the spinal cord inside [Ozawa et al. 2004]. If the spinal cord is compressed, the *pia mater* helps restore the spinal cord to its original shape and configuration after decompression.

Despite these layers of protection, the spinal cord is still vulnerable to injury from compression (such as from bulging intervertebral discs) or swelling. In addition to these mechanical protections, there is also a barrier between the blood supply and the spinal cord. This protects the spinal cord from potentially harmful substances in the bloodstream, but can also prevent potentially therapeutic drugs from entering the spinal cord.

3.6 Conclusions

The soft tissue structures of the spine provide flexibility, mobility, and connectivity. The intervertebral discs are specialized structures that allow for the large loads and varied motions of the spine. The annulus fibrosus, nucleus pulposus, and end plates of the intervertebral disc act in concert to absorb and distribute loads in complex combinations of bending, shear, torsion, compression, and tension. However, the intervertebral discs lose flexibility and mobility with age and degeneration as a result of decreases in mechanical properties and alterations to structure and composition. The ligaments of the spine provide reinforcement to the spinal column, preventing excessive motions which might damage the other soft tissue structures of the spine. The highly organized structure of these ligaments contributes to their mechanical function in the spine. These soft tissues, along with the vertebral bones, protect the fragile spinal cord, a soft tissue that provides motor control and sensory perception to the rest of the body. Although the intervertebral discs and ligaments are tough, flexible tissues—and the spinal cord has many protections—these soft tissues are susceptible to injury and degeneration, and healing and repair in these tissues are difficult to accomplish.

3.7 References

Acaroglu, E. R., J. C. Iatridis, and L. A. Setton (1995). "Degeneration and Aging Affect the Tensile Behavior of Human Lumbar Anulus Fibrosus," *Spine* 20:2690–2701.

Adams, M. A., N. Bogduk, K. Burton, and P. Dolan (2002). *The Biomechanics of Back Pain*. Edinburgh: Churchill Livingstone.

Anderson, P. A., and J. P. Rouleau (2004). "Intervertebral Disc Arthroplasty," *Spine* 29:2779–2786.

Antoniou, J., T. Steffen, and F. Nelson (1996). "The Human Lumbar Intervertebral Disc: Evidence for Changes in the Biosynthesis and Denaturation of the Extracellular Matrix with Growth, Maturation, Ageing, and Degeneration," *J. Clin. Invest.* 98:996–1003.

Ayotte, D. C., K. Ito, and S. Tepic (2001). "Direction-dependent Resistance to Flow in the Endplate of the Intervertebral Disc: An Ex Vivo Study," *J. Orthop. Res.* 19:1073–1077.

Battie, M. C., T. Videman, and K. Gill (1991). "1991 Volvo Award in Clinical Sciences. Smoking and Lumbar Intervertebral Disc Degeneration: An MRI Study of Identical Twins," *Spine* 16:1015–1021.

Battie, M. C., T. Videman, and E. Parent (2004). "Lumbar Disc Degeneration: Epidemiology and Genetic Influences," *Spine* 29:2679–2690.

Beattie, P. F., and S. P. Meyers (1998). "Magnetic Resonance Imaging in Low Back Pain: General Principles and Clinical Issues," *Phys. Ther.* 78:738–753.

Benneker, L. M., P. F. Heini, and M. Alini (2005). "2004 Young Investigator Award Winner: Vertebral Endplate Marrow Contact Channel Occlusions and Intervertebral Disc Degeneration," *Spine* 30:167–173.

Bernick, S., and R. Cailliet (1982). "Vertebral End-plate Changes with Aging of Human Vertebrae," *Spine* 7:97–102.

Bilston, L. E., and L. E. Thibault (1996). "The Mechanical Properties of the Human Cervical Spinal Cord In Vitro," *Ann Biomed. Eng.* 24:67–74.

Boos, N., S. Weissbach, and H. Rohrbach (2002). "Classification of Age-related Changes in Lumbar Intervertebral Discs: 2002 Volvo Award in Basic Science," *Spine* 27:2631–2644.

Brinckmann, P., W. Frobin, and E. Hierholzer (1983). "Deformation of the Vertebral Endplate Under Axial Loading of the Spine," *Spine* 8:851–856.

Buckwalter, J. A. (1995). "Aging and Degeneration of the Human Intervertebral Disc," *Spine* 20:1307–1314.

Buckwalter, J. A., S. D. Boden, and D. R. Eyre (2000b). "Intervertebral Disk Aging, Degeneration, and Herniation," in J. A. Buckwalter, T. A. Einhorn, and S. R. Simon, (eds.), *Orthopaedic Basic Science.* American Academy of Orthopaedic Surgeons.

Buckwalter, J., V. C. Mow, and S. D. Boden (2000a). "Intervertebral Disc Structure, Composition, and Mechanical Function," in J. A. Buckwalter, T. A. Einhorn, and S. R. Simon (eds.), *Orthopaedic Basic Science.* pp. 547–556, American Academy of Orthopaedic Surgeons.

Buckwalter, J. M. J. (1996). "Intervertebral Disk Degeneration and Back Pain," in G. Weinstein (ed.), *Low Back Pain.* American Academy of Orthopaedic Surgeons.

Cassidy, J. J., A. Hiltner, and E. Baer (1989). "Hierarchical Structure of the Intervertebral Disc," *Connective Tissue Research* 23:75–88.

Coventry, M. B., R. K. Ghormley, and J. W. Kernohan (1945a). "The Intervertebral Disc: Its Microscopic Anatomy and Pathology, Part I: Anatomy, Development, and Physiology," *J. Bone Joint Surg.* 27:105–112.

Coventry, M. B., R. K. Ghormley, and J. W. Kernohan (1945b). "The Intervertebral Disc: Its Microscopic Anatomy and Pathology, Part II: Changes in the Intervertebral Disc Concomitant with Age," *J. Bone Joint Surg.* 27:233–247.

Ebara, S., J. C. Iatridis, and L. A. Setton (1996). "Tensile Properties of Nondegenerate Human Lumbar Anulus Fibrosus," *Spine* 21:452–461.

Edwards, W. T., Y. Zheng, and L. A. Ferrara (2001). "Structural Features and Thickness of the Vertebral Cortex in the Thoracolumbar Spine," *Spine* 26:218–225.

Elliott, D. M., and L. A. Setton (2001). "Anisotropic and Inhomogeneous Tensile Behavior of the Human Anulus Fibrosus: Experimental Measurement and Material Model Predictions," *J. Biomech. Eng.* 123:256–263.

Eyre, D. R. (1979). "Biochemistry of the Intervertebral Disc," *Int. Rev. Connect. Tissue Res.* 8:227–291.

Eyre, D. R., and H. Muir (1976). "Types I and II Collagens in Intervertebral Disc: Interchanging Radial Distributions in Annulus Fibrosus," *Biochem. J.* 157:267–270.

Frank, C. B., S. L. Woo, and T. Andriacchi (1988). "Normal Ligament: Structure, Function, and Composition," in S. L. Y. Woo and J. A. Buckwalter (eds.), *Injury and Repair of the Musculoskeletal Soft Tissues.* American Academy of Orthopaedic Surgeons.

Frymoyer, J. W., and W. L. Cats-Baril (1991). "An Overview of the Incidences and Costs of Low Back Pain," *Ortho. Clin. North Am.* 22:263–271.

Fujita, Y., N. A. Duncan, and J. C. Lotz (1997). "Radial Tensile Properties of the Lumbar Annulus Fibrosus Are Site and Degeneration Dependent," *J. Orthop. Res.* 15:814–819.

Goupille, P., M. I. Jayson, and J. P. Valat (1998). "Matrix Metalloproteinases: The Clue to Intervertebral Disc Degeneration," *Spine* 23:1612–1626.

Grant, J. P., T. R. Oxland, and M. F. Dvorak (2001). Mapping the Structural Properties of the Lumbosacral Vertebral Endplates," *Spine* 26:889–896.

Guerin, H. A. L., and D. M. Elliott (2005a). "The Role of Fiber-Matrix Interactions in a Nonlinear Fiber-Reinforced Strain Energy Model of Tendon," *J. Biomech. Eng.* 127(2):345–350.

Guerin, H. L., and D. M. Elliott (2005b). "Degeneration Affects the Fiber Reorientation of Human Annulus Fibrosus Under Tensile Load," *J. Biomech.* (in press).

Haughton, V. (2004). "Medical Imaging of Intervertebral Disc Degeneration: Current Status of Imaging," *Spine* 29:2751–2756.

Hickey, D. S., and D. W. Hukins (1980). "X-ray Diffraction Studies of the Arrangement of Collagenous Fibres in Human Fetal Intervertebral Disc," *J. Anat.* 131: 81–90.

Hormel, S. E., and D. R. Eyre (1991). "Collagen in the Aging Human Intervertebral Disc: An Increase in Covalently Bound Fluorophores and Chromophores," *Biochim. Biophys. Acta.* 1078:243–250.

Hukins, D. W., and J. R. Meakin (2000). "Relationship Between Structure and Mechanical Function of the Tissues of the Intervertebral Joint," *A. Zool.* 40: 42–52.

Iatridis, J. C., and I. ap Gwynn (2004). "Mechanisms for Mechanical Damage in the Intervertebral Disc Annulus Fibrosus," *J. Biomech.* 37:1165–1175.

Iatridis, J. C., S. Kumar, and R. J. Foster (1999). "Shear Mechanical Properties of Human Lumbar Annulus Fibrosus," *J. Orthop. Res.* 17:732–737.

Iatridis, J. C., L. A. Setton, and R. J. Foster (1998). "Degeneration Affects the Anisotropic and Nonlinear Behaviors of Human Annulus Fibrosus in Compression," *J. Biomech.* 31:535–544.

Iatridis, J. C., L. A. Setton, and M. Weidenbaum (1997). "Alterations in the Mechanical Behavior of the Human Lumbar Nucleus Pulposus with Degeneration and Aging," *J. Orthop. Res.* 15:318–322.

Iatridis, J. C., M. Weidenbaum, and L. A. Setton (1996). "Is the Nucleus Pulposus a Solid or a Fluid? Mechanical Behaviors of the Nucleus Pulposus of the Human Intervertebral Disc," *Spine* 21:1174–1184.

Ichihara, K., T. Taguchi, and I. Sakuramoto (2003). Mechanism of the Spinal Cord Injury and the Cervical Spondylotic Myelopathy: New Approach Based on the Mechanical Features of the Spinal Cord White and Gray Matter," *J. Neurosurg. Spine* 99:278–285.

Johannessen, W., and D. M. Elliott (2005). "Effects of Degeneration on the Biphasic Material Properties of Human Nucleus Pulposus in Confined Compression," *Spine* 30:E724–E729.

Johannessen, W., E. J. Vresilovic, and J. R. Mills (2005). "Effect of Nucleotomy on Tension-Compression Behavior of the Intervertebral Disc," in *Transactions of the Orthopaedic Research Society.*

Johnstone, B., and M. T. Bayliss (1995). "The Large Proteoglycans of the Human Intervertebral Disc: Changes in Their Biosynthesis and Structure with Age, Topography, and Pathology," *Spine* 20:674–684.

Kastelic, J., I. Pally, and E. Baer (1980). "A Structural Mechanical Model for Tendon Crimping," *J. Biomech.* 13:887–893.

Kurowski, P., and A. Kubo (1986). "The Relationship of Degeneration of the Intervertebral Disc to Mechanical Loading Conditions on Lumbar Vertebrae," *Spine* 11:726–731.

Lynch, H. A., W. Johannessen, and J. P. Wu (2003). "Effect of Fiber Orientation and Strain Rate on the Nonlinear Uniaxial Tensile Material Properties of Tendon," *J. Biomech. Eng.* 125:726–731.

Marchand, F., and A. M. Ahmed (1990). Investigation of the Laminate Structure of Lumbar Disc Anulus Fibrosus," *Spine* 15:402–410.

Masuda, K., T. R. Oegema Jr., and H. S. An (2004). "Growth Factors and Treatment of Intervertebral Disc Degeneration," *Spine* 29:2757–2769.

McNally, D. S., and M. A. Adams (1992). "Internal Intervertebral Disc Mechanics As Revealed by Stress Profilometry," *Spine* 17:66–73.

Meakin, J. R., T. W. Redpath, and D. W. Hukins (2001). "The Effect of Partial Removal of the Nucleus Pulposus from the Intervertebral Disc on the Response of the Human Annulus Fibrosus to Compression," *Clinical Biomechanics* 16:121–128.

Nachemson, A., and J. M. Morris (1964). "In Vivo Measurements of Intradiscal Pressure," *Journal of Bone and Joint Surgery* 46A:1077–1092.

Nerlich, A. G., E. D. Schleicher, and N. Boos (1997). "1997 Volvo Award Winner in Basic Science Studies: Immunohistologic Markers for Age-related Changes of Human Lumbar Intervertebral Discs," *Spine* 22:2781–2795.

Neumann, P., L. A. Ekstrom, and T. S. Keller (1994). "Aging, Vertebral Density, and Disc Degeneration Alter the Tensile Stress-strain Characteristics of the Human Anterior Longitudinal Ligament," *J. Orthop. Res.* 12:103–112.

Neumann, P., T. S. Keller, and L. Ekstrom (1992). "Mechanical Properties of the Human Lumbar Anterior Longitudinal Ligament," *J. Biomech.* 25:1185–1194.

Oegema, T. R. Jr. (1993). "Biochemistry of the Intervertebral Disc," *Clin. Sports Med.* 12:419–439.

Osti, O. L., and D. E. Cullum (1994). "Occupational Low Back Pain and Intervertebral Disc Degeneration: Epidemiology, Imaging, and Pathology," *Clin. J. Pain* 10: 331–334.

Osti, O. L., B. Vernon-Roberts, and R. Moore (1992). "Annular Tears and Disc Degeneration in the Lumbar Spine: A Post-mortem Study of 135 Discs," *J. Bone Joint Surg. Br.* 74:678–682.

Ozawa, H., T. Matsumoto, and T. Ohashi (2004). "Mechanical Properties and Function of the Spinal Pia Mater," *J. Neurosurg. Spine* 1:122–127.

Park, P., H. J. Garton, and V. C. Gala (2004). "Adjacent Segment Disease After Lumbar or Lumbosacral Fusion: Review of the Literature," *Spine* 29:1938–1944.

Pearce, R. H. (1993). "Morphologic and Chemical Aspects of Aging," in J. A. Buckwalter, V. M. Goldberg, and S. L. Woo (eds.), *Musculoskeletal Soft-Tissue Aging: Impact on Mobility*. Rosemont, IL: American Academy of Orthopaedic Surgeons.

Perey, O (1957). "Fracture of the Vertebral End-plate in the Lumbar Spine: An Experimental Biochemical Investigation," *Acta Orthop. Scand.* 1–101.

Quapp, K. M., and J. A. Weiss (1998). "Material Characterization of Human Medial Collateral Ligament," *Journal of Biomechanical Engineering* 120:757–763.

Roberts, S., J. Menage, and J. P. Urban (1989). "Biochemical and Structural Properties of the Cartilage End-plate and Its Relation to the Intervertebral Disc," *Spine* 14:166–174.

Roughley, P. J. (2004). "Biology of Intervertebral Disc Aging and Degeneration: Involvement of the Extracellular Matrix," *Spine* 29:2691–2699.

Runza, M., R. Pietrabissa, and S. Mantero (1999). "Lumbar Dura Mater Biomechanics: Experimental Characterization and Scanning Electron Microscopy Observations," *Anesth. Analg.* 88:1317–1321.

Seroussi, R. E., M. H. Krag, and D. L. Muller (1989). "Internal Deformations of Intact and Denucleated Human Lumbar Discs Subjected to Compression, Flexion, and Extension Loads," *J. Orthop. Res.* 7:122–131.

Setton, L. A., and J. Chen (2004). Cell Mechanics and Mechanobiology in the Intervertebral Disc," *Spine* 29:2710–2723.

Shimer, A. L., R. C. Chadderdon, and L. G. Gilbertson (2004). "Gene Therapy Approaches for Intervertebral Disc Degeneration," *Spine* 29:2770–2778.

Spivak, J. M. (1998). "Degenerative Lumbar Spinal Stenosis," *J. Bone Joint Surg. Am.* 80:1053–1066.

Stokes, I. A., and J. C. Iatridis (2004). "Mechanical Conditions That Accelerate Intervertebral Disc Degeneration: Overload Versus Immobilization," *Spine* 29:2724–2732.

Urban, J. P., S. Holm, and A. Maroudas (1982). "Nutrition of the Intervertebral Disc: Effect of Fluid Flow on Solute Transport," *Clin. Orthop.* 296–302.

Urban, J. P., S. Smith, and J. C. Fairbank (2004). "Nutrition of the Intervertebral Disc," *Spine* 29:2700–2709.

Wilke, H. J., P. Neef, and M. Caimi (1999). "New In Vivo Measurements of Pressures in the Intervertebral Disc in Daily Life," *Spine* 24:755–762.

Woo, S. L., G. A. Johnson, and B. A. Smith (1993). "Mathematical Modeling of Ligaments and Tendons," *J. Biomech. Eng.* 115: 468–473.

Woo, S. L. Y., K. N. An, and C. B. Frank (2000). "Anatomy, Biology, and Biomechanics of Tendon and Ligament," in J. A. Buckwalter, T. A. Einhorn, and S. R. Simon (eds.), *Orthopaedic Basic Science.* American Academy of Orthopaedic Surgeons.

Yin, L., and D. M. Elliott (2004). "A Biphasic and Transversely Isotropic Mechanical Model for Tendon: Application to Mouse Tail Fascicles in Uniaxial Tension," *Journal of Biomechanics* 37:907–916.

Review Questions

1. The intervertebral discs and ligaments:
   a) Impart flexibility and mobility to the spine
   b) Protect the spinal cord
   c) Connect the vertebrae
   d) All of the above

2. Daily activities such as walking, running, driving, or lifting expose the intervertebral discs to:
   a) Compression and tension
   b) Bending and torsion
   c) Shear
   d) All of the above

3. The predominant collagen in the nucleus pulposus is:
   a) Type I collagen
   b) Type II collagen
   c) Type IX collagen
   d) None of the above

4. Nucleus pulposus pressurization arises from:
   a) Osmotic ion imbalance with the surrounding fluid
   b) Constraint from the surrounding annulus fibrosus and nucleus pulposus
   c) Water
   d) All of the above

5. Aggrecan, the major proteoglycan in the nucleus pulposus, is comprised of:
   a) Brush-like proteoglycans aggregated along a hyaluronan molecule
   b) Long negatively charged hyaluronan chain molecules
   c) Glycosaminoglycans attached to water molecules
   d) All of the above

6. Compression of the intervertebral disc results in:
   a) A decrease in pressure in the nucleus pulposus, which attracts water into the tissue
   b) Repressurization due to loss of fluid
   c) An increase in pressure in the nucleus pulposus, with an outflow of water to equilibrate pressure
   d) All of the above

7. The mechanical properties of the nucleus pulposus are:
   a) Direction dependent because of highly organized collagen fibers
   b) Solid-like, with high stiffness to withstand compression
   c) Isotropic because of the random organization of nucleus pulposus components
   d) All of the above

8. The annulus fibrosus is:
   a) Comprised of type II collagen fibers that are oriented in concentric bands
   b) Organized into concentric layers, with the collagen fibers of each layer oriented at alternating angles
   c) Made up of type I collagen fibers oriented parallel to the length of the spine to provide tensile load bearing in that direction
   d) All of the above

9. Axial compression of the intervertebral disc results in:
   a) Radial bulging of the nucleus pulposus
   b) Circumferential tension in the outer annulus fibrosus
   c) Axial compression in the inner annulus fibrosus
   d) All of the above

10. Annulus fibrosus tensile mechanical properties are greatest in the:
    a) Circumferential direction because tensile loads are greatest in that direction
    b) Inner annulus fibrosus due to a greater percentage of type I collagen there
    c) Posterior of the intervertebral disc as a result of highly organized collagen fiber structure
    d) Axial direction because of the angled, lamellar structure

11. Viscoelasticity in the annulus fibrosus may be caused by:
    a) High loads
    b) Collagen fiber uncrimping
    c) Water or friction between collagen fibers and the proteoglycan matrix
    d) All of the above

12. The end plates of the intervertebral disc:
    a) Provide a pathway for nerves to enter the intervertebral disc
    b) Distribute pressure across the area of the intervertebral disc
    c) Provide greatest resistance to failure
    d) All of the above

13. Loss of nucleus pulposus water content as a result of intervertebral disc degeneration causes:
    a) Increase in shear mechanical properties
    b) Altered load distribution in the annulus fibrosus
    c) Bulging inward of the inner annulus fibrosus
    d) All of the above

14. Intervertebral disc degeneration causes:
    a) Loss of disc height
    b) Altered loading patterns on vertebral bodies and facet joints
    c) Loss of demarcation between the nucleus pulposus and annulus fibrosus
    d) All of the above

15. The anterior longitudinal ligament:
    a) Resists hyperflexion of the spine
    b) Is comprised of type I collagen fibers oriented parallel to the length of the spine
    c) Is connected to each vertebrae and intervertebral disc of the spine
    d) All of the above

16. The spinal cord is protected from injury by:
    a) Mechanical properties that can withstand high loads
    b) Three soft tissue layers and the bones of the vertebrae
    c) Myelination
    d) All of the above

Chapter 4

Biomechanics of Vertebral Bone

Tony M. Keaveny[1,2] *and Jenni M. Buckley*[1]
(1) Orthopaedic Biomechanics Laboratory, Department
of Mechanical Engineering, The University of
California, Berkeley, CA
(2) Department of Bioengineering, The University
of California, Berkeley, CA

4.1 Introduction

Research on the biomechanics of vertebral trabecular bone is still intensely active, due in large part to the interest in providing improved estimates of osteoporotic fracture risk and assessment of new drug treatments for osteoporosis. Detailed knowledge of the biomechanical behavior of vertebral bone is also required in order to design robust implants. Design of orthopaedic implants for the spine is particularly challenging because vertebral trabecular bone is so weak and the cortices are so thin. As a result, failure of the bone-implant system often originates in the bone. The problem is compounded because the bone properties vary so much across individuals and over time and with disease. The development of minimally invasive surgical repair techniques for vertebral fractures such as vertebroplasty and kyphoplasty also invites biomechanical analysis of vertebral trabecular bone and the whole vertebral body in order to refine those procedures. Similarly, computational models are now being used to refine and indeed develop designs of new implants for the spine. In this chapter, we address first the biomechanics of human vertebral trabecular bone, including discussion of such topics as aging, disease, and repetitive loading. We then address the behavior of the whole vertebra, including discussion of the role of the cortical shell, intervertebral disc, and posterior elements. We finish by addressing noninvasive assessment techniques of whole vertebral strength. In the interest of focus, we have limited our attention to the thoraco lumbar vertebra.

4.2 Trabecular Bone

4.2.1 Trabecular Bone Composition and Microstructure

Trabecular bone—also referred to as cancellous bone—is the spongy, porous type of bone that is found at the ends of all long bones, and within flat and irregular bones such as the sternum, pelvis, and spine (Figure 4.1). The microstructural struts or individual *trabeculae* that make up a specimen of trabecular bone are composed of *trabecular tissue* material. The trabeculae enclose a 3D interconnected open porous space, resulting in a cellular solid [Gibson and Ashby 1997] type of material. The pores are filled with bone marrow and cells *in vivo*, which are thought to have little mechanical role except perhaps in high-energy trauma. The scale of these pores is on the order of 1 mm, and the scale of the trabecular thickness is about an order of magnitude lower. We are concerned mostly with the behavior of small specimens of trabecular bone, on

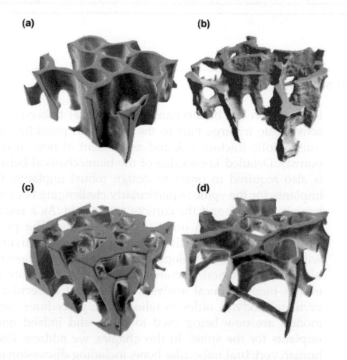

Fig. 4.1.

Volume rendering (20-micron resolution) of bovine proximal tibial (a), human proximal tibial (b), human femoral neck (c), and human vertebral (d) trabecular bone. All specimens have the same bulk dimensions (3 × 3 × 1 mm³).

the order of 5 to 10 mm in dimension, a scale at which most effects of the microstructure can be averaged to produce continuum-like behavior [Harrigan et al. 1988; Zysset, Goulet, and Hollister 1998]. The trabecular microstructure is typically oriented such that there is a "grain" direction along which mechanical stiffness and strength are greatest, resulting in anisotropic material behavior. In the vertebral body, the principal material orientation is along the inferior-superior direction. The trabecular tissue material itself is morphologically similar to cortical bone (an anisotropic composite of hydroxyapatite, collagen, water, and trace amounts of other proteins), but is arranged in "packets" of lamellar bone [Choi and Goldstein 1992]. Thus, trabecular bone is classified from an engineering materials perspective as a composite, anisotropic, open porous cellular solid. Like many biological materials, it displays time-dependent behavior, as well as damage susceptibility during cyclic loading.

4.2.2 Stress-Strain Behavior

The stress-strain curve for vertebral trabecular bone (Figure 4.2) resembles that of many conventional engineering materials. There is an initial linear portion (indeed it is slightly nonlinear [Morgan et al. 2001], but this is usually neglected in whole bone structural analyses), a yield region in which the tissue begins to fail, and then a post-yield region in which the load-carrying capacity of the tissue remains constant, falls off, or abruptly ends with fracture. The behaviors in tension and compression are different, mostly in the post-yield regions. Although generally trabecular bone is weaker in tension than compression, this effect is quite small for the spine because of its low density and can often be neglected. Fracture occurs at apparent strains of about 1.5% for tensile loading [Kopperdahl and Keaveny 1998], whereas prolonged but slightly reduced load-carrying capacity is sustained after the ultimate point for compressive loading.

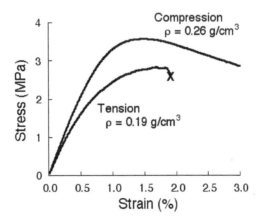

Fig. 4.2.

Stress-strain curve for vertebral trabecular bone in tension and compression. The X represents fracture. *(From Kopperdahl et al. [1998] with permission.)*

Table 4.1.
Mean (±SD) values of compressive modulus and ultimate stress for vertebral trabecular bone. Note that the modulus values from Kopperdahl and Keaveny are much higher than in the other studies because the effects of end artifacts were minimized in Kopperdahl and Keaveny.

Study	Age Range	Modulus (MPa)	Ultimate Stress (MPa)
Mosekilde et al. [Mosekilde, Mosekilde, and Danielsen 1987]	15–87	67 ± 45	2.4 ± 1.6
Hansson et al. [Hansson, Keller, and Panjabi 1987]	71–84	22.8 ± 15.5	1.55 ± 1.11
Kopperdahl and Keaveny [Kopperdahl and Keaveny 1998]	32–65	291 ± 113	2.23 ± 0.95

The ultimate strain in compression is about the same as it is in tension [Kopperdahl and Keaveny 1998].

4.2.3 Elastic Modulus and Strength: Heterogeneity and Aging

A critical issue that distinguishes trabecular bone from conventional engineering materials is its substantial heterogeneity, which leads to wide variations in mechanical properties.[1] In the vertebra, this heterogeneity results primarily from underlying variations in bone volume fraction (defined as the ratio of the volume of actual tissue to the bulk volume), which ranges from about 0.05 to 0.25. As a result, elastic modulus can vary by more than an order of magnitude, from as low as 50 MPa to over 700 MPa. The strength, most often characterized by the ultimate stress, is typically about one-hundredth of the elastic modulus. It varies from less than about 0.5 MPa to about 5 MPa. These different properties can occur in different portions of the vertebral body but more substantially across different individuals. While different measures of strength are often reported, the strong correlation between yield and ultimate strengths (Figure 4.3) indicates that this distinction is not critical because one can easily be inferred from the other.

---

1. Because trabecular bone spans multiple length scales, it is important to distinguish between mechanical behavior at the level of the whole specimen—the *apparent properties*—as opposed to that at the level of individual trabeculae (the *tissue properties*). Thus, for example, we talk of apparent versus tissue modulus for trabecular bone for the whole specimen and trabecular tissue, respectively. Unless noted otherwise, we refer to material properties at the apparent level.

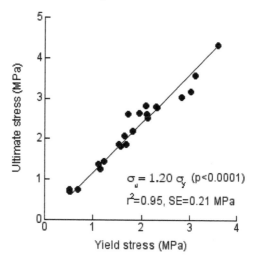

Fig. 4.3.

Correlation between yield and ultimate strength for vertebral trabecular bone. *(From Crawford et al. [2003], with permission.)*

Large changes in mechanical properties occur with aging. Based on cross-sectional observation studies in cadavers, ultimate stress in vertebral trabecular bone is reduced on average by almost 11% per decade from ages 20 to 100, although strength does not appear to decrease in any significant manner until after about age 30 (Figure 4.4) [Mosekilde and Mosekilde 1986; Mosekilde, Mosekilde, and Danielsen 1987]. It should be noted, however, that age is not a very specific predictor of mechanical properties because at any given age there is substantial scatter in the data across multiple specimens. Thus, at age 60 (for example) individuals can have bone more typical of a 35-year-old or a 100-year-old (see Figure 4.4). Because of this, estimates of bone strength are best made from measures of density or bone volume fraction.

Because of the substantial heterogeneity of trabecular bone, factors such as age and sex need to be designated when discussing the specifics of the mechanical properties of vertebral trabecular bone (i.e., trabecular bone from an aged female is typically much different than that from a young male). This heterogeneity is a key concept in trabecular bone biomechanics. It has direct relevance to fields such as tissue engineering in which the ideal goal would be to replace damaged trabecular bone with a substitute having appropriate mechanical properties specific to that individual. This heterogeneity is even more pronounced across sites. Trabecular bone from the vertebra is among the weakest in the human skeleton, being 5 to 10 times weaker than in the femoral neck region, for example [McCalden, McGeough, and Court-Brown 1997; Morgan and Keaveny 2001; Mosekilde, Mosekilde, and Danielsen 1987]. Thus, an

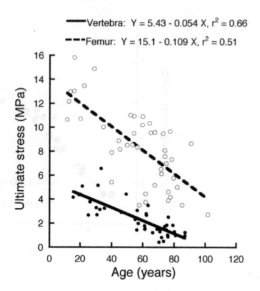

Fig. 4.4.

Dependence of compressive strength on age for human vertebral and proximal femoral trabecular bone cores. (*Redrawn, based on data from [Mosekilde and Mosekilde 1986] and [McCalden, McGeough, and Court-Brown 1997].*)

implant designed for the relatively dense bone of the proximal femur may be not optimal for the vertebra, and vice versa.

4.2.4 Anisotropy

Vertebral trabecular bone is anisotropic in both modulus and strength [Galante, Rostoker, and Ray 1970; Mosekilde, Mosekilde, and Danielsen 1987], although the extent of anisotropy is quite modest. Mean values of strength and modulus of human vertebral bone in the superior-inferior direction have been reported to be higher than those in the transverse direction by factors of 2.8 and 3.4, respectively [Mosekilde, Mosekilde, and Danielsen 1987]. A complete set of anisotropic elastic constants has been reported using micro-CT-based finite element models to compute the elastic constants [Ulrich et al. 1999], an innovative approach because direct mechanical testing to obtain all elastic constants is extremely difficult for such delicate material as vertebral trabecular bone.

4.2.5 Density-mechanical Property Relations

The best single predictor of modulus and strength properties for trabecular bone is its bone volume fraction or the density (see Table 4.2). Apparent density

Table 4.2.

Power-law regressions between ultimate stress (σ in MPa) and apparent density (ρ in g/cm^3) for compressive loading of human lumbar vertebral trabecular bone specimens.

Study	Cadavers		Specimens	$\sigma = a\rho^b$		
	Number	Age	Number	a	b	r^2
Hansson et al. [Hansson, Keller, and Panjabi 1987]	3	71–84	231	50.3	2.24	0.76
Mosekilde et al. [Mosekilde, Mosekilde, and Danielsen 1987]	42	15–87	40	24.9	1.80	0.83
Kopperdahl and Keaveny [Kopperdahl and Keaveny 1998]§	11	32–65	22	33.2	1.53	0.68

§0.2% offset yield stress is reported instead of ultimate stress because the latter was not measured.

is the product of the bone volume fraction and the tissue density, the latter being approximately constant at about 2.0 g/cm^3.

As it turns out, the failure behavior of trabecular bone is remarkably simple if failure is characterized by measures of strain. It has long been noticed that there is a strong linear correlation between the stress at which trabecular bone fails and the corresponding elastic modulus [Brown and Ferguson 1980; Fyhrie and Schaffler 1994; Goldstein et al. 1983; Keaveny et al. 1994] (Figure 4.5). Because the ratio of yield stress to modulus is the yield strain, this correlation suggests that failure strains for trabecular bone are relatively constant. Indeed, in experiments of direct measures of strains at failure it has been found that the failure strains for human vertebral trabecular bone have only a slight, if any, dependence on density [Kopperdahl and Keaveny 1998], although failure strains can vary across sites [Morgan and Keaveny 2001]. For elderly human vertebral trabecular bone, the mean (±SD) compressive yield strain of 0.84 ± 0.06% is statistically significant but only slightly higher than the tensile yield strain of 0.78 ± 0.04% in tension [Kopperdahl and Keaveny 1998; Morgan and Keaveny 2001]. Results from testing of bovine bone have shown evidence of isotropy of yield strains [Chang et al. 1999; Turner 1989]. Thus, it is often sufficient to assume a single strain value for failure of human vertebral trabecular bone, regardless of orientation or sign of loading. The simplicity of such a strain-based description of failure is an important concept in trabecular bone biomechanics. It implies, for example, that if the elastic properties of trabecular bone are known the strength can be estimated with a high degree of accuracy, regardless of the bone density, for any loading axes based only on the yield strain. Further, plots of strain can indicate regions of failure regardless of bone density [Kopperdahl, Roberts, and Keaveny 1999; Silva, Keaveny, and Hayes 1998] (Figure 4.6). This greatly simplifies interpretation of results from finite element analyses that use different modulus values for each element in the model.

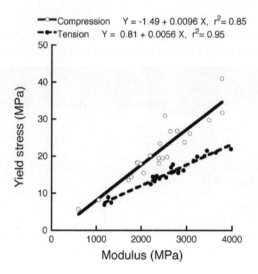

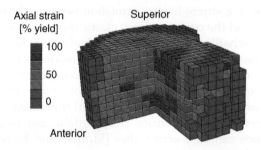

Fig. 4.5.

Yield stress versus modulus for bovine tibial trabecular bone, loaded in an on-axis configuration in tension and compression. (*From [Keaveny et al. 1994] with permission.*)

Fig. 4.6.

The strain distribution within a vertebral body at whole-bone ultimate force. This is a voxel-based finite element model of a T10 from an 82-year-old female subjected to uniform compressive force along the superior end plate. The end plates have been transected and a section has been removed for illustrative purposes.

4.2.6 Post-yield and Damage Behavior

Damage and repair of individual trabeculae are now recognized as normal physiologic processes [Burr et al. 1997; Hansson and Roos 1981] that tend to increase with age [Fazzalari et al. 1998; Hahn et al. 1995; Mori et al. 1997] and that may have clinical and biological relevance. Such damage has been proposed to increase osteoporotic fracture risk [Burr et al. 1997; Fyhrie and Schaffler 1994; Keaveny, Wachtel, and Kopperdahl 1999], act as a stimulus for

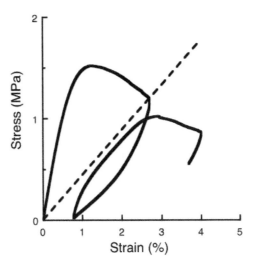

Fig. 4.7.

Load-unload-reload "post-yield" behavior of human vertebral trabecular bone. For multiple specimens, the secant modulus (dashed line) is statistically similar to the slope of the main linear region
in the reloading curve, and the initial slope of the reloading curve is statistically similar to the
modulus of the initial loading cycle. (*From [Keaveny, Wachtel, and Kopperdahl 1999] with permission.*)

remodeling [Pugh, Rose, and Radin 1973], and occur during implantation of
prostheses, particularly in the elderly spine where the bone is very fragile
[Keaveny, Wachtel, and Kopperdahl 1999].

When human vertebral trabecular bone—as well as the whole vertebral body
[Kopperdahl, Pearlman, and Keaveny 2000]—is loaded past its yield point, it
unloads to a non-zero residual strain at zero stress, reloads with a modulus
equal to its initial modulus, but quickly has a reduced modulus that equals that
value of a perfectly damaging material [Keaveny, Wachtel, and Kopperdahl
1999] (Figure 4.7). Residual strains of over 1.0% strain occur after compressive
loading of up to 3.0% strain, and increase in a slightly nonlinear fashion with
increasing total applied strain [Keaveny, Wachtel, and Kopperdahl 1999].
Osteoporotic spine fractures are defined in terms of permanent deformations
(see 4.11) [Jiang et al. 2004], but many fractures are not associated with any specific traumatic event [Cooper et al. 1992; Myers, Wilson, and Greenspan 1996].
Thus, it is possible that isolated overloads (or perhaps prolonged static or cyclic
loading) that do not cause overt fracture do cause subtle but cumulative permanent deformations. It has been suggested that vertebral "morphology" fractures are not really fractures at all [Kleerekoper and Nelson 1992; Nelson,
Kleerekoper, and Peterson 1994; Ziegler, Scheidt-Nave, and Leidig-Bruckner
1996]. This provides a plausible etiology for the gradual development of clinical fractures over a number of years [Kopperdahl, Pearlman, and Keaveny
2000]. This hypothesis remains to be tested.

The reductions in modulus and strength that occur for reloading after
monotonic overloading are substantial, depend strongly on the magnitude of

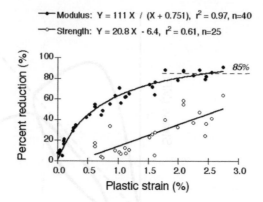

Fig. 4.8.

Dependence of percent stiffness and modulus reduction on level of initial applied "plastic" strain for vertebral trabecular bone cores from bodies. Plastic strain was defined as the total applied strain minus the 0.2% offset yield strain. (*From [Keaveny et al. 1999] with permission.*)

the applied strain, but are mostly independent of volume fraction. In an experiment performed on machined specimens of human vertebral trabecular bone [Keaveny, Wachtel, and Kopperdahl 1999], modulus reductions (between the intact Young's and the residual moduli) were over 85% for applied plastic strains of up to 3.0% (Figure 4.8). Using concepts of continuum damage mechanics for brittle materials [Krajcinovic and Lemaitre 1987], these modulus reductions can be interpreted as quantitative measures of effective mechanical damage in the specimen. Thus, a modulus reduction of 85% corresponds to 85% damage from a mechanical perspective.

At the trabecular tissue level, examination of the physical damage that occurs with overloading has confirmed that subtle damage within trabeculae (versus fracture of entire trabeculae) can cause large reductions in apparent modulus [Wachtel and Keaveny 1997]. Consistent with this, Fyhrie and Schaffler [1994] reported that for human vertebral specimens loaded in compression to 15% strain the primary mechanism of failure was microscopic cracking rather than overt fracture of individual trabeculae. Complete fracture of trabeculae was confined to elements oriented transversely to the loading direction. Laser scanning confocal microscopy [Fazzalari et al. 1998] has shown the staining associated with cross-hatch shear bands and the more diffuse [Vashishth et al. 2000] staining observed with basic fuchsin included "ultra-microcracks" about 10 microns in length. The implication is that cracking can occur at very small scales. Yeh and Keaveny [2001] have shown with finite element modeling that unless trabecular tissue fractures at very low strains—which is unlikely—microdamage (versus microfracture) is the most plausible explanation for the large apparent level reductions in mechanical properties after overloads. One practical implication of these findings is that after a nonfracturing overload damaged trabecular bone may appear to be radiographically normal but can have severely reduced mechanical properties. This may explain why a history of previous fractures is a strong risk factor for subsequent vertebral osteoporotic fractures [Black et al. 1999] and why there is an increased risk of repeat fractures in patients treated for vertebral fractures [Kim et al. 2004] (presumably the adjacent vertebra was also damaged in the event that caused the primary fracture).

4.2.7 Cyclic and Time-dependent Loading

Failure in response to cyclic loading is important both clinically and biologically. Clinically, cyclic loading and its associated damage and strain accumulation likely weaken vertebrae [Burr et al. 1997; Kopperdahl, Pearlman, and Keaveny 2000; Tehranzadeh, Serafini, and Pais 1989; White and Panjabi 1990] and may be associated with loosening of implants [Bauer and Schils 1999; Taylor and Tanner 1997]. Biologically, understanding the cyclic behavior of vertebral trabecular bone may provide insight into remodeling patterns in the spine. Microfractures of individual trabeculae and callus formations are commonly seen in human vertebrae (Cheng et al. 1997; Hahn et al. 1995; Hansson and Roos 1981]. More subtle intratrabecular microdamage also exists *in vivo* [Fazzalari et al. 1998; Mori et al. 1997; Vashishth et al. 2000; Wenzel, Schaffler, and Fyhrie 1996]. One likely source of this damage is from cyclic loading during habitual activities, accentuated perhaps by occasional overloads. Because cortical bone remodeling may be initiated by fatigue damage [Bentolila et al. 1998; Burr et al. 1985; Martin 2000; Mori and Burr 1993; Prendergast and Huiskes 1996] it is possible that fatigue loading also acts as a stimulus for remodeling in trabecular bone.

Standard S-N curves, using nondimensional measures of stress, have now been reported for human vertebral trabecular bone [Haddock et al. 2004] that can serve as input into whole bone and bone-implant structural analyses of the human vertebra. These data indicate that the compressive strength of devitalized vertebral trabecular bone can be reduced by up to 70% after 10^6 cycles of loading. There is a classical power law relation between the ratio of stress to initial modulus and the number of cycles to failure, N_f (Figure 4.9). The statistical regression from the log transformations (±standard errors) and the corresponding power law relation is as follows:

$$Log_{10}N_f = -[17.3 \pm 3.22] - [8.54 \pm 1.37] - Log_{10}(\sigma/E_0) \quad (r^2 = 0.54, n = 35)$$

$$N_f = 4.57 \times 10^{-18}(\sigma/E_0)^{-8.54}$$

According to this power law relation, cyclic loading at σ/E_0 levels of 0.003, 0.005, and 0.007 causes failure of human vertebral trabecular bone to occur *on average* at 16044, 205, and 12 cycles, respectively. During cyclic loading, creep strains—defined as translation of the stress-strain curve along the strain axis— also occur, indicating a shortening of the specimen. Loss of modulus can also occur, indicative of microdamge mechanisms.

One limitation with the current data for cyclic loading of human vertebral trabecular bone is the high level of loads used. It is unlikely that human bone

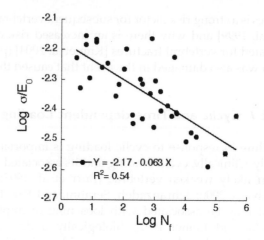

Fig. 4.9.
S-N type plot of human vertebral trabecular bone. The applied stress σ has been normalized by the initial modulus E_0. (From [Haddock et al. 2004] with permission.)

is subjected to such high levels of habitual loads, and thus extrapolation is required for most applications. In interpreting the literature on creep or fatigue for trabecular bone, it should also be noted that any *in vitro* experiments preclude biological healing, and thus the resulting fatigue S-N or creep stress-time curves might best be considered as lower bounds on the specimen life (i.e., we can expect a longer life if biological healing of the fatigue or creep related damage occurs). However, it has been suggested that osteoclastic resorption during the remodeling process can in some situations reduce strength if the resulting resorption cavities serve as significant stress concentrations [Martin et al. 1997]. If that is the case, the *in vitro* fatigue characteristics may well represent upper bounds on the *in vitro* fatigue life. Clearly, this is an area deserving of more research.

4.3 Mechanical Behavior of the Vertebral Body

4.3.1 Anatomy of a Vertebra

A vertebra consists of four principal structural components: the end plates, the centrum, the cortical shell (all parts of the vertebral body), and the posterior elements. The end plates, which are located along the inferior and superior surfaces of the vertebral body, are composed of cortical bone that varies in thickness between 0.4 and 0.8 mm [Edwards et al. 2001; Silva, Keaveny, and Hayes 1994] (Figure 4.10). Endplate thickness depends on spinal level and position on the end plate [Edwards et al. 2001]. The lower lumbar vertebrae have the thickest end plates, and the central portion of the end plate is generally thinner than

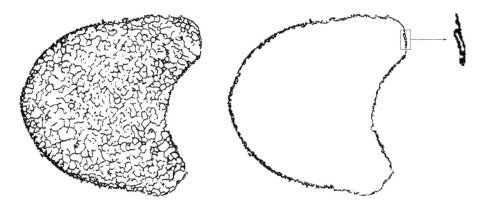

Fig. 4.10.

A transverse plane cross section through a human lumbar vertebral body, taken from a micro-CT scan and illustrating the thin, porous nature of the cortical shell. (*From [Eswaran et al. 2006] with permission.*)

the periphery [Edwards et al. 2001]. Similarly, the failure load and stiffness of the end plate varies with axial position and across the end plate [Grant, Oxland, and Dvorak 2001]. Using a mechanical indenter, Grant, Oxland, and Dvorak [2001] showed that the posterolateral regions of the end plate are stronger than the interior and that for a given vertebra the inferior end plate is generally stronger than the superior end plate. As a structural component, the end plate deforms in response to the stresses imposed by the intervertebral disc [Brinckmann, Biggemann, and Hilweg 1989], and this deformation transfers load to the underlying trabecular bone. Schmorl's nodes, which are herniations of the intervertebral disc through the end plate, may develop as a result of trauma. It is currently unclear if end plate failure always occurs with *in vivo* vertebral failure or if it is possible to have failure of only the underlying bone. The end plate, which is porous—particularly in the interior region [Edwards et al. 2001]—also serves as a nutrient pathway by allowing for material transport between the vertebral body and the adjacent intervertebral disc [Ohshima et al. 1989; Urban and McMullin 1988].

The trabecular centrum is the principal load-bearing component of the vertebra [Hansson, Roos, and Nachemson 1980; McBroom et al. 1985; Mosekilde and Mosekilde 1986; Yoganandan et al. 1988]. The density of the trabecular bone within the centrum varies with location in the centrum [Cody et al. 1991; Keller et al. 1989; McBroom et al. 1985] and spinal level [Brinckmann, Biggemann, and Hilweg 1989; Edmondston et al. 1997; Hansson, Roos, and Nachemson 1980], decreasing caudally between T1 and L3 [Singer et al. 1995].

Direct [Edwards et al. 2001; Silva, Keaveny, and Hayes 1994] and microcomputed tomography (CT) [Bayraktar et al. 2004] measurements of the cortical shell indicate that the shell thickness is approximately 0.3 to 0.4 mm. The shell is thickest near the end plates and thinnest at the mid-axial plane [Edwards et al. 2001]. Clinical resolution CT scans tend to overestimate the thickness of the shell by a factor of two or more [Prevrhal et al. 2002; Silva, Keaveny, and Hayes 1994]. The mechanical properties of the cortical shell are thought to be comparable to cortical bone at other anatomic sites [Reilly and Burstein 1975; Turner et al. 1999]. Using nanoindentation, Roy et al. [1999] found the elastic modulus of the shell to be 16.9 ± 3.2 GPa in the transverse direction and 18.1 ± 2.7 GPa in the axial direction (mean $\pm$ st. dev). They also found that although the mechanical properties of the shell are similar to cortical bone the microstructure (particularly on the endosteal surface) is more representative of condensed trabeculae [Mosekilde 1993; Roy et al. 1999; Silva, Keaveny, and Hayes 1994]. The load-carrying capacity of the shell is currently unclear and remains a topic of interest, given its potentially important clinical role.

The posterior elements are bony processes that extend from the posterior aspect of the vertebral body. Two pairs of facet (apophyseal) joints connect the vertebra to the adjacent vertebrae in the inferior and superior directions. In the lower thoracic and lumbar spine, the facets resist transverse shear force and restrict excessive motion in torsion and extension [Adams and Hutton 1983]. We discuss the biomechanical role of the posterior elements, as well as the intervertebral disc and the cortical shell in more detail in material following.

4.3.2 Vertebral Fractures

Vertebral fractures are commonly grouped into three morphological cases: anterior wedge, biconcavity, and compression fractures (Figure 4.11) [Eastell et al. 1991; Jiang et al. 2004]. Wedge fractures are the most common, constituting over half of all vertebral fractures [Eastell et al. 1991]. Osteoporotic vertebral fractures are an important clinical problem [Melton et al. 1992; Ray et al. 1997]. They typically develop from T6 to L3 [Cooper et al. 1992; Melton and Wahner 1989], with the most frequently fractured vertebrae located at T8, T9, and L1 [Cooper et al. 1992] (Figure 4.12). Unlike osteoporotic hip fractures, which are attributable to a fall in approximately 90% of all cases [Cummings et al. 1994; Grisso et al. 1991; Michelson et al. 1995], many osteoporotic vertebral fractures result from what can be considered nontraumatic loading conditions [Cooper et al. 1992; Myers, Wilson, and Greenspan 1996]. For example, in a clinical study of 341 elderly individuals presenting with vertebral fractures only 39% of the fractures were attributable to trauma, such as motor vehicle accidents and falls (from any height) [Cooper et al. 1992]. In general, vertebral fractures are difficult to diagnose because they may be initially asymptomatic, can be classified in different ways [Jiang et al. 2004], and often do not present as a sudden discrete fracture [Cooper et al. 1992]. One poorly understood biomechanical issue is whether or not these changes in vertebral geometry alter the loads acting on the vertebral body due to the resulting change in kinematics—and if so to what extent. This is of clinical interest because new treatments are now available that can help restore the height of fractured vertebral bodies [Baroud et al. 2004; Sandhu and Khan 2002]. Questions have also been raised about whether or not deformity "fractures" are really fractures [Kleerekoper and Nelson 1992;

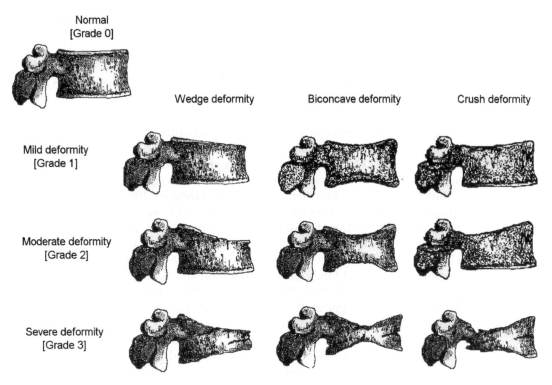

Fig. 4.11.
Clinical classification of different vertebral fracture types based on the deformed shape. Anterior wedge fractures are vertebral deformities in which the anterior height is less than the posterior height, whereas biconcavity fractures exhibit comparable anterior and posterior heights and a lesser midsagittal height [Eastell et al. 1991; Smith-Bindman et al. 1991]. Crush fractures result in a mean vertebral body height that is less than normal for that vertebral level and that of the surrounding vertebrae [Eastell et al. 1991; Smith-Bindman et al. 1991]. (*From [Riggs and Melton 1995] with permission.*)

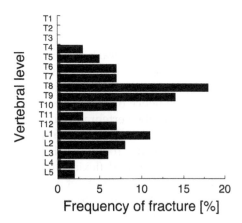

Fig. 4.12.
Prevalence of vertebral fractures at each vertebral level in the thoroco-lumbar spine. Data was taken from a study of 341 individuals diagnosed with vertebral fractures. (*Adapted from [Cooper et al. 1992] with permission.*)

Nelson, Kleerekoper, and Peterson 1994; Ziegler, Scheidt-Nave, and Leidig-Bruckner 1996].

4.3.3 Strength Properties Under Static Loading Conditions and Effects of Bone Density and Area

The compressive strength of human thoroco lumbar vertebrae ranges from about 2 kN for specimens having low bone density and small cross-sectional areas to about 8 kN for specimens having high bone density and large cross-sectional areas [Brinckmann, Biggemann, and Hilweg 1989; Cheng et al. 1997; Ebbesen et al. 1999; Eriksson, Isberg, and Lindgren 1989; Moro et al. 1995; Mosekilde and Mosekilde 1990; Singer et al. 1995]. Across individuals, variations in vertebral strength are quite well explained (r^2 approximately 0.50 to 0.65) by variations in average bone density [Brinckmann, Biggemann, and Hilweg 1989; Cheng et al. 1997; Ebbesen et al. 1999; Edmondston et al. 1997; Eriksson, Isberg, and Lindgren 1989; Hansson and Roos 1981; Lochmuller et al. 2002; McBroom et al. 1985; Mosekilde and Mosekilde 1986; Mosekilde and Mosekilde 1990; Singer et al. 1995; Veenland et al. 1997]. Within individuals, vertebral compressive strength increases caudally from T1 to L5 at a rate of approximately 200 N per segment, mostly due to the increase in vertebral cross-sectional area [Edmondston et al. 1994; Singer et al. 1995]. Other determinants of vertebral compressive strength include the regional distribution of bone mineral density [Cody et al. 1991; McBroom et al. 1985] and geometry of the vertebra [Brinckmann, Biggemann, and Hilweg 1989; Cheng et al. 1997; Singer et al. 1995] (i.e., minimum transverse plane cross-sectional area). When combined with bone density, these measures can account for 65 to 90% of the variation in compressive vertebral strength (Brinckmann, Biggemann, and Hilweg 1989; Cheng et al. 1997; Cody et al. 1991], although the success of the predictive power seems to depend on the particular variables used, the sample size in the experiment, and the demographics (age, sex, and so on) of the test specimens (Tables 4.3 and 4.4). The bone density and disc condition can also affect the fracture type. For example, it was found that for uniform compressive loading of cadaveric vertebral bodies wedge fractures tended to occur with low bone density and degenerated discs, whereas central fractures tended to occur with higher bone density and healthier discs [Hansson and Roos 1981].

Due to the prevalence of anterior wedge fractures, it is also relevant to consider the strength of the vertebra for loading conditions that mimic such *in vitro* activities as forward bending. Although the mechanical response of cadaver spinal motion segments (bone-disc-bone complexes but no muscles) under combined compression and flexion has been well investigated [Adams et al. 1994; Panjabi et al. 1994; Schultz et al. 1979; Tencer, Ahmed, and Burke 1982], the main outcome variable in these studies has been related to measures of deformation of the motion segment, rather than strength of the vertebra. It is not clear at this juncture exactly what type of stresses develop along the end plate for forward bending activities and thus it is difficult to prescribe *in vitro* stress boundary conditions in experiments on isolated vertebrae. Experiments

Table 4.3.

Coefficients of determination (r^2) for linear regressions between DXA bone mineral density and *ex vivo* vertebral strength.

Study	Cadavers		Specimens		r^2
	Number	Age	Number	Type	
Eriksson et al. [Eriksson, Isberg, and Lindgren]	19	59–94	73	Isolated vertebrae (L1-L4)*	0.23 0.55
Cheng et al.	62	68 ± 16+	62	Isolated vertebrae (L3)*	0.64 0.44 0.61
Moro et al.	11	48–87	11	Bone-disc complexes (T10-L4)**	0.69
Lochmuller et al.	126	76 ± 11 (M)+ 82 ± 9 (F)+	378	Bone-disc complexes (T5-L4)**	0.62 0.48

+Mean age ± st.dev.
*Isolated vertebra = vertebral body only, no posterior elements, bone loaded via rigid platens.
**Bone-disc complex = bone-disc-bone-disc-bone, bone at each end embedded in grips.

using pressure-tipped catheters within the disc have shown that the stresses that develop within the disc—and thus imparted to the end plate—depend on the state of the degeneration of the disc and the degree of forward bending. These experiments also show that the center of pressure shifts anteriorly for forward bending [Adams et al. 1994; Horst and Brinckmann 1981]. However, there is conflicting evidence as to whether physiological flexion from neutral spinal position results in a uniform pressure distribution across the end plate [Adams et al. 1994] or a nonuniform distribution that is more heavily concentrated toward the anterior aspect [Horst and Brinckmann 1981]. Determining the exact nature of the pressure distribution along the end plate—and its dependence on disc health and spinal posture—is an area of current research.

Results from the few studies in which bending moments were applied directly to a vertebral body have provided some unique insight in possible *in vitro* failure mechanisms (Figure 4.13). In one experiment in which combined compression and forward bending was applied to isolated vertebral bodies—all with metastatic lesions—and vertebral strength was the outcome, it was found that the contribution from the applied bending moment to the calculated maximum strains on the vertebral surface was about three times that from the applied compressive force [Whealan et al. 2000]. Although these results clearly suggest the importance of bending as an *in vitro* failure mechanism, the magnitude of the applied bending moment was quite large in these tests (exceeding 50 Nm based on reported regressions in that study). In a finite element study that compared the response of the vertebra to pure compression versus pure bending [Crawford and Keaveny 2004], it was found that although measures

Table 4.4.

Coefficients of determination (r^2) for linear regressions between vertebral strength and volumetric trabecular density as measured by QCT.

| Study | Cadavers | | Specimens | | r^2 |
	Number	Age	Number	Type	
Edmondston et al.	16	29–88	250	Isolated vertebrae (T1-L5)*	0.36
Brinckmann et al.	53	19–79	98	Motion segments (T1-L5)***	0.38 0.64†
Eriksson et al.	19	59–94	73	Isolated vertebrae (L1-L4)*	0.23 0.55†
McBroom et al.	26	63–99	40	Isolated vertebrae (L1,L3)*	0.46
Ebbesen et al.	101	18–96	101	Isolated vertebrae (L3)*	0.86 0.61†
Cheng et al.	62	68 ± 16+	62	Isolated vertebrae (L3)*	0.44 0.61†
Mosekilde et al.	30	43–95	30	Isolated vertebrae (L3,L2)*	0.52
Eckstein et al.	126	79 ± 11+	39	Bone-disc complexes (T3–L5)**	0.66

*Isolated vertebra = vertebral body only, no posterior elements.
**Bone-disc complex = bone-disc-bone-disc-bone.
***Motion segment = bone-disc-bone.
+mean age ± st.dev.
VTD = volumetric bone mineral density.
AT = transverse plane cross-sectional area.
†VTD × AT.

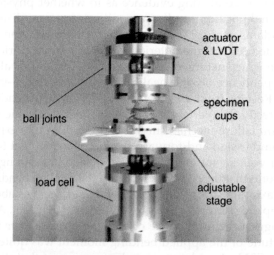

Fig. 4.13.

A biomechanical testing apparatus for conducting combined axial compression and anterior bending tests on human lumbar motion segments. The ball joints may be adjusted to apply 10 degrees (5 degrees each) of flexion.

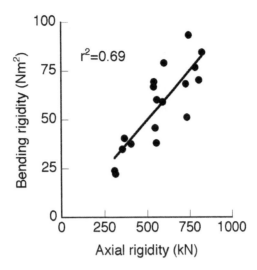

Fig. 4.14.

The relationship between vertebral stiffness in compression and anterior bending. These results were obtained from finite element analyses of 13 vertebrae. (*From [Crawford and Keaveny 2004] with permission.*)

of the compressive versus bending rigidities were quite well correlated (Figure 4.14, $r^2 = 0.69$) there remained appreciable scatter. In some instances, vertebrae displayed similar compressive characteristics but very different bending characteristics. The width of the vertebra in the AP direction was most influential on such differences in characteristics. This suggests that some individuals may have "normal" vertebrae in terms of resistance to compressive loads, but may be vulnerable to bending type loads. The clinical relevance of these findings remains to be seen.

4.3.4 Effects of Aging and Disease

Substantial changes occur to the vertebra with aging. Vertebral body strength decreases by about 12% per decade from ages 25 to 85 [Mosekilde and Mosekilde 1990] (Figure 4.15). It is thought that these changes are due to a loss of bone density, which is offset in part by subtle increases in bone size [Mosekilde and Mosekilde 1986]. The vertebra experiences changes in both trabecular and cortical bone mineral density with age [Greenspan, Maitland-Ramsey, and Myers 1996; Hannan, Felson, and Anderson 1992; Steiger et al. 1992], and there is some evidence that the loss of the peripheral bone in the vertebra is not as pronounced biomechanically as the loss of the trabecular bone at the center of the vertebra [Mosekilde and Mosekilde 1990]. Aging is also accompanied by osteoarthritic changes around the disc and end plates (formation of osteophytes, and so on) [Antonacci et al. 1997; Vernon-Roberts and Pirie 1977], including substantial disc degeneration. There are also likely adaptive

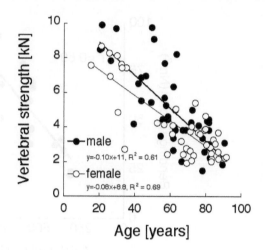

Fig. 4.15.

Vertebral strength versus age for L2 vertebral bodies from 90 individuals, ranging in age from 15 to 91 years old. (*Adapted from [Mosekilde and Mosekilde 1990] with permission.*)

alterations of the bone within the vertebra in response to these changes [Keller et al. 1989]. Degenerative changes in the adjacent intervertebral discs also affect the structure of the vertebra. For example, using regional indentation tests on the end plates of cadaveric vertebrae it was found that the strength in the central region of the superior end plate was associated with increased disc degeneration [Grant, Oxland, and Dvorak 2001]. Presumably, with disc degeneration load is shunted to the periphery of the vertebra, leading to a stress shielding type adaptive response in the central end plate. Vertebrae adjacent to degenerated discs have more uniform distributions of bone mineral density than do vertebra adjacent to healthy discs, which tend to have a higher bone density in the posterocentral region [Keller et al. 1989].

4.3.5 Damage and Fatigue

Whereas most biomechanical studies on vertebral strength have measured the response to monotonic loads, the vertebra is subjected to and may fail under cyclic or prolonged loads *in vitro*. Vertebrae may also fail *in vitro* at relatively low loads if damaged previously by isolated, nonfracturing overloads. Damage refers to the reduction in vertebral strength and stiffness that occurs upon reloading after the specimen has been overloaded past its elastic region (Figure 4.16). As with trabecular bone cores (Figures 4.7 and 4.8), the reduction in whole vertebral stiffness and strength after an isolated single overload is highly dependent on magnitude of the applied strain, with larger strain values resulting in greater reductions regardless of bone density [Kopperdahl, Pearlman, and Keaveny 2000]. Localized regions of damage may form within the trabecular centrum, and the effect of this localized damage on the whole bone

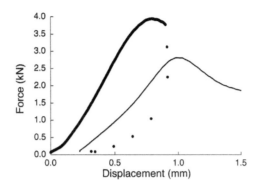

Fig. 4.16.
The behavior of a typical vertebral body subjected to a compressive overload and then reload. The thick line is the original loading path and the thin line is the reloading path. Note that the strength and stiffness during reloading are less than during the initial loading. (*From [Kopperdahl, Pearlman, and Keaveny 2000] with permission.*)

behavior is most pronounced when damage occurs in regions of high strain energy density [Kopperdahl, Roberts, and Keaveny 1999].

The response of the whole vertebral body to cyclic loading has been characterized experimentally but the data are relatively sparse despite the potential importance of this failure mechanism. Outcome parameters from these tests, such as the number of cycles to failure and the change in stiffness, have been shown to correlate with bone mineral content [Hanson, Keller, and Spengle 1987], bone mineral density in the posterior region of the centrum [McCubbrey et al. 1995], and age [Hansson, Keller, and Spengler 1987]. Cyclic loading tests on lumbar motion segments have indicated two general failure mechanisms: a gradual creep-like increase in mean displacement and rapid crack propagation from the cortical shell to the interior of the vertebral body [Liu et al. 1983]. The lumbar vertebra is thought to be susceptible to fatigue failure under normal daily activities [Brinckmann, Biggeman, and Hilweg 1988; Hanson, Keller, and Spengler 1987; Myers and Wilson 1997]. For example, using cadaver lumbar motion segments, Brinckmann et al. [1988] applied compressive forces of only 30% of the estimated static strength of the vertebra for up to 5,000 cycles—equivalent to about two weeks of exercise—and found that the probability of fatigue failure was 36%. At cyclic loading to 70% of the estimated static strength, the probability of failure increased to 92%. *In vivo*, bone remodeling is thought to repair damage induced by cyclic loading. Thus, the cadaver data probably represent a worst-case scenario in terms of risk of fracture (but see previous comments on this issue).

4.3.6 Role of the Cortical Shell

The structural role of the cortical shell is a controversial research topic. Experimental studies in which the shell was removed [McBroom et al. 1985; Rockoff,

Sweet, and Bleustein 1969; Yoganandan et al. 1988] have shown that the shell supports anywhere from 10 [McBroom et al. 1985] to 75% [Rockoff, Sweet, and Bleustein 1969] of the axial compressive load. Some of this variation may be attributed to differences in experimental techniques and the small sample sizes typically used, and thus these findings are difficult to reconcile.

Finite element models developed from clinical resolution CT scans have also been used to determine the structural role of the shell [Faulkner, Cann, and Hasegawa 1991; Liebschner et al. 2003; Silva, Keaveny, and Hayes 1997]. Using this technique, the load-carrying capacity of the cortical shell has been found to be anywhere from 12 [Faulkner, Cann, and Hasegawa 1991] to 75% [Silva, Keaveny, and Hayes 1997] of the total compressive load. Several issues arise when generating finite element models of the cortical shell from clinical-resolution CT scans [Silva, Keaveny, and Hayes 1994]. Because the in-plane dimensions of the scan are on the order of 1 mm and the thickness of the shell is approximately 0.35 mm [Bayraktar et al. 2004; Silva, Keaveny, and Hayes 1994], the thickness of the shell is generally overestimated in the finite element models. Furthermore, the cortical shell is typically modeled as a thin layer of hexahedral elements [Liebschner et al. 2003; Silva, Keaveny, and Hayes 1997] that is adhered to the peripheral surface trabecular centrum. This modeling strategy creates two independent load paths through the vertebral body: one through the cortical shell and the other through the centrum. A recent study using micro-CT-based finite element models [Bayraktar et al. 2004] has suggested that these load paths are not independent and there is a mechanical interaction between the shell and the centrum. Finite element investigations have also suggested that the axial load supported by the shell depends on the boundary conditions imposed by the disc on the end plate [Homminga et al. 2001; Silva, Keaveny, and Hayes 1997]. Using a generic finite element model of a lumbar vertebra, Silva et al. [1997] found that when a "stepped" pressure distribution is imposed on the end plate (simulating a higher pressure in a healthy disc nucleus) the shell supported 5% of the total force acting on the vertebral body. When a uniform pressure distribution was imposed on the end plate (simulating a degenerated disc), the shell supported 24% of the total load. Using patient-specific QCT-based finite element models of lumbar vertebrae that were surrounded by generic discs, Homminga et al. [2001] also found that disc degeneration affected the structural role of the shell, with the shell supporting approximately 50% of the axial load for a healthy disc and 75% for a degenerated disc. Overall, it appears that the shell may take a substantial portion of the load at the mid-vertebral transverse cross section, but the trabecular centrum seems to take the most load close to the end plates.

4.3.7 Role of the Posterior Elements

The two load transfer paths through the vertebrae are the adjacent discs (which transfer load through the vertebral body) and the facet joints and posterior ligaments, which transfer load through the posterior elements. Although the posterior elements—particularly the facet joints [Adams and Hutton 1983; Asano et al. 1992; Lin, Liu, and Adams 1978; McGlashen et al. 1987; Schendel et al. 1993; Sharma, Langrana, and Rodriguez 1995; Shirazi-Adl 1994; Shirazi-Adl, Ahmed, and Shrivastava 1986]—have been shown to play a significant role in torsion, transverse shear, and extension, it has been well established that the disc carries the majority of the load for compression loading [Adams and Hutton 1983; Asano et al. 1992; Hongo et al. 1999; Lin, Liu, and Adams 1978; Schendel et al. 1993; Shirazi-Adl 1994; Tencer, Ahmed, and Burke 1982]. For anterior bending, cadaver studies have shown that the facet joints again play only a minor role in load transfer [Adams and Hutton 1983; Lin, Liu, and Adams 1978]. However, the ligaments spanning the posterior elements (specifically, the supraspinous, the interspinous, the ligamentum flavum, and capsular ligaments) have been shown to play an important role in resisting *large* flexion moments [Adams, Green, and Dolan 1994; Cripton et al. 2000; Lin, Liu, and Adams 1978; McGlashen et al. 1987; Pintar et al. 1992; Schendel et al. 1993; Sharma, Langrana, and Rodriguez 1995; Shirazi-Adl 1994; Shirazi-Adl, Ahmed, and Shrivastava 1986].

The role of the posterior elements in determining vertebral strength is still a topic of investigation. Although numerous studies suggest that less than 10% of the net compressive load is transferred through the posterior elements under physiologic compression [Adams and Hutton 1983; Asano et al. 1992; Hongo et al. 1999; Lin, Liu, and Adams 1978; Schendel et al. 1993; Shirazi-Adl 1994; Tencer, Ahmed, and Burke 1982], the structural role of the posterior elements under loads that are large enough to induce vertebral failure has not been assessed. Additionally, there is clearly an interaction between disc health, loading mode, and load transfer through the posterior elements. Using intradiscal pressure measurements, Pollintine et al. [2004] suggested that the posterior elements support less than 10% of the axial load through the spine when the surrounding discs are healthy. When the discs are degenerated, the role of the posterior elements depended on loading mode, with the posterior elements supporting as much as 40% of the load in compression and less than 10% in anterior bending [Pollintine et al. 2004]. Although the results of this study suggest that the posterior elements may play a significant structural role in some cases, the net loads on the spine were well below those needed to induce vertebral fracture. Thus, the role of the posterior elements in influencing vertebral strength is still under investigation.

4.3.8 Role of the Intervertebral Disc

The stresses the vertebra experiences *in vivo* along its end plates depend on the level of degeneration of the adjacent discs. A healthy disc has a gelatinous nucleus pulposus that is capable of migrating along the end plate under bending-type activities [Iatridis et al. 1996]. In contrast, the nucleus of a degenerated disc can become quite similar to the annulus fibrosis material [Iatridis et al. 1997], no longer capable of migration. The state of stress within the intervertebral disc *in situ* has been investigated using pressure tipped catheters inserted into the disc ("stress profilometry") [Adams, McNally, and Dolan 1994;

McNally and Adams 1992; Ranu, Denton, and King 1979], strain gauges imbedded beneath the end plate [Horst and Brinckmann 1981], and pressure-sensitive film placed beneath the disc [van Dieen et al. 2001]. For example, using an array of pressure sensors embedded under the end plate the axial stress distribution within the nucleus of a healthy lumbar intervertebral disc was found to be uniform both for axial compression and anterior bending [Horst and Brinckmann 1981]. However, for a degenerated disc under axial compression the stress profile was uniform [Horst and Brinckmann 1981], whereas for anterior bending it was asymmetric with a sharp peak anteriorly [Horst and Brinckmann 1981]. Using a generic finite element model of a bone-disc complex, Kurowski and Kubo [1986] found that healthy discs preferentially load the interior of the centrum in axial compression, whereas degenerated discs load the cortical shell. In anterior bending, disc degeneration has been shown to increase the percentage of the net load supported by the anterior region of the vertebral body [Horst and Brinckmann 1981]. The results of these experimental studies suggest that there is an interaction between disc health and loading mode in determining the stress state within the vertebra.

There is also an interaction between disc health and bone mineral density in determining vertebral strength. *Ex vivo* compressive tests of lumbar vertebrae have shown that vertebrae with normal bone density that are surrounded by healthy discs predominantly fail via central end plate ruptures, whereas wedge-type fractures were more common in low-density vertebrae with degenerated discs [Hansson and Roos 1981]. Furthermore, recent finite element studies [Homminga et al. 2001; Polikeit, Nolte, and Ferguson 2003] have suggested that disc degeneration reduces the risk of vertebral fracture for osteoporotic vertebrae but does not affect fracture risk for healthy vertebrae. Despite the insight gained from these studies, it is not yet established with experiments whether or not the state of disc degeneration actually affects the strength of the vertebra independent of any influence of bone density [Hansson and Roos 1981].

4.4 Noninvasive Vertebral Strength Assessment

Three techniques have been developed to noninvasively assess whole vertebral strength, all using some form of X-ray-based imaging. Dual-energy X-ray absorptiometry (DEXA, or DXA) is a 2D imaging technique that involves passing an X-ray beam through the vertebra to a single detector. An "areal" measure of bone mineral density (BMD, units g/cm^2) is obtained by dividing the bone mineral content by the area of a standardized region of interest. Clinically, DXA scans are performed in the anterior-posterior direction because this maximizes precision in repeated scanning. The resulting BMD measurements reflect the density of the trabecular centrum as well as the cortical shell and posterior elements. Despite these limitations, DXA is currently the clinical standard for bone density assessment in the diagnosis of osteoporosis. Correlations between measured compressive strength of cadaveric vertebrae versus BMD are modest, with r^2 values in the range 0.62 to 0.69 (Table 4.3).

Quantitative computed tomography (QCT) is another X-ray-based method of bone density assessment, but it is 3D in nature. A calibration phantom is also used to convert the grayscale data (Hounsfield units) into calibrated measures of bone mineral density. QCT provides a true measure of volumetric bone mineral density (units g/cm^3) and can isolate the trabecular bone from the cortical shell, end plates, and posterior elements. The posterior elements are generally not included in QCT volumetric bone density assessment because the region of interest is typically confined to the central portion of the vertebral bone, avoiding the shell and end plates. Further analysis of the QCT scans can produce measures of vertebral geometry, such as cross-sectional area and total volume. Correlations between measured compressive strength of cadaveric vertebrae versus QCT volumetric bone mineral density are weak in comparison with DXA, with r^2 values in the range 0.23 to 0.66 (Table 4.4). However, direct comparisons between DXA and QCT for vertebral strength prediction have indicated that both techniques are about the same in terms of r^2 values if the QCT metric includes both density and cross-sectional area (compare Tables 4.3 and 4.4) [Cheng et al. 1997; Eriksson, Isberg, and Lindgren 1989; Singer et al. 1995].

QCT-based finite element models—which are generated from the QCT scans—are a promising alternative to standard densitometric techniques in predicting *in vivo* fracture risk because they biomechanically integrate all the information in the QCT scan with loading conditions and material property-density distributions [Crawford and Keaveny 2004; Crawford, Cann, and Keaveny 2003; Faulkner, Cann, and Hasegawa 1991; Homminga et al. 2001]. Although the QCT-based finite element technique has been used for over a decade in orthopedic research to study the mechanical behavior of the femur [Cody et al. 1999; Keyak et al. 1990, 1995, 1998; Lengsfeld et al. 1998], skull [Camacho et al. 1997], and vertebra [Bozic et al. 1994; Faulkner, Cann, and Hasegawa 1991; Homminga et al. 2001; Martin et al. 1998], its use as a tool for clinical vertebral strength assessment is rather new [Crawford and Keaveny 2004; Crawford, Cann, and Keaveny 2003; Faulkner, Cann, and Hasegawa 1991]. Much of this may be attributed to recent technological advances, specifically the development of more powerful computers and faster CT scanning techniques. Also, there has been much work done on characterizing trabecular bone material properties—specifically principal modulus and yield strength—using QCT [Kopperdahl, Morgan, and Keaveny 2002] (Figure 4.17). QCT-based finite element models have shown excellent potential in predicting *ex vivo* vertebral compressive strength [Crawford, Cann, and Keaveny 2003; Faulkner, Cann, and Hasegawa 1991] (Figure 4.18). Faulkner et al. [1991] found that QCT voxel-based finite element models of lumbar vertebrae, when implemented clinically, could better discriminate between osteoporotic and non-osteoporotic individuals than bone density alone. In a later study, Crawford, Cann, and Keaveny [2003] found that finite element model predictions of cadaveric vertebral strength performed better ($r^2 = 0.86$) than both the product of QCT-BMD and transverse plane cross-sectional area ($r^2 = 0.65$, $p = 0.030$) and QCT-BMD alone ($r^2 = 0.53$, $p = 0.027$) (Figure 4.19). This new technique is currently undergoing clinical evaluation given its great promise in the laboratory.

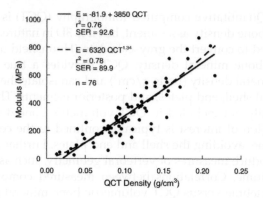

Fig. 4.17.

Trabecular bone principal elastic modulus was well predicted by either linear or power law models using mineral density measured using quantitative computed tomography as the independent variable. SER = standard error of the regression. These data were derived from tests on 76 specimens taken from 32 cadavers (19 male, 13 female; age: mean = 70.1 y.o., SD = 16.8 y.o., range = 20–91 y.o.). (*From [Kopperdahl, Morgan, and Keaveny 2002] with permission.*)

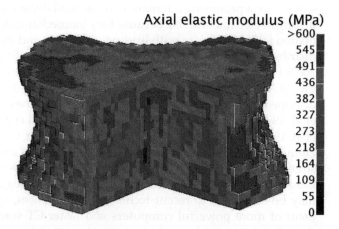

Fig. 4.18.

A QCT-based finite element model from a representative human lumbar vertebra (L1, 73 y.o. female). The distribution of axial elastic moduli is also shown, and the top end plate and a wedge-shaped portion of the vertebral body are removed for illustrative purposes. (*From [Crawford, Cann, and Keaveny 2003] with permission.*)

4.4.1 *In Vivo* Fracture Risk Prediction

Although DXA and QCT measures of bone mineral density are quite well correlated with *ex situ* vertebral compressive strength, these techniques are not strong predictors of whether an individual will suffer an osteoporotic vertebral fracture *in vivo* [Cummings, Bates, and Black 2002; National Osteoporosis Foundation 1998; Ott 1991]. The important distinction between bone strength assess-

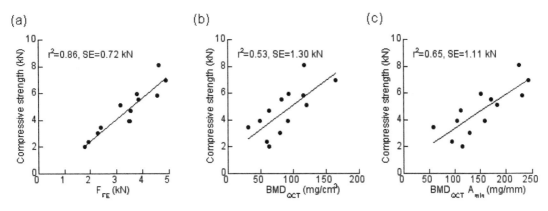

Fig. 4.19.

Predictions of *ex situ* vertebral compressive strength using (a) QCT-based finite element models, (b) QCT-BMD, (c) QCT-BMD adjusted for minimum transverse plane cross-sectional area. QCT-based finite element models better predict vertebral strength than the QCT-BMD measures. (*From [Crawford, Cann, and Keaveny 2003] with permission.*)

ment and fracture risk prediction is that the latter, which represents the true clinical endpoint in terms of osteoporotic fractures, includes measures of both bone strength and the *in vivo* loads that act on the bone [Hayes 1991; Myers and Wilson 1997]. *In vivo* loading conditions are difficult to predict because they depend on such factors as the individual's body mass index (weight normalized by height), level of physical activity, propensity to fall, presence of preexisting vertebral fractures, and the health of the intervertebral disc. Thus, it remains to be seen from clinical studies if improved bone strength assessment tools such as QCT-based finite element models do indeed improve clinical fracture risk prediction over what is currently achievable by DXA.

One important phenomenon to consider in the meanwhile is that current anti-resorptive drug therapies work so well—typically producing decreases in fracture incidence of up to 60% [Bates, Black, and Cummings 2002; Cummings et al. 2002; Delmas and Seeman 2004]. Presumably, these treatments affect only the strength of the bone and not the loads acting on the bone. This indicates that the fracture risk is not dominated by the loading conditions, because if they were one would expect treatment-induced changes in bone strength to have a smaller clinical effect. As a result, there is substantial interest in understanding the mechanisms of vertebral strength and improving methods to noninvasively monitor treatment effects. The material discussed in this chapter provides an excellent basis for understanding these issues.

4.5 Acknowledgments

The authors acknowledge support from the National Institutes of Health (grant AR49828) and a graduate student fellowship from the University of California,

Berkeley. The authors would also like to thank Bethany Baumbach for editorial assistance.

4.6 References

Adams, M. A., and W. C. Hutton (1983). "The Mechanical Function of the Lumbar Apophyseal Joints," *Spine* 8:327–330.

Adams, M. A., T. P. Green, and P. Dolan (1994). "The Strength in Anterior Bending of Lumbar Intervertebral Discs," *Spine* 19:2197–2203.

Adams, M. A., D. S. McNally, and P. Dolan (1996). "Stress Distributions Inside Intervertebral Discs: The Effects of Age and Degeneration," *Journal of Bone and Joint Surgery. British Volume* 78:965–972.

Adams, M. A., D. S. McNally, H. Chinn, and P. Dolan (1994). "Posture and the Compressive Strength of the Lumbar Spine," *Clinical Biomechanics* 9:5–14.

Antonacci, M. D., D. S. Hanson, A. Leblanc, and M. H. Heggeness (1997). "Regional Variation in Vertebral Bone Density and Trabecular Architecture Are Influenced by Osteoarthritic Change and Osteoporosis," *Spine* 22:2393–2401; discussion 2392–2401.

Asano, S., K. Kaneda, S. Umehara, and S. Tadano (1992). "The Mechanical Properties of the Human L4–5 Functional Spinal Unit During Cyclic Loading: The Structural Effects of the Posterior Elements," *Spine* 17:1343–1352.

Baroud, G., R. Falk, et al. (2004). "Experimental and Theoretical Investigation of Directional Permeability of Human Vertebral Cancellous Bone for Cement Infiltration," *Journal of Biomechanics* 37:189–196.

Bates, D. W., D. M. Black, and S. R. Cummings (2002). "Clinical Use of Bone Densitometry: Clinical Applications," *Jama-Journal of the American Medical Association* 288:1898–1900.

Bauer, T. W., and J. Schils (1999). "The Pathology of Total Joint Arthroplasty: II. Mechanisms of Implant Failure," *Skeletal Radiology* 28:483–497.

Bayraktar, H. H., M. F. Adams, et al. (2004). *Micromechanics of the Human Vertebral Body.* Trans. Orthop. Res. Soc. San Francisco.

Bentolila, V., T. M. Boyce, et al. (1998). "Intracortical Remodeling in Adult Rat Long Bones After Fatigue Loading," *Bone* 23:275–281.

Black, D. M., N. K. Arden, et al. (1999). "Prevalent Vertebral Deformities Predict Hip Fractures and New Vertebral Deformities But Not Wrist Fractures," Study of Osteoporotic Fractures Research Group. *Journal of Bone and Mineral Research* 14:821–828.

Bozic, K. J., J. H. Keyak, et al. (1994). "Three-dimensional Finite Element Modeling of a Cervical Vertebra: An Investigation of Burst Fracture Mechanism," *Journal of Spinal Disorders & Techniques* 7:102–110.

Brinckmann, P., M. Biggeman, and D. Hilweg (1988). "Fatigue Fracture of Human Lumbar Vertebrae," *Clinical Biomechanics* 3:S1–S23.

Brinckmann, P., M. Biggemann, and D. Hilweg (1989). "Prediction of the Compressive Strength of Human Lumbar Vertebrae," *Spine* 14:606–610.

Brown, T. D., and A. B. Ferguson (1980). "Mechanical Property Distributions in the Cancellous Bone of the Human Proximal Femur," *Acta Orthopaedic Scandinavica* 51:429–437.

Burr, D. B., M. R. Forwood, et al. (1997). "Bone Microdamage and Skeletal Fragility in Osteoporotic and Stress Fractures," *Journal of Bone and Mineral Research* 12:6–15.

Burr, D. B., R. B. Martin, M. B. Schaffler, and E. L. Radin (1985). "Bone Remodeling in Response to In Vivo Fatigue Microdamage," *Journal of Biomechanics* 18:189–200.

Camacho, D. L., R. H. Hopper, G. M. Lin, and B. S. Myers (1997). "An Improved Method for Finite Element Mesh Generation of Geometrically Complex Structures with Application to the Skullbase," *Journal of Biomechanics* 30:1067–1070.

Chang, W. C. W., T. M. Christensen, T. P. Pinilla, and T. M. Keaveny (1999). "Isotropy of Uniaxial Yield Strains for Bovine Trabecular Bone," *Journal of Orthopaedic Research* 17:582–585.

Cheng, X. G., P. H. F. Nicholson, et al. (1997a). "Prevalence of Trabecular Microcallus Formation in the Vertebral Body and the Femoral Neck," *Calcified Tissue International* 60:479–484.

Cheng, X. G., P. H. F. Nicholson, et al. (1997b). "Prediction of Vertebral Strength in Vitro by Spinal Bone Densitometry and Calcaneal Ultrasound," *Journal of Bone and Mineral Research* 12:1721–1728.

Choi, K., and S. A. Goldstein (1992). "A Comparison of the Fatigue Behavior of Human Trabecular and Cortical Bone Tissue," *Journal of Biomechanics* 25:1371–1381.

Cody, D. D., S. A. Goldstein, M. J. Flynn, and E. B. Brown (1991). "Correlations Between Vertebral Regional Bone Mineral Density (rBMD) and Whole Bone Fracture Load," *Spine* 16:146–154.

Cody, D. D., G. J. Gross, et al. (1999). "Femoral Strength Is Better Predicted by Finite Element Models Than QCT and DXA," *Journal of Biomechanics* 32:1013–1020.

Cooper, C., E. J. Atkinson, W. M. O'Fallon, and L. J. Melton (1992). "Incidence of Clinically Diagnosed Vertebral Fractures: A Population-based Study in Rochester, Minnesota, 1985–1989," *Journal of Bone and Mineral Research* 7:221–227.

Crawford, R. P., and T. M. Keaveny (2004). "Relationship Between Axial and Bending Behaviors of the Human Thoracolumbar Vertebra," *Spine* 29:2248–2255.

Crawford, R. P., C. E. Cann, and T. M. Keaveny (2003). "Finite Element Models Predict In Vitro Vertebral Body Compressive Strength Better Than Quantitative Computed Tomography," *Bone* 33:744–750.

Cripton, P. A., G. M. Jain, R. H. Wittenberg, and L. P. Nolte (2000). "Load-sharing Characteristics of Stabilized Lumbar Spine Segments," *Spine* 25:170–179.

Cummings, S. R., D. Bates, and D. M. Black (2002). "Clinical Use of Bone Densitometry: Scientific Review," *Jama-Journal of the American Medical Association* 288:1889–1897.

Cummings, S. R., D. B. Karpf, et al. (2002). "Improvement in Spine Bone Density and Reduction in Risk of Vertebral Fractures During Treatment with Antiresorptive Drugs," *American Journal of Medicine* 112:281–289.

Cummings, S. R., R. Marcus, et al. (1994). "Does Estimating Volumetric Bone Density of the Femoral Neck Improve the Prediction of Hip Fracture? A Prospective Study," Study of Osteoporotic Fractures Research Group. *Journal of Bone and Mineral Research* 9:1429–1432.

Delmas, P. D., and E. Seeman (2004). "Changes in Bone Mineral Density Explain Little of the Reduction in Vertebral or Nonvertebral Fracture Risk with Anti-resorptive Therapy," *Bone* 34:599–604.

Eastell, R., S. L. Cedel, et al. (1991). "Classification of Vertebral Fractures," *Journal of Bone and Mineral Research* 6:207–215.

Ebbesen, E. N., J. S. Thomsen, et al. (1999). "Lumbar Vertebral Body Compressive Strength Evaluated by Dual-energy X-ray Absorptiometry, Quantitative Computed Tomography, and Ashing," *Bone* 25:713–724.

Eckstein, F., M. Fischbeck, et al. (2004). "Determinants and Heterogeneity of Mechanical Competence Throughout the Thoracolumbar Spine of Elderly Women and Men," *Bone* 35:364–374.

Edmondston, S. J., K. P. Singer, et al. (1994). "The Relationship Between Bone Mineral Density, Vertebral Body Shape and Spinal Curvature in the Elderly Thoracolumbar Spine: An In Vitro Study," *British Journal Radiology* 67:969–975.

Edmondston, S. J., K. P. Singer, et al. (1997). "Ex Vivo Estimation of Thoracolumbar Vertebral Body Compressive Strength: The Relative Contributions of Bone Densitometry and Vertebral Morphometry," *Osteoporos International* 7:142–148.

Edwards, W. T., Y. G. Zheng, L. A. Ferrara, and H. A. Yuan (2001). "Structural Features and Thickness of the Vertebral Cortex in the Thoracolumbar Spine," *Spine* 26:218–225.

Eriksson, S. A., B. O. Isberg, and J. U. Lindgren (1989). "Prediction of Vertebral Strength by Dual Photon Absorptiometry and Quantitative Computed Tomography," *Calcified Tissue International* 44:243–250.

Eswaran, S. K., A. Gupta, M. F. Adams, and T. M. Keaveny (2006). "Cortical and Trabecular Load Sharing in the Human Vertebral Body," *Journal of Bone and Mineral Research* 21:307–314.

Faulkner, K. G., C. E. Cann, and B. H. Hasegawa (1991). "Effect of Bone Distribution on Vertebral Strength: Assessment with Patient-specific Nonlinear Finite Element Analysis," *Radiology* 179:669–674.

Fazzalari, N. L., M. R. Forwood, et al. (1998a). "Assessment of Cancellous Bone Quality in Severe Osteoarthrosis: Bone Mineral Density, Mechanics, and Microdamage," *Bone* 22:381–388.

Fazzalari, N. L., M. R. Forwood, et al. (1998b). "Three-dimensional Confocal Images of Microdamage in Cancellous Bone," *Bone* 23:373–378.

Fyhrie, D. P., and M. B. Schaffler (1994). "Failure Mechanisms in Human Vertebral Cancellous Bone," *Bone* 15:105–109.

Galante, J., W. Rostoker, and R. D. Ray (1970). "Physical Properties of Trabecular Bone," *Calcified Tissue Research* 5:236–246.

Gibson, L. J., and M. F. Ashby (1997). *Cellular Solids: Structures and Properties.* Oxford: Pergamon Press.

Goldstein, S. A., D. L. Wilson, D. A. Sonstegard, and L. S. Matthews (1983). "The Mechanical Properties of Human Tibial Trabecular Bone As a Function of Metaphyseal Location," *Journal of Biomechanics* 16:965–969.

Grant, J. P., T. R. Oxland, and M. F. Dvorak (2001). "Mapping the Structural Properties of the Lumbosacral Vertebral End Plates," *Spine* 26:889–896.

Greenspan, S. L., L. Maitland-Ramsey, and E. Myers (1996). "Classification of Osteoporosis in the Elderly Is Dependent on Site-specific Analysis," *Calcified Tissue International* 58:409–414.

Grisso, J. A., J. L. Kelsey, et al. (1991). "Risk Factors for Falls As a Cause of Hip Fracture in Women," The Northeast Hip Fracture Study Group. *New England Journal of Medicine* 324:1326–1331.

Haddock, S. M., and O. C. Yeh, et al. (2004). "Similarity in the Fatigue Behavior of Trabecular Bone Across Site and Species," *Journal of Biomechanics* 37:181–187.

Hahn, M., M. Vogel, et al. (1995). "Microcallus Formations of the Cancellous Bone: A Quantitative Analysis of the Human Spine," *Journal of Bone and Mineral Research* 10:1410–1416.

Hannan, M. T., D. T. Felson, and J. J. Anderson (1992). "Bone Mineral Density in Elderly Men and Women: Results from the Framingham Osteoporosis Study," *Journal of Bone and Mineral Research* 7:547–553.

Hansson, T., and B. Roos (1981a). "Microcalluses of the Trabeculae in Lumbar Vertebrae and Their Relation to the Bone Mineral Content," *Spine* 6:375–380.

Hansson, T., and B. Roos (1981b). "The Relation Between Bone-Mineral Content, Experimental Compression Fractures, and Disk Degeneration in Lumbar Vertebrae," *Spine* 6:147–153.

Hansson, T. H., T. S. Keller, and M. M. Panjabi (1987b). "A Study of the Compressive Properties of Lumbar Vertebral Trabeculae: Effects of Tissue Characteristics," *Spine* 12:56–62.

Hansson, T. H., T. S. Keller, and D. M. Spengler (1987a). "Mechanical Behavior of the Human Lumbar Spine: II. Fatigue Strength During Dynamic Compressive Loading," *Journal of Orthopaedic Research* 5:479–487.

Hansson, T., B. Roos, and A. Nachemson (1980). "The Bone Mineral Content and Ultimate Compressive Strength of Lumbar Vertebrae," *Spine* 5:46–55.

Harrigan, T. P., M. Jasty, R. W. Mann, and W. H. Harris (1988). "Limitations of the Continuum Assumption in Cancellous Bone," *Journal of Biomechanics* 21: 269–275.

Harvinder, S., M. D. Safdar, and N. Khan (2002). "Vertebral Fractures and Vertebroplasty," *http://www.spineuniverse.com/displayarticle.php/article1464.html?source=google* (accessed 01/07/2002).

Hayes, W. (1991). "Biomechanics of Cortical and Trabecular Bone: Implications for Assessment of Fracture Risk," in V. Mow and W. Hayes (eds). *Basic Orthopaedic Biomechanics*. New York: Raven Press, Ltd.

Homminga, J., H. Weinans, et al. (2001). "Osteoporosis Changes the Amount of Vertebral Trabecular Bone At Risk of Fracture But Not the Vertebral Load Distribution," *Spine* 26:1555–1561.

Hongo, M., E. Abe, et al. (1999). "Surface Strain Distribution on Thoracic and Lumbar Vertebrae Under Axial Compression. The Role in Burst Fractures," *Spine* 24:1197–1202.

Horst, M., and P. Brinckmann (1981a). "Measurement of the Distribution of Axial Stress on the End plate of the Vertebral Body," *Spine* 6:217–232.

Horst, M., and P. Brinckmann (1981b). "1980 Volvo Award in Biomechanics: Measurement of the Distribution of Axial Stress on the End-plate of the Vertebral Body," *Spine* 6:217–232.

Iatridis, J. C., L. A. Setton, M. Weidenbaum, and V. C. Mow (1997). "Alterations in the Mechanical Behavior of the Human Lumbar Nucleus Pulposus with Degeneration and Aging," *Journal of Orthopaedic Research* 15:318–322.

Iatridis, J. C., M. Weidenbaum, L. A. Setton, and V. C. Mow (1996). "Is the Nucleus Pulposus a Solid or a Fluid? Mechanical Behaviors of the Nucleus Pulposus of the Human Intervertebral Disc," *Spine* 21:1174–1184.

Jiang, G., R. Eastell, N. A. Barrington, and L. Ferrar (2004). "Comparison of Methods for the Visual Identification of Prevalent Vertebral Fracture in Osteoporosis," *Osteoporos International* 15:887–896.

Keaveny, T. M., E. F. Wachtel, and D. L. Kopperdahl (1999). "Mechanical Behavior of Human Trabecular Bone After Overloading," *Journal of Orthopaedic Research* 17:346–353.

Keaveny, T. M., E. F. Wachtel, C. M. Ford, and W. C. Hayes (1994). "Differences Between the Tensile and Compressive Strengths of Bovine Tibial Trabecular Bone Depend on Modulus," *Journal of Biomechanics* 27:1137–1146.

Keller, T. S., T. H. Hansson, et al. (1989). "Regional Variations in the Compressive Properties of Lumbar Vertebral Trabeculae: Effects of Disc Degeneration," *Spine* 14:1012–1019.

Keyak, J. H., I. Y. Lee, S. A. Rossi, and H. B. Skinner (1995). "Prediction of Femoral Fracture Load and Location Using CT Scan-derived Finite Element Models," *Tranactruns of the Orthopedic Research Society* 20:457.

Keyak, J. H., J. M. Meagher, H. B. Skinner, and C. D. Mote Jr. (1990). "Automated Three-dimensional Finite Element Modelling of Bone: A New Method," *Journal of Biomedical Engineering* 12:389–397.

Keyak, J. H., S. A. Rossi, K. A. Jones, and H. B. Skinner (1998). "Prediction of Femoral Fracture Load Using Automated Finite Element Modeling," *Journal of Biomechanics* 31:125–133.

Kim, S. H., H. S. Kang, J. A. Choi, and J. M. Ahn (2004). "Risk Factors of New Compression Fractures in Adjacent Vertebrae After Percutaneous Vertebroplasty," *Acta Radiologica* 45:440–445.

Kleerekoper, M., and D. A. Nelson (1992). "Vertebral Fracture or Deformity?," *Calcified Tissue International* 50:5–6.

Kopperdahl, D. L., and T. M. Keaveny (1998). "Yield Strain Behavior of Trabecular Bone," *Journal of Biomechanics* 31:601–608.

Kopperdahl, D. L., E. F. Morgan, and T. M. Keaveny (2002). "Quantitative Computed Tomography Estimates of the Mechanical Properties of Human Vertebral Trabecular Bone," *Journal of Orthopaedic Research* 20:801–805.

Kopperdahl, D. L., J. L. Pearlman, and T. M. Keaveny (2000). "Biomechanical Consequences of an Isolated Overload on the Human Vertebral Body," *Journal of Orthopaedic Research* 18:685–690.

Kopperdahl, D. L., A. D. Roberts, and T. M. Keaveny (1999). "Localized Damage in Vertebral Bone Is Most Detrimental in Regions of High Strain Energy Density," *Journal of Biomechanical Engineering* 121:622–628.

Krajcinovic, D., and J. Lemaitre (1987). *Continuum Damage Mechanics: Theory and Applications*. New York: Springer Verlag.

Kurowski, P., and A. Kubo (1986). "The Relationship of Degeneration of the Intervertebral Disc to Mechanical Loading Conditions on Lumbar Vertebrae," *Spine* 11:726–731.

Lengsfeld, M., J. Schmitt, et al. (1998). "Comparison of Geometry-based and CT Voxel-based Finite Element Modelling and Experimental Validation," *Medical Engineering & Physics Journal* 20:515–522.

Liebschner, M. A., D. L. Kopperdahl, W. S. Rosenberg, and T. M. Keaveny (2003). "Finite Element Modeling of the Human Thoracolumbar Spine," *Spine* 28:559–565.

Lin, H. S., Y. K. Liu, and K. H. Adams (1978). "Mechanical Response of the Lumbar Intervertebral Joint Under Physiological (Complex) Loading," *Journal of Bone and Joint Surgery American* 60:41–55.

Liu, Y. K., G. Njus, J. Buckwalter, and K. Wakano (1983). "Fatigue Response of Lumbar Intervertebral Joints Under Axial Cyclic Loading," *Spine* 8:857–865.

Lochmuller, E. M., D. Burklein, et al. (2002). "Mechanical Strength of the Thoracolumbar Spine in the Elderly: Prediction from In Situ Dual-energy X-ray Absorptiometry, Quantitative Computed Tomography (QCT), Upper and Lower Limb Peripheral QCT, and Quantitative Ultrasound," *Bone* 31:77–84.

Lochmuller, E. M., R. Muller, et al. (2003). "Can Novel Clinical Densitometric Techniques Replace or Improve DXA in Predicting Bone Strength in Osteoporosis at the Hip and Other Skeletal Sites?," *Journal of Bone and Mineral Research* 18:906–912.

McBroom, R. J., W. C. Hayes, et al. (1985). "Prediction of Vertebral Body Compressive Fracture Using Quantitative Computed Tomography," *Journal of Bone and Joint Surgery* 67-A:1206–1214.

McCalden, R. W., J. A. McGeough, and C. M. Court-Brown (1997). "Age-related Changes in the Compressive Strength of Cancellous Bone: The Relative Importance of Changes in Density and Trabecular Architecture," *Journal of Bone and Joint Surgery. American Volume* 79:421–427.

McCubbrey, D. A., D. D. Cody, et al. (1995). "Static and Fatigue Failure Properties of Thoracic and Lumbar Vertebral Bodies and Their Relation to Regional Density," *Journal of Biomechanics* 28:891–899.

McGlashen, K. M., J. A. Miller, A. B. Schultz, and G. B. Andersson (1987). "Load Displacement Behavior of the Human Lumbo-sacral Joint," *Journal of Orthopaedic Research* 5:488–496.

McNally, D. S., and M. A. Adams (1992). "Internal Intervertebral Disc Mechanics as Revealed by Stress Profilometry," *Spine* 17:66–73.

Martin, H., J. Werner, et al. (1998). "Noninvasive Assessment of Stiffness and Failure Load of Human Vertebrae from CT-data," *Biomedical Technology (Berl)* 43:82–88.

Martin, R. B (2000). "Toward a Unifying Theory of Bone Remodeling," *Bone* 26:1–6.

Martin, R. B., V. A. Gibson, et al. (1997). "Residual Strength of Equine Bone Is Not Reduced by Intense Fatigue Loading: Implications for Stress Fracture," *Journal of Biomechanics* 30:109–114.

Melton, L. J., and H. W. Wahner (1989). "Defining Osteoporosis [editorial]," *Calcified Tissue International* 45:263–264.

Melton, L. J., E. A. Chrischilles, et al. (1992). "Perspective. How Many Women Have Osteoporosis?," *Journal of Bone and Mineral Research* 7:1005–1010.

Michelson, J. D., A. Myers, et al. (1995). "Epidemiology of Hip Fractures Among the Elderly: Risk Factors for Fracture Type," *Clinical Orthopedic and Related Research* 311:129–135.

Morgan, E. F., and T. M. Keaveny (2001). "Dependence of Yield Strain of Human Trabecular Bone on Anatomic Site," *Journal of Biomechanics* 34:569–577.

Morgan, E. F., O. C. Yeh, W. C. Chang, and T. M. Keaveny (2001). "Nonlinear Behavior of Trabecular Bone at Small Strains," *Journal of Biomechanical Engineering* 123:1–9.

Mori, S., and D. B. Burr (1993). "Increased Intracortical Remodeling Following Fatigue Damage," *Bone* 14:103–109.

Mori, S., R. Harruff, W. Ambrosius, and D. B. Burr (1997). "Trabecular Bone Volume and Microdamage Accumulation in the Femoral Heads of Women with and Without Femoral Neck Fractures," *Bone* 21:521–526.

Moro, M., A. T. Hecker, M. L. Bouxsein, and E. R. Myers (1995). "Failure Load of Thoracic Vertebrae Correlates with Lumbar Bone Mineral Density Measured by DXA," *Calcified Tissue International* 56:206–209.

Mosekilde, L. (1993). "Vertebral Structure and Strength *In Vivo* and *In Vitro*," *Calcified Tissue International* 53:S121–S126.

Mosekilde, L., and L. Mosekilde (1986). "Normal Vertebral Body Size and Compressive Strength: Relations to Age and to Vertebral and Iliac Trabecular Bone Compressive Strength," *Bone* 7:207–212.

Mosekilde, L., and L. Mosekilde (1990). "Sex Differences in Age-related Changes in Vertebral Body Size, Density and Biomechanical Competence in Normal Individuals," *Bone* 11:67–73.

Mosekilde, L., S. M. Bentzen, G. Ortoft, and J. Jorgensen (1989). "The Predictive Value of Quantitative Computed Tomography for Vertebral Body Compressive Strength and Ash Density," *Bone* 10:465–470.

Mosekilde, L., L. Mosekilde, and C. C. Danielsen (1987). "Biomechanical Competence of Vertebral Trabecular Bone in Relation to Ash Density and Age in Normal Individuals," *Bone* 8:79–85.

Myers, E. R., and S. E. Wilson (1997). "Biomechanics of Osteoporosis and Vertebral Fracture," *Spine* 22:25S–31S.

Myers, E. R., S. E. Wilson, and S. L. Greenspan (1996). "Vertebral Fractures in the Elderly Occur with Falling and Bending," *Journal of Bone and Mineral Research* 11:S355.

National Osteoporosis Foundation (1998). "Osteoporosis: Review of the Evidence for Prevention, Diagnosis and Treatment and Cost-effectiveness Analysis," *Osteoporosis International* 8:S7–S80.

Nelson, D. A., M. Kleerekoper, and E. L. Peterson (1994). "Reversal of Vertebral Deformities in Osteoporosis: Measurement Error or Rebound," *Journal of Bone and Mineral Research* 9:977–982.

Ohshima, H., H. Tsuji, et al. (1989). "Water Diffusion Pathway, Swelling Pressure, and Biomechanical Properties of the Intervertebral Disc During Compression Load," *Spine* 14:1234–1244.

Ott, S. M. (1991). "Methods of Determining Bone Mass," *Journal of Bone and Mineral Research* 6 Suppl. 2:S71–S76; discussion S83–84.

Panjabi, M. M., T. R. Oxland, I. Yamamoto, and J. J. Crisco (1994). "Mechanical Behavior of the Human Lumbar and Lumbosacral Spine as Shown by Three-dimensional Load-displacement Curves," *Journal of Bone and Joint Surgery American* 76:413–424.

Pintar, F. A., J. F. Cusick, et al. (1992). "The Biomechanics of Lumbar Facetectomy Under Compression-flexion," *Spine* 17:804–810.

Polikeit, A., L. P. Nolte, and S. J. Ferguson (2003). "The Effect of Cement Augmentation on the Load Transfer in an Osteoporotic Functional Spinal Unit: Finite Element Analysis," *Spine* 28:991–996.

Pollintine, P., P. Dolan, J. H. Tobias, and M. A. Adams (2004). "Intervertebral Disc Degeneration Can Lead to 'Stress-shielding' of the Anterior Vertebral Body: A Cause of Osteoporotic Vertebral Fracture?," *Spine* 29:774–782.

Prendergast, P. J., and R. Huiskes (1996). "Microdamage and Osteocyte-lacuna Strain in Bone: A Microstructural Finite Element Analysis," *Journal of Biomechanical Engineering* 118:240–246.

Prevrhal, S., J. Fox, J. A. Shepherd, and H. Genant (2003). "Accuracy of CT-based Thickness Measurement of Thin Structures: Modeling of Limited Spatial Resolution in All Three Dimensions," *Medical Physics* 30:1–8.

Pugh, J. W., R. M. Rose, and E. L. Radin (1973). "A Possible Mechanism of Wolff's Law: Trabecular Microfractures," *Archives Internationales de Physiologie et de Biochimic* 81:27–40.

Ranu, H. S., R. A. Denton, and A. I. King (1979). "Pressure Distribution Under an Intervertebral Disc: An Experimental Study," *Journal of Biomechanics* 12:807–812.

Ray, N. F., J. K. Chan, M. Thamer, and L. J. Melton (1997). "Medical Expenditures for the Treatment of Osteoporotic Fractures in the United States in 1995: Report from the National Osteoporosis Foundation," *Journal of Bone and Mineral Research* 12:24–35.

Reilly, D. T., and A. H. Burstein (1975). "The Elastic and Ultimate Properties of Compact Bone Tissue," *Journal of Biomechanics* 8:393–405.

Riggs, B. L., and L. J. Melton (1995). *Osteoporosis: Etiology, Diagnosis, and Management.* Philadelphia: Lippincott-Raven.

Rockoff, S. D., E. Sweet, and J. Bleustein (1969). "The Relative Contribution of Trabecular and Cortical Bone to the Strength of Human Lumbar Vertebrae," *Calcified Tissue Research* 3:163–175.

Roy, M. E., J. Y. Rho, et al. (1999). "Mechanical and Morphological Variation of the Human Lumbar Vertebral Cortical and Trabecular Bone," *Journal of Biomedical Materials Research* 44:191–197.

Schendel, M. J., K. B. Wood, et al. (1993). "Experimental Measurement of Ligament Force, Facet Force, and Segment Motion in the Human Lumbar Spine," *Journal of Biomechanics* 26:427–438.

Schultz, A. B., D. N. Warwick, M. H. Berkson, and A. L. Nachemson (1979). "Mechanical Properties of Human Lumbar Spine Motion Segments. Part I: Responses in Flexion, Extension, Lateral Bending, and Torsion," *Journal of Biomechanical Engineering* 101:46–52.

Sharma, M., N. A. Langrana, and J. Rodriguez (1995). "Role of Ligaments and Facets in Lumbar Spinal Stability," *Spine* 20:887–900.

Shirazi-Adl, A. (1994). "Biomechanics of the Lumbar Spine in Sagittal/Lateral Moments," *Spine* 19:2407–2414.

Shirazi-Adl, A., A. M. Ahmed, and S. C. Shrivastava (1986). "A Finite Element Study of a Lumbar Motion Segment Subjected to Pure Sagittal Plane Moments," *Journal of Biomechanics* 19:331–350.

Silva, M. J., T. M. Keaveny, and W. C. Hayes (1994). "Direct and Computed Tomography Thickness Measurements of the Human Lumbar Vertebral Shell and Endplate," *Bone* 15:409–414.

Silva, M. J., T. M. Keaveny, and W. C. Hayes (1997). "Load Sharing Between the Shell and Centrum in the Lumbar Vertebral Body," *Spine* 22:140–150.

Silva, M. J., T. M. Keaveny, and W. C. Hayes (1998). "Computed Tomography-based Finite Element Analysis Predicts Failure Loads and Fracture Patterns for Vertebral Sections," *Journal of Orthopaedic Research* 16:300–308.

Singer, K., S. Edmondston, et al. (1995). "Prediction of Thoracic and Lumbar Vertebral Body Compressive Strength: Correlations with Bone Mineral Density and Vertebral Region," *Bone* 17:167–174.

Smith-Bindman, R., S. R. Cummings, P. Steiger, and H. K. Genant (1991). "A Comparison of Morphometric Definitions of Vertebral Fracture," *Journal of Bone and Mineral Research* 6:25–34.

Steiger, P., S. R. Cummings, et al. (1992). "Age-related Decrements in Bone Mineral Density in Women over 65," *Journal of Bone and Mineral Research* 7:625–632.

Taylor, M., and K. E. Tanner (1997). "Fatigue Failure of Cancellous Bone: A Possible Cause of Implant Migration and Loosening," *Journal of Bone and Joint Surgery British* 79:181–182.

Tehranzadeh, J., A. N. Serafini, and M. J. Pais (1989). *Avulsion and Stress Injuries of the Musculoskeletal System.* New York: Karger.

Tencer, A. F., A. M. Ahmed, and D. L. Burke (1982). "Some Static Mechanical Properties of the Lumbar Intervertebral Joint, Intact and Injured," *Journal of Biomechanical Engineering* 104:193–201.

Turner, C. H. (1989). "Yield Behavior of Bovine Cancellous Bone," *Journal of Biomechanical Engineering* 111:256–260.

Turner, C. H., J. Rho, et al. (1999). "The Elastic Properties of Trabecular and Cortical Bone Tissues Are Similar: Results from Two Microscopic Measurement Techniques," *Journal of Biomechanics* 32:437–441.

Ulrich, D., B. Van Rietbergen, A. Laib, and P. Rueegsegger (1999). "The Ability of Three-dimensional Structural Indices to Reflect Mechanical Aspects of Trabecular Bone," *Bone* 25:55–60.

Urban, J. P., and J. F. McMullin (1988). "Swelling Pressure of the Lumbar Intervertebral Discs: Influence of Age, Spinal Level, Composition, and Degeneration," *Spine* 13:179–187.

van Dieen, J. H., I. Kingma, et al. (2001). "Stress Distribution Changes in Bovine Vertebrae Just Below the Endplate After Sustained Loading," *Clinical Biomechanics (Bristol, Avon)* 16 Suppl. 1:S135–S142.

Vashishth, D., J. Koontz, et al. (2000). "In Vivo Diffuse Damage in Human Vertebral Trabecular Bone," *Bone* 26:147–152.

Veenland, J. F., T. M. Link, et al. (1997). "Unraveling the Role of Structure and Density in Determining Vertebral Bone Strength," *Calcified Tissue International* 61:474–479.

Vernon-Roberts, B., and C. J. Pirie (1977). "Degenerative Changes in the Intervertebral Discs of the Lumbar Spine and Their Sequelae," *Rheumatol Rehabil* 16:13–21.

Wachtel, E. F., and T. M. Keaveny (1997). "Dependence of Trabecular Damage on Mechanical Strain," *Journal of Orthopaedic Research* 15:781–787.

Wenzel, T. E., M. B. Schaffler, and D. P. Fyhrie (1996). "In Vivo Trabecular Microcracks in Human Vertebral Bone," *Bone* 19:89–95.

Whealan, K. M., S. D. Kwak, et al. (2000). "Noninvasive Imaging Predicts Failure Load of the Spine with Simulated Osteolytic Defects," *Journal of Bone and Joint Surgery American* 82:1240–1251.

White, A. A., and M. M. Panjabi (1990). *Clinical Biomechanics of the Spine*. Philadelphia: Lippincott.

Yeh, O. C., and T. M. Keaveny (2001). "The Relative Roles of Microdamage and Microfracture in the Mechanical Behavior of Trabecular Bone," *Journal of Orthopaedic Research* 19:1001–1007.

Yoganandan, N., J. B. Myklebust, et al. (1988). "Functional Biomechanics of the Thoracolumbar Vertebral Cortex," *Clinical Biomechanics* 3:11–18.

Ziegler, R., C. Scheidt-Nave, and G. Leidig-Bruckner (1996). "What Is a Vertebral Fracture?," *Bone* 18:169S–177S.

Zysset, P. K., R. W. Goulet, and S. J. Hollister (1998). "A Global Relationship Between Trabecular Bone Morphology and Homogenized Elastic Properties," *Journal of Biomechanical Engineering* 120:640–646.

Chapter 5

Musculature Actuation and Biomechanics of the Spine

Peter A. Cripton, Ph.D.; Shannon G. Kroeker, M.A.Sc.; and Amy Saari, B.Sc. (Eng.)

Division of Orthopaedic Engineering Research,
Departments of Mechanical Engineering and Orthopaedics,
University of British Columbia

5.1 Spine Muscles

5.1.1 Anatomy and Physiology

Muscles of the back can be classified into superficial, intermediate, or deep groups. Spinal column stability and movement is attributed primarily to the deep muscles of the back, although all muscle groups contribute to these functions to some extent. Deep muscles run the entire length of the spinal column from the pelvis to the skull and consist of several subgroups. The spinotransverse (Figure 5.1) and suboccipital (Figure 5.2) muscle groups are concerned with the extension, rotation, and stability of the axis (C2), atlas (C1), and skull. The erector spinae (Figure 5.3) and transversospinalis groups are involved with extension, rotation, and stability of the spinal column during motion. Two series of short segmental postural muscles, the interspinalis and intertransversarii, are involved with stability of contiguous vertebrae during motion.

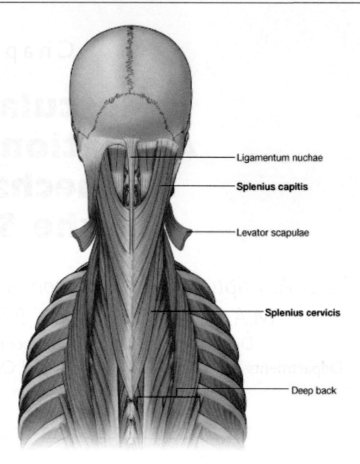

Fig. 5.1.
Milestones in the evolutions of clinical islet transplantation.

Additionally, the psoas and longus colli assist in the motion and stability of the spine from the anterior.

Two muscles make up the spinotranverse group (Figure 5.1). The splenius capitis arises from the inferior part of the ligamentum nuchae and the spinous processes of C7 to T4 and inserts on the mastoid process and along the lateral third of the superior nuchal line. The splenius cervicis originates on the spinous processes of T3 to T6 and inserts on the transverse processes of C1 to C3. Both muscles provide the same action: engaged bilaterally they extend the neck and unilateral contractions rotate the head.

The suboccipital muscles connect the atlas vertebra (C1), axis (C2), and base of the skull (Figure 5.2). There are four muscles in this group. Together, they provide stability and movement to the atlanto-axial and atlanto-occipital joints. The rectus capitis posterior major and minor muscles connect the spinous processes of the axis and atlas respectively to the occipital bone. The insertion

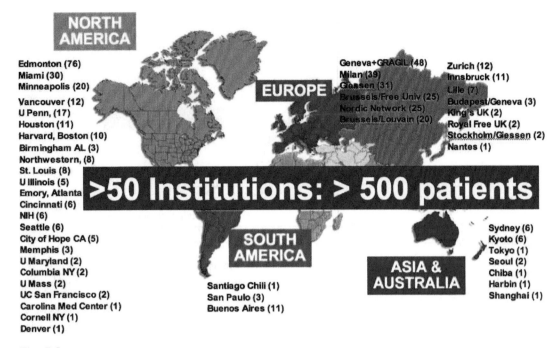

Fig. 5.2.

Islet Transplant Activity 1999–2005. More than 500 islet transplants have been performed in over 50 international centres in recent years.

point is lateral to their origin, enabling the muscle to produce both extension and some rotation of the joint. Obliquus capitis superior runs from the transverse process of the atlas to the occipital bone, providing extension and lateral bending. Oliquus capitis inferior originates on the spinous process of C2 and inserts of the transverse process of C1 and contributes to rotation of the head.

The largest group of the deep muscles is the erector spinae (Figure 5.3). The functions of this group include the extension and lateral bending of the spinal column and rotation of the head. The entire group has a common origin at the thoraco lumbar fascia, which is connected to the posterior sacrum, iliac crest, and the spinous and transverse processes of T11 to L5. The muscle mass arising from this common origin divides into three columns of muscle in the upper lumbar region. Each column is further divided by region. The most lateral muscle is the iliocostalis muscle. The lumbar and thoracic regions have insertion points at the angles of the ribs. The thoracic region also inserts on the transverse process of C7. The cervical region inserts on the transverse processes of C4 to C6. Medial to iliocostalis is the longissimus muscle. This is the largest of the erector spinae muscles and is again divided into three regions. The thoracic and cervical regions of this muscle insert on the transverse process of all the

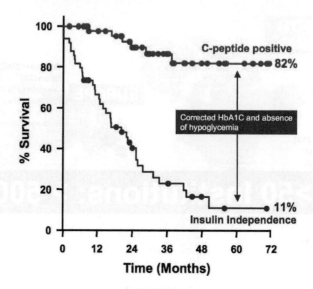

Fig. 5.3.
Outcomes five years after islet transplantation at the University of Alberta. Discrepancy between maintenance of persistent endogenous transplant C-peptide secretion vs loss of insulin independence at five years post islet transplantation.

thoracic and cervical vertebrae excluding C1. The capitis portion of the longissimus inserts on the posterior margin of the mastoid process. The most medial muscle of the erector spinae group is the spinalis muscle, which connects the spinous processes of adjacent vertebrae. In addition to sharing the common origin of the group, it has origins at the spinous processes of T10 to L2 and C7, as well as at the inferior part of the ligamentum nuchae. It inserts on the spinous processes of T1 to T8 and C2. Spinalis capitis blends with semispinalis as the muscle approaches the skull.

Deep to the erector spinae muscles is the transversospinalis group. These muscles run upward between the transverse and spinous processes of two individual vertebrae. There are three types of muscles in this group that are defined by their length. The semispinalis are the longest and the most superficial. Individual muscles cross four to six vertebrae from origin to insertion. The most inferior origin is at T10, with the most superior insertion on the occipital bone. Multifidus muscles run deep to the semispinalis, with each muscle spanning two to four vertebrae. They are present along the entire length of the spinal column, originating most inferiorly on the sacrum and iliac crest and inserting as high as C2. Multifidus muscles are most developed in the lumbar region. The deepest of the transversospinalis group are the rotatores, which span one or two vertebrae. Like the multifidus these muscles are present along the entire length of the column. They are most developed in the thoracic region. The three types of muscles work together to extend, rotate, or bend the spinal column.

The segmental postural muscles involved with spine stability are the inter-spinalis and the intertransversarii. The interspinalis muscles attach the spinous processes of adjacent vertebrae on either side of the interspinous ligament. Interspinalis provides extension between contiguous vertebrae. The intertrans-versarii muscles connect the transverse processes of adjacent vertebrae. Inter-transversarii are found throughout the length of the spinal column but are poorly developed in the thoracic region. Eccentric contractions of bilateral muscles provide stability between contiguous vertrebrae during movement. Unilateral contractions result in bending movement.

In addition to the posterior muscles there are two anterior muscles generally associated with stabilization and movement of the spine in the cervical and lumbar region. In the cervical region the longus colli has slight control over rotation and flexion of the cervical spine. This long flat muscle on the anterior side of the vertebral bodies is composed of three portions: the superior oblique, inferior oblique, and vertical portion. It originates at the body of T3 and inserts at the anterior tubercle of the axis. Along its length it inserts on the bodies of C1 to C3 and the transverse processes of C3 to C6. In the lumbar region psoas muscles, which lie anteriorly on either side of the spine, assist in flexion and lateral bending of the lumbar spine as well as balance while sitting. Psoas major arises from the transverse processes of the lumbar spine as well as from the bodies of T12 to L5 and their corresponding intervertebral discs. Psoas minor lies against the anterior surface of psoas major. It arises from the bodies of T12 and L1 and their respective intervertebral disc. It inserts onto the ilio-pectineal eminence and the iliac fascia as a long flat tendon.

The most fundamental structure of skeletal muscle is the myofilament, a structure made of either myosin or actin proteins. The interaction of the two types of myofilament causes muscle contraction. Both types of myofilaments are packed together in structures called sarcomeres, creating a striated myo-fibril. Several myofibrils in turn are packed together to form muscle fibers. The length and number of fibers in a muscle vary depending on the physiologic demands of the muscle.

Muscles consist of two parts: the belly and the tendons. The belly of a muscle is made predominantly of muscle fibers. The arrangement of the fibers influ-ences the amount of force the muscle is capable of applying and the amount of possible contraction. The maximum force a muscle can exert is proportional to the physiological cross-sectional area. This is the cross-sectional area of the muscle perpendicular to the direction of the muscle fibers. In muscles where a high force is needed, the fibers lie at an angle to the line of action. This is the pennation angle. The fibers in a pennated muscle are shorter than the length of the muscle, which reduces the distance the muscle can contract.

5.1.2 Muscle Biomechanics

Muscle contraction is initiated by impulse from motor neurons. A neuron can branch into many axons, each ending on a muscle fiber. The motor neuron and all of the fibers it supplies are a motor unit. A single muscle can consist of hundreds of motor units. Regulation of muscle force is controlled by the size and number of motor units recruited and by the frequency of the applied nerve impulse.

Muscle forces occur in two forms: active and passive force. An active force is generated through muscle stimulation by motor neurons causing contraction, whereas passive forces occur when the muscle is stretched beyond its resting length independent of its level of contraction. The active and passive muscle forces work together to produce the total force in the muscle, as shown in Figure 5.4. A single muscle fiber generates its greatest active force at resting length when the passive force component is negligible. The active component of force decreases and the passive component increases as the muscle fiber is stretched beyond its resting length.

The force that can be produced by a muscle is plotted versus muscle velocity in Figure 5.5. In concentric contraction, the muscle is shortening and the applied load must be less than that maximum force the muscle is capable of generating. There is an inverse relationship between the velocity at which a muscle shortens and the force applied to it during concentric contraction: the rate of contraction increases as the external applied load decreases. Eccentric contraction or active lengthening of a muscle occurs when the applied load exceeds the muscle's capacity for static load resulting in muscle lengthening. A greater applied load results in an increased rate of lengthening. Muscle can be characterized in terms of its force-velocity and force-displacement behaviors simultaneously and in this case a 3D surface relating the three variables is appropriate (see Figure 5.6).

5.2 Spinal Loading Estimation Techniques

5.2.1 Basics

The foregoing sections have established that the spine is acted on by many muscles; that the force produced by these muscles is a complex function of muscle activation level, muscle length, and velocity of the muscle shortening or lengthening; and that these muscles are organized in complex orientations with respect to the spine. The loads on the spine are also affected by the weight of the body segments being supported above the spinal level being considered. If the spinal loading situation under consideration involves movement, the dynamic effects associated with accelerating and decelerating the moving components of the body will also affect the spinal loading. If the motions are rapid (as they often are required to be for industrial material handling tasks), the dynamic effects may result in considerable increases in spinal loading [Dolan et al. 1999; Granata and Marras 1995]. These dynamic effects will be approximately proportional to Newton's second law for translation (Force = mass * acceleration) and rotation (Torque = mass moment of inertia * angular acceleration). Both static equilibrium and motion of the spine can result from the coordinated activation of many individual muscles and groups of muscles. At the

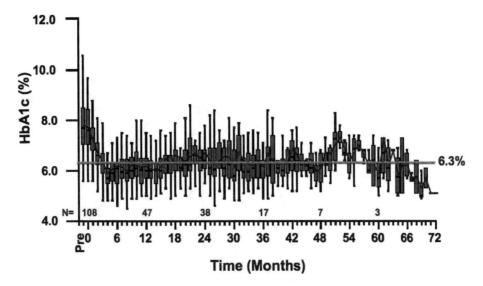

Fig. 5.4.
Correction of HbA$_{1c}$ by successful islet transplantation in insulin independent recipients.

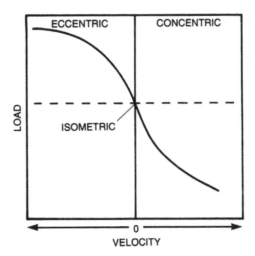

Fig. 5.5.
Simplified relationship of applied load versus rate of change in length (velocity) of a muscle. (Pitman and Peterson 1989)

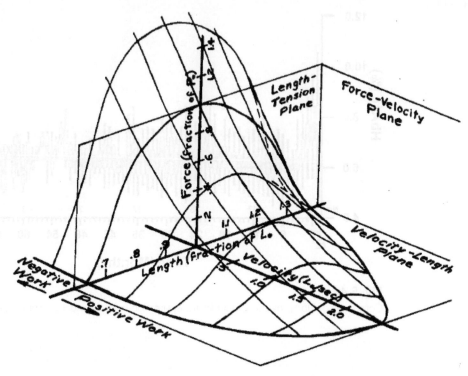

Fig. 5.6.
Three dimensional representation of the force-velocity-length relationship for a muscle under maximum activation. (Winter 2005)

level of the lower abdomen, it is noteworthy that the lumbar spine is the only component of the human skeleton that can counteract the tension produced in the many muscles that cross this area of the body. Human muscles can only produce tension, and at virtually all levels of the human spine (Figure 5.7) this tension results in considerable magnitudes of compression in the spine. It is also noteworthy to point out that the function of the muscles located posterior to the spine (such as the erector spinae) is to maintain body posture, counteract trunk flexion, or to withstand loads held anterior to the body. Due to the posterior placement of the spine within the body, these posterior muscles have relatively small moment arms (Figure 5.7), and this results in very large compressive forces being produced in response to sagittal plane loading even when small external loads are applied.

During general motions of the body, the resulting mechanical loads at the spine are 3D in nature (Figure 5.8). The most common and constant mechanical force experienced by the spine during everyday activities is compression, and for this reason most discussions of spinal loading focus almost exclusively on compression. It is important to recognize that any posture or motion of the spine will likely also include some shear forces and bending moments at

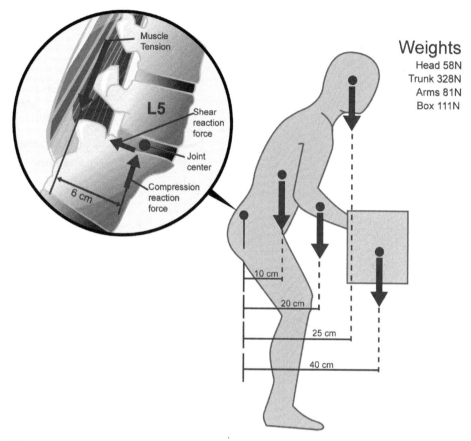

Fig. 5.7.
Simplified diagram of the forces present in the spine during lifting. The small moment arm (characterized as 6 cm in the upper left figure) over which the posterior muscles act result in very high compression forces in the spine.

the spine in addition to the compressive force. (Figure 5.7 demonstrates the anterior-posterior shear force present at the L5-S1 level of the spine.) This is especially true for asymmetric loading with respect to the sagittal plane, such as motion or lifting tasks that involve lateral bending or twisting movements of the trunk [Granata and Marras 1995]. The natural lordotic (cervical and lumbar spines) and kyphotic (thoracic spine) curvatures of the spine dictate that even a pure nonvarying compression applied to the spine will result in varying levels of segmental shear force as the spinal level of interest is varied.

A quantitative understanding of the mechanical loads acting on the spine during activities of daily living has been eagerly sought by biomechanical engineers and clinical scientists for several decades. Many researchers in this area feel that this information holds the key to understanding such important issues

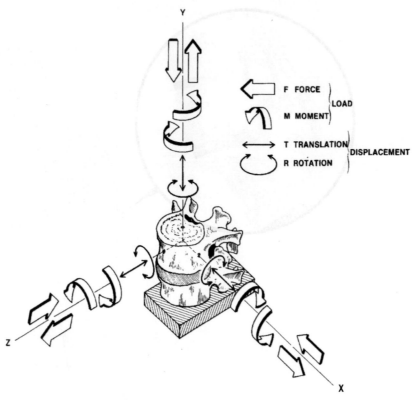

Fig. 5.8.

Spinal co-ordinate system proposed by White and Panjabi. (White and Panjabi 1990) General three dimensional spine motion is indicated by the thin arrows and comprises anterior/posterior, lateral, and cranial-caudal translation as well as rotation in all three anatomic planes (sagittal, frontal, and coronal). Similarly, the general three dimensional spinal loading is illustrated by the thick arrows and includes three forces (anterior/posterior (z) and lateral (x) shear force, and axial compression or tension (y)) and three moments (right and left axial torsion (y), flexion extension (x), and lateral bending (z))

as low back pain, occupational back injury, the etiology of intervertebral disc and spine degeneration, osteoporotic spine fractures, and the appropriate design of implantable surgical devices used in the spine such as posterior instrumentation systems or interbody fusion devices. The techniques used to address the question of spine loading have included purely theoretical mathematical models (such as linked segment or finite element models), combined mathematical models and experimental data (such as linked segment models with electromyographic [EMG] data) and purely experimental approaches (such as implantable telemetric load sensors or the measurement of the pressure within intervertebral discs). These approaches will be summarized in the following sections.

5.2.2 Mathematical Models

Many researchers have attempted to estimate the mechanical loads experienced by the spine using mathematical models, including models using both analytical and numerical approaches [Bernhardt et al. 1999; Cholewicki and McGill 1994; Dolan et al. 1990; Gagnon, Lariviere, and Loisel 2001; Granata and Marras 1995; Hughes et al. 1994; McGill and Norman 1986; Moroney, Schultz, and Miller 1988; Nussbaum and Chaffin 1996; Schultz and Andersson 1981]. The problem of determining the mechanical loads experienced by the spine involves using the principles of static equilibrium (for stationary postures) or dynamics (for slow or fast movement) to calculate the loads in the spine. In this approach, the body is often represented by a number of rigid segments that represent the various parts of the body such as the head, thorax, arms, legs, and so on (Figure 5.9). The segments are connected by defined joints that generally have approximately the same degrees of freedom as the anatomic joints they represent (i.e., planar pin joints for the knee, ball-in-socket joints for the hip, and so on). These models are often referred to as linked-segment models.

Classically, a cross section of the body through the spinal level of interest is considered (Figure 5.10) and the model is constructed by considering all of the body segments above or below the cross section to be the system under consideration. The equations of static equilibrium or the dynamic equations of motion are then written for the various segments of the half body under study. The resulting forces at the spine and at each muscle are then calculated from these equations (Figure 5.10). If the spinal loads for a movement are desired, the movement will be studied with video cameras or other means to track the positions of the body segments during the movement.

This procedure is more complicated than it may at first appear because neither the muscle forces nor the reaction forces at the spine are normally known at the time of the analysis. This results in an indeterminate mathematical formulation because the number of unknowns generally far exceeds the number of equations available for solution. The number of equations available for solution for a single 3D representation of a cross section in static equilibrium is six (three force equations and three moment equations). The number of unknown muscle and spine reaction forces is 13. Various methods have been utilized to allow simplification of the indeterminate system to render it determinate such that mathematical solutions could be obtained. These methods can generally be classified as either reduction or mathematical optimization [Collins 1995].

In the reduction method, the number of unknown parameters at the cross section of interest is reduced by making simplifying assumptions until the number of unknowns is equal to or less than the number of static equilibrium equations or equations of dynamic motion. Some of the assumptions made in the reduction method are assigning several muscle groups to a single activation pattern [Dolan et al. 1999] or assuming that specific muscles can be neglected in the analysis (as in assuming the single muscle force illustrated in

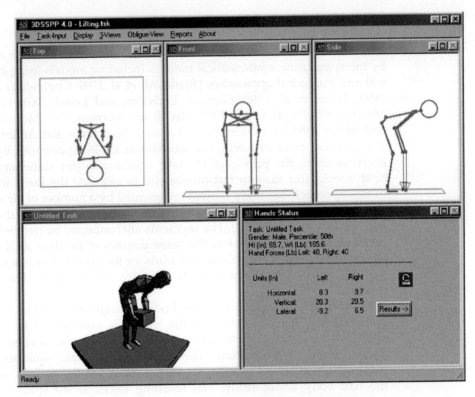

Fig. 5.9.
A screen capture from a commercially available occupational biomechanics analysis program (University of Michigan 3D Static Strength Prediction Program™). The top three images depict three views of the linked segment model positioned for a particular lifting task. At lower left is a humanoid representation of the lifting task and the image at lower right indicates the position and magnitudes of the resultant loads applied to each hand that correspond to the task.

Figure 5.7) or assuming a monotonic relationship between EMG signal and muscle force [Dolan et al. 1999, 2001; Gagnon, Lariviere, and Loisel 2001; Granata and Marras 1995]. The three most common spine loading models published to date can be characterized as (1) EMG-assisted, (2) optimization, and (3) EMG-assisted optimization. These techniques are described in material following.

EMG figures prominently in many mathematical modeling approaches to understand spine loading. EMG relies on electrodes placed over a muscle on the skin or inserted into a muscle (indwelling electrodes) to measure the electrical activity of a muscle. Muscle contraction is signalled by the motor neurons and this results in a momentary depolarization of the muscle fibers. This depolarization is associated with a small voltage known as a muscle action potential, and this voltage is measured by the EMG electrodes. The EMG

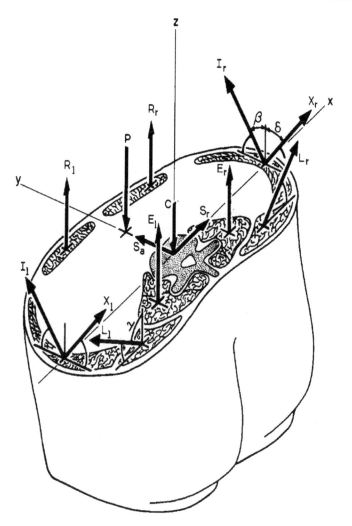

Fig. 5.10.
Cross-section through a lumbar level showing the forces acting on the cross-section due to muscles (I, X, L, E, R), intra-abdominal pressure (P), and spine loads (compression C and shear S). (Schultz et al. 1982)

voltage is known to be monotonically related to muscle force, but it is extremely difficult to use changes in EMG voltage to quantitatively estimate muscle force. The muscle force estimation is affected by length of the muscle fibers, velocity of the muscle contraction (Figure 5.6), the cross-sectional area of the muscle, the level of activation of the muscle, and the extent to which the muscle is stretched beyond its resting length (resulting in the production of passive force in the muscle).

EMG-Assisted

Despite the reported difficulties in relating muscle force to EMG level, several groups have developed, evaluated, and reported spinal loading models based on the premise that muscle force could be accurately related to EMG if velocity, cross-sectional area, muscle length, passive force, and the maximum EMG signal obtained at a particular electrode location were considered. The force prediction models often take the following form [Chaffin, Andersson and Martin 1999; Cholewicki, McGill, and Norman 1995]:

$$F_{muscle} = \left[G \times \frac{EMG}{EMG_{max}} \times f(length) \times f(velocity) \times \sigma_{max} PCSA \right] + F_P$$

Here, F_{muscle} is the force in the muscle, G is a gain or error term (which accounts for electrode conditions, crosstalk, and other unknown factors that may be affecting the force versus EMG relationship), EMG/EMG_{max} is the EMG signal measured normalized by the maximum EMG signal that the subject could produce at that electrode location, $f(length)$ and $f(velocity)$ are scaling factors taking into account the muscle length and velocity versus force relationships, σ_{max} is the maximum muscle stress (force/area), $PCSA$ is the muscle physiologic cross-sectional area, and F_P is the passive muscle force that occurs when the muscle is stretched beyond its resting length (Figure 5.4). A common gain (G) is calculated for the entire time period of the task by comparing the reaction bending moments about the spine that are created based on the EMG signals and the F_{muscle} formula with those that result from an inverse dynamics analysis of the linked segment model undergoing the motions and accelerations measured with a camera or other motion analysis system [Cholewicki, McGill, and Norman 1995; Gagnon, Lariviere, and Loisel 2001; Granata and Marras 1995; McGill and Norman 1986, 1995]. The differences between the moments from the inverse dynamics analysis and that from the EMG signals are normally minimized using a least squares regression over the entire task studied. One strength of the EMG-assisted approach is that it accurately incorporates the so-called co-contraction of agonist and antagonist muscles (muscles on opposing sides of the joint) often observed in EMG recordings of subjects. This approach suffers from inaccuracies introduced by simplified models of the musculoskeletal anatomy of the trunk and limitations in the number of electrodes that can be effectively deployed to measure EMG [Cholewicki, McGill, and Norman 1995; Gagnon, Lariviere, and Loisel 2001]. It is noteworthy that this method minimizes the errors in the moment constraint equations but does not require the moments predicted using the EMG approach to exactly equal the moments obtained from the inverse dynamics analysis.

Mathematical Optimization Techniques

The second common technique used to solve indeterminate spine loading problems involves using the techniques of mathematical optimization. [Choi 2003; Cholewicki, McGill, and Norman 1995; Gagnon, Lariviere, and Loisel 2001; Hughes, Bean, and Chaffin 1995; Moroney, Schultz, and Miller 1988; Nussbaum, Chaffin, and Rechtien 1995; Schult, and Andersson 1981; Shea et al. 1995]. With optimization, additional mathematical constraints are introduced to the problem (through identification of a so-called objective function) until the number of unknowns is reduced to the extent that the problem becomes solvable. Some examples of objective functions used include minimizing spine compression force, minimizing muscle stress in all muscles, minimizing the square of muscle power, and minimizing the total value of muscle force [Granata and Marras 1995].

Additional mathematical constraint equations are often applied to further constrain the mathematical solution toward those considered relevant. Common constraints include static or dynamic equilibrium conditions, conditions to ensure the muscle cannot generate nonphysiologic force, and the assumption that each muscle can produce tension only (i.e., muscles cannot sustain compression) [Cholewicki, McGill, and Norman 1995; Gagnon, Lariviere, and Loisel 2001; Schultz et al. 1982].

Most frequently two consecutive mathematical optimizations are applied. The first minimizes muscle force or stress while maintaining equilibrium. The second optimization uses the solution from the first optimization to establish the maximum force that each muscle can apply and then finds the solution for muscle forces that minimizes the spine compression (Figure 5.10) [Cholewicki, McGill, and Norman 1995; Gagnon, Lariviere, and Loisel 2001; Schultz et al. 1983]. The first objective to minimize muscle force results in activation of the joint agonist (prime mover) muscles. The second objective to minimize joint compression results in muscles with the largest moment arms being recruited first, muscles with the next largest moment arms being identified second, and so on [Cholewicki, McGill, and Norman 1995].

An advantage of this approach is that it is relatively straightforward to collect data because there is no need to collect EMG data. The most often cited disadvantage of this method is that many of the applied objective functions are driven toward optimum solutions in which there is no co-contraction of muscles [Hughes, Bean, and Chaffin 1995]. This directly contradicts EMG data from actual subjects performing the tasks modeled. Hughes, Bean, and Chaffin [1995] have modified the double optimization problem by applying so-called Karush-Kuhn-Tucker multipliers, which raise the lower bound for muscle stress on each of the muscle stresses (found to be inactive but known to be active based on EMG data). Using this approach, Hughes et al. have established that physiological co-contraction can significantly raise the mechanical loads predicted by double linear optimization models.

EMG-Assisted Optimization Models

EMG-assisted optimization (EMGAO) was first proposed by Cholewicki and colleagues in 1994. It combines the two previous approaches in order to address the lack of co-contraction inherent with pure optimization approaches to spine loading and to address difficulties and nonlinearities inherent in calculating muscle force based on EMG data. This method starts with muscle forces derived from the EMG-assisted approach and modifies the individual muscle force gains such that an exact match between the moments computed using the muscle forces and those obtained from the inverse dynamics analysis is obtained. The modification of the individual muscle force gains is carried out by performing a mathematical optimization with a quadratic objective function that requires the minimization of the gain applied to each muscle while simultaneously balancing the 3D moment equations at L4-L5 [Cholewicki and McGill 1994; Cholewicki, McGill, and Norman 1995]. Cholewicki et al. [1995] compared the lumbar spine loads calculated using optimization alone, EMG-assisted, and EMGAO and concluded that both EMG-assisted and EMGAO resulted in significantly higher L4–L5 joint compression force than did the optimization method alone. The advantage of this method is that it closely matches EMG activation patterns recorded from subjects and exactly satisfies the 3D concordance between the L4–L5 spinal moments as obtained from inverse dynamic analysis of the linked segment model and the moments calculated based on the geometries and activation patterns of the muscles included in the model.

5.2.3 Telemetric Load Sensors on Spine Implants

An instrument that has the capacity to take measurements and wirelessly send the results to another component is known as a telemetric device. Some of the first uses of a telemetric device *in vivo* include implantation to measure properties such as temperature, pressure, pH [Mackay 1968], and loads in hip implants [Bergmann et al. 1988]. Telemetric devices were later used to measure muscle potentials [Herberts et al. 1968] and to perform as pacemakers [Holcomb, Glenn, and Sato 1969]. Since these developments, they have been implanted in load-bearing devices for the spine, thus facilitating measurement of spinal loads and bending moments [Graichen, Bergmann, and Rohlmann 1996; Rohlmann et al. 1995]. With this information, research can be accomplished to evaluate the differences in spinal loads between static and dynamic activities of daily living, such as the spinal loads while walking in comparison to those while sitting [Rohlmann et al. 2001]. This information can also be used to evaluate the effectiveness of ergonomic devices and treatment methods for spine deformities, diseases, and compromises to the structure.

Nachemson et al. [1971] applied telemetry to measure loads in Harrington distraction rods used to correct scoliosis (Figure 5.11). In this particular study, four patients with idiopathic scoliosis were implanted with a telemetric device during their first surgery. The telemetric device was composed of a force-gauging pressductor (a transformer with a zero reading in the absence of mechanical load), an internal power transfer coil, and an internal transmitter [Nachemson and Elfstrom 1971]. Electromagnetic induction was generated through the interaction of an external and implanted power transfer coil. This produced the electrical energy necessary to power the transmitter and the pressductor. Load measurements were taken during distraction; during lifts and turns of the patient; while the patient coughed; while the patient wore a Milwaukee brace; and while the patient lay in the supine position. From this data, Nachemson et al. [1971] were able to assess the patient transport methods, the effectiveness of the Milwaukee brace, the size of the pillow used during recovery, and several other factors thought to affect patient recovery. (See Figure 5.11.)

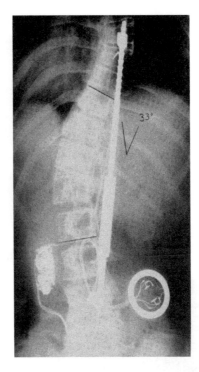

Fig. 5.11.
Radiograph showing an implanted telemetric Harrington distraction rod. (Nachemson and Elfstrom 1971)

More recently, spinal fixators have been implanted with telemetric devices [Graichen, Bergmann, and Rohlmann 1996]. Rohlmann et al. [1995, 2000] have published several papers using this method to evaluate the differences in spinal loads in the thoracic and lumbar spine during activities of daily living. In contrast to the study performed by Nachemson et al. [1971] in which only the axial loads were measured, Rohlmann et al.'s instrumented spinal fixators are able to measure three force components and three moments using six semiconductor strain gauges. Together, the strain gauges, an eight-channel telemetric unit, and a coil were inserted into the longitudinal threaded rod of the internal fixator by Dick [1987] (Figure 5.12). Electron-beam welding was used to create an airtight seal, which is essential when using these devices *in vivo* in order to maintain biocompatibility and function of the fixator. Extensive development, evaluation, and validation of the device was published in 1993 and 1994 [Rohlmann, Bergmann, and Graichen 1994; Rohlmann et al. 1993]. Accuracy tests were performed with known loads applied individually along each axis [Rohlmann, Bergmann, and Graichen 1994]. In the axial direction, there was a 5% error calculated with the maximum applied load. The loads in the remaining two directions had an error of less than 2%. A 1% error was evident between the measured bending moment and the actual moment applied to the fixator when the vertebral bodies were loaded axially by forces between 50 and 150 N. (See Figure 5.12.)

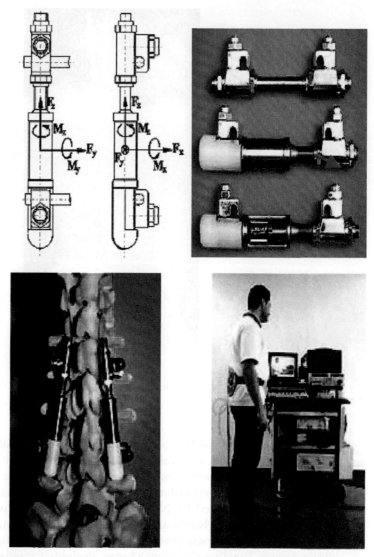

Fig. 5.12.
The telemetric spinal fixator developed by Rohlmann and colleagues. (Rohlmann et al. 2000) Top right: the Dick fixator was modified with strain gauges to sense the six-axis loads (shown in right-most fixator with arrow) and a telemetric device to transmit the six-axis loads to a receiver unit (the light colored components on the caudal end of each fixator). Top left: The orientation of the co-ordinate system incorporated into the fixator. Bottom left: The fixators are mounted on a lum-bosacral spine model. Bottom right: The telemetric receiver is shown on a patient with an implanted telemetric device.

The coordinate system used to evaluate the data is fixed to the implant (Figure 5.12). The X axis runs parallel approximately laterally. The Z axis runs longitudinally toward the cranium. The Y axis lies perpendicular to these axes, pointing approximately anteriorly [Rohlmann et al. 1995]. This device is implanted internally onto the spine of the patient using standard surgical techniques. A flat coil and antenna are attached externally to the patient's back (Figure 5.12). These activate the spinal implants. As the patient performs certain activities or holds a particular position, fixator loads are collected together with a video camera recording of their motion (which is later synchronized with the telemetry signals) [Rohlmann, Bergmann, and Graichen 1994].

The results and comparisons obtained through data from the instrumented internal spinal fixators are dependent on the pathological indication for surgery, the surgical procedure (compression or distraction), the load magnitude, factors such as body weight and material properties of the vertebra and surrounding soft tissues, and the level of fusion [Rohlmann et al. 1995, 2000, 2001].

A recent development in the measurement of spinal loads with the use of telemetry has emerged with micro-electromechanical systems (MEMS) technology. Although it has not been used for this purpose to date, some investigators are exploring the feasibility of implanting MEMS technology into a device called the smart disc implant [Ferrara 2005]. The smart disc, equipped with MEMS technology, would have the ability to detect changes in the natural disc condition and perform specific operations to adapt to changes in loads, moments, strains, and pressures. The biocompatibility of MEMS pressure sensors has been evaluated for *in vivo* cervical and lumbar spine in goats [Ferrara et al. 2003]. Due to their microscale dimensions, using MEMS to measure *in vivo* loads will likely be less invasive to the surrounding tissue.

An interbody spinal implant has been developed by Ledet et al. [2005] with the goal of collecting *in vivo* spine load data. It was designed to collect strain data as well as to act as an interbody spacer allowing for interbody fusion. A telemetric implant with 16 strain gauges was placed in the L4-L5 disc space of two baboons to record compressive loads transferred through the spine. To protect the implant, it was coated in conformal expoxy and Parylene C [Cookson Electronics, London, England]. Similar to data collection for the spinal fixation device in humans, data was recorded and synchronized to a video recording of the baboon activities [Ledet et al. 2005]. The use of animal models that closely approximate the human spine—such as the baboon [Tominaga et al. 1995] used by Ledet et al.—would allow the results to be applied to the human spine. Such information could be applied to further understand and evaluate human *in vivo* spinal loads.

A disadvantage to using spinal implants with telemetric transmitters—whether posterior [Rohlmann, Bergmann, and Graichen 1994, 1997, 2000; Rohlmann et al. 1993, 1996, 2001] or anterior [Ledet et al. 2000]—is apparent when the loads carried by the implant are considered. The implant is only able to measure the loads transferred through it, not those transferred through the spine [Rohlmann et al. 1995]. Because our knowledge regarding the correlation between the loads carried by the implant and the spine is incomplete it is difficult to relate these loads to exact *in vivo* spine loads. Recent advances in this area that combine the telemetric data with *in vitro* spine data are improving this situation [Rohlmann et al. 1997, 2000; Wilke et al. 2003]. Subsequent to Rohlmann et al.'s studies, in which the *in vivo* fixator loads were measured [Rohlmann et al. 1997], Wilke et al. [2003] incorporated this information into an *in vitro* analysis to determine *in vivo* spine loads for patients equipped with a fixator. The opportunity to evaluate the changes in load through the fixators allows us to infer similar trends in the spine. Discrepancies between the loads measured by the fixator and those traveling through the spine may be addressed with the incorporation of MEMS and telemetric devices, which allow direct measurement of spine tissue loads in the vicinity of the telemetric implants.

Despite the previously mentioned disadvantage, telemetric devices provide several advantages and opportunities to advance our knowledge in the area of spine biomechanics. These devices allow a greater range of activities to be evaluated as opposed to intradiscal pressure measurements, in that no part of the device transits the skin. The information obtained through this technology allows direct loads to be measured. This information can be used to verify or identify weaknesses in other methods for determining spinal loads, such as mathematical models or the use of intradiscal pressure needles. This data also sheds significant light on the basic biomechanics of the surgical devices that measure the load (i.e., posterior fixators and interbody implants).

5.2.4 Intradiscal Pressure Studies

Intervertebral discs are fibrocartilaginous cushions in the spine, which absorb shock and allow spinal motion. They consist of an annulus fibrosus and a nucleus pulposus. The annulus is a tough collagen based encasement organized in concentric rings around the nucleus. The nucleus contains a large amount of water to form a gel-like material that resists compression. The hydrostatic pressure of the nucleus has been shown to be linearly related to the forces acting on the spine at that level (Figure 5.13). Numerous studies have focused on measuring this pressure *in vitro* and *in vivo* in the lumbar [Adams, McNally, and Dolan 1996; Fye et al. 1998; McNally et al. 1996; Nachemson 1981; Sato, Kikuchi, and Yonezawa 1999; Wilke et al. 1999] and cervical spine [Cripton, Dumas, and Nolte 2001; Pospiech et al. 1999]. (See Figure 5.13.)

5.2.4.1 Lumbar

In the 1960s and 1970s a series of studies on intervertebral disc pressure in the lumbar spine were conducted *in vitro* and *in vivo* by Nachemson et al. [1960, 1964, 1966, 1981]. They used a custom designed needle-based transducer [Nachemson 1960]. This consisted of a 1.1-mm-diameter needle with a sealed end and a small opening on the side (Figure 5.14). Polyethelene tubing was used to create a diaphragm. The needle was filled with water and connected to an electromanometer. The needle was inserted posterolaterally into the L3 or L4 intervertebral disc in volunteers or cadaveric specimens. *In vitro* experiments focused on developing the pressure transducer and the relationship between

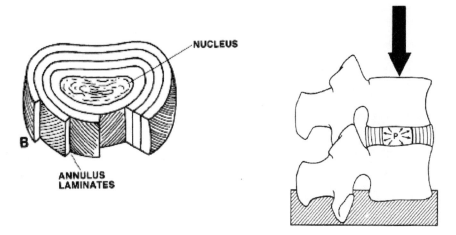

Fig. 5.13.
An intervertebral disc consists of a nucleus and an annulus. The annulus is made up of many concentric layers of fibrous tissue. Under compression the nucleus is pressurized which results in outward bulging of the disc and end plates. (White and Panjabi 1990)

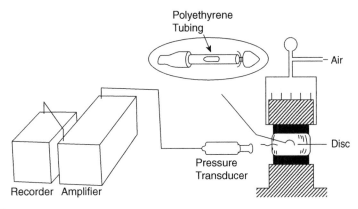

Fig. 5.14.
Schematic of the pressure transducer and associated set up used by Nachemson et al. to measure intradiscal pressures in cadavaric specimens. (Nachemson 1981)

axial compression and intradiscal pressure. In the *in vivo* studies, subjects were asked to perform various tasks (though each subject did not perform all the tasks). These tasks include holding 4.5 or 11.4 kg, performing a Valsalva maneuver, standing, sitting, and reclining [Nachemson 1966, 1981; Nachemson and Morris 1964]. The cross-sectional area of the disc was determined using biplanar roentgenograms and was used together with the *in vitro* experiments to determine the force acting on the disc. Nachemson [1981] reported a proportional relationship between the measured intradiscal pressure and the force acting on the spine. He found that the measured pressure is 1.5 times the expected pressure as calculated from the applied force and measured disc area. (See Figure 5.14.)

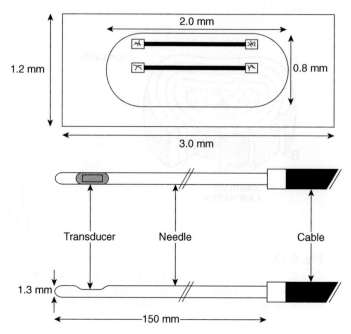

Fig. 5.15.

Schematic diagrams of the sensor and needle mount developed by McNally et al. (McNally, Adams, and Goodship 1992)

Since the completion of Nachemson's work there have been many studies on *in vitro* lumbar disc pressures [Cunningham et al. 1997; Fye et al. 1998; McNally, Adams, and Goodship 1992; Wilke et al. 1996]. McNally et al. [1992] designed and validated a new pressure transducer to measure intradiscal pressure under compression and flexion/extension. Their pressure transducer was a needle-based device. They used a 1.3-mm needle with a 1.2 × 3-mm window cutout covered by a membrane instrumented with strain gauges (Figure 5.15). Testing included applying 4,000 N of axial compression and 12 degrees flexion to 8 degrees extension to cadaveric lumbar spine specimens. They subsequently extended this device for use to obtain "stress profiles" by mounting it to a device that allowed them to measure stress in the disc while drawing the sensor through a disc at a controlled rate [McNally and Adams 1992]. Further work by the group examined the differences in stress profiles between degenerative and normal discs *in vivo* [McNally et al. 1996].

Wilke and colleagues [1996] evaluated the influence of simulated muscle force on the L4/5 disc pressure in a human cadaveric lumbar spine specimen. Muscle forces were applied by attaching cables to the L4 vertebra at the anatomical insertion points of five pairs of muscles. Specimens were tested with various musculature conditions: no musculature, single muscle activation (80 N applied load per pair), and all muscles activated. Pure moments of 3.75 N were applied to the specimen under each condition to produce flexion/extension, lateral bending, and axial rotation motions. Pressures were measured using a 6-mm-long 1.2-mm-diameter transducer containing a micropressure sensor. This was inserted into the nucleus pulposus using a guide tube.

In 1999, Wilke et al. revisited the concept of measuring intervertebral disc pressure *in vivo* (Figure 5.16). This study recorded the disc pressure over the course of 24 hours in one volunteer. A similar device to that used in their *in vitro* studies was inserted into the L4/5 intervertebral disc. Wires were led out of the body to a transmitting device on a belt. The data was collected telemetrically at 200 Hz. The volunteer performed various activities such as lifting tasks, sitting, and climbing stairs. Also in 1999, Sato et al. conducted *in vivo* tests on eight healthy volunteers and 28 patients with back problems [Sato, Kikuchi, and Yonezawa 1999]. The participants were asked to assume eight common body positions while the intradiscal pressure was measured using a needle-based pressure transducer (1.2-mm diameter).

5.2.4.2 Cervical

In contrast to the extensive body of work on lumbar disc pressure data, similar data related to the cervical discs is extremely limited. Only one reported study on the *in vivo* cervical disc pressures was found [Hattori et al. 1981]. This study used a needle-type pressure transducer to measure pressures during common movements of the neck. The transducer used strain gauges mounted on a diaphragm at the tip of the needle. Discs between C3 and C6 were tested in volunteers in supine and neutral postures and in flexion/extension, rotation, and lateral bending motions.

Pospiech and colleagues reported cervical disc pressures *in vitro* in 1999. Their goal was to determine normal values for cervical disc pressures under simulated muscle forces in intact cervical spines as well as in a fused specimen. Cervical musculature was recreated by three pairs of cables attached at muscle insertion points on C4 and 5. A force of 10 N was applied to each cable. Each specimen was tested with and without muscle forces as well as after a discectomy and fusion of C4/5. Testing involved applying an axial load of 10 N and pure moments of 0.5 Nm to the cervical spine to produce flexion/extension, axial rotation, and bending motions. Pressures were measured in the intervertebral discs above and below the discectomy level using a pressure transducer mounted on a 1.3-mm-diameter needle.

The majority of disc pressure studies have been conducted using a needle-based transducer design. Cripton et al. [2001] pointed out that the small size and anatomy of cervical discs made the study of intradiscal pressure technically challenging. In particular, there is a danger of negatively affecting the specimen biomechanics, through contact between the vertebrae and the needle, with the traditional needle-based pressure transducers. They developed a technique using a unique disc-shaped pressure sensor that was inserted via a guide tube into the nucleus in various functional cervical spine units. The sensor had a diameter of 1.5 mm and a thickness of 0.3 mm (Figure 5.17). It was implanted into the nucleus with only three 0.26-mm-diameter wires passing through the annulus. They used this device to measure cervical disc pressures under axial loading. The specimens were compressed at 10 N/s to a maximum of 800 N.

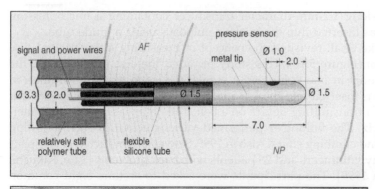

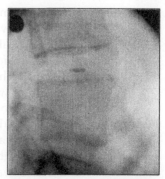

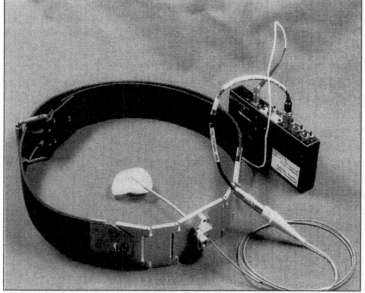

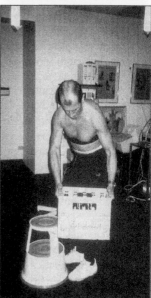

Fig. 5.16.

Details of experimental set up from Wilke et al. (Wilke et al. 1999) Clockwise from upper left: Schematic of implanted sensor; radiograph showing implant in the subject's L4/5 disc; subject performing lifting task; harness and transmitter worn by the subject.

5.3 Spinal Loads During Various Activities

5.3.1 Thoraco Lumbar and Lumbar

5.3.1.1 Intradiscal Pressure

Nachemson compiled his group's *in vivo* tests in a 1981 paper. These studies measured disc pressures in the lumbar spine during daily activities. Wilke and colleagues [1999] summarized Nachemson's results and compared them to their more recent *in vivo* lumbar disc pressure results (Figure 5.18). Comparison of these two sets of results shows some discrepancies in the relative pres-

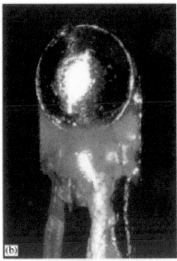

Diameter=1.5 mm
Thickness=0.3 mm

Fig. 5.17.
Intradiscal pressure sensor used by Cripton et al. (Cripton, Dumas, and Nolte 2001) to measure *in vitro* cervical disc pressures.

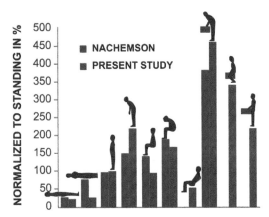

Fig. 5.18.
Modified results of Wilke et al. and Nachemson's *in vivo* intradiscal pressures in the lumbar spine during common activities. Present study refers to the work by Wilke et al. (Wilke et al. 1999) The 2000 N spinal load called out is the approximate value for a 50th percentile male.

sures such as an increase in pressure between sitting and standing in Wilke's results and a decrease in Nachemson's. Sato et al. [1999] report results slightly lower then those reported by Wilke et al. in their healthy participants. The intradiscal pressures measured in the degenerative discs were lower than in the healthy discs.

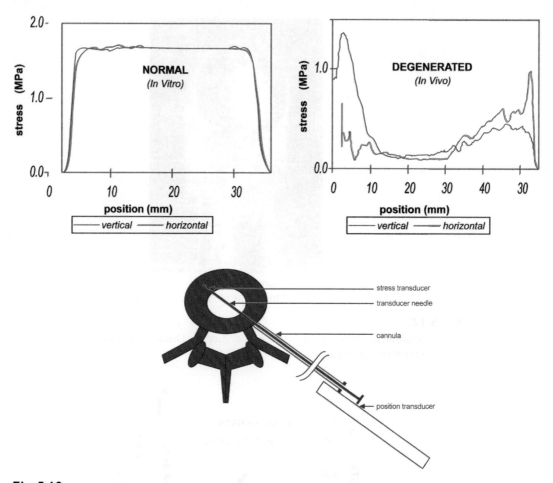

Fig. 5.19.

Stress profiles of cadaveric discs as measured by McNally et al. (McNally et al. 1996) The degenerative disc on the right shows two regions of stress concentration. The normal disc on the left has a smooth profile. The stress profilometry apparatus is shown schematically at the bottom of the figure.

Of interest from the *in vitro* intradiscal pressure studies are the results from McNally et al. [1992]. This group examined the effect of the condition of the disc on the pressure profile through the disc cross section in a posterior lateral to anterior posterior direction. They found that normal discs had a more consistent pressure along the profile, whereas the degenerative discs had multiple regions of pressure concentrations (Figure 5.19). Similar results were seen for degenerated discs *in vivo* in patients [McNally et al. 1996].

5.3.1.2 Telemetric Load Cells on Spine Implants

Rohlmann et al. [1994] pioneered the adaptation of the AO Dick fixator [Dick 1987] into a telemetric device capable of measuring, and transmitting transcutaneously, complete 3D reaction loads (three forces and three moments) at each fixator. The impact of specific exercises that have been implemented to accelerate healing and to avoid overloading the spine can be assessed using this information in order to help reduce further complications such as implant fracture or screw loosening. Development of this device has provided a means to assess *in vivo* fixator loads for walking, standing, sitting, activating specific muscles, load carrying, and jumping [Rohlmann, Bergmann, and Graichen 1997, 1999; Rohlmann, Graichen, and Bergmann 2000; Rohlmann et al. 1998, 2000, 2001].

In a series of their studies, Rohlmann et al. implanted the AO fixator into ten patients. Each patient had a fixator that bridged either two discs in the lower thoracic spine or in the lumbar spine. The patients also had anterior interbody fusion (AIF) with bone grafts. This last procedure increased the fixator loads for most patients [Rohlmann et al. 2000]. The loads in the fixators were measured telemetrically one to three times a week while the patient remained hospitalized, and subsequently only once a month [Rohlmann, Bergmann, and Graichen 1999; Rohlmann, Graichen, and Bergmann 2000; Rohlmann et al. 2000, 2001].

Measurements gathered for activities such as sitting, standing, walking, lying in the supine position, and lifting an extended leg while lying in the supine position demonstrated that the most prominent loads through the spinal fixator were a result of the axial force and bending moments. The transverse force and torsional moments were relatively small compared to these. Axial forces in the fixator registered an average of 25 N in tension and 240 N in compression. Patients with bridged thoracic vertebrae had lower compression forces than patients with bridged lumbar vertebrae. It took approximately 150 days after the anterior interbody fusion for the loads to remain constant. It was also observed that once bony fusion had occurred there was no decrease in the implant loads. As a result, implant loads cannot be used as an indicator for bony fusion [Rohlmann et al. 2000].

Another study by Rohlmann et al. [1997] was designed specifically to analyze the loads through the fixator during walking (Figure 5.20). Only two patients participated in this study. Their implant loads were measured every four weeks while walking at three different speeds. Although they did not record the exact speeds, they were classified as slow, normal, and fast. However, this may not be significant because there was little effect on the spinal loads due to a change in walking speed. They did note, however, that the length and strength of each step had a slight influence on the implant loads [Rohlmann, Bergmann, and Graichen 1997].

Loads were also collected for sitting in several different types of seats: stool, chair, office chair, bench, physiotherapy ball, knee stool, and a stool with a padded wedge. Similar to the results for walking speed, the type of seat had little effect on the implant loads. The loads between sitting on a bench versus on a knee stool were the only results that demonstrated a significant difference in seat type on spinal implant loads. However, the inclination of the seat back influenced the implant loads. As the angle of inclination was decreased from the upright position, the loads decreased. The difference between standing up

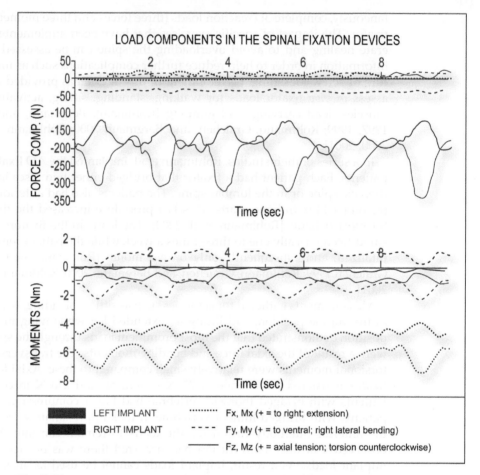

Fig. 5.20.

Loads in the telemetric Dick fixator as a function of time during walking for 59 year old female patient with the fixator affixed between the L2 and L4 vertebrae. (Rohlmann, Bergmann, and Graichen 1997) This reading was taken approximately four weeks after anterior interbody fusion between the L2 and L4 vertebrae. The caption at the bottom identifies the various load components and the meaning of positive signals. The corresponding implant co-ordinate system is also illustrated in Figure 12.

and sitting down was also considered. An evaluation of the implant loads between these two positions showed that only a moderate increase in spinal loads was present when standing [Rohlmann et al. 2001].

Contradictory results were seen using an interbody spinal implant in baboons [Ledet et al. 2005]. This difference is likely due to the fact that the Dick fixator device is positioned within the posterior column of the spine, whereas the interbody implant lies within the anterior column and thus plays a more significant role in the compressive load-sharing behavior of the spine [Cripton et al. 2000].

The impact of load carrying has been another area of concern regarding implant loads, especially while a patient is healing after spine surgery. The loads while carrying various weights were measured by Rohlmann et al. [2000]. It was found that carrying weights in each hand induced less force than walking. Additionally, holding a load caused smaller bending moments than walking. In all exercises performed while carrying loads, only a small amount of the added external force was compensated for by the implants [Rohlmann, Graichen, and Bergmann 2000].

The analyses made possible by measuring implant loads assist with determining which positions and activities put the implant at highest risk for failure, such as screw breakage. The results have also indicated that although the implants may not be at risk during certain activities the additional load supported by the spine may present a threat. The loads through the spine could potentially affect the healing process at the implant due to an increase in risk for bone sintering and correction loss [Rohlmann, Graichen, and Bergmann 2000]. It is important to keep in mind when interpreting these results that the loads through the spinal fixators are not only different between patients but differ in the direction of change (i.e., compression versus tension). These dissimilarities occur due to differences in bone quality, indication for surgery, the surgery performed, patient health and weight, and level of fusion [Rohlmann et al. 2000, 2001]. Additionally, the measured loads will change with healing as the bone graft is resorbed and as muscle strength increases while the muscles heal from the effects of surgery [Rohlmann et al. 2000]. Temporal changes in the loads measured can also be indicative of problems with the implant, such as screw breakage or implant loosening (Figure 5.21). [Rohlmann et al. 2000]. (See Figure 5.21.)

Rohlmann and colleagues have also specifically examined the effect of muscle activation on the fixator loads (Figure 5.22) [Rohlmann et al. 1998]. They concluded that muscles greatly influence the implant loads. In particular, muscles were found to prevent tension in the spine when the patient is hanging from the hands or feet.

5.3.1.3 Mathematical Models

EMGAO models are currently considered the most accurate because they have the highest concordance to observed EMG patterns and exactly satisfy the moment equilibrium equations required for static equilibrium or dynamic motion. EMG-assisted, EMGAO, and optimization methods were computed and compared for the lumbar spine by Cholewicki et al. [1995], for isometric exertions, and by Gagnon et al. [2001] for dynamic trunk flexion exertions. The individual muscle forces for a typical exertion from the Cholewicki study are presented in Table 5.1. The muscle forces predicted using the EMG-assisted and EMGAO techniques were generally in close agreement but both differed considerably from the optimization solution. The optimization solution also

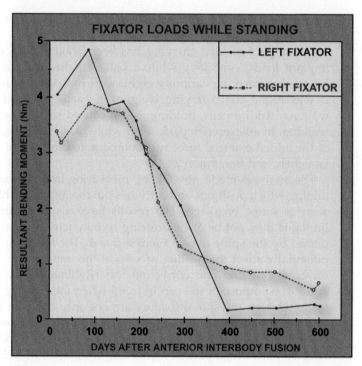

Fig. 5.21.

Comparison of the temporal change in right and left fixator loads while standing for one patient after anterior interbody fusion. (Rohlmann et al. 2000) This figure illustrates how data of this type can be used to monitor the implant's function and identify problems such as implant fracture or loosening. This record was markedly different from the other patients in the study in the rate and extent of the decrease in implant loads. Upon implant revision it was determined that both pedicle screws on the left side were loose. This may be the reason for the significantly lower loads in the left implant beginning at 390 days.

predicted zero tension for several muscles, some of which would likely be active during a real-world isometric effort of this type (as was predicted with the EMG and EMGAO methods). The L4-L5 compression values for the three models are presented in Figure 5.23. Again, the optimization model gives considerably different values for joint compression than the EMG-assisted and EMGAO methods. The joint compression predicted using EMGAO increased with increasing isometric moment in all directions tested (flexion, extension, lateral bending). The maximum spine compressions were approximately 7.0 kN.

Gagnon et al. [2001] presented a graphical comparison of muscle forces predicted using the optimization and EMGAO modeling technique for dynamic trunk flexion moments (Figure 5.24). A much more physiologically reasonable muscle activation pattern (including co-activation) was predicted using the EMGAO method of solution. The muscle forces calculated with the EMGAO

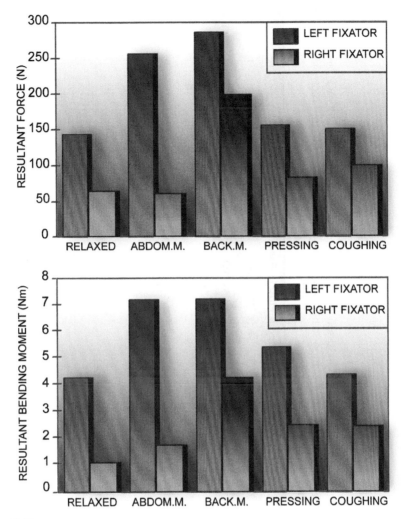

Fig. 5.22.
Effect of muscle activation on fixator force (top) and moment (bottom) loads. (Rohlmann et al. 1998) These loads were recorded after for an AIF in a 59-year-old female patient with the fixator affixed and anterior interbody bone graft between the L2 and L4 vertebrae.

method were significantly higher for each muscle than were the optimization solution results.

The resulting L4-L5 compression and shear force reaction loads for McGill and Norman's [1986] EMG-assisted model of sagittal plane lifting tasks are presented in Table 5.2, where they are also indexed to the mass lifted and the dynamic hand force. For lifts between 27 and 91 kg, the L4-L5 moment ranged from 298 to 449 Nm. The spinal compression ranged from 5,571 to almost 9,000 N.

Table 5.1.
Predicted muscle forces and joint compression forces at L4-L5 using EMG-assisted (EMG), EMG-assisted optimization (EMGAO), and double linear optimization (OPTIM, first minimize muscle stress then minimize spine compression) [Cholewicki, McGill, and Norman 1995]. This is a typical result for a single subject at the maximal isometric efforts.

Muscle	Cross Sectional Area (cm²)	Extension			Flexion			Lat. Bend. L		
		EMG	EMGAO	OPT	EMG	EMGAO	OPT	EMG	EMGAO	OPT
R. rect. abd.	10.0	47	45	0	505	528	315	149	131	286
L. rect. abd.	10.0	68	71	0	633	696	315	474	371	286
R. ext. obl. 1	10.0	90	78	0	449	431	315	175	210	286
L. ext. obl. 1	10.0	40	46	0	317	363	315	521	298	269
R. ext. obl. 2	9.0	76	72	0	378	384	283	147	138	257
L. ext. obl. 2	9.0	34	36	0	267	292	284	438	354	257
R. int. obl. 1	9.0	133	149	163	445	474	59	208	124	0
L. int. obl. 1	9.0	134	117	126	492	454	0	393	560	257
R. int. obl. 2	8.0	117	133	0	390	444	252	183	84	0
L. int. obl. 2	8.0	117	101	0	432	419	252	345	446	229
R. Pars. lum. 1	9.0	303	289	227	96	87	0	68	82	0
L. Pars. lum. 1	9.0	315	326	227	91	88	0	120	133	0
R. Pars. lum. 2	10.0	335	321	252	107	96	0	75	91	0

The heading above the data groups reads: **Predicted Muscle Forces (N)**

L. Pars. lum. 2	10.0	349	362	252	101	97	0	133	147	286
R. Pars. lum. 3	11.0	371	374	277	118	111	0	84	87	0
L. Pars. lum. 3	11.0	386	380	277	112	105	0	147	182	315
R. Pars. lum. 4	12.0	426	459	302	135	134	0	96	80	0
L. Pars. lum. 4	12.0	443	406	302	129	116	0	169	237	343
R. iliolum.	6.0	113	115	151	160	151	0	50	51	0
L. iliolum.	6.0	162	157	151	67	62	0	43	55	172
R. long. thor.	8.0	149	154	202	210	200	0	66	68	0
L. long. thor.	8.0	213	204	202	88	80	0	57	75	201
R. quad. lum.	5.0	196	177	126	62	57	0	44	53	0
L. quad. lum.	5.0	203	222	126	59	61	0	77	70	143
R. lat. dors.5	4.0	105	115	101	88	88	0	91	76	0
L. lat. dors.5	4.0	145	131	101	115	101	0	82	118	114
R. multifid.1	2.8	102	91	71	32	28	0	23	31	0
L. multifid.1	2.8	106	116	71	31	31	0	40	38	0
R. multifid.2	2.8	99	99	71	32	29	0	22	25	0
L. multifid.2	2.8	103	103	71	30	28	0	39	48	0
R. psoas 1	4.4	74	70	0	249	239	139	117	122	0
L. psoas 1	4.4	75	79	111	276	288	139	220	207	126

Continued

Table 5.1. *Continued*

| | | Predicted Muscle Forces (N) | | | | | | | | |
| | | Extension | | | Flexion | | | Lat. Bend. L | | |
Muscle	Cross Sectional Area (cm²)	EMG	EMGAO	OPT	EMG	EMGAO	OPT	EMG	EMGAO	OPT
R. psoas 2	4.4	74	71	0	249	240	139	117	118	0
L. psoas 2	4.4	75	79	19	275	287	139	220	212	126
R. psoas 3	4.4	74	71	0	249	241	126	116	119	0
L. psoas 3	4.4	75	78	0	275	286	71	220	210	126
R. psoas 4	4.4	74	70	0	249	236	0	117	124	0
L. psoas 4	4.4	75	79	0	275	285	0	220	211	126
RMS difference*	0.00	0.08	0.78	0.00	0.07	1.00	0.00	0.23		2.72
L4/L5 compression (N)	5,806	5,780	3,984	7,458	7,515	3,010	5,397	5,305		4,022
Generated moments (Nm)†	Ext./flex		194			−191			−70	
	R/L bend		−4			9			−142	
	R/L twist		−4			−2			21	

*RMS difference between the muscle force estimates and the EMG predicted forces.
†The sign convention is such that the moments generated in the trunk extension direction, twisting to the left and lateral bending to the right, are positive.

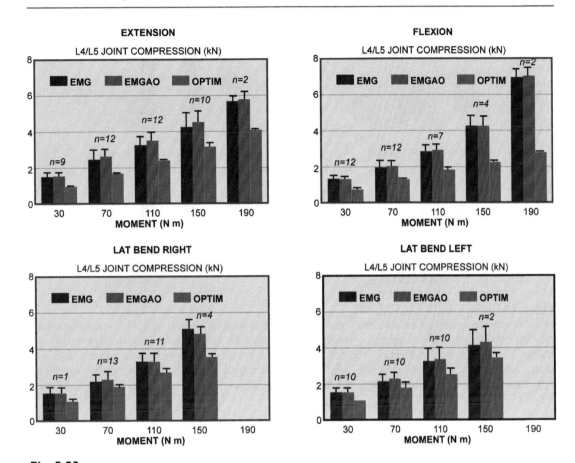

Fig. 5.23.

Results for spinal compression at L4-L5 using EMG-assisted (EMG), EMG-assisted optimization (EMGAO) and double linear optimization (OPTIM, first minimize muscle stress then minimize spine compression). (Cholewicki, McGill, and Norman 1995) Average values and one standard deviation are given. Between 2 and 13 subjects underwent maximal isometric efforts in flexion/extension and lateral bending. The subjects were restrained with belts to prevent movement. An isometric task was used in this study in order to reduce confounding effects related to muscle's dependence on length and velocity.

5.3.2 Cervical

5.3.2.1 Disc Pressure

Hattori and colleagues' [1981] results for the cervical intradiscal pressures *in vivo* do not differentiate between disc levels. Using Nachemson's relationship between intradiscal pressure and applied force, it is possible to estimate the forces in the spine from Hattori's disc pressure data (Figure 5.25).

Pospiech et al. [1999] reported intradiscal pressures *in vitro* in the C3/4 and C5/6 discs both with and without simulated musculature undergoing flexibility testing (see Table 5.3). A maximum disc pressure of 0.86 MPa was seen

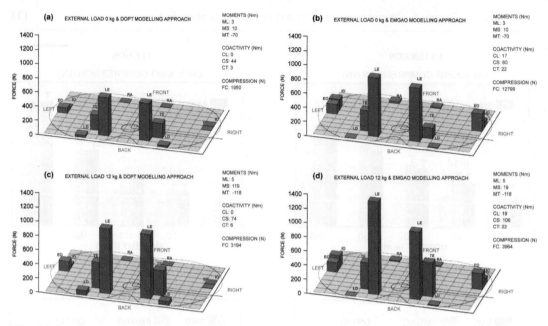

Fig. 5.24.
Modified graphs representing individual trunk muscles at the L5/S1 level for a typical subject at near maximal spine moment during trunk flexion. (Gagnon, Lariviere, and Loisel 2001) The subject was undergoing trunk flexion with and without a 12 kg load as indicated. The L5-S1 spine compression (F_c) is given for each case and results are presented for both double optimization (DOPT) and EMG-assisted optimization (EMGAO). The muscles modeled are rectus abdominus (RA), internal oblique (IO), external oblique (EO), lumbar erector spinae (LE), thoracic erector spinae (TE), and latissimus dorsi (LD).

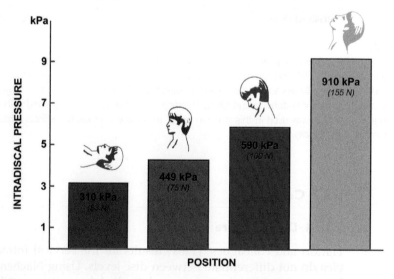

Fig. 5.25.
Cervical intradiscal pressures as measured by Hattori et al. (Hattori et al. 1981) and as presented by White and Panjabi. (White and Panjabi 1990) The corresponding force (given in Newtons in brackets) can be estimated using Nachemson's relationship (Nachemson 1981) between measured intradiscal pressure and applied compressive force. Disc dimensions were taken from Pooni et al. (Pooni et al. 1986)

Table 5.2.

Hand load and L4-L5 compression, moment, and shear data for the EMG-assisted model developed by McGill and Norman [McGill and Norman 1986]. Three subjects performed six sagittal plane lifts of masses as presented in the table.

Lift Trial	Load Mass (kg)	Dynamic Hand Force (N)	L4-L5 Moment (Nm)	L4-L5 Compression (N)	Compression* Reduction (%)	L4-L5 Shear (N)	Shear* Reduction (%)
1	27.3	832	449	7,296	25	612	52.1
2	27.3	749	384	6,787	19.5	39	46.3
3	77.3	913	364	6,149	23.9	350	67.8
4	77.3	894	364	6,060	25.3	618	39.7
5	54.5	739	332	5,709	22.9	268	71.0
6	54.5	707	331	5,571	23.8	304	67.9
1	45.5	1,197	306	6,485	11.5	963	25.0
2	45.5	1,134	300	6,518	8.7	1,197	2.8
3	90.9	1,097	298	6,264	9.1	1,065	15.8
4	90.9	1,185	395	7,534	16.0	1,272	17.1
5	68.2	1,163	302	7,014	5.7	934	26.9
6	68.2	1,136	290	6,557	4.3	1,105	11.1
1	45.5	970	421	7,894	17.1	618	45.6
2	45.5	897	353	6,624	17.8	190	81.5
3	90.9	1,297	438	8,195	17.4	905	32.8
4	90.9	1,316	431	8,921	8.9	843	34.1
5	72.7	1,319	417	8,327	12.8	640	49.5
6	72.7	1,219	471	8,862	16.5	678	50.9
Subject/ trial totals					16.2		42.5

*The compression and shear reduction values refer to the difference between forces predicted by this model and forces predicted by former models that presumed the erector musculature to run parallel to the line of compression and through a 5-cm moment arm.

Table 5.3.

Intradiscal pressure values for an intact cervical spine with and without simulated musculature [Pospiech et al. 1999].

	Without Simulated Musculature		With Simulated Musculature	
	C3/4 (MPa)	C5/6 (MPa)	C3/4 (MPa)	C5/6 (MPa)
Flexion/extension	0.32	0.23	0.36	0.64
Axial rotation	0.25	0.17	0.35	0.86
Lateral bending	0.16	0.16	0.32	0.56

during flexion under simulated musculature in the C5/6 disc. These results show significant increase in disc pressures with the addition of musculature for all motions.

Cripton et al. [2001] found a linear relationship between applied compressive load and measuring pressure under axial loading (Figure 5.26). They hypothesized a "rule of thumb" for disc pressure under compression load in the cervical spine is approximately 3.75 MPa per 1,000 N of compression. In contrast, the rule of thumb for lumbar discs is approximately 1 MPa per 1,000 N of compression.

5.3.2.2 Mathematical Models

Compared to the situation for the thoraco lumbar spine, the number of biomechanical models focused on the cervical spine is extremely limited. Only one double optimization model (first minimize muscle intensity then minimize spinal compression at level C4) [Moroney, Schultz, and Miller 1988] and one EMGAO model were identified in our literature search [Choi 2003]. Both of these models are focused on isometric neck muscle contractions.

The prediction of individual muscle forces from Moroney et al. [1988] is presented in Table 5.4. The shear force and compression reaction forces are presented in Table 5.5. The maximum compression force occurred under extension (1,164 N), and a spinal compression of 122 N was predicted for the relaxed posture.

The corresponding joint reaction forces at C4/5 for Choi's EMGAO cervical spine model [Choi 2003] is presented in Table 5.6. It is noteworthy that the EMGAO Choi model predicts higher muscle forces than does the pure optimization Moroney model. This is expected based on the earlier results presented for the lumbar spine. The EMGAO C4/5 compression results range from 941 N for lateral bending to 1,626 N in flexion. It is also noteworthy that in contrast to the Moroney model the EMGAO model predicts higher compression loads in flexion than in extension.

Table 5.4.

Average (SD) calculated muscle forces for the double optimization (first minimize muscle intensity and then spinal compression) cervical spine model presented by Moroney, Schultz, and Miller [1988]. Fourteen subjects performed maximum isometric cervical spine exertions.

Muscle Equivalent	Relaxed	Attempted Left Twist	Attempted Left Bend	Attempted Extension	Attempted Flexion
L Platysma		23 (8)	19 (11)		19 (14)
R Platysma					19 (14)
L Infrahyoid		72 (25)	60 (35)		62 (45)
R Infrahyoid		68 (30)	41 (45)		62 (45)
L SCM			140 (83)		145 (106)
R SCM		170 (58)	68 (47)		145 (106)
L Longi		31 (11)	26 (15)		26 (19)
R Longi					26 (19)
L Scal. ant.		42 (15)	35 (20)		36 (27)
R Scal. ant.					36 (27)
L Scal. med.	3 (1)	45 (15)	37 (22)	39 (17)	
R Scal. med.	3 (1)			39 (17)	
L Long. cerv.	2 (1)	29 (10)	24 (14)	26 (11)	
R Long. cerv.	2 (1)			26 (11)	
L Levator scap.	8 (4)	2 (3)	106 (62)	116 (51)	
R Levator scap.	8 (4)	14 (14)		116 (51)	
L Multifidus	3 (1)			42 (19)	
R Multifidus	3 (1)	47 (16)	39 (23)	42 (19)	
L Semispin. cerv.	7 (3)		2 (8)	96 (42)	
R Semispin. cerv.	7 (3)			96 (42)	
L Semispin. cap.	9 (4)	96 (22)	111 (57)	127 (56)	
R Semispin. cap.	9 (4)			127 (56)	
L Splenius cerv.	1 (1)	17 (6)	14 (8)	15 (7)	
R Splenius cerv.	1 (1)			15 (7)	
L Splenius cap.	4 (2)	68 (23)	56 (33)	61 (27)	
R Splenius cap.	4 (2)			61 (27)	
L Trapezius	5 (2)			73 (32)	
R Trapezius	5 (2)	81 (29)	5 (9)	73 (32)	

Standard deviation are in parentheses.
L, left; R, right.

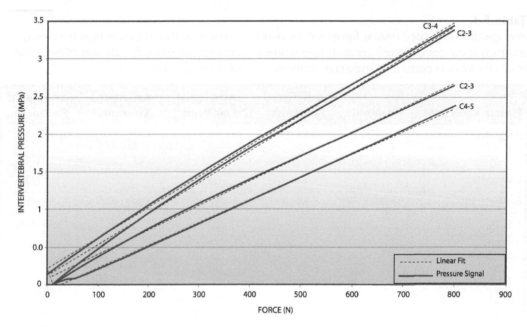

Fig. 5.26.
Disc pressure and associated linear regression fits, plotted as a function of applied compression. (Cripton, Dumas, and Nolte 2001)

Table 5.5.
Average (SD) calculated C4 reaction forces for the double optimization (first minimize muscle intensity and then spinal compression) cervical spine model presented by Moroney, Schultz, and Miller [1988]. Fourteen subjects performed maximum isometric cervical spine exertions.

Exercise	Lateral Shear (N)	Anteroposterior Shear (N)	Compression (N)
Relaxed	0 (0)*	−2 (1)	122 (36)
Left twist	33 (8)	70 (24)	778 (228)
Extension	0 (0)	135 (69)	1,164 (494)
Flexion	0 (0)	31 (63)	558 (375)
Left bending	125 (58)	93 (59)	758 (422)

*Standard deviations in parentheses.

Table 5.6.

Average (±SD) C4/C5 calculated spinal compression forces from the EMGAO cervical spine model presented by Choi [2003]. The forces are given as total or subdivided into co-contraction and task or agonist force. Values are given between 25 and 100% of maximal isometric contractions. The results are averages from 10 subjects.

Plane and Direction of Moment	25%	50%	75%	100%
Sagittal plane				
Extension				
Compression from total muscle forces	305 ± 58	620 ± 95	946 ± 177	1,338 ± 195
Compression from task muscle forces	284 ± 39	568 ± 57	851 ± 89	1,135 ± 121
Compression from co-contraction	21 ± 12	52 ± 22	95 ± 40	203 ± 98
Flexion				
Compression from total muscle forces	342 ± 125	698 ± 209	1,107 ± 271	1,626 ± 301
Compression from task muscle forces	231 ± 41	461 ± 79	692 ± 105	923 ± 173
Compression from co-contraction	111 ± 38	237 ± 89	415 ± 182	703 ± 212
Frontal plane				
L. lat. bending				
Compression from total muscle forces	218 ± 95	449 ± 151	623 ± 174	941 ± 215
Compression from task muscle forces	160 ± 28	320 ± 55	436 ± 87	641 ± 108
Compression from co-contraction	58 ± 25	129 ± 59	187 ± 89	300 ± 125
R. lat. bending				
Compression from total muscle forces	231 ± 115	470 ± 140	727 ± 161	1,013 ± 178
Compression from task muscle forces	162 ± 35	324 ± 61	487 ± 85	649 ± 113
Compression from co-contraction	69 ± 34	146 ± 67	240 ± 103	364 ± 154

5.4 References

Adams, M. A., D. S. McNally, and P. Dolan (1996). "Stress Distributions Inside Intervertebral Discs: The Effects of Age and Degeneration," *The Journal of Bone and Joint Surgery* 78:965–972.

Bergmann, G., F. Graichen, et al. (1988). "Multichannel Strain Gauge Telemetry for Orthopaedic Implants," *Journal of Biomechanics* 21:169–176.

Bernhardt, P., H. J. Wilke, et al. (1999). "Multiple Muscle Force Simulation in Axial Rotation of the Cervical Spine," *Clinical Biomechanics* (*Bristol, Avon*) 14:32–40.

Chaffin, D. B., G. B. J. Andersson, and B. J. Martin (1999). *Occupational Biomechanics.* New York: John Wiley and Sons.

Choi, H. (2003). "Quantitative Assessment of Co-contraction in Cervical Musculature," *Med. Eng. Phys.* 25:133–140.

Cholewicki, J., and S. M. McGill (1994). "EMG Assisted Optimization: A Hybrid Approach for Estimating Muscle Forces in an Indeterminate Biomechanical Model," *J. Biomech.* 27:1287–1289.

Cholewicki, J., S. M. McGill, and R. W. Norman (1995). "Comparison of Muscle Forces and Joint Load from an Optimization and EMG-assisted Lumbar Spine Model: Towards Development of a Hybrid Approach," *J. Biomech.* 28:321–331.

Collins, J. J. (1995). "The Redundant Nature of Locomotor Optimization Laws," *J. Biomech.* 28:251–267.

Cripton, P. A., G. A. Dumas, and L. Nolte (2001). "A Minimally Disruptive Technique for Measuring Intervertebral Disc Pressure In Vitro: Application to the Cervical Spine," *J. Biomech.* 34:545–549.

Cripton, P. A., G. M. Jain, R. H. Wittenberg, and L. P. Nolte (2000). "Load-sharing Characteristics of Stabilized Lumbar Spine Segments," *Spine* 25:170–179.

Cunningham, B. W., Y. Kotani, et al. (1997). "The Effect of Spinal Destabilization and Instrumentation on Lumbar Intradiscal Pressure: An In Vitro Biomechanical Analysis," *Spine* 22:2655–2663.

Dick, W. (1987). "The Fixateur Interne as a Versatile Implant for Spine Surgery," *Spine* 12:882–900.

Dolan, P., I. Kingma, et al. (1999). "Dynamic Forces Acting on the Lumbar Spine During Manual Handling. Can They Be Estimated Using Electromyographic Techniques Alone?," *Spine* 24:698–703.

Dolan, P., I. Kingma, et al. (2001). "An EMG Technique for Measuring Spinal Loading During Asymmetric Lifting," *Clin. Biomech. (Bristol, Avon)* 16 Suppl. 1:S17–S24.

Drake, R., W. Vogl, and W. Adam (2005). *Gray's Anatomy for Students*. Philadelphia: Elsevier/Churchill Livingstone.

Ferrara, L. (2005). "The Smart Intervertebral Disc," in R. Guyer and J. Zigler (eds.). *Spinal Arthroplasty: A New Era in Spine Care*. St. Louis: Quality Medical Publishing.

Ferrara, L. A., et al. (2003). "An In Vivo Biocompatibility Assessment of MEMS Materials for Spinal Fusion Monitoring," *Biomedical Microdevices* 5:297–302.

Fye, M. A., E. P. Southern, M. M. Panjabi, and J. Cholewicki (1998). "Quantitative Discomanometry: Technique and Reproducibility In Vitro," *Journal of Spinal Disorders* 11:335–340.

Gagnon, D., C. Lariviere, and P. Loisel (2001). "Comparative Ability of EMG, Optimization, and Hybrid Modelling Approaches to Predict Trunk Muscle Forces and Lumbar Spine Loading During Dynamic Sagittal Plane Lifting," *Clin. Biomech. (Bristol, Avon)* 16:359–372.

Graichen, F., G. Bergmann, and A. Rohlmann (1996). "Patient Monitoring System for Load Measurement with Spinal Fixation Devices," *Med. Eng. Phys.* 18:167–174.

Granata, K. P., and W. S. Marras (1995). "An EMG-assisted Model of Trunk Loading During Free-dynamic Lifting," *J. Biomech.* 28:1309–1317.

Hattori, S., H. Oda, S. Kawai, and Ube-Shi (1981). "Cervical Intradiscal Pressure in Movements and Traction of the Cervical Spine," *Zeitschrift fur Orthopadie* 119:568–569.

Herberts, P., R. Kadefors, E. Kaiser, and I. Petersen (1968). "Implantation of Microcircuits for Myo-electric Control of Prostheses," *J. Bone Joint Surg. Br.* 50:780–791.

Holcomb, W. G., W. W. Glenn, and G. Sato (1969). "A Demand Radiofrequency Cardiac Pacemaker," *Med. Biol. Eng.* 7:493–499.

Hughes, R. E., J. C. Bean, and D. B. Chaffin (1995). "Evaluating the Effect of Co-contraction in Optimization Models," *J. Biomech.* 28:875–878.

Hughes, R. E., D. B. Chaffin, S. A. Lavender, and G. B. Andersson (1994). "Evaluation of Muscle Force Prediction Models of the Lumbar Trunk Using Surface Electromyography," *J. Orthop. Res.* 12:689–698.

Ledet, E. H., B. L. Sachs, et al. (2000). "Real-time In Vivo Loading in the Lumbar Spine: Part 1. Interbody Implant: Load Cell Design and Preliminary Results," *Spine* 25:2595–2600.

Ledet, E. H., M. P. Tymeson, et al. (2005). "Direct Real-time Measurement of In Vivo Forces in the Lumbar Spine," *Spine J.* 5:85–94.

McGill, S. M., and R. W. Norman (1986). "Partitioning of the L4–L5 Dynamic Moment into Disc, Ligamentous, and Muscular Components During Lifting," *Spine* 11:666–678.

Mackay, R. S. (1968). *Bio-medical Telemetry. Sensing and Transmitting Biological Information from Animals and Man.* New York: John Wiley.

McNally, D. S., and M. A. Adams (1992). "Internal Intervertebral Disc Mechanics as Revealed by Stress Profilometry," *Spine* 17:66–73.

McNally, D. S., M. A. Adams, and A. E. Goodship (1992). "Development and Validation of a New Transducer for Intradiscal Pressure Measurement," *J. Biomed. Eng.* 14:495–498.

McNally, D. S., I. M. Shackleford, A. E. Goodship, and R. C. Mulholland (1996). "In Vivo Stress Measurement Can Predict Pain on Discography," *Spine* 21:2580–2587.

Moroney, S. P., A. B. Schultz, and J. A. Miller (1988). "Analysis and Measurement of Neck Loads," *J. Orthop. Res.* 6:713–720.

Nachemson, A. L. (1960). "Lumbar Intradiscal Pressure," *Acta Orthopaedica Scandinavica* Supplementum 43:1–104.

Nachemson, A. L. (1966). "The Load on Lumbar Disks in Different Positions of the Body," *Clinical Orthopaedics and Related Research* 45:107–122.

Nachemson, A. L. (1981). "Disc Pressure Measurements," *Spine* 6:93–97.

Nachemson, A., and G. Elfstrom (1971). "Intravital Wireless Telemetry of Axial Forces in Harrington Distraction Rods in Patients with Idiopathic Scoliosis," *J. Bone Joint Surg Am.* 53:445–465.

Nachemson, A. L., and J. M. Morris (1964). "In Vivo Measurements of Intradiscal Pressure: Discometry, Method for the Determination of Pressure in the Lower Lumbar Discs," *Journal of Bone and Joint Surgery. American Volume* 46-A:1077–1092.

Nussbaum, M. A., and D. B. Chaffin (1996). "Development and Evaluation of a Scalable and Deformable Geometric Model of the Human Torso," *Clin. Biomech. (Bristol, Avon)* 11:25–34.

Nussbaum, M. A., D. B. Chaffin, and C. J. Rechtien (1995). "Muscle Lines-of-action Affect Predicted Forces in Optimization-based Spine Muscle Modeling," *J. Biomech.* 28:401–409.

Pitman, M. I., and L. Peterson (1989). "Biomechanics of Skeletal Muscle," in M. Nordin and V. H. Frankel (eds.). *Basic Biomechanics of the Muskuloskeletal System.* (2d ed.). Philadelphia: Lea & Febiger.

Pooni, J. S., D. W. Hukins, et al. (1986). "Comparison of the Structure of Human Intervertebral Discs in the Cervical, Thoracic and Lumbar Regions of the Spine," *Surg. Radiol. Anat.* 8:175–182.

Pospiech, J., D. Stolke, H. J. Wilke, and L. E. Claes (1999). "Intradiscal Pressure Recordings in the Cervical Spine," *Neurosurgery* 44:379–384.

Rohlmann, A., G. Bergmann, and F. Graichen (1994). "A Spinal Fixation Device for In Vivo Load Measurement," *J. Biomech.* 27:961–967.

Rohlmann, A., G. Bergmann, and F. Graichen (1997). "Loads on an Internal Spinal Fixation Device During Walking," *Journal of Biomechanics* 30:41–47.

Rohlmann, A., G. Bergmann, and F. Graichen (1999). "Loads on Internal Spinal Fixators Measured in Different Body Positions," *Eur. Spine. J.* 8:354–359.

Rohlmann, A., F. Graichen, and G. Bergmann (2000). "Influence of Load Carrying on Loads in Internal Spinal Fixators," *J. Biomech.* 33:1099–1104.

Rohlmann, A., U. Arntz, F. Graichen, and G. Bergmann (2001). "Loads on an Internal Spinal Fixation Device During Sitting," *J. Biomech.* 34:989–993.

Rohlmann, A., G. Bergmann, F. Graichen, and H. M. Mayer (1995). "Telemeterized Load Measurement Using Instrumented Spinal Internal Fixators in a Patient with Degenerative Instability," *Spine* 20:2683–2689.

Rohlmann, A., G. Bergmann, F. Graichen, and H. M. Mayer (1998). "Influence of Muscle Forces on Loads in Internal Spinal Fixation Devices," *Spine* 23:537–542.

Rohlmann, A., G. Bergmann, F. Graichen, and U. Weber (1997). "Comparison of Loads on Internal Spinal Fixation Devices Measured In Vitro and In Vivo," *Med. Eng. Phys.* 19:539–546.

Rohlmann, A., G. Bergmann, F. Graichen, and U. Weber (2000). Changes in the Loads on an Internal Spinal Fixator After Iliac-Crest Autograft," *J. Bone Joint Surg. Br.* 82:445–449.

Rohlmann, A., L. E. Claes, et al. (2001). "Comparison of Intradiscal Pressures and Spinal Fixator Loads for Different Body Positions and Exercises," *Ergonomics* 44:781–794.

Rohlmann, A., O. Eick, G. Bergmann, and F. Graichen (1993). "Measuring Loads with the Aid of an Instrumented Internal Spinal Fixation Device," *Biomedizinische Technik* 38:255–259.

Rohlmann, A., F. Graichen, U. Weber, and G. Bergmann (2000). "2000 Volvo Award Winner in Biomechanical Studies: Monitoring In Vivo Implant Loads with a Telemeterized Internal Spinal Fixation Device," *Spine* 25:2981–2986.

Rohlmann, A., S. Neller, et al. (2001). "Effect of an Internal Fixator and a Bone Graft on Intersegmental Spinal Motion and Intradiscal Pressure in the Adjacent Regions," *Eur. Spine. J.* 10:301–308.

Rohlmann, A., L. H. Riley, G. Bergmann, and F. Graichen (1996). "In Vitro Load Measurement Using an Instrumented Spinal Fixation Device," *Med. Eng. Phys.* 18:485–488.

Sato, K., S. Kikuchi, and T. Yonezawa (1999). "In Vivo Intradiscal Pressure Measurement in Healthy Individuals and in Patients with Ongoing Back Problems," *Spine* 24:2468–2474.

Schultz, A. B., and G. B. Andersson (1981). "Analysis of Loads on the Lumbar Spine," *Spine* 6:76–82.

Schultz, A. B., G. B. Andersson, et al. (1982). "Analysis and Measurement of Lumbar Trunk Loads in Tasks Involving Bends and Twists," *J. Biomech.* 15:669–675.

Schultz, A. B., K. Haderspeck, D. Warwick, and D. Portillo (1983). "Use of Lumbar Trunk Muscles in Isometric Performance of Mechanically Complex Standing Tasks," *J. Orthop. Res.* 1:77–91.

Shea, M., W. T. Edwards, A. A. White III, and W. C. Hayes (1995). "Optimization Technique for the Calculation of In Vitro Three-dimensional Vertebral Motion," *J. Biomech. Eng.* 117:366–369.

Tominaga, T., C. A. Dickman, V. K. Sonntag, and S. Coons (1995). "Comparative Anatomy of the Baboon and the Human Cervical Spine," *Spine* 20:131–137.

White, A. A., and M. M. Panjabi (1990). *Clinical Biomechanics of the Spine.* New York: J. B. Lippincott Company.

Wilke, H. J., P. Neef, et al. (1999). "New In Vivo Measurements of Pressures in the Intervertebral Disc in Daily Life," *Spine* 24:755–762.

Wilke, H. J., A. Rohlmann, et al. (2003). "ISSLS Prize Winner: A Novel Approach to Determine Trunk Muscle Forces During Flexion and Extension: A Comparison of Data from an In Vitro Experiment and In Vivo Measurements," *Spine* 28:2585–2593.

Wilke, H. J., S. Wolf, et al. (1996). "Influence of Varying Muscle Forces on Lumbar Intradiscal Pressure: An In Vitro Study," *Journal of Biomechanics* 29:549–555.

Winter, D. A. (2005). *Biomechanics and Motor Control of Human Movement*. Hoboken: John Wiley and Sons.

Chapter 6

Spine Disorders: Implications for Bioengineers

Vijay K. Goel, Koichi Sairyo,
Sri Lakshmi Vishnubhotla,
Ashok Biyani, and Nabil Ebraheim
Spine Research Center, Department of Bioengineering,
University of Toledo, and Department of Orthopedic
Surgery, Medical University of Ohio, Toledo, Ohio

6.1 Introduction

Normal function of the human spine is possible due to a complex interaction of its components (i.e., vertebrae, ligaments, discs, rib cage, and muscles). Age, trauma, spinal disorders, and a host of other parameters can disrupt this interaction to an extent that in certain cases surgery may be required to restore normal function. This chapter describes several spinal disorders from a mechanical perspective. An understanding of these disorders can assist in the design and development of spinal instrumentation. As biomechanics begins to be intertwined with tissue engineering, a better understanding of the particular disorders may also provide insight into "biological" solutions.

6.2 Scoliosis

Scoliosis is the structural deformity of the spine in the frontal plane. The usual vertical orientation of the spine in the frontal plane is disturbed, leading to a lateral curvature of spine [Goel and Weinstein 1980]. Cobb's angle measures the degree of scoliosis [Martinez-Lozano 2001]. (See Figure 6.1.) Identifying the particular curve pattern and location is essential to making treatment decisions, which may include nonsurgical options such as orthoses and braces. The curve patterns of idiopathic scoliosis are called "primary" and "compensatory," each with specific meanings. "Primary curve" refers to the curve that is larger in magnitude, more rigid on supine side bending (side bending in the supine posture), and generally having more cosmetic deformity. "Compensatory curves" are those that are smaller in magnitude and more flexible on supine side bending. The curves are always named for the location of the apex of the curve being discussed. Idiopathic scoliosis assumes five classical curve patterns: right thoracic, thoracolumbar, lumbar, double primary, and double thoracic primary.

● *Right thoracic curve*: This curve typically extends from T5 or T6 to T11 or T12, with the apex at T8 or T9 [Goel and Weinstein 1980] (Figure 6.2). There is a compensatory curve in the lumbar region, which is usually smaller but may be nearly equal in magnitude to the primary thoracic curve. In the latter case, it must be differentiated from the double primary curve by assessment of

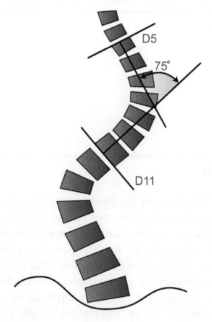

Fig. 6.1.
Measurement of Cobb's angle [Martinex-Lozano 2001].

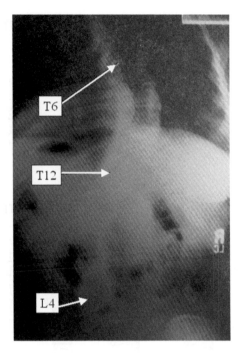

Fig. 6.2.
Radiograph of right thoracic curve [Goel and Weinstein 1980].

flexibility of the lumbar curve. When the patient is in a forward bending position, the rib deformity will be considerably greater than the lumbar deformity.

- *Thoracolumbar curve*: The curve extends from about T8 to L3, with apex at T12
  or L1, or the T12-L1 disc space.
- *Lumbar curve*: This curve typically extends from about T11 to L4. It may be in
  either direction but is more commonly to the left. The thoracic compensatory
  curve is smaller in magnitude than the primary lumbar curve.
- *Double primary curve*: This curve pattern has a right thoracic curve that usually
  extends from T5 to T12 and a left lumbar curve from T12 to L4. This pattern
  has two rigid curves. On forced supine side bending, both curves will correct
  to about the same degree.
- *Double thoracic primary curve*: This curve pattern has two primary curves, but
  both are in the thoracic region. The upper one is to the left, extending from
  about T2 to T5, whereas the lower one is to the right (from T5 to T10). The upper
  left thoracic curve is the more difficult to control and produces the most cosmetic deformity.

A number of investigators have reported on the incidence of these curve patterns among patients with scoliosis. Although the incidence varies from one
study to the next, certain trends prevail. The right thoracic curve pattern is the
most common, followed by the double primary, thoracolumbar, and lumbar
curve patterns.

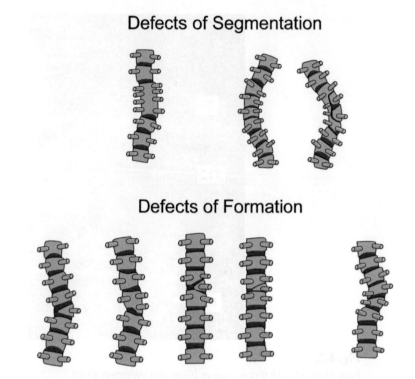

Fig. 6.3.
Classification of congenital scoliosis [McMaster 2001].

The abnormal curvature may be due to developmental abnormalities (congenital scoliosis) or may be without any obvious cause (idiopathic scoliosis). The scoliosis may also combine with neuromuscular disease. Also, among the elderly population the degeneration of the spine could be responsible for scoliosis. Overall, idiopathic scoliosis comprises about 70% of all cases.

About 80% of congenital scoliosis cases arise from defects of segmentation and defects of formation (Figure 6.3). In the defects of segmentation, bilateral failure of segmentation is unlikely to show clinical problems, because the scoliotic curve rarely exceeds 20 degrees. Unilateral failure of segmentation invariably progresses to a severe curve, which requires surgical intervention. On average, the rate of curve growth is about 5 degrees a year. However, presence of one or more hemivertebrae on the convex side can lead to a very severe curve, in that the hemivertebrae have greater potential for longitudinal growth. In severe cases the curve can be more than 60 degrees at the age of 4. If left untreated, the child will become extremely deformed, with concurrent respiratory impairment. There are four subtypes of the hemivertebrae, according to the pathology and its relationship to the adjacent vertebra (Figure 6.3) [McMaster 2001]. Fully segmented is the most common, and semisegmented is less common. Nonsegmented and incarcerated subtypes are rare. The semisegmented, nonsegmented, and incarcerated hemivertebrae may not require surgical intervention, because they do not usually progress to severe scoliotic curves. A fully segmented hemivertebra has a normal disc space between adjacent vertebrae, permitting longitudinal growth to occur. Unlike most defects of the segmentation type, this subtype does not typically cause a severe cosmetic deformity, as the amount of combined vertebral rotation is small. The curve usually increases at a rate of 1 to 2 degrees a year.

A unilateral unsegmented bar with contralateral hemivertebrae at the same level frequently requires surgical intervention. The purpose of the surgery is to balance spinal growth by retarding the growth on the convex side. Early diagnosis is very important, because early on the curve is not severe and prophylactic surgery is possible. The progression of congenital scoliosis can be anticipated based on the remaining amount of spinal growth, the type and site of vertebral anomaly, and the degree of growth imbalance it may produce. Another goal of the treatment procedure is to prevent curve deterioration.

The precise etiology of idiopathic scoliosis is largely an unknown entity. Several factors have been implicated: heredity, genetics, neuromotor mechanisms, connective tissue problems, muscular disorders, and hormonal system dysfunction [Hadley-Miller, Mims, and Milewicz 1994; Harrington 1997; Machida et al. 1993; Miller 2001; Riseborough and Wynn-Davies 1973; Sahlstrand, Ortengren, and Nachemson 1978; Sahlstrand, Petruson, and Ortengren 1979; Salehi et al. 2002; Spencer and Eccles 1976; Yamada 1984; Yamamoto et al. 1982].

Idiopathic scoliosis may be termed infantile (0 to 3 years), juvenile (4 to 9 years), and adolescent (10 years to maturity), depending on the age at the onset. Infantile idiopathic scoliosis has some unique features. About 90% of the cases show left thoracic curve, and it is more predominant in males [Jevtic 2001; Scott and Morgan 1955]. Scott and Morgan [1955] reported that approximately 90% of these curves were self-limited and resolved spontaneously. On the other hand, double structural curves with a thoracic component tend to be progressive in nature. Also, right-sided thoracic curves in females have a worse prognosis [Thompson and Bentley 1980]. The RVAD (rib-vertebral angle difference) measurement has been used for understanding its progression [Mehta 1972] (Figure 6.4). If the value is greater than 20 degrees, the scoliosis may increase. On the other hand, the curve is likely to resolve spontaneously when it measures less than 20 degrees. Mehta [1972] also noted that the phase of the rib head can serve as a predictor for progression of the scoliotic curve. Phase I means that on AP radiograph a rib at the convex side does not overlap the vertebral body, and in phase II it overlaps. When the apical rib head shows phase II, the curve may continue to progress.

Juvenile idiopathic scoliosis occurs between the ages of 4 and 10 years, with about 70% of cases progressive and requiring surgical intervention [Lenke and Dobbs 2004]. Unlike the infantile type, juvenile scoliosis is unlikely to resolve spontaneously.

The adolescent idiopathic scoliosis has been classified based on (1) the curve type (1 through 6), (2) lumbar spine modifier (A, B, C), and (3) a thoracic modifier (−, N, +) [Lenke et al. 2001, 2002]. The lumbar modifier is based on the position of the lumbar apex in relation to the center sacral vertical line (CSVL). The

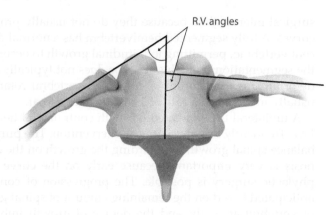

Fig. 6.4.
Measurement of RV angle [Mehta et al. 1972].

sagittal thoracic modifier is based on the upright lateral radiograph and measured from the superior end plate of T5 to the inferior end plate of T12. When this measurement is less than 10 degrees, the sagittal modifier is indicated as (–). When the measurement is between 10 and 40 degrees, it is designated as (N), and (+) is assigned to cases with angles over 40 degrees. Based on these findings, there can be 42 different classifications (not 48, because all type 5 and 6 curves should only have C lumbar modifier).

For infantile and juvenile type scoliosis, surgery is recommended when the curve exceeds 45 to 50 degrees [Lenke and Dobbs 2004]. Fusion may impede growth over time. The amount of potential shortening after spinal fusion may be predicted as 0.07 times the number of segments fused times the number of years of growth remaining. Among different surgical options, instrumentation without spinal fusion or limited fusion is considered only for younger children (less than 8 years old). In such cases, the rod is lengthened every 6 to 12 months and replaced as additional length is needed. This allows for continued growth of the spine and delays the formal spinal fusion until closer to skeletal maturity [Lenke and Dobbs 2004; Moe et al. 1984].

Although the concept of this procedure is ideal, complications (including hook displacements, rod breakages, laminar fracture, and wound infection) have been reported [Blakemore et al. 2001; Klemme et al. 1997; Mineiro and Weinstein 2002]. Also, the children need multiple surgeries under general anesthesia. Thus, there is a need to develop more appropriate instrumentation/procedures (e.g., gradual lengthening techniques such as Ilizarov's method for long bones, as well as developing more reliable techniques for holding hooks to laminae). In 1998, Takaso et al. developed a remote-controlled rod instrumentation system that may be lengthened at the will of the surgeon [Takaso et al. 1998].

For adolescent scoliotic patients, surgical treatment is considered when the curve exceeds 50 degrees [Lenke and Dobbs 2004]. The goal of this strategy is to fuse the major and structural minor curve. Recently, a minimally invasive technique using thoracoscopes has been applied to scoliosis surgery and is

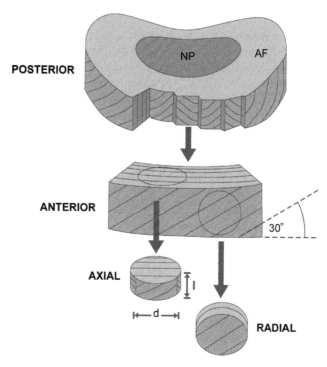

Fig. 6.5.
Structure of the intervertebral disc [website].

gaining wider acceptance among surgeons [Al-Sayyad, Crawford, and Wolf 2004; Lieberman et al. 2000; Newton et al. 2005; Puttlitz and Lenke 2003].

6.2.1 Intervertebral Disc

The intervertebral discs make up approximately one-third of the total spinal column's length [Cassar-Pullicino 1998]. Each disc consists of a tough cartilaginous annulus fibrosis and a jelly-like nucleus pulposus. The discs, along with the osseous end plates, form the main articulation between vertebral bodies. The annulus fibrosis is a composite of ground substance and matrix (Figure 6.5). The matrix basically consists of layers of type I collagen fibers oriented at various angles. The nucleus pulposus is made up of water, type II collagen, proteoglycans, and other components (such as elastin, fibronectin, tenascin, growth factors, enzymes, and cytokines). The presence of these components in the disc directly influences its mechanical properties and physiological functions. The disc is almost avascular except for the outermost layers of annulus. Thus, the intervertebral disc derives nutrition from diffusion of solutes through the end plates and outer annulus [Urban, Smith, and Fairbank 2004].

Any load through the spinal column is transmitted to the intervertebral disc from the vertebral body. Under loading, the nucleus pulposus acts like a fluid-filled bag and swells under pressure due to the hydrophilic nature of the proteoglycans. In this manner, a circumferential tension is applied to the annulus, converting it to a load-bearing structure. The whole construct acts as a shock absorber for the spine such that there is no high-spot loading at any point. This also allows for complex motion to occur. The amount of water in the nucleus varies throughout the day, depending on activity. Hence, the intervertebral discs play an essential role in mobility and load transfer through the spinal column.

6.2.2 Intervertebral Disc Disease

Intervertebral disc disease is a broad term used to describe alteration of the biomechanical properties of the disc through degenerative disease. The exact pathogenesis of the degenerative process is still unknown [An, Thonar, and Masuda 2003]. It has been suggested that disc degeneration might be predetermined genetically [Ala-Kokko 2002], occurs due to aging, or may be caused by overloading or underloading [Drerup et al. 1999; Luoma et al. 2000; Stokes and Iatridis 2004]. Loss of nutrition to the disc may also be an important factor in disc degeneration [Urban, Smith, and Fairbank 2004]. It is likely that almost any abnormal loading condition (including overload and immobilization) can lead to adaptive changes that may in turn lead to the degeneration of the disc. Studies evaluating all the previously cited factors as causes of disc degeneration are needed to understand the reason and progress of disc degeneration.

Once degeneration sets in, the intervertebral disc goes through a cascade of degenerative changes that result in biomechanical alteration of load transfer through the disc, in turn causing changes in the mechanical properties and composition of the tissue. Structural disorganization of the intervertebral disc along with loss in proteoglycans stemming from degeneration causes the hydrostatic mechanism to fail. There are different ways a degenerated disc can lead to low back pain, depending on if the degeneration occurs in the nucleus pulposus or the annulus (Figure 6.6).

A degenerated annulus can have fissures that consist of microscopic fragmentation of individual fibers. Annular tears at the corners of the vertebral body separating the annulus from the end plates (due to age, wear, and tear), concentric cracks, cavities, and radiating ruptures are also seen [Ferguson and Steffen 2003]. Disc bulging may occur due to decrease in the radial tensile strength of the annulus. Degeneration of the nucleus occurs following loss of water content leading to collagenation of the nucleus. This results in an increase of the elastic modulus of the nucleus.

Nucleus degeneration combined with annular degeneration may cause disc herniation into the spinal canal, causing low back pain due to nerve pinching. Thinning of the disc and loss of disc height are also seen in a degenerated disc. This loss of disc height combined with gradual ossification of the end plate and protrusion of the disc tissue causes stenosis, which again leads to back pain. Thompson grading is a five-category grading scheme for assessing gross morphology of midsagittal sections of human lumbar intervertebral disc

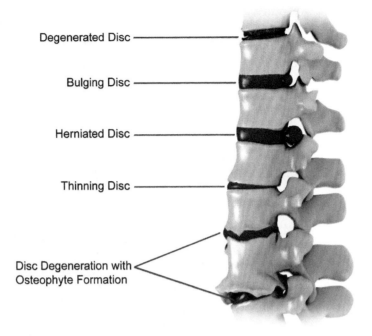

Degenerated Disc ———————

Bulging Disc ———————

Herniated Disc ———————

Thinning Disc ———————

Disc Degeneration with
Osteophyte Formation

Fig. 6.6.
Intervertebral disc disease [website].

[Thompson et al. 1990]. The Thompson grading scale may be used to identify the level of disc degeneration as a function of the gain in water content in the annulus with a corresponding loss of water content in the nucleus.

6.2.3 Imaging

Imaging the intervertebral disc can help diagnose the origin of discogenic low back pain. Before the advent of the recent imaging techniques, plain radiographs or invasive techniques such as discography were used to determine whether a patient was a candidate for surgery. Plain radiographs (usually the initial imaging because they are inexpensive) when taken in flexion/extension and oblique directions show the disc space height and changes in the end plates.

Magnetic resonance imaging (MRI) and computed tomography (CT) are noninvasive imaging methods used to evaluate disc degenerative disease [An et al. 2004]. In a MRI image the anatomical features such as disc height, tears in the annulus, fissures in the nucleus, and the level of hydration in the nucleus can be assessed. Jevtic [2001] described the MR depiction of various discovertebral lesions. Tanaka et al. [2001] have shown correlation between Thompson grading of the intervertebral disc degeneration and MRI images (Figure 6.7).

One of the major disadvantages of MRI is that previously placed instrumentation may cause an imaging artifact due to the metal [Brennan and

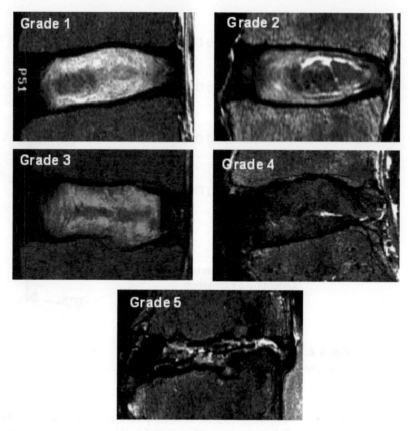

Fig. 6.7.
MRI Images of intervertebral disc with disc degeneration from grades I to V. [Tanaka et al. 2001]

Lauryssen 2000]. In such cases myelogram with postmyelographic computed tomography (CT myelogram) can be used.

Plain radiographs, CT images, and MR images do not differentiate abnormal asymptomatic from symptomatic painful disc levels. It is difficult to determine if the changes in the disc are related to aging or due to disc degeneration [Cassar-Pullicino 1998]. Various MR-based functional imaging strategies such as dynamic computed tomography, dynamic/functional magnetic resonance imaging, diffusion imaging, and magnetic resonance spectroscopy are potential techniques to give a more clinical and biomechanical basis for the cause of the disc degeneration [Haughton 2004].

6.2.4 Treatment Modalities

Low back pain due to disc degeneration is treated with conservative treatment in early stages. However, surgery is the preferred option for advanced disc disease where there is no pain relief with conservative therapy. Two common procedures intended to relieve back pain due to disc disease are discectomy and decompression of the segment. Discectomy involves surgically removing the painful disc. Decompression surgery is performed to relieve nerve impingement. This involves taking out part of the posterior spine (e.g., laminectomy, facetectomy) to make some space for the nerve. However, decompression causes instability at the operated segment and additional surgery, typically fusion or spinal arthrodesis, is required to restore the stability.

6.2.5 Spinal Arthrodesis

Spinal fusion surgery has been one of the gold standards for treatment of disc disease. Fusion surgery is based on the concept that instability causes pain and hence restricting the mobility will reduce the pain. The main aim of a spinal fusion surgery is to correct deformity, restore disc height, and provide stability to the particular spinal segment. The early spinal fusion surgeries involved removing the pain-causing part of the disc and filling the space by placing a fusion graft. These fusion grafts were generally taken from the hip or from loose bone chips. In recent years the evolution of interbody fusion devices (cages/spacers) has changed the approach to spinal fusion. The modern-day spinal fusion surgery often involves placing an interbody cage device filled with graft material into the site. Posterior instrumentation such as a rigid pedicle screw system is used to rigidly fix the segment to reduce the mobility, which should encourage bony fusion. Many spacer designs have been developed in different shapes with different materials. Over the years, various surgical approaches for fusion have been adopted, including posterior and posterolateral fusion as well as anterior interbody fusion and posterior lumbar interbody fusion [Lee and Langrana 2004].

Facet joint fixation for restoring stability after fusion has gained some popularity recently because it is less invasive than pedicle screw fixation systems. Phillips et al. [2004] conducted a biomechanical study using spine specimens for the use of translaminar facet screws with a standalone cage. They found that supplementing the standalone cage with a facet joint fixation enhanced the stability of the motion segment under low compressive preload conditions. Beaubien et al. [2004] also performed a cadaveric study with translaminar facet screws in comparison to pedicle screws and reported that the stability offered by the fixation systems was similar.

Fusion surgery, however, has some drawbacks, including adjacent-level degeneration and the potential need for a secondary surgery if the first surgery fails. Adjacent-level degeneration may occur because fusion surgery makes the spinal segment rigid, which in turn causes abnormal loading patterns through the segment. Radiographic fusion success has been reported to be in the 90 to 95% range. However, the clinical success rate of fusion is only about 50 to 70% [Viscogliosi, Viscogliosi, and Viscogliosi 2004].

Several long-term follow-up studies of cervical and lumbar fusion procedures as reported by Throckmorton et al. [2003] suggest that adjacent segment degeneration and adjacent segment disease are common. However, they could not conclude if the findings were the result of the spinal fusion due to rigid motion segment or if they are just the natural progression of degenerative disease.

6.2.6 Dynamic Stabilization

This is a relatively new concept and is intended for use in young patients who are in the early stages of disc degeneration. The aim is to unload the intervertebral disc partially so that more physiological loads may pass through it. A primary advantage of a typical dynamic stabilization system is the ease of the surgical procedure as compared to a fusion surgery. A proposed use of dynamic stabilization systems is in a decompression surgery, whereby the level adjacent to the fusion is fitted with a dynamic system in the hope of avoiding adjacent-level degeneration. In principle, dynamic stabilization devices are fully reversible and thus may represent an early-stage procedure to preserve the disc.

There are two types of dynamic stabilization systems: interspinous spacers and pedicle-screw-based systems. Interspinous spacers are intended to treat lumbar spinal stenosis and disc herniation. Their mode of action is to distract an affected spinal segment by placing it in a slightly flexed position, thus decompressing the nerve root to relieve pain.

Swanson et al. [2003] conducted an *in vitro* test to measure the effect of interspinous spacers on the intervertebral disc pressures and concluded that there was no change in adjacent-level disc pressures and that at the level of instrumentation the disc pressure decreased. In addition, an international clinical study found that postoperative MRI images of patients implanted with the Wallis interspinous spacer showed increased hydration at the treated level in almost 50% of patients [Viscogliosi, Viscogliosi, and Viscogliosi 2004].

Pedicle-screw-based dynamic stabilization systems can be used standalone or in conjunction with fusion to treat disc herniation and spinal stenosis. Clinical trials, performed using the pedicle-screw-based system Dynesys indicate that the device was effective for the treatment of degenerative disc disease and therefore a viable alternative to fusion. However, complications such as screw loosening were seen in some patients. Grob et al. [2005] reported on a clinical study with 50 patients implanted with Dynesys and found that only half the patients had improvement with restored functional capabilities. FEM study comparing both rigid and dynamic stabilization systems showed that partial loading through the disc remains in a dynamic stabilization system [Vishnubhotla et al. 2005].

6.2.7 Arthroplasty

The main goal of spinal arthroplasty is to restore normal mobility to the degenerated segment and to restore disc height. In recent years, spinal arthroplasty has gained interest due to some of the outcomes of fusion surgery, including adjacent-level degeneration and restriction of the mobility of the patient. A total disc replacement surgery involves removing the pain-causing disc, replacing it with a mechanical device that mimics normal spine kinematics. Indications for a total disc replacement (TDR) surgery include advanced stage of disc disease, multiple-level discectomy, or as a secondary procedure after a failed fusion surgery. The TDR devices approved or under study today are either metal-on-metal or metal-on-polyethylene designs. The various artificial discs that have evolved for cervical spine include the Prestige, Bryan and the Prodisc. Lumbar spine TDRs include the Charité, Prodisc II, and Maverick [Anderson and Rouleau 2004].

In an early clinical trial comparing fusion with disc replacement, Delamarter et al. [2003] indicated that disc replacement patients reported significantly less pain and disability. McAfee et al. [2003] reported on 60 prospective randomized cases in the United States for one-level discogenic pain. A third of the cases underwent fusion and the other two-thirds received a Charité disc replacement [McAfee et al. 2003]. They used functional outcome measurements and found that the results following TDR were comparable to fusion.

Complications observed after implantation of up to 127 months after implantation of Charité artificial disc included degeneration of other lumbar discs, facet joint arthrosis at the same or other levels, and subsidence of the prosthesis [van Ooij, Oner, and Verbout 2003]. The precise surgical implantation of the device is of primary concern because improper placement could cause abnormal load distribution through the segment. The subsidence of the artificial disc is also an issue that needs to be further studied and followed, as is the issue of wear debris. Hallab et al. [2003] conducted a study that highlighted the association between spinal implants' particulate wear debris and increased potential for osteolysis. More such studies are required to definitively report on the association between wear debris and osteolysis in the spine.

6.2.8 Nucleus Replacement Technologies

These technologies are intended to restore disc height and maintain normal biomechanical behavior, including range of motion. The indications for use of a nucleus replacement device are loss of disc height and disc herniation in patients who have relatively healthy discs and for whom fusion might be an excessive treatment. The contraindications for nucleus replacement are excessive loss of disc height and incompetent annulus and spondylolysis of grade higher than 1.

The advantage of using these devices is the ease of surgery when compared to fusion or total disc replacement. In the actual surgery, the annulus is retained and the herniated or degenerated material is removed. The posterior approach is most commonly used and the artificial nucleus is placed using the recommended technique for the device (e.g., distraction for proper disc height, pressurized injection, and so on). In the different designs proposed, a variety of materials are being used, including polymers, ceramics, injectable fluids, and hydrogels. Some designs, such as hydrogel-based concepts, allow for fluid transfer as well as swelling under hydrostatic pressure, thereby permitting the devices to behave in principle more like the natural nucleus. Jin et al. [2003] conducted a six-month clinical follow-up study on one such device, the PDN (prosthetic disc nucleus), to evaluate its efficacy in the treatment of disc herniation and concluded that implantation of the PDN restored disc heights and showed good functional and clinical results. A few of the complications arising from using these devices are device migration, failure, and dislocation. For example, Klara and Ray [2002] modified the design of the PDN device and the surgical procedure to mitigate potential migration. They also reported that after these changes the outcomes improved significantly. Only a small percentage of patients required revision surgery.

6.2.9 Annulus Repair Technology

Annulus repair consists of mechanical solutions to reinforce the annulus. Current technology uses autograft tissue or polymers to create a sealing mechanism. This technology can in principle be used along with nucleus replacement surgery in an attempt to avoid recurrent herniation. Holekamp et al. [2002] studied, using *in vitro* and finite element studies, the effects of changing mechanical properties of a disc sealant on the range of motion of the spinal segment. They found that a disc sealant increased the rotational resistance of the treated level as compared to the resistance following just an annulotomy.

6.2.10 Disc Regeneration

The previously cited treatment modalities for disc degeneration do not guarantee long-term pain relief or the need for revision surgeries. Fusion reduces mobility of the segment and reduces the pain to some extent, but induces abnormal stresses at the adjacent segments (which might cause degeneration at those levels). In TDR surgeries or nucleus replacement surgeries there is always a possibility of device failure, subsidence and migration, and other unforeseen complications. However, considering the prevalence of low back pain in the young population regenerating the disc may provide the best option in the future. Hence, the ideal approach to treat intervertebral disc degeneration is to find a way to regenerate the tissue and cells. Mochida et al. [2005] reported that nucleus pulposus has an important role in preserving overall disc structure, like the annulus fibrosis cells. They also concluded that injecting nucleus pulposus cells slowed disc degeneration. They have stated that the cavity for nucleus pulposus was advantageous in retaining transplanted cells. However, many factors come into play, such as the extent of disc degeneration and extent of loss of height. If the patient has a chronic back pain, the regeneration of cells might not be the best approach.

   An et al. have described the methods by which the disc can be regenerated in early, intermediate, and advanced stages of disc disease [An, Thonar, and Masuda 2003]. They state that injecting growth factors such as OP-1 will induce regeneration of the disc. For advanced stages, the cells or tissues that carry specific genes can be introduced. They have also conducted animal studies to show that injection of the growth factors initiated regeneration.

Another approach to regenerate nucleus is to implant cell-seeded collagen-based scaffolds in the disc space [Long et al. 2005]. Long et al. have stated that further studies need to be made for the factors for optimization of the cells within the scaffold, which include growth factors and hydrostatic loading. Annulus repair and regeneration is an evolving area aimed at preventing recurrent disc herniation as a standalone or after nucleus replacement. This is done by regenerating type II collagen at a specific site.

6.2.11 Facet Degeneration

The facet joint along with the disc forms a three-joint complex and plays an important part in maintaining the stability of the segment. A facet joint replacement or arthroplasty replaces the degenerated facets with an articulating prosthesis that imitates the motion of the natural facet joint, thus preserving motion. Early clinical trials with facet joint replacements are just beginning to appear in the literature. Additional biomechanical studies will aid in understanding the overall load transfer patterns [Shaw et al. 2005].

6.3 Osteoporosis

Osteoporosis is the most prevalent metabolic bone disease. Although decrease in bone mass is the hallmark of osteoporosis, alterations in bone marrow quality and the rate of bone turnover may also be present. The decrease in bone mass can occur in the cancellous region (as an increase in porosity) and/or in the cortical bone. In 1994, a study group of the World Health Organization (WHO) proposed that osteoporosis in white women be operationally defined as a bone mineral density (BMD) level 2.5 SD below the mean for young women. Osteoporosis is divided into primary and secondary types [Bono and Einhorn 2003]. Primary osteoporosis is further classified into two subtypes: type I, postmenopausal osteoporosis, and type II, senile osteoporosis. Peak bone mass is achieved around 20 years of age, and thereafter bone mass continuously decreases. The rate of decrease varies among genders: 0.3% per year in males versus 0.5% in females. However, in females during the first five years after menopause the rate in decrease can be as high as 6% per year [Riggs and Melton 1992]. Postmenopausal osteoporosis mostly manifests itself as a loss in trabecular bone, whereas in senile osteoporosis both cortical and trabecular bone are affected [Riggs and Melton 1983].

From a mechanical perspective, the strength of osteoporotic vertebra is low and therefore presents a challenge for stabilization using instrumentation (e.g., anchoring of pedicle screws) [Cook et al. 2004; Renner et al. 2004; Yuan et al. 1994]. The fusion rate is also adversely affected. The decrease in bone mass over time can lead to collapse of the vertebral body height in the anterior region, leading to osteoporotic kyphosis. Although some osteoporotic fractures can be treated with hyperextension braces and bed rest, posterolateral fusion with segmental instrumentation and iliac crest graft in addition to brace may be indicated in some cases [Liew and Simmons 1998]. Such an aggressive intervention, however, may be contraindicated in many patients with vertebral compression fractures due to comorbidities found in the typically elderly population prone to such fractures. Education, adequate nutrition, and strengthening exercises along with hormone therapy (such as use of bisphosphonates, etidronate, and alendronate) are also important in preventing fractures and/or increasing bone mineral density.

Relatively few candidates are able to survive an open surgical reconstruction following a vertebral compression fracture (VCF). This led interventional neuroradiologists in France to develop vertebroplasty to stabilize and to strengthen the osteoporotic collapsed vertebral bodies. In vertebroplasty, bone cement is percutaneously injected into the fractured body [Galibert et al. 1987]. Vertebroplasty has been reported to provide a good clinical outcome in terms of reducing fracture pain [Barr et al. 2000; Evans et al. 2003; Jenson et al. 1997]. However, the technique suffers from several shortcomings. These primarily include that vertebroplasty cannot address the spinal kyphotic deformity, and that it has the concomitant complication of cement leaks through the fracture clefts or the venous sinuses because the cement is injected under pressure [Harrington 2001; Padovani et al. 1999; Ryu et al. 2002]. To overcome some of these limitations of vertebroplasty, kyphoplasty was developed. Kyphoplasty is an advanced technique used to treat osteoporotic or osteolytic painful vertebral compression fractures. Using a specially designed cannula into the vertebral body and an inflatable bone tamp, the collapsed end plates are elevated to their original heights, while creating a cavity to be filled with bone cement. By this maneuver, the height of anterior wall and the sagittal alignment of the spine may be restored, providing patients with both cosmetic and functional improvements. Unlike vertebroplasty, in the kyphoplasty technique bone cement can be injected without pressure. Thus, leakage of bone cement into the spinal canal has been rarely reported [Garfin, Yuan, and Reiley 2001; Ledlie and Renfro 2003; Lieberman et al. 2001; Liew and Simmons 1998; Togawa et al. 2003]. Since the first kyphoplasty was performed in 1998 [Garfin, Yuan, and Reiley 2001], presently over 150,000 patients in the United States have had kyphoplasty for over 175,000 fractures. Over 90% of patients reported significant pain relief.

6.3.1 Osteoporotic Compression Fracture

The National Osteoporosis Foundation estimates that over 100 million people worldwide, and nearly 30 million in the United States, are at risk to develop fragility fractures secondary to osteoporosis. In the United States, there are an estimated 700,000 pathological vertebral body compression fractures each year, with more than a third of such cases reporting chronic pain. The cost for treatment of osteoporotic fracture is estimated to reach $15 billion annually.

BMD is one of the most important determinants of vertebral fracture risk. Roughly, it has been considered that risk of fracture increases twofold with one standard deviation (1 SD) reduction in BMD. Melton et al. [1998] showed total hip BMD was the strongest predictor of fracture risk in women (odds ratio per 1 SD decline, 2.4), whereas wrist BMD was best for men (odds ratio per 1 SD decline, 1.5). Theoretically, the BMD in the lumbar region should be the most predictive value. However, BMD value of the lumbar region is not suitable for understanding age-related bone loss of the spine due to the effects of osteoarthritic sclerotic changes and osteophytes that are often present in the lumbar region [Jones et al. 1995; Masud et al. 1993; Orwoll, Oviatt, and Mann 1990; Reid et al. 1991].

Osteoporotic fractures are most prevalent in females, in that their BMD is always lower than that of males and because of postmenopausal-related architectural changes in the cancellous bone. The presence of a kyphotic deformity is a strong risk factor for the vertebral fracture [Kayanja, Togawa, and Lieberman 2005; Keller et al. 2003]. After adjusting for BMD, weight, and other covariates, white and Hispanic women were found to have the highest risk for fracture (relative risk, RR 1.0 [reference group] and 0.95; 95% CI, 0.76, 1.20, respectively), followed by Native Americans (RR, 0.87; 95% CI, 0.57, 1.32), blacks (RR, 0.52; 95% CI, 0.38, 0.70), and Asian Americans (RR, 0.32; 95% CI, 0.15, 0.66) [Barrett-Connor et al. 2005]. Although black women had the highest BMD levels and Asian women had the lowest BMD levels, these two groups had a similar low risk of fracture, and may reflect musculoskeletal factors other than BMD that are important in fracture prediction. Patients with kyphotic deformities due to osteoporotic compression fractures sometimes experience physical, emotional, and social limitations [Cook et al. 1993; Cortet et al. 1999; Ettinger et al. 1992; Leidig et al. 1990; Leidig-Bruckner et al. 1997]. Women whose deformities were more than 4 SD away from the average had a 1.9 times higher risk of moderate to severe back pain and 2.6 times higher risk of disability involving the back. Also, they were 2.5 times more likely to have lost greater than or equal to 4 cm in height. Although the actual mechanism is unclear, some investigations indicate that the changes in BMD may be related to back extensor weakness [Sinaki et al. 1996].

Others have speculated that the relative weakness of the extensor muscles may increase the possibility of compressing the vertebral body [Beimborn and Morrissey 1988; Ettinger et al. 1992; Limburg et al. 1991]. It is well known that severe thoracic deformity with scoliosis impairs pulmonary function. Thus, one can assume that thoracic spinal deformation due to osteoporotic compression fracture may lead to reduced pulmonary function. If the pulmonary function is impaired due to kyphotic deformation after compression fracture, one may speculate that in such patients mortality rates should be higher. Although the mechanism is unclear, several authors have found that vertebral fractures were associated with increased cancer mortality [Kado et al. 1999]. Kado et al. [1999] hypothesized that some cytokines, which are released from malignant neoplasms, may affect skeletal metabolism and be mediators of bone loss. Furthermore (as described in the next section), bisphosphonate is an anti-cancer drug as well as a drug for osteoporosis. Thus, one can assume that the underlying pathogenesis of vertebral fractures and that of cancer spread may have a common denominator.

6.4 Cancer: Metastatic Spine Tumor

The spinal column is one of the most common sites of cancer metastasis [Wong, Fornasier, and MacNab 1990]. Seventy percent of the spine tumors are reported in the thoracic region, with 20% in the lumbar spine and 10% in the cervical spine region. In 1986, Harrington classified the metastatic spinal tumor into five categories: (1) no significant neurologic involvement, (2) involvement of bone without collapse or instability, (3) major neurologic impairment (sensor or motor) without significant involvement of bone, (4) vertebral collapse with pain resulting from mechanical causes or instability, but with no significant neurologic compromise, and (5) vertebral collapse or instability combined with major neurologic impairment. The clinical problems of spine metastasis are pain and neurological deficit. Treatment includes chemotherapy, radiation therapy, and surgery. According to Harrington, patients in category 4 or 5 are candidates for surgical intervention.

The surgical treatment of spinal metastasis is still controversial. In patients who have an expected survival period of more than two years, the goal for surgery should be long-term local control. For such patients, a palliative surgery such as decompression and fusion without total resection of tumor is not appropriate because after palliative surgery (largely intra-lesional resection) the rate of local recurrence appears to be very high. Oncologic concepts should be taken into account for long-term local control, such as total en-bloc spondylectomy (Figure 6.8). For example, the entire vertebrae can be removed by posterior approach [Tomita et al. 1994, 1997, 2001]. The total en-bloc spondylectomy can lead to a complete loss of spinal stability, in that the vertebral bone and surrounding ligaments are removed with tumor, especially in case the bone graft does not heal/fuse. There is thus a need to establish a method to surely obtain bone union of the grafted materials, which might include the use of growth factors such as BMP at the corpectomized space.

For pain management of the spine metastasis, radiotherapy has widely been conducted. When radiotherapy is not effective, surgical intervention is considered as described previously. Other than spinal reconstruction fusion surgery, recently minimally invasive spinal procedures such as vertebroplasty and kyphoplasty have been used to reduce pain [Barr et al. 2000; Lieberman and Reinhardt 2003; Levine et al. 2000; Weill et al. 1996]. Good indications for these procedures include poor surgical candidates with disabling pain secondary to a pathologic thoracic or lumbar vertebral fracture without epidural compression. For both vertebroplasty and kyphoplasty, bone cement type material is placed into the collapsed vertebral body through the pedicles percutaneously. In the treatment of osteoporotic fractures, complete relief of symptoms has been reported for 90% of patients, whereas in the treatment of osteolytic bone metastases the results have been slightly poorer (about an 80% success rate). It has

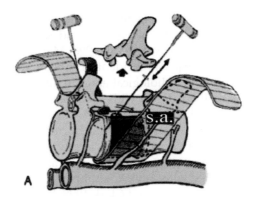

Fig. 6.8.
Surgical technique of the en-bloc spondyloctomy [Tomita et al. 1997].

also been reported that complication rates in patients with metastasis are higher than those of osteoporotic patients. The reported rates of complication are 1.3% in osteoporosis and 10% in metastatic disease.

Traditionally, conservative treatment using drugs for patients with metastatic spinal tumor have mainly focused on pain control using opioids or NSAIDS. Recently, more aggressive drug treatment has been realized for spine metastasis patients, using bisphosphonate. Bisphosphonates bind preferentially to bone at sites of active bone metabolism, are released from the bone matrix during bone resorption, and potently inhibit osteoclast activity and survival, thereby reducing osteoclast-mediated bone resorption. Furthermore, more recently bisphosphonates have been reported to have direct anti-cancer effects, indicating that the role of this drug may continue to expand [Green 2004].

An anti-VEGF (vascular endotherial growth factor) antibody drug, bevacizumab has a possibility to be used for bone metastasis for the future. Angiogenesis is essential for the growth of most malignant tumor and their subsequent metastasis. The VEGF plays the most important role in its angiogenesis. Thus, a variety of therapeutic strategies aimed at blocking VEGF or its receptor signaling system are currently being developed. Bevacizumab is one such drug and is the most advanced in clinical development and has shown promising results in clinical trials. Presently, there is no report on this drug for spinal metastasis. However, this class of drugs may be effective in treating bone metastatic tumors at some point in the future.

6.5 Rheumatoid Arthritis

The prevalence of rheumatoid arthritis (RA) worldwide has been estimated to be 1 to 2% of the population. In the United States, rheumatoid arthritis affects over 2 million patients [Linos et al. 1980]. It is the most common inflammatory disorder of the cervical spine. The incidence of cervical involvement in RA has been reported to vary between 25 and 80% [Cabot and Becker 1978; Casey and Crockard 1995; Fujiwara et al. 1998; Matthews 1974; Pellicci et al. 1981; Reiter and Boden 1998]. The incident of myelopathy has not been correlated to the incidence of the radiological abnormality. Based on the prospective follow-up analysis of 106 patients with rheumatoid arthritis, Pellicci et al. [1981] found cervical spine involvement in 80% of patients at the final follow-up. However, only 36% showed neurological abnormalities at that time.

The types of cervical spine involvement seen in rheumatoid arthritis, in decreasing order of frequency, include anterior atlanto-axial subluxation (AAS), AAS combined with subaxial subluxation (SAS), isolated SAS, and vertical sub-luxation (VS) [Ballard and Clark 1998; Boden and Clark 1998]. From these data sets, various rationales with respect to certain musculoskeletal structures have been developed in support of the radiographic findings. Most believe that inflammatory destruction via synovitis of the atlantal transverse ligament leads to AP instability of the atlanto-axial joint [Boos et al. 1997; Etter et al. 1991]. The manifestation of this instability is anterior subluxation of the atlas on the axis. Erosion of the odontoid process is frequently coincident with the development of AAS.

Protrusion of the odontoid process posteriorly into the spinal canal can result in clinical symptoms or signs such as suboccipital pain and myelopathy. Further progression of the disease involves loss of alar and capsular ligament integrity (in addition to further destruction of the transverse ligament) and advanced osseous erosion of the odontoid process. Finally, loss of atlanto-occipital and atlanto-axial articulation integrity via joint surface destruction and atlantal lateral mass erosion and osteolysis leads to cranial settling or basilar invagination of the odontoid process. Occipitalization of the atlas has been shown to result in irreversible paralysis and death.

Radiographic diagnostic criteria have been developed as descriptors of existence and advancement of anterior atlanto-axial subluxation. One of the most commonly used criteria—posterior atlanto-dental interval (PADI) (Figure 6.9)—measures the distances between the atlas and the odontoid process on flexion lateral views [Boden et al. 1993]. The determination of PADI involves constructing a line that connects the centroids of the anterior and posterior rings of the atlas on a lateral plain radiograph at maximal flexion. PADI is then measured as the distance between the posterior surface of the odontoid process and the anterior surface of the posterior ring of the atlas. Most studies define the existence of AAS when the PADI is less than or equal to 14 mm [Boden et al. 1993]. PADI less than 14 (mm) yields a 97% sensitivity for detecting patients with paralysis [El-Khoury et al. 1980].

To evaluate vertical subluxation (VS), the Ranawat value—or the distance between the center of the pedicles of axis to a line connecting the anterior and posterior arch of the atlas—is measured [Ranawat et al. 1979]. A distance less than 13 mm indicates the presence of VS. Redlund-Johnell's (RJ) occipito-atlanto-axial index is also used as an indicator of VS. The RJ index is measured by the distance from McGregor's line to the sagittal midpoint at the base of the axis. A value of less than 33 (mm) for males and less than 27 (mm) for females

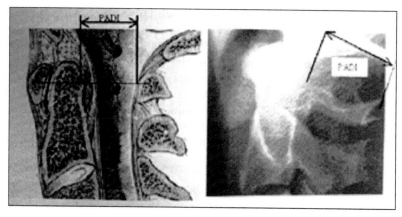

Fig. 6.9.
Measurement of PADI [Puttlitz 1999].

is considered indicative of VS. In the subaxial cervical spine, subluxation (SS) is defined when the displacement of the superior on the inferior vertebra is more than 3 mm on radiographs with the patient in flexion or extension posture.

There are essential indications for surgery: persistent intractable pain and neurological deficits. Most of the neck pain can be controlled by medication. However, when the pain progresses to intractable pain surgery is considered. Once neurological deficit occurs, the surgical intervention is clearly indicated. Although challenging but not essential from the patients' perspective, cervical instability without neurological deficit and minimal pain is also an indication for surgery. For such patients, prophylactic fusion surgery with or without decompression should decrease the possibility of the neurological involvement. However, there is a risk of added morbidity and mortality due to surgery.

In terms of surgical management for AAS, different strategies to fix the atlanto-axial complex can be found in the literature. Arthrodesis procedures involving the entire craniovertebral junction are difficult and require skillful intervention. Stabilization of the craniovertebral junction is not common. However, its importance for treating rheumatoid-arthritis-associated lesions, fractures, and tumors cannot be underestimated. These procedures are extremely dangerous in that the risk of neural or vascular compromise due to the lesion itself or during implementation of the fusion-promoting hardware is significant. Surgical intervention seeks to fuse the affected areas, thus maintaining safe spatial relationships between the osseous and neural structures. To achieve a solid fusion one must provide rigid fixation in the immediate postoperative period—where, in the limit, motion is eliminated.

Commonly available fixation techniques to stabilize the atlanto-axial complex are posterior wiring procedures (Brooks fusion [1978], Gallie fusion [1939], McGraw's technique [1973]), interlaminar clamps (Halifax) [Cybulski et al. 1988], and transarticular screw [Magerl and Seeman 1986]—either alone or in combination. Currently, the most commonly used technique is Magerl's

C1-C2 transarticular screwing with posterior wiring procedures. However, this technique is associated with a risk of vertebral artery injury [Coric et al. 1996; Gluf, Schmidt, and Apfelbaum 2005]. Approximately 20% of patients indicating atlanto-axial arthrodesis have anatomic variations in the path of the vertebral artery and in the osseous anatomy on at least one side and may not be suitable candidates for transarticular screw placement [Jun 1998; Madawi et al. 1997]. For alternative technique, recently, the use of C1 lateral mass and C2 pedicle screw have been considered [Goel and Laheri 1994; Harms and Melcher 2001]. This technique, compared to the transarticular screwing, has a lower risk of vertebral artery injury.

6.6 Trauma: Whiplash Injury

Whiplash, also called neck sprain or neck strain, is an injury of the soft tissues of the neck. According to the Quebec Task Force on Whiplash-Associated Disorders, whiplash may be defined as "an acceleration-deceleration mechanism of energy transfer to the neck which may result from rear-end or side impact, predominately in motor vehicle accidents, and from other mishaps" [Spitzer et al. 1995]. The energy transfer may result in bony or soft tissue injuries (whiplash injuries), which may in turn lead to a wide variety of clinical manifestations (whiplash-associated disorders, WADs). During whiplash the cervical spine undergoes compression from below as the trunk is forced upward toward the head. As a result it deforms in a sigmoid shape with lower segments forced into extension and upper segments forced into flexion. In the process, the anterior ends of the vertebral bodies separate while the zygapophyeseal joints are impacted. In addition to soft tissue damage, severe whiplash can also injure the intervertebral joints, discs, ligaments, cervical muscles, and nerve roots. The Quebec Task Force on Whiplash-Associated Disorders has categorized the WAD into four grades [Spitzer et al. 1995] (Table 6.1). Most of the whiplash patients have grade 1 or 2 WAD, these being attributed to soft tissue injuries. Thus, this chapter focuses on these two grades with reference to symptom and treatment.

Whiplash injury is essentially a benign condition. It is considered that 80% of patients recover, and the remaining 20% have residual symptoms [Bogduc 2000; Radanov, Sturzenegger, and DiStefano 1995] such as headaches and neck pain. On the other hand, the incidence of patients with chronic pain varies between 4 and 55% [Barnsley, Lord, and Bogduk 1994; Bunketorp, Nordholm, and Carlsson 2002; Carette 1994; Deans et al. 1987; Hildingsson and Toolanen 1990; Radanov, Sturzenegger, and DiStefano 1995]. Hildingsson and Toolanen [1990] reviewed 93 cases with a car-accident soft-tissue injury of the cervical spine prospectively. At follow-up, on an average of 2 years after the accident 42% had recovered completely, 15% had minor discomfort, and 43% had discomfort sufficient to interfere with their capacity for work. Bunketorp et al. [2002] reported a 17-year follow-up for 121 patients with whiplash and found 55% of them had residual disorders referable to the original accident.

Table 6.1.

The Quebec Task Force on whiplash associated disorders (WAD) classification scheme. Spilzer et al. [1995] findings.

Grade	Injury and Symptoms	Signs
1	Probable muscle sprain. Neck stiffness only.	No tenderness and normal range of motion. Normal reflexes and muscle strength in the limbs.
2	Probable muscle and/or ligament sprain. Any combination of neck pain with or without back pain, jaw pain, jaw locking, jaw clicking, limb numbness, dizziness.	Paraspinal tenderness and restricted spine range of motion. Normal reflexes and muscle strength in the limbs.
3	Probable disc protrusion with nerve root impingement. Neck pain, often arm pain or numbness.	Abnormal reflexes and/or muscle weakness, often with sensory changes in a dermatomal pattern suggesting nerve root impingement (typically due to disc protrusion).
4	Cervical fracture and/or dislocation. Neck pain, possibly neurological symptoms in limbs, urinary incontinence due to spinal cord involvement.	Possible hyperreflexia, positive Babinal's sign, motor weakness and sensory changes suggesting spinal cord injury. Radiograph reveals fracture and/or dislocation.

Factors that affect the long-term outcome include female gender, older age, and larger number of dependents, marital status, and not being employed full time. Associated collision-related factors appear to be greater severity of collision, rotated or inclined head position at the time of impact, occupancy in a truck or bus, being a passenger, moving vehicle, not using a seat belt, and non-rear-end collision. Associated clinical factors seem to be initial neck pain and headache intensity, neck pain on palpation, muscle pain, radiating pain or numbness, impaired neck movement, symptoms of radicular deficit, symptoms of nausea, and vision difficulties. More recently, Treleaven et al. [2003] measured the cervical joint position error of whiplash patients with or without dizziness. In patients with dizziness, the joint position error was greater and the authors concluded that cervical mechanoreceptor dysfunction combined with whiplash can be a cause of dizziness. Segal et al [2003] reviewed 83 whiplash patients and found that 55.4% of patients complained of tinnitus and 81.3% showed an acoustic-trauma-like hearing impairment. The underlying injury mechanisms are not clear and warrant additional investigation.

Because whiplash (in WAD 1 or 2) usually only causes damage to the soft tissues of the neck, it is difficult to diagnose the damage on plain radiographs. However, abnormal alignment on radiograph can be a sign of soft tissue damage as the degree of soft tissue swelling can be estimated from retro-pharyngeal space at C3 and retro-tracheal space at C6 [Sun 2000]. The abnormal alignment is indicated by loss of lordosis, local kyphosis, minor sub-luxation, and widening of the interspinous space (fanning). Soft tissue damage can be seen on MRIs as well, especially on T2-weighted images—where ligamentous tears with hemorrhage are visible as high-signal-intensity areas. When neurological signs of patients suggest spinal cord injury or radiculopathy, even though it is rare (WAD 3 or 4 cases), MRI is also the most useful diagnostic tool [Ferrari 2002].

For the initial treatment after the event, historical protocol recommends rest for 10 to 14 days in combination with soft collars. However, recent clinical studies suggest that the rest and motion restrictions are detrimental and may slow down the healing process [Borchgrevink et al. 1998; McKinney, Dornan, and Ryan 1989; Mealy, Brennan, and Fenelon 1986; Rosenfeld, Gunnarsson, and Borenstein 2000; Rosenfeld et al. 2003]. Rosenfeld et al. [2003] concluded, based on their three-year follow-up of a prospective randomized trial in 97 whiplash patients, that active intervention is more effective in reducing pain intensity and sick leave (and in retaining total range of motion) than a standard intervention.

6.6.1 Whiplash-related Infant Injury (Shaken Baby Syndrome)

Guthkelch, a neurosurgeon, reported in 1971 subdural hematoma as a feature of the "battered child syndrome" and postulated that the brain injury was caused by shaking. He wrote that the "relatively large head and puny neck muscles" render the infant particularly vulnerable to whiplash injury. Most life-threatening cases of abusive head trauma in children aged less than two years were associated with shaken baby syndrome [Bruce and Simmerman 1989]. The sequence of events in shaken baby syndrome is initiated by a violent whiplash-type shaking [Blumenthal 2002] (Figure 6.10). The pivotal movement of the head during shaking causes a stretch injury at the craniocervical junction [Geddes et al. 2001; Shannon et al. 1998]. This produces breathing difficulty or apnea. The ensuing hypoxia and shock cause hypoxic ischemic cerebral injury. Further brain damage occurs as a consequence of cerebral edema, intracranial hypertension, and a fall in cerebral perfusion pressure. Recently, diffusion-weighted magnetic resonance imaging (DWIMRI) has assumed an important role in the diagnosis of shaken baby syndrome [Biousse et al. 2002]. It demonstrates cerebral ischemia within minutes of onset and can distinguish between acute and chronic infarction.

6.6.2 Spondylolisthesis

Spondylolisthesis is a forward slip of one vertebra with respect to the inferior vertebra (Figure 6.11). It can occur in children and adults, although the mechanisms are quite different. A brief description of both follows.

6.6.3 Degeneraive (Adult) Spondylolisthesis

This disorder affects both the bony and soft tissue elements of a motion segment [Farfan, Osteria, and Lamy 1976; Inoue et al. 1988; Steffee and Sitkowski 1988].

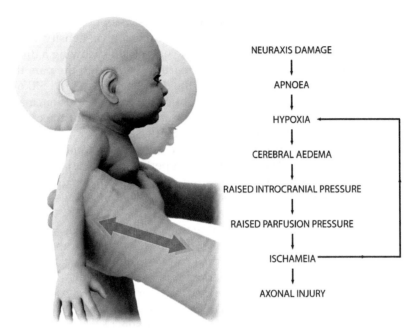

NEURAXIS DAMAGE
↓
APNOEA
↓
HYPOXIA ←
↓
CEREBRAL AEDEMA
↓
RAISED INTROCRANIAL PRESSURE
↓
RAISED PARFUSION PRESSURE
↓
ISCHAMEIA
↓
AXONAL INJURY

Fig. 6.10.
Mechanism of shaken baby syndrome [Blumenthal 2002].

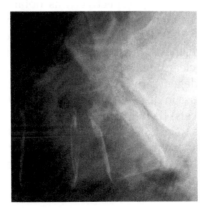

Fig. 6.11.
L5 isthmic spondylolisthesis [Sairyo et al. 2006].

The bony changes observed in the facets are spur formation (osteophytes) around the facets, loose body in the joint, and fracture of the articular surface [Inoue et al. 1988]. Soft-ray roentgenography of the transverse sections of the cadaver spines has revealed a reorientation of the facet joints in a more sagittal direction [Inoue et al. 1988]. The facet angle varied 59 ± 15 degrees in degenerative spondylolisthesis cases as opposed to 40 ± 9.2 degrees in the control group of patients. A comparison of density of the bone bilaterally reveals the calcification of bone on one side showing a different and asymmetric radial pattern. The pseudoarthrosis through the pars that are usually very thin is found to accompany the disorder [Steffee and Sitkowski 1988]. Fibrillation of the articular cartilage, often to complete erosion, may be present as well. The yellow (posterior longitudinal) ligament and the capsule facing the canal are calcified or hypertrophied [Steffee and Sitkowski 1988]. The annulus in this region also becomes thick. The anterior iliolumbar ligamentous complex is stretched and consequently is hypertrophied. The joint capsule on one side may become loose, and under strain the joint is opened up. The degenerative process also alters the disc structure and its function. The gelatinous nucleus pulposus is replaced by the fibrosus tissue [Kirkaldy-Willis et al. 1978]. Circumferential tears in the posterolateral region of the annulus may appear and it is believed that in some cases disc herniation follows. From this point on, further minor mechanical trauma in conjunction with biochemical and immunologic factors ultimately leads to a marked loss in disc height. The annulus bulges around the circumference of the disc. Further loss of the content of the disc results in resorption of the disc. The narrow space between the vertebral bodies is occupied by a small amount of fibrous tissue. Osteophytes also may form.

These degenerative changes ultimately lead to spondylolisthesis [Inoue et al. 1988; Kaneda et al. 1986; Kirkaldy-Willis et al. 1978]. The L4-5 motion segment seems to be the most affected level, followed by the L5-S1 and L3-4 levels. Average percent slip and slip angle at the slipped level are 14.0 ± 7.8 and −2 ± 12.0 degrees, respectively, as obtained from radiographs. The absolute value of the anterior slip (translation) may vary from 2 to 13 mm (average 6.7 mm). Despite a knowledge of the changes associated with the degenerative spondylolisthesis, the exact sequence of changes that leads to spondylolisthesis is not clear [Steiner and Micheli 1985]. The most widely accepted theory is that the degenerative spondylolisthesis begins with disc degeneration (progressive loss in disc height) followed by the breakage of the posterior bony elements (facets) [Feffer et al. 1985; Jensen et al. 1997; Kirkaldy-Willis et al. 1978]. This leads to instability and rotary strain. Because biological tissue is known to respond to external loads, the structural changes associated with the disorder suggest that certain elements of the motion segment must experience large loads during the degenerative process. Biomechanical studies may help identify those structures and provide indirect evidence for or against the proposed theory.

Conservative management of the disorder includes a large number of modalities ranging from nothing to plaster body jackets [Steiner and Micheli 1985]. The literature also shows a wide variation in success rates. There is a general agreement for the surgical indications in the treatment of spondylolisthesis [Klara and Ray 2002]. The strongest indication that surgery is required is persistent pain unresponsive to conservative treatment. The primary aim of the surgery is to remove the pressure from the neural elements whether in the central canal or spinal nerve root canal. Decompressive surgery alone may be a cause of instability. Degenerative spondylolisthesis may develop after laminectomy and extensive facetectomies, especially in younger patients. (This is less likely to happen in the older age group of patients.) The clinical literature suggests excellent results with decompressive surgery and fusion *in situ*. However, some surgeons feel that the vertebra continues to slip forward and many patients continue to have discomfort despite a bony fusion [DeWald et al. 1981; Feffer et al. 1985; Steffe and Sitkowski 1988]. These authors believe that the pain is due to the compression of the L5 root between the L5 pedicle and the thickened, almost vertical, face of the annulus. The *in situ* fusion is incapable of relieving pain in these types of patients. Midline decompression with fusion may resolve pain.

The major problem with this approach, according to these authors, is how to maintain stability until the bone has healed [Kaneda et al. 1986]. The maintenance of proper anatomic relations at the involved levels may be achieved with the use of appropriate spinal instrumentation. This approach has recently gained a boost due to the availability of several fixation devices. These devices are strong enough to resist large loads imposed at the lower lumbar region. Many studies show successful results, but some complications are also reported. For example, the spinal instrumentation is observed to maintain the surgical correction only for a short while; the correction is lost by the follow-up evaluation [Kaneda et al. 1986]. The spinal devices, in the absence of structures that are responsible for maintaining the stability of the spine, are exposed to abnormal loads. The loss of correction over time may be attributed to this factor. Instrumentation failure/loosening has also been observed. Clinical follow-ups also suggest that segments adjacent to the stabilized segment(s) may show degenerative change with time.

6.6.4 Isthmic (Pediatric) Spondylolisthesis

This lumbar spondylolysis arises from stress fracture at the pars interarticularis [Sairyo et al. 2003, 2005; Wiltse 1975]. The incidence has been reported to be about 6% in the entire population [Fredrickson et al. 1984]. Using 3D finite element (FE) methods [Sairyo et al. 2005] of intact lumbar spine (L3-S1), the stress distribution at various structures was calculated during the full range of lumbar spine motion. These studies suggest that the pars interarticularis exhibited the highest stress. However, the stress during extension and rotation was higher than any other motion, indicating these two motions may play a role in the stress fracture.

Traditionally, isthmic spondylolisthesis is diagnosed by the Scottish terrier collar sign on the oblique projection of plain radiograph. However, the stage when it is obvious on the plain radiograph is likely to be the terminal (pseudoarthrosis) stage. CT scan and scintigram have been used to provide an earlier diagnosis. MRI has also begun to be used for early diagnosis [Sairyo et al. 2005]. MRI has the additional advantage of avoiding radiation, which is an important consideration in the pediatric population. The high signal on T2-weighted MR images of pedicle is reported to be a good indicator. Figure 6.12 demonstrates an example of CT and MRI of early-stage spondylolysis. Both

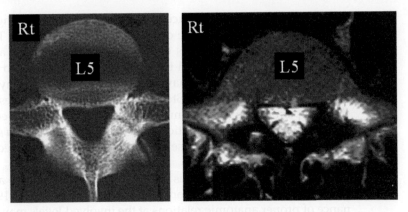

Fig. 6.12.
CT and MRI of early stage of L5 spondylolysis [Sairyo et al. 2006].

right and left sides of pars show early-stage spondylolysis on CT, and the adjoining pedicles show high signal. Also using MRI, other pediatric lumbar disorders—such as apophyseal bony ring fracture and herniated nucleus pulposus—can be diagnosed. At early and progressive stages, the defects still have a possibility for bony healing with conservative treatment [Fujii et al. 2004; Sys et al. 2001]. Therefore, for patients in these stages conservative treatment to obtain bony healing is planned.

6.7 References

Ala-Kokko, L. (2002). "Genetic Risk Factors for Lumbar Disc Disease," *Ann. Med.* 34:42–47.

Alini, M., W. Li, P. Markovic, et al. (2003). "The Potential and Limitations of a Cell-seeded Collagen/Hyaluronan Scaffold to Engineer an Intervertebral Disc-like Matrix," *Spine* 28:446–454.

Al-Sayyad, M. J., A. H. Crawford, and R. K. Wolf (2004). "Early Experiences with Video-assisted Thoracoscopic Surgery: Our First 70 Cases," *Spine* 29:1945–1951.

An, H. S., E. J. Thonar, and K. Masuda (2003). "Biological Repair of Intervertebral Disc," *Spine* 28(15 Suppl.):S86–S92.

An, H. S., P. A. Anderson, V. M. Haughton, et al. (2004). "Disc Degeneration: Summary." *Spine* 29:2677–2678.

An, H. S., S. D. Boden, J. Kang, et al. (2003). "Emerging Techniques for Treatment of Degenerative Lumbar Disc Disease," *Spine* 28(15 Suppl.):S24–S25.

Anderson, P. A., and J. P. Rouleau (2004). "Intervertebral Disc Arthroplasty," *Spine* 29:2779–2786.

Ballard, W. T., and C. R. Clark (1998). "Fractures of the Dens," in C. R. Clark (ed.), *The Cervical Spine*. Philadelphia: Lippincott-Raven.

Barnsley, L., S. Lord, and N. Bogduk (1994). "Whiplash Injury," *Pain* 58:283–307.

Barr, J. D., M. S. Barr, T. J. Lemley, and R. M. McCann (2000). "Percutaneous Vertebroplasty for Pain Relief and Spinal Stabilization," *Spine* 25:923–928.

Barrett-Connor, E., E. S. Siris, L. E. Wehren, et al. (2005). "Osteoporosis and Fracture Risk in Women of Different Ethnic Groups," *J. Bone Miner. Res.* 20:185–194.

Beaubien, B. P., A. A. Mehbod, P. M. Kallemeier, et al. (2004). "Posterior Augmentation of an Anterior Lumbar Interbody Fusion: Minimally Invasive Fixation *Versus* Pedicle Screws In Vitro," *Spine* 29:E406–E412.

Beimborn, D. S., and M. C. Morrissey (1988). "A Review of the Literature Related to Trunk Muscle Performance," *Spine* 13:655–660.

Biousse, V., D. Y. Suh, N. J. Newman, et al. (2002). "Diffusion-weighted Magnetic Resonance Imaging in Shaken Baby Syndrome," *Am. J. Ophthalmol.* 133:249–255.

Blakemore, L. C., P. V. Scoles, C. Poe-Kochert, and G. H. Thompson (2001). "Submuscular Isola Rod with or Without Limited Apical Fusion in the Management of Severe Spinal Deformities in Young Children: Preliminary Report," *Spine* 26:2044–2048.

Blumenthal, I. (2002). "Shaken Baby Syndrome," *Postgrad. Med. J.* 78:732–735.

Boden, S. D. (1994). "Rheumatoid Arthritis of the Cervical Spine: Surgical Decision Making Based on Predictors of Paralysis and Recovery," *Spine* 19:2275–2280.

Boden, S. D., and C. R. Clark (1998). "Rheumatoid Arthritis of the Cervical Spine," in C. R. Clark (ed.), *The Cervical Spine*. Philadelphia: Lippincott-Raven.

Boden, S. D., L. D. Dodge, H. H. Bohlman, and G. R. Rechtine (1993). "Rheumatoid Arthritis of the Cervical Spine: A Long-term Analysis with Predictors of Paralysis and Recovery," *J. Bone Joint Surg. Am.* 75:1282–1297.

Bogduc, N. (2000). "An Overview of Whiplash," in N. Yogananadan and F. A. Pintar (eds.), *Frontiers of Whiplash Trauma*. Amsterdam: IOS Press.

Bono, C. M., and T. A. Einhorn (2003). "Overview of Osteoporosis: Pathophysiology and Determinants of Bone Strength," *Eur. Spine J.* 12 Suppl. 2:S90–S96.

Boos, N., R. Khazim, R. W. Kerslake, et al. (1997). "Atlanto-axial Dislocation Without Fracture: Case Report of an Ejection Injury," *J. Bone Joint Surg. Br.* 79:204–205.

Borchgrevink, G. E., A. Kaasa, D. McDonagh, et al. (1998). "Acute Treatment of Whiplash Neck Sprain Injuries: A Randomized Trial of Treatment During the First 14 Days After a Car Accident," *Spine* 23:25–31.

Brennan, J., and C. Lauryssen (2000). "Current Indications for Posterior Lumbar Interbody Fusions," *Semin. Neuro.* 11.

Brooks, A. L., and E. B. Jenkins (1978). "Atlanto-axial Arthrodesis by the Wedge Compression Method," *J. Bone Joint Surg. Am.* 60:279–284.

Bruce, D. A., and R. A. Zimmerman (1989). "Shaken Impact Syndrome," *Pediatr. Ann.* 18:482–484.

Buck, J. E. (1970). "Direct Repair of the Defect in Spondylolisthesis: Preliminary Report," *J. Bone Joint Surg. Br.* 52:432–437.

Bunketorp, L., L. Nordholm, and J. Carlsson (2002). "A Descriptive Analysis of Disorders in Patients 17 Years Following Motor Vehicle Accidents," *Eur. Spine J.* 11:227–234.

Cabot, A., and A. Becker (1978). "The Cervical Spine in Rheumatoid Arthritis," *Clin. Orthop. Relat. Res.* 131:130–140.

Carette, S. (1994). "Whiplash Injury and Chronic Neck Pain," *N. Engl. J. Med.* 330:1083–1084.

Casey, A. T., and A. Crockard (1995). "In the Rheumatoid Patient: Surgery to the Cervical Spine," *Br. J. Rheumatol.* 34:1079–1086.

Casey, A. T., H. A. Crockard, and J. Stevens (1997). "Vertical Translocation. Part II. Outcomes After Surgical Treatment of Rheumatoid Cervical Myelopathy," *J. Neurosurg.* 87:863–869.

Cassar-Pullicino, V. N. (1998). "MRI of the Ageing and Herniating Intervertebral Disc," *Eur. J. Radiol.* 27:214–228.

Clark, C. R., D. D. Goetz, and A. H. Menezes (1989). "Arthrodesis of the Cervical Spine in Rheumatoid Arthritis," *J. Bone Joint Surg. Am.* 71:381–392.

Cook, D. J., G. H. Guyatt, J. D. Adachi, et al. (1993). "Quality of Life Issues in Women with Vertebral Fractures Due to Osteoporosis," *Arthritis Rheum.* 36:750–756.

Cook, S. D., S. L. Salkeld, T. Stanley, et al. (2004). "Biomechanical Study of Pedicle Screw Fixation in Severely Osteoporotic Bone," *Spine J.* 4:402–408.

Coric, D., C. L. Branch Jr., J. A. Wilson, and J. C. Robinson (1996). "Arteriovenous Fistula as a Complication of C1-2 Transarticular Screw Fixation: Case Report and Review of the Literature," *J. Neurosurg.* 85:340–343.

Cortet, B., E. Houvenagel, F. Puisieux, et al. (1999). "Spinal Curvatures and Quality of Life in Women with Vertebral Fractures Secondary to Osteoporosis," *Spine* 24:1921–1925.

Cotton, A., F. Dewatre, B. Cortet, et al. (1996). "Percutaneous Vertebroplasty for Osteolytic Metastases and Myeloma: Effects of the Percentage of Lesion Filling and the Leakage of Methyl Methacrylate at Clinical Follow-up," *Radiology* 200:525–530.

Cybulski, G. R., J. L. Stone, R. M. Crowell, et al. (1988). "Use of Halifax Interlaminar Clamps for Posterior C1-C2 Arthrodesis," *Neurosurgery* 22:429–431.

Dandy, D. J., and M. J. Shannon (1971). "Lumbosacral Subluxation (Group I Spondylolisthesis)," *J. Bone Joint Surg. [Br]* 53:578–595.

Deans, G. T., J. N. Magalliard, M. Kerr, and W. H. Rutherford (1987). "Neck Sprain: A Major Cause of Disability Following Car Accidents," *Injury* 18:10–12.

Delamarter, R. B., D. M. Fribourg, L. E. Kanim, and H. Bae (2003). "ProDisc Artificial Total Lumbar Disc Replacement: Introduction and Early Results from the United States Clinical Trial," *Spine* 28:S167–S175.

DeWald, R. L., M. M. Faut, R. F. Taddonio, and M. G. Neuwirth (1981). "Severe Lumbosacral Spondylolisthesis in Adolescents and Children: Reduction and Staged Circumferential Fusion," *J. Bone Joint Surg. Am.* 63:619–626.

Drerup, B., M. Granitzka, J. Assheuer, and G. Zerlett (1999). "Assessment of Disc Injury in Subjects Exposed to Long-term Whole-body Vibration," *Eur. Spine J.* 8:458–467.

El-Khoury, G. Y., M. H. Wener, A. H. Menezes, et al. (1980). "Cranial Settling in Rheumatoid Arthritis," *Radiology* 137:637–642.

Etter, C., M. Coscia, H. Jaberg, and M. Aebi (1991). "Direct Anterior Fixation of Dens Fractures with a Cannulated Screw System," *Spine* 16:S25–S32.

Ettinger, B., D. M. Black, M. C. Nevitt, et al. (1992). "Contribution of Vertebral Deformities to Chronic Back Pain and Disability: The Study of Osteoporotic Fractures Research Group," *J. Bone Miner. Res.* 7:449–456.

Evans, A. J., M. E. Jensen, K. E. Kip, et al. (2003). "Vertebral Compression Fractures: Pain Reduction and Improvement in Functional Mobility After Percutaneous Polymethylmethacrylate Vertebroplasty Retrospective Report of 245 Cases," *Radiology* 226:366–372.

Farfan, H. F. (1980). "The Pathological Anatomy of Degenerative Spondylolisthesis: A Cadaver Study," *Spine* 5:412–418.

Farfan, H. F., V. Osteria, and C. Lamy (1976). "The Mechanical Etiology of Spondylolysis and Spondylolisthesis," *Clin. Orthop.* 117:40–55.

Feffer, H. L., S. W. Wiesel, J. M. Cuckler, and R. H. Rothman (1985). "Degenerative Spondylolisthesis: To Fuse or Not to Fuse," *Spine* 10:287–289.

Ferguson, S. J., and T. Steffen (2003). "Biomechanics of the Aging Spine," *Eur. Spine J.* 12(Suppl. 12):S97–S103.

Ferrari, R. (2002). "Prevention of Chronic Pain After Whiplash," *Emerg. Med. J.* 19:526–530.

Fleisch, H. (2002). "Development of Bisphosphonates," *Breast Cancer Res.* 4:30–34.

Fredrickson, B. E., D. Baker, W. J. McHolick, et al. (1984). "The Natural History of Spondylolysis and Spondylolisthesis," *J. Bone Joint Surg. Am.* 66:699–707.

Friberg, S. (1939). "Studies on Spondylolisthesis," *Acta. Chir. Scand.* 55.

Fujii, K., S. Katoh, K. Sairyo, et al. (2004). "Union of Defects in the Pars Interarticularis of the Lumbar Spine in Children and Adolescents: The Radiological Outcome After Conservative Treatment," *J. Bone Joint Surg. Br.* 86:225–231.

Fujiwara, K., M. Fujimoto, H. Owaki, et al. (1998). "Cervical Lesions Related to the Systemic Progression in Rheumatoid Arthritis," *Spine* 23:2052–2056.

Galibert, P., H. Deramond, P. Rosat, and D. Le Gars (1987). [Preliminary note on the treatment of vertebral angioma by percutaneous acrylic vertebroplasty]. *Neurochirurgie* 33:166–168.

Gallie, W. (1939). "Fractures and Dislocations of the Cervical Spine," *Am. J. Surg.* 46:495–499.

Gamradt, S. C., and J. C. Wang (2005). "Lumbar Disc Arthroplasty," *Spine J.* 5:95–103.

Garfin, S. R., H. A. Yuan, and M. A. Reiley (2001). "New Technologies in Spine: Kyphoplasty and Vertebroplasty for the Treatment of Painful Osteoporotic Compression Fractures," *Spine* 26:1511–1515.

Geddes, J. F., and J. Plunkett (2004). "The Evidence Base for Shaken Baby Syndrome," *BMJ* 328:719–720.

Geddes, J. F., A. K. Hackshaw, G. H. Vowles, et al. (2001). "Neuropathology of Inflicted Head Injury in Children: I. Patterns of Brain Damage," *Brain* 124(Pt. 7):1290–1298.

Gluf, W. M., M. H. Schmidt, and R. I. Apfelbaum (2005). "Atlantoaxial Transarticular Screw Fixation: A Review of Surgical Indications, Fusion Rate, Complications, and Lessons Learned in 191 Adult Patients," *J. Neurosurg. Spine* 2:155–163.

Goel, A., and V. Laheri (1994). "Plate and Screw Fixation for Atlanto-axial Subluxation," *Acta Neurochir. (Wien)* 129:47–53.

Goel, V. K., and J. N. Weinstein (1980). *Clinical Biomechanics of the Lumbar Spine*. Boca Raton: CRC Press.

Goel, A., K. I. Desai, and D. P. Muzumdar (2002). "Atlantoaxial Fixation Using Plate and Screw Method: A Report of 160 Treated Patients," *Neurosurgery* 51:1351–1356; discussion 1356–1357.

Green, J. R. (2004). "Bisphosphonates: Preclinical Review," *Oncologist* 9(Suppl. 14):3–13.

Grob, D., A. Benini, A. Junge, and A. F. Mannion (2005). "Clinical Experience with the Dynesys Semirigid Fixation System for the Lumbar Spine," *Spine* 30:324–331.

Guthkelch, A. N. (1971). "Infantile Subdural Haematoma and Its Relationship to Whiplash Injuries," *Br. Med. J.* 2:430–431.

Hadley-Miller, N., B. Mims, and D. M. Milewicz (1994). "The Potential Role of the Elastic Fiber System in Adolescent Idiopathic Scoliosis," *J. Bone Joint Surg. Am.* 76:1193–1206.

Hallab, N. J., B. W. Cunningham, and J. J. Jacobs (2003). "Spinal Implant Debris-Induced Osteolysis," *Spine* 28:S125–S138.

Harms, J., and R. P. Melcher (2001). "Posterior C1-C2 Fusion with Polyaxial Screw and Rod Fixation," *Spine* 26:2467–2471.

Harrington, K. D. (1986). "Impending Pathologic Fractures from Metastatic Malignancy: Evaluation and Management," *Instr. Course Lect.* 35:357–381.

Harrington, K. D. (2001). "Major Neurological Complications Following Percutaneous Vertebroplasty with Polymethylmethacrylate: A Case Report," *J. Bone Joint Surg. Am.* 83A:1070–1073.

Harrington, P. R. (1977). "The Etiology of Idiopathic Scoliosis," *Clin. Orthop.* 126:17–25.

Haughton, V. (2004). "Medical Imaging of Intervertebral Disc Degeneration," *Spine* 29:2751–2756.

Hildingsson, C., and G. Toolanen (1990). "Outcome After Soft-tissue Injury of the Cervical Spine: A Prospective Study of 93 Car-accident Victims," *Acta Orthop. Scand.* 61:357–359.

Holekamp, S., V. Goel, N. Ebraheim, and H. Kuroki (2005). "The Effect of Material Properties on Annulotomy Sealant Biomechanics." The 51st Annual Meeting of Orthopedic Research Society. Washington, D.C.

Ikata, T., R. Miyake, S. Katoh, et al. (1996). "Pathogenesis of Sports-related Spondylolisthesis in Adolescents: Radiographic and Magnetic Resonance Imaging Study," *Am. J. Sports Med.* 24:94–98.

Inoue, S., T. Watanabe, S. Goto, K. Takahashi, et al. (1988). "Degenerative Spondylolisthesis: Pathophysiology and Results of Anterior Interbody Fusion," *Clin. Orthop. Relat. Res.* 227:90–98.

James, J. I., G. C. Lloyd-Roberts, and M. F. Pilcher (1959). "Infantile Structural Scoliosis," *J. Bone Joint Surg. Br.* 41B:719–735.

Jensen, M. E., A. J. Evans, J. M. Mathis, et al. (1997). "Percutaneous Polymethylmethacrylate Vertebroplasty in the Treatment of Osteoporotic Vertebral Body Compression Fractures: Technical Aspects," *Am. J. Neuroradiol.* 18:1897–1904.

Jevtic, V. (2001). "Magnetic Resonance Imaging Appearances of Different Discovertebral Lesions," *Eur. Radio.* 11:1123–1135.

Jin, D., D. Qu, L. Zhao, et al. (2003). "Prosthetic Disc Nucleus (PDN) Replacement for Lumbar Disc Herniation: Preliminary Report with Six Months Follow-up," *J. Spinal. Disord. Tech.* 16:331–337.

Jones, G., T. Nguyen, P. N. Sambrook, et al. (1995). "A Longitudinal Study of the Effect of Spinal Degenerative Disease on Bone Density in the Elderly," *J. Rheumatol.* 22:932–936.

Jun, B. Y. (1998). "Anatomic Study for Ideal and Safe Posterior C1-C2 Transarticular Screw Fixation," *Spine* 23:1703–1707.

Kado, D. M., W. S. Browner, L. Palermo, et al. (1999). "Vertebral Fractures and Mortality in Older Women: A Prospective Study," Study of Osteoporotic Fractures Research Group. *Arch. Intern. Med.* 159:1215–1220.

Kajiura, K., S. Katoh, K. Sairyo, et al. (2001). "Slippage Mechanism of Pediatric Spondylolysis: A Biomechanical Study Using Immature Calf Spine," *Spine* 26:2208–2213.

Kaneda, K., H. Kazama, S. Satoh, and M. Fujiya (1986). "Follow-up Study of Medial Facetectomies and Posterolateral Fusion with Instrumentation in Unstable Degenerative Spondylolisthesis," *Clin. Orthop. Relat. Res.* 203:159–167.

Kayanja, M. M., D. Togawa, and I. H. Lieberman (2005). "Biomechanical Changes After the Augmentation of Experimental Osteoporotic Vertebral Compression Fractures in the Cadaveric Thoracic Spine," *Spine J.* 5:55–63.

Keller, T. S., D. E. Harrison, C. J. Colloca, et al. (2003). "Prediction of Osteoporotic Spinal Deformity," *Spine* 28:455–462.

Kirkaldy-Willis, W. H., J. H. Wedge, K. Yong-Hing, and J. Reilly (1978). "Pathology and Pathogenesis of Lumbar Spondylosis and Stenosis," *Spine* 3:319–328.

Klara, P. M., and C. D. Ray (2002). "Artificial Nucleus Replacement, Clinical Experience," *Spine* 27:1374–1377.

Klemme, W. R., F. Denis, R. B. Winter, et al. (1997). "Spinal Instrumentation Without Fusion for Progressive Scoliosis in Young Children," *J. Pediatr. Orthop.* 17:734–742.

Konz, R. J., V. K. Goel, L. J. Grobler, et al. (2001). "The Pathomechanism of Spondylolytic Spondylolisthesis in Immature Primate Lumbar Spines: In Vitro and Finite Element Assessments," *Spine* 26:E38–E49.

Laurent, L. E. (1958). "Spondylolisthesis," *Acta Orthop. Scand.* 27(Suppl. 35):1–45.

Laurent, L. E., and S. Einola (1961). "Spondylolisthesis in Children and Adolescents," *Acta Orthop. Scand.* 31:45–64.

Ledlie, J. T., and M. Renfro (2003). "Balloon Kyphoplasty: One-year Outcomes in Vertebral Body Height Restoration, Chronic Pain, and Activity Levels," *J. Neurosurg.* 98:36–42.

Leidig, G., H. W. Minne, P. Sauer, et al. (1990). "A Study of Complaints and Their Relation to Vertebral Destruction in Patients with Osteoporosis," *J. Bone Miner. Res.* 8:217–229.

Leidig-Bruckner, G., H. W. Minne, C. Schlaich, et al. (1997). "Clinical Grading of Spinal Osteoporosis: Quality of Life Components and Spinal Deformity in Women with Chronic Low Back Pain and Women with Vertebral Osteoporosis," *J. Bone Miner. Res.* 12:663–675.

Lee, C. K., and N. A. Langrana (2004). "A Review of Spinal Fusion for Degenerative Disc Disease: Need for Alternative Treatment Approach of Disc Arthroplasty?," *Spine J.* 4(Suppl. 6):173S–176S.

Lenke, L. G. (2003). "Anterior Endoscopic Discectomy and Fusion for Adolescent Idiopathic Scoliosis," *Spine* 28(Suppl. 15):S36–S43.

Lenke, L. G., and M. B. Dobbs (2004). "Idiopathic Scoliosis," in J. W. Frywoyer and S. W. Wiesel (eds.), *The Adult and Pediatric Spine* (3d ed.). Philadelphia: Lippincott Williams & Wilkins.

Lenke, L. G., R. R. Betz, D. Clements, et al. (2002). "Curve Prevalence of a New Classification of Operative Adolescent Idiopathic Scoliosis: Does Classification Correlate with Treatment?," *Spine* 27:604–611.

Lenke, L. G., R. R. Betz, J. Harms, et al. (2001). "Adolescent Idiopathic Scoliosis: A New Classification to Determine Extent of Spinal Arthrodesis," *J. Bone Joint Surg. Am.* 83A:1169–1181.

Levine, S. A., L. A. Perin, D. Hayes, and W. S. Hayes (2000). "An Evidence-based Evaluation of Percutaneous Vertebroplasty," *Manag. Care* 9:56–63.

Lieberman, I. H., and M. K. Reinhardt (2003). "Vertebroplasty and Kyphoplasty for Osteolytic Vertebral Collapse," *Clin. Orthop. Relat. Res.* 415:S176–S186.

Lieberman, I. H., S. Dudeney, M. K. Reinhardt, and G. Bell (2001). "Initial Outcome and Efficacy of Kyphoplasty in the Treatment of Painful Osteoporotic Vertebral Compression Fractures," *Spine* 26:1631–1638.

Lieberman, I. H., R. R. Kuzhupilly, M. K. Reinhardt, and W. J. Davros (2001). "Three-dimensional Computed Tomographic Volume Rendering Techniques in Endoscopic Thoracoplasty," *Spine J.* 1:390–394.

Lieberman, I. H., P. T. Salo, R. D. Orr, and B. Kraetschmer (2000). "Prone Position Endoscopic Transthoracic Release with Simultaneous Posterior Instrumentation for Spinal Deformity: A Description of the Technique," *Spine* 25:2251–2257.

Liew, S. M., and E. D. Simmons Jr. (1998). "Thoracic and Lumbar Deformity: Rationale for Selecting the Appropriate Fusion Technique (Anterior, Posterior, and 360-degree)," *Orthop. Clin. North Am.* 29:843–858.

Limburg, P. J., M. Sinaki, J. W. Rogers, et al. (1991). "A Useful Technique for Measurement of Back Strength in Osteoporotic and Elderly Patients," *Mayo Clin. Proc.* 66:39–44.

Linos, A., J. W. Worthington, W. M. O'Fallon, and L. T. Kurland (1980). "The Epidemiology of Rheumatoid Arthritis in Rochester, Minnesota: A Study of Incidence, Prevalence, and Mortality," *Am. J. Epidemiol.* 111:87–98.

Long, R., K. Sairyo, V. K. Goel, et al. (2005). "Biological Evaluation of Gelfoam as a Bioabsorbable Scaffold for Nucleus Pulposus Cells," 32nd Annual Meeting of International Society of Study for the Lumbar Spine. New York, NY.

Luoma, K., H. Riihimaki, R. Luukkonen, et al. (2000). "Lumbar Disc Degeneration in Relation to Occupation," *Spine* 25:487–492.

McAfee, P. C., I. L. Fedder, S. Saiedy, et al. (2003). "SB Charité Disc Replacement, Report of 60 Prospective Randomized Cases in a U.S. Center," *J. Spinal. Disord. Tech.* 16:424–433.

McGraw, R. W., and R. M. Rusch (1973). "Atlantoaxial Arthrodesis," *J. Bone Joint Surg. Br.* 55:482–489.

McKinney, L. A., J. O. Dornan, and M. Ryan (1989). "The Role of Physiotherapy in the Management of Acute Neck Sprains Following Road-traffic Accidents," *Arch. Emerg. Med.* 6:27–33.

McMaster, M. J. (2001). "Congenital Scoliosis," in S. L. Weinstein (ed.), *The Pediatric Spine* (2d ed.). Philadelphia: Lippincott Williams & Wilkins.

Machida, M., J. Dubousset, Y. Imamura, et al. (1993). "An Experimental Study in Chickens for the Pathogenesis of Idiopathic Scoliosis," *Spine* 18:1609–1615.

Machida, M., J. Dubousset, Y. Imamura, et al. (1994). "Pathogenesis of Idiopathic Scoliosis: SEPs in Chickens with Experimentally Induced Scoliosis and in Patients with Idiopathic Scoliosis," *J. Pediatr. Orthop.* 14:329–335.

Machida, M., J. Dubousset, Y. Imamura, et al. (1995). "Role of Melatonin Deficiency in the Development of Scoliosis in Pinealectomised Chickens," *J. Bone Joint Surg. Br.* 77:134–138.

Madawi, A. A., A. T. Casey, G. A. Solanki, et al. (1997). "Radiological and Anatomical Evaluation of the Atlantoaxial Transarticular Screw Fixation Technique," *J. Neurosurg.* 86:961–968.

Magerl, F., and P-S. Seemann (1986). "Stable Posterior Fusion of the Atlas and Axis by Transarticular Screw Fixation," in I. P. Kehr and A. Weidner (eds.), *Cervical Spine.* Wien, New York: Springer-Verlag.

Martinez-Lozano, A. G. (2001). "Radiographic Measurements," in S. L. Weinstein (ed.), *The Pediatric Spine* (2d ed.). Philadelphia: Lippincott Williams & Wilkins.

Masud, T., S. Langley, P. Wiltshire, et al. (1993). "Effect of Spinal Osteophytosis on Bone Mineral Density Measurements in Vertebral Osteoporosis," *BMJ* 307:172–173.

Masuda, A., K. Sairyo, V. K. Goel, et al. (2005). "Forward Slippage in Pediatric Spines Following Spondylolysis: Role of Stresses in the Growth Plate," 32nd Annual Meeting of International Society of Study for the Lumbar Spine. New York, NY.

Mathews, J. A. (1974). "Atlanto-axial Subluxation in Rheumatoid Arthritis: A 5-year Follow-up Study," *Ann. Rheum. Dis.* 33:526–531.

Mealy, K., H. Brennan, and G. C. Fenelon (1986). "Early Mobilization of Acute Whiplash Injuries," *Br. Med. J. (Clin. Res. Ed.)* 292:656–657.

Mehta, M. H. (1972). "The Rib-vertebra Angle in the Early Diagnosis Between Resolving and Progressive Infantile Scoliosis," *J. Bone Joint Surg. Br.* 54:230–243.

Melton, L. J. III, E. J. Atkinson, M. K. O'Connor, et al. (1998). "Bone Density and Fracture Risk in Men," *J. Bone Miner. Res.* 13:1915–1923.

Miller, N. H. (2001). "Adolescent Idiopathic Scoliosis: Etiology," in S. L. Weinstein (ed.), *The Pediatric Spine* (2d ed.). Philadelphia: Lippincott Williams & Wilkins.

Mineiro, J., and S. L. Weinstein (2002). "Subcutaneous Rodding for Progressive Spinal Curvatures: Early Results," *J. Pediatr. Orthop.* 22:290–295.

Mochida, J. (2005). "New Strategies for Disc Repair: Novel Preclinical Trials," *J. Orthop. Sci.* 10:112–118.

Moe, J. H., K. Kharrat, R. B. Winter, and J. L. Cummine (1984). "Harrington Instrumentation Without Fusion Plus External Orthotic Support for the Treatment of Difficult Curvature Problems in Young Children," *Clin. Orthop. Relat. Res.* 185: 35–45.

Neva, M. H., R. Myllykangas-Luosujarvi, H. Kautiainen, and M. Kauppi (2001). "Mortality Associated with Cervical Spine Disorders: A Population-based Study of 1666 Patients with Rheumatoid Arthritis Who Died in Finland in 1989," *Rheumatology (Oxford)* 40:123–127.

Newton, P. O., K. K. White, F. Faro, and T. Gaynor (2005). "The Success of Thoracoscopic Anterior Fusion in a Consecutive Series of 112 Pediatric Spinal Deformity Cases," *Spine* 30:392–398.

Orwoll, E. S., S. K. Oviatt, and T. Mann (1990). "The Impact of Osteophytic and Vascular Calcifications on Vertebral Mineral Density Measurements in Men," *J. Clin. Endocrinol. Metab.* 70:1202–1207.

Padovani, B., O. Kasriel, P. Brunner, and P. Peretti-Viton (1999). "Pulmonary Embolism Caused by Acrylic Cement: A Rare Complication of Percutaneous Vertebroplasty," *Am. J. Neuroradiol.* 20:375–377.

Pellicci, P. M., C. S. Ranawat, P. Tsairis, and W. J. Bryan (1981). "A Prospective Study of the Progression of Rheumatoid Arthritis of the Cervical Spine," *J. Bone Joint Surg. Am.* 63:342–350.

Phillips, F. M., B. Cunningham, G. Carandang, et al. (2004). "Effect of Supplemental Translaminar Facet Screw Fixation on the Stability of Stand-alone Anterior Lumbar Interbody Fusion Cages Under Physiologic Compressive Preloads," *Spine* 29:1731–1736.

Phillips, F. M., E. Ho, M. Campbell-Hupp, et al. (2003). "Early Radiographic and Clinical Results of Balloon Kyphoplasty for the Treatment of Osteoporotic Vertebral Compression Fractures," *Spine* 28:2260–2265.

Picetti, G. D., and D. Pang (2004). "Thoracoscopic Techniques for the Treatment of Scoliosis," *Childs. Nerv. Syst.* 20:802–810.

Puttlitz, C. M. (1999). "*A Biomechanical Investigation of C0-C1-C2*," PhD thesis. University of Iowa.

Radanov, B. P., M. Sturzenegger, and G. Di Stefano (1995). "Long-term Outcome After Whiplash Injury: A 2-year Follow-up Considering Features of Injury Mechanism and Somatic, Radiologic, and Psychosocial Findings," *Medicine (Baltimore)* 74:281–297.

Ranawat, C. S., P. O'Leary, P. Pellicci, et al. (1979). "Cervical Spine Fusion in Rheumatoid Arthritis," *J. Bone Joint Surg. Am.* 61:1003–1010.

Ray, C. D. (2002). "The PDN Prosthetic Disc-nucleus Device," *Eur. Spine. J.* 11(Suppl. 12):S137–S142.

Reid, I. R., M. C. Evans, R. Ames, and D. J. Wattie (1991). "The Influence of Osteophytes and Aortic Calcification on Spinal Mineral Density in Postmenopausal Women," *J. Clin. Endocrinol. Metab.* 72:1372–1374.

Reiter, M. F., and S. D. Boden (1998). "Inflammatory Disorders of the Cervical Spine," *Spine* 23:2755–2766.

Renner, S. M., T. H. Lim, W. J. Kim, et al. (2004). "Augmentation of Pedicle Screw Fixation Strength Using an Injectable Calcium Phosphate Cement as a Function of Injection Timing and Method," *Spine* 29:E212–E216.

Riggs, B. L., and L. J. Melton III (1983). "Evidence for Two Distinct Syndromes of Involutional Osteoporosis," *Am. J. Med.* 75:899–901.

Riggs, B. L., and L. J. Melton III (1992). "The Prevention and Treatment of Osteoporosis," *N. Engl. J. Med.* 327:620–627.

Riseborough, E. J., and R. Wynne-Davies (1973). "A Genetic Survey of Idiopathic Scoliosis in Boston, Massachusetts," *J. Bone Joint Surg. Am.* 55:974–982.

Rosenfeld, M., R. Gunnarsson, and P. Borenstein (2000). "Early Intervention in Whiplash-associated Disorders: A Comparison of Two Treatment Protocols," *Spine* 25:1782–1787.

Rosenfeld, M., A. Seferiadis, J. Carlsson, and R. Gunnarsson (2003). "Active Intervention in Patients with Whiplash-associated Disorders Improves Long-term Prognosis: A Randomized Controlled Clinical Trial," *Spine* 28:2491–2498.

Ryu, K. S., C. K. Park, M. C. Kim, and J. K. Kang (2002). "Dose-dependent Epidural Leakage of Polymethylmethacrylate After Percutaneous Vertebroplasty in Patients with Osteoporotic Vertebral Compression Fractures," *J. Neurosurg.* 96:56–61.

Sahlstrand, T., R. Ortengren, and A. Nachemson (1978). "Postural Equilibrium in Adolescent Idiopathic Scoliosis," *Acta Orthop. Scand.* 49:354–365.

Sahlstrand, T., B. Petruson, and R. Ortengren (1979). "Vestibulospinal Reflex Activity in Patients with Adolescent Idiopathic Scoliosis: Postural Effects During Caloric Labyrinthine Stimulation Recorded by Stabilometry," *Acta Orthop. Scand.* 50:275–281.

Sairyo, K., V. K. Goel, L. J. Grobler, et al. (1998). "The Pathomechanism of Isthmic Spondylolisthesis: A Biomechanical Study in Immature Calf Spine," *Spine* 23:1442–1446.

Sairyo, K., V. K. Goel, A. Masuda, et al. (2005). "Biomechanical Rationale of Endoscopic Decompression for Lumbar Spondylolysis as an Effective Minimally Invasive Procedure: A Study Based on the Finite Element Analysis," *Minim. Invasive Neurosurg.* 48(2):119–122.

Sairyo, K., S. Katoh, T. Ikata, et al. (2001). "Development of Spondylolytic Olisthesis in Adolescents," *Spine J.* 1:171–175.

Sairyo, K., S. Katoh, S. Komatsubara, et al. (2005). "Spondylolysis Fracture Angle in Children and Adolescents on CT Indicates the Facture Producing Force Vector: A Biomechanical Rationale," *Internet J. Spine Surg.* (in press).

Sairyo, K., S. Katoh, T. Sakamaki, et al. (2003). "Three Successive Stress Fractures at the Same Vertebral Level in an Adolescent Baseball Player," *Am. J. Sports Med.* 31: 606–610.

Sairyo, K., S. Katoh, T. Sakamaki, et al. (2004). "Vertebral Forward Slippage in Immature Lumbar Spine Occurs Following Epiphyseal Separation and Its Occurrence Is Unrelated to Disc Degeneration: Is the Pediatric Spondylolisthesis a Physis Stress Fracture of Vertebral Body?," *Spine* 29:524–527.

Sairyo, K., S. Katoh, T. Sasa, et al. (2005). "Athletes with Unilateral Spondylolysis Are at Risk of Stress Fracture at the Contralateral Pedicle and Pars Interarticularis," *Am. J. Sports Med.* 33:580–590.

Sairyo, K., S. Katoh, Y. Takata, et al. (2006). "MRI Signal Changes of the Pedicle as an Indicator for Early Diagnosis of Spondylolysis in Children and Adolescents: A Clinical and Biomechanical Study," *Spine* 31:206–211.

Sakamaki, T., S. Katoh, and K. Sairyo (2002). "Normal and Spondylolytic Pediatric Spine Movements with Reference to Instantaneous Axis of Rotation," *Spine* 27:141–145.

Sakamaki, T., K. Sairyo, S. Katoh, et al. (2003). "The Pathogenesis of Slippage and Deformity in the Pediatric Lumbar Spine: A Radiographic and Histologic Study Using a New Rat In Vivo Model," *Spine* 28:645–650.

Salehi, L. B., M. Mangino, M. S. De Serio, et al. (2002). "Assignment of a Locus for Autosomal Dominant Idiopathic Scoliosis (IS) to Human Chromosome 17p11," *Hum. Genet.* 111:401–404.

Scott, J. C., and T. H. Morgan (1955). "The Natural History and Prognosis of Infantile Idiopathic Scoliosis," *J. Bone Joint Surg. Br.* 37B:400–413.

Segal, S., E. Eviatar, L. Berenholz, et al. (2003). "Hearing Loss After Direct Blunt Neck Trauma," *Otol. Neurotol.* 24:734–737.

Seitsalo, S., K. Osterman, and H. Hyvarinen (1991). "Progression of Spondylolisthesis in Children and Adolescents," *Spine* 16:417–421.

Shannon, P., C. R. Smith, J. Deck, et al. (1998). "Axonal Injury and the Neuropathology of Shaken Baby Syndrome," *Acta Neuropathol. (Berl.)* 95:625–631.

Shaw, M., V. K. Goel, S. Vadapalli, et al. (2005). "Development of Artificial Facets: Biomechanical Perspective. The 51st Annual Meeting of Orthopedic Research Society. Washington, D.C.

Sinaki, M., E. Itoi, J. W. Rogers, et al. (1996). "Correlation of Back Extensor Strength with Thoracic Kyphosis and Lumbar Lordosis in Estrogen-deficient Women," *Am. J. Phys. Med. Rehabil.* 75:370–374.

Spencer, G. S., and M. J. Eccles (1976). "Spinal Muscle in Scoliosis. Part 2. The Proportion and Size of Type 1 and Type 2 Skeletal Muscle Fibres Measured Using a Computer-controlled Microscope," *J. Neurol. Sci.* 30:143–154.

Spitzer, W. O., M. L. Skovron, L. R. Salmi, et al. (1995). "Scientific Monograph of the Quebec Task Force on Whiplash-Associated Disorders: Redefining "Whiplash" and Its Management," *Spine* 20(Suppl. 8):1S–73S.

Steffee, A. D., and D. J. Sitkowski (1988). "Posterior Lumbar Interbody Fusion and Plates," *Clin. Orthop. Relat. Res.* 227:99–102.

Steiner, M. E., and L. J. Micheli (1985). "Treatment of Symptomatic Spondylolysis and Spondylolisthesis with the Modified Boston Brace," *Spine* 10:937–943.

Stokes, I. A. F., and J. C. Iatridis (2004). "Mechanical Conditions That Accelerate Intervertebral Disc Degeneration: Overload *Versus* Immobilization," *Spine* 29:2724–2732.

Sun, Z. (2000). *Emergency Management for Whiplash Injuries.* N. Yogananadan and F. A. Pintar (eds.). Amsterdam: IOS Press.

Swanson, K. E., D. P. Lindsey, K. Y. Hsu, et al. (2003). "The Effects of an Interspinous Implant on Intervertebral Disc Pressures," *Spine* 28:26–32.

Sys, J., J. Michielsen, P. Bracke, et al. (2001). "Nonoperative Treatment of Active Spondylolysis in Elite Athletes with Normal X-ray Findings: Literature Review and Results of Conservative Treatment," *Eur. Spine J.* 10:498–504.

Takaso, M., H. Moriya, H. Kitahara, et al. (1998). "New Remote-controlled Growing-rod Spinal Instrumentation Possibly Applicable for Scoliosis in Young Children," *J. Orthop. Sci.* 3:336–340.

Tanaka, N., H. S. An, T. H. Lim, et al. (2001). "The Relationship Between Disc Degeneration and Flexibility of the Lumbar Spine," *Spine J.* 1:47–56.

Thompson, J. P., R. H. Pearce, M. T. Schechter, et al. (1990). "Preliminary Evaluation of a Scheme for Grading the Gross Morphology of the Human Intervertebral Disc," *Spine* 15:411–415.

Thompson, S. K., and G. Bentley (1980). "Prognosis in Infantile Idiopathic Scoliosis," *J. Bone Joint Surg. Br.* 62B:151–154.

Throckmorton, T. W., A. S. Hilibrand, G. A. Mencio, et al. (2003). "The Impact of Adjacent Level Disc Degeneration on Health Status Outcomes Following Lumbar Fusion," *Spine* 28:2546–2550.

Togawa, D., T. W. Bauer, I. H. Lieberman, and S. Takikawa (2003). "Histologic Evaluation of Human Vertebral Bodies After Vertebral Augmentation with Polymethyl Methacrylate," *Spine* 28:1521–1527.

Tomita, K., N. Kawahara, H. Baba, et al. (1994). "Total En Bloc Spondylectomy for Solitary Spinal Metastases," *Int. Orthop.* 18:291–298.

Tomita, K., N. Kawahara, H. Baba, et al. (1997). "Total En Bloc Spondylectomy: A New Surgical Technique for Primary Malignant Vertebral Tumors," *Spine* 22:324–333.

Tomita, K., N. Kawahara, T. Kobayashi, et al. (2001). "Surgical Strategy for Spinal Metastases," *Spine* 26:298–306.

Treleaven, J., G. Jull, and M. Sterling (2003). "Dizziness and Unsteadiness Following Whiplash Injury: Characteristic Features and Relationship with Cervical Joint Position Error," *J. Rehabil. Med.* 35:36–43.

Urban, J. P., S. Smith, and J. C. Fairbank (2004). "Nutrition of the Intervertebral Disc," *Spine* 29:2700–2709.

van Ooij, A., F. C. Oner, and A. J. Verbout (2003). "Complications of Artificial Disc Replacement: A Report of 27 Patients with the SB Charite Disc," *J. Spinal Disord. Tech.* 16:369–383.

Viscogliosi, A. G., J. J. Viscogliosi, and M. R. Viscogliosi (2004). *Beyond Total Disc: The Future of Spine Surgery.* New York: Viscogliosi Bros.

Vishnubhotla, S., V. Goel, J. Walkenhorst, et al. (2005). "Biomechanical Advantages of Using Dynamic Stabilization over Rigid Stabilization," 32nd Annual Meeting of International Society of Study for the Lumbar Spine. New York, NY.

Weill, A., J. Chiras, J. M. Simon, et al. (1996). "Spinal Metastases: Indications for and Results of Percutaneous Injection of Acrylic Surgical Cement," *Radiology* 199: 241–247.

Wiltse, L. L., H. Widell Jr., and D. W. Jackson (1975). "Fatigue Fracture: The Basic Lesion Is Isthmic Spondylolisthesis," *J. Bone Joint Surg. Am.* 57:17–22.

Wong, D. A., V. L. Fornasier, and I. MacNab (1990). "Spinal Metastases: The Obvious, the Occult, and the Impostors," *Spine* 15:1–4.

Yamada, K., H. Yamamoto, Y. Nakagawa, et al. (1984). "Etiology of Idiopathic Scoliosis," *Clin. Orthop.* 184:50–57.

Yamamoto, H., T. Tani, G. D. MacEwen, and R. Herman (1982). "An Evaluation of Brainstem Function as a Prognostication of Early Idiopathic Scoliosis," *J. Pediatr. Orthop.* 2:521–528.

Yuan, H. A., S. R. Garfin, C. A. Dickman, and S. M. Mardjetko (1994). "A Historical Cohort Study of Pedicle Screw Fixation in Thoracic, Lumbar, and Sacral Spinal Fusions," *Spine* 19(Suppl. 20):2279S–2296S.

Chapter 7

Historical Review of Spinal Instrumentation for Fusion: Rods, Plates, Screws, and Cages

Marta L. Villarraga, Ph.D.[1,2]
(1) Exponent, Inc. Philadelphia, PA
(2) Drexel University, Philadelphia, PA

The objective of this chapter is to trace the history and development of implant technologies that have led to techniques currently used to stabilize and fuse the spine. For a more in-depth historical account of the evolution of spine surgery, various references are available in textbooks and other publications [Albertone, Naderi, and Benzel 2005; Houten 2005; Moftakhar and Trost 2004; Mohan and Das 2003; Omeis et al. 2004; Singh et al. 2004]. This chapter covers the history of spine instrumentation starting with posterior applications for the thoraco lumbar and lumbo-sacral spine, including Harrington and Luque, and then continuing with anterior instrumentation for the thoraco lumbar spine. Then a historical review of intervertebral cages is presented. The chapter ends with a review of instrumentation for both posterior and anterior approaches for the cervical spine.

7.1 Thoraco Lumbar and Lumbo-Sacral

7.1.1 Posterior Instrumentation

In this section we first review the posterior application of spinal instrumentation for the treatment of fractures and other pathologies, excluding scoliosis.

The second section reviews the historical development of posterior implants for the treatment of scoliosis, which is where Drs. Harrington and Luque made their contributions.

7.1.1.1 Applications for Treatment of Fractures and Other Pathologies

Internal fixation for the posterior aspect of the spine was first reported in 1891 by Hadra when he documented the use of wires around the spinous processes for treating Pott's disease [Hadra 1891]. Pott's disease is manifested as a partial destruction of vertebral bodies, usually caused by a tuberculosis infection and often producing curvature of the spine. At that time, the use of simple loops of wire around the spinous processes were indicated for use in lumbar operations, and were described as being "sufficient, as the latter stand nearly horizontally, and slipping is therefore not expected." Soon after, in 1911, Hibbs described an operation for treating progressive spinal deformities in three patients in which he proposed utilizing a "bony bridge" to prevent kyphosis and to provide a cantilever support to the deformed spine [Hibbs 1911]. The proposed bony bridges were created by fracturing off the spinous processes from the vertebrae, sliding them caudally to touch the inferior vertebral body processes, and suturing them in place. These were meant to achieve fusion. With time, this operation became known as the Hibbs technique.

In 1948, King reported the use of facet screws in the lumbo-sacral spine and indicated that he had been using them for eight years [King 1948]. The screws were placed through the lateral articulations (facets) with the goal of eliminating prolonged patient immobilization in plaster. Of the series of 45 patients reported at this time, only 9.1% had indications of pseudarthrosis. In 1949, Thompson and Ralston reported a pseudarthrosis rate of 55.1% following spinal fusion in a group of patients in which some type of internal fixation (i.e., a stainless steel machine screw) was utilized across each of the facet joints [Thompson and Ralston 1949]. Holdsworth and Hardy reported in 1953 the use of posterior plates attached to one or more spinous processes to treat fracture dislocations in the thoraco lumbar spine [Holdsworth 1970; Holdsworth and Hardy 1953]. They indicated that in cases when the spinous processes were damaged, the plate fixation could be achieved via the lamina. They reported that the fixation was effective for 8 to 12 weeks, at which time the spine would be reportedly stable enough via fusion of the vertebral bodies. The reduction was well maintained, with no reported displacements.

The approach of posterior instrumentation evolved to the point that in 1970 Dr. Roy-Camille of Paris reported the use of spine instrumentation (plates, screws) on the posterior aspect of the lumbar and lumbo-sacral spine by inserting screws through the pedicles and facet joints [Roy-Camille, Roy-Camille, and Demeulenaere 1970]. The exploitation of the pedicle as an attachment site is generally credited to this application, which was first used by Dr. Roy-Camille in 1963 but not reported until his 1970 publication [Houten 2005]. At this time, various curvatures and lengths of plates made of cobalt chrome alloy or stainless steel were offered for posterior use [Roy-Camille, Saillant, and Mazel 1986]. The plates available had 5 to 15 holes located every 1.3 cm. As part of this initial series, Dr. Roy-Camille reported on the quality of the fixation and indicated that the long-term results demonstrated a low incidence of complications [Roy-Camille, Roy-Camille, and Demeulenaere 1970].

Posterior stabilization of the cervical and lumbar spine using the Daab plate was reported in 1984 by Bostman et al. The Daab plate was originally developed in the 1960s by Janusz Daab from Poland for treatment of acute unstable fractures. This one-piece implant looked like an elongated H, was made of low-carbon vacuum-melted stainless steel, and was available in three lengths: 60, 80, or 120 mm. The plate was placed longitudinally in the coronal plane and fixed by pinching the ends around the spinous processes.

In the early 1980s, Dr. Steffee made the use of pedicle screws popular in the United States with his design of segmental spine plates fixed with pedicle screws [Biscup and Sitkowski 1986; Stambough 1997]. This design evolved from a standard AO plate with fixed holes to that of a plate with slots that included a "nest" to permit the solid fixation of a tapered nut. The pedicle screws he presented were modified cancellous bone screws, and primarily designed to be made out of titanium. In his initial publication, he presented five detailed case reports from a group of 120 patients that had been operated on with this system as part of an ongoing clinical trial. In this group, 89% of the patients achieved a clinical rating of 4 out of 5, which was indicative of a good result with few activity limitations and only mild discomfort. Table 7.1 presents a summary of characteristics of the main categories of posterior instrumentation for the treatment of thoraco lumbar trauma in 1977.

7.1.1.2 Applications for Scoliosis: Deformity Correction

In 1941, the Research Committee of the American Orthopaedic Association conducted a study to review the methods and results of treating scoliosis, by following the treatment of 425 patients with idiopathic scoliosis. In summary, the study found that implantation without fusion resulted in complete loss of correction after the external support was discontinued, but correction by a turnbuckle jacket and subsequent fusion yielded better results than any other type of treatment. This study traced the importance of promoting fusion during deformity correction to achieve better results.

In 1973, Dr. Harrington reported the historical development of his instrumentation, noting that in 1953 he used screws to fix vertebral facets in a corrected position on polio patients who were displaying an increase in scoliosis. He described how this surgery was gratifying for the patient, but indicated that the results were somewhat shortlived in that loss of the correction was usually seen within 6 to 12 months [Houten 2005]. With the evident failure of that approach came the birth of internal fixation for scoliosis. In this approach, hooks were used on the posterior elements and nuts were placed on threaded rods to adjust corrective forces. Dr. Harrington then went on to utilize combinations of compression and distraction hooks with rods made of stainless steel. He made the instrumentation with the help of a local orthotist the night before each surgery. With the aid of some research funds he obtained in 1954, Dr. Harrington started an investigation in which he developed

Table 7.1.

Summary of characteristics of posterior instrumentation for the treatment of thoraco-lumbar trauma. (Reproduced from Stambough 1997.)

Types of Posterior Instruments*	Spinal Fixation	Number Fixation	Length	Additional Fixation	Biomechanics	Sagittal Plane Restoration	Middle Column Correction	Peculiar Complications
Harrington (square end)	Hook lamina	2 per rod	2 or 3 above, 2 or 3 below	Spinous process, sublaminal wires, rod sleeves	Distraction at end of rod	++	Yes	Overdistraction
Luque rod segmental spinal instrumentation	Wire rod lamina	Every level	2 or 3 above, 2 or 3 below	Transverse loaders	Translation	++++	No	Sublaminar wire passage, long term sublaminar wire sequelae
Multiple hook rod constructs laminar (Cotrel-Dubousset, instrumentation Isola, Texas Scottish Rite Hospital)	Hook lamina	Multiple	1 or 2 below, 2 or 3 above	Transverse loaders	Distraction, compression, translation	++++	Yes	Forcible correction, neuorinjury +/-, laminar fracture
Transpedicle screw fixation with plate or rod linkage**	Screw bone	Every level	1 below, 1 or 2 above	Transverse loaders	Distraction, compression, translation	+++	Yes (may require anterior strut graft)	Nerve root injury

*All systems commercially available have cross linkage available.
**Transpedicle screw fixation is the only posterior system allowing fixation of all three columns (anterior, middle, posterior), compared with only posterior column fixation for the remainder.

instrumentation to treat 50 scoliotic patients. He designed longer rods with a ratchet adjustment.

Unfortunately, there were complications with this instrumentation, with evident fractures of the rods and disengagement of the hooks, both of which led to the loss of the original scoliotic correction. In addition, the use of distraction as the only means of correction resulted in the loss of the normal sagittal curvature (lordosis), leading to what was referred to as "flat back syndrome" [Houten 2005]. Moreover, patients were required to be braced immediately postoperatively, which was not optimal for all cases. Given these drawbacks and failures, Dr. Harrington proposed that a fusion be superimposed within the extent of the instrumentation to preserve the correction. With the use of his instrumentation began the true modern era of spinal instrumentation.

To improve the performance of the Harrington instrumentation over the next 20 years, many changes took place on the hook design and to the technique to combine distraction and compression. Additionally, a greater understanding was gained of the increased fatigue endurance the implants had to withstand prior to the fusion mass being well developed. By 1960, the instrumentation was being considered for manufacturing by Zimmer Manufacturing Co. (Warsaw, IN), and the technique was presented before the national meeting of the American Academy of Orthopedic Surgeons.

In 1963, Dr. Harrington reported on the correction and internal fixation of scoliosis using spine instrumentation with devices made of SMO 18-8 stainless steel and rods ranging from 3-3/4 to 15-3/4 inches in length. The rods (3/16 inch and 1/8 inch in diameter) were designed with a ratchet system, allowing progressive distraction of the two vertebrae engaged by hooks at either end of the rod. The implants were designed with the goal of exerting a corrective force on the scoliotic curvature by using distraction on the concave side and compression on the convex side. In this report, he shared his experience based on implanting the instrumentation in 129 patients over a period of eight years [Harrington 1963]. A Harrington rod with hooks is shown in Figure 7.1. In 1963, Dr. Harrington presented his experience on 200 scoliotic patients treated with his instrumentation.

Throughout the next decade, evolutions took place in the surgical technique utilizing the Harrington instrumentation, but no changes were made to the design of the implants [Dickson and Harrington 1973]. Results reported in 1979 on the clinical use of Harrington instrumentation to treat 207 scoliotic patients between 1963 and 1974 indicated that age and preoperative curve magnitude were significant variables that could be related to the amount of surgical correction obtained and the maintenance of that correction [Curtis et al. 1979]. Fractures of Harrington rods due to fatigue loading were reported in the literature in the 1970s [Sturz et al. 1979]. In 1980, Erwin et al. presented a review of 2,016 patients fitted between 1961 and 1974 with Harrington rods to determine the incidence of fracture in distraction and compression rods. This clinical review showed a much lower incidence of rod fracture (2.1% compared to 12.5%) in patients in which autogenous bone graft was used compared to the group in which none was used. All fractured rods analyzed showed signs of fatigue failure.

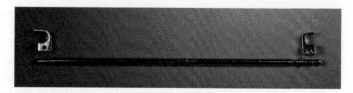

Fig. 7.1.
Harrington rod with hooks after being *in vivo* for 13.5 years. It was removed due to indications of back pain and pseudarthrosis.

New advances in posterior spinal instrumentation came about in the mid 1970s in response to difficulties encountered with the Harrington system. Dr. Luque from Mexico proposed segmental spinal instrumentation (SSI) for internal fixation in the correction of scoliosis [Houten 2005; Luque 1982, 1986]. His approach proposed utilizing 316 stainless steel rods (3/16-inch diameter and 50 cm long) cut to size, pre-bent, and placed along the posterior aspect of the spine, with an L shape at the end to prevent their migration. The pre-bent parallel convex and concave rods were placed with one being cephalad and the other being caudad on either side of the posterior spine. In addition, 316 stainless steel wire loops (1.22-mm diameter) were placed sublaminarly (underneath the lamina) at each vertebral level (Figure 7.2). In this "segmental" approach, the number of fixation points was increased as a means of lessening the force placed on each individual location, while providing correction without postoperative immobilization [Hitchon and Follett 1995].

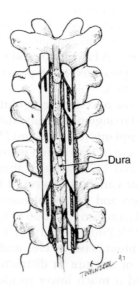

Fig. 7.2.
Luque instrumentation. (*Reprinted from Hitchon et al. 1995 with permission from Thieme Medical Publishers.*)

Dr. Luque reported on a series of 65 consecutive patients operated with his technique, and followed up for a period of 12 to 25 months. In this group, the average loss of correction was 1.5 degrees to 2%. At the time, the advantages he noted for his technique were that not only was it a satisfactory method for correction, but it needed no external fixation and led to rapid and efficient arthrodesis (fusion) [Luque 1982]. Dr. Luque also proposed the use of this technique for the treatment of fractures in the thoraco lumbar spine to afford immediate rigid internal fixation and permit mobilization without external support [Luque, Cassis, and Ramirez-Wiella 1982]. Specifically, he indicated that his instrumentation was capable of fixing each vertebra in a three-point system (as seen from the sagittal plane) with rods and wiring at each lamina, while utilizing the disc as the third point of fixation.

Despite the advantages noted with this new instrumentation, there were still reports in the literature of neurological complications after the manipulation or passage of sublaminar wires [Johnston et al. 1986; Mohan and Das 2003]. In response to concerns of possible neurological injury with sublaminar wires [Geremia et al. 1985], Dr. Drummond [1984] developed a button-wire implant to be anchored on the base of the spinous process at the thickest and strongest part of this location. The round button (8-mm diameter and 0.8 mm thick) was fabricated from 316L stainless steel and the wire was 16- or 18-gauge stainless steel. In a report of clinical experience with this implant, he reviewed 30 cases treated for idiopathic scoliosis that had been followed up for an average of 12 months, and indicated encouraging results with no findings of spinous process failure to that point.

In the mid 1980s, Drs. Cotrel and Dubousett reported on their design of a new set of posterior instrumentation they named Cotrel-Duboussett (CD), to be used for surgical fixation of the scoliotic spine and for fracture treatment [Bennett 1995; Cotrel and Dubousset 1984; Cotrel, Dubousset, and Guillaumat 1988]. The instrumentation was composed of two parallel stainless steel cylindrical rods (1/4 inch) [Houten 2005], with diamond-shaped asperities made to be pre-bent. These were attached to hooks (available in various types) placed on the lamina or pedicles and locked by bolts, or attached to pedicle screws with a closed or open configuration. The screws were only used in the lumbar or lumbo-sacral region. This system provided for a unique mechanism for deformity correction by allowing rod rotation during implantation. Transverse bars (devices for transverse traction, DTTs) were also part of this system, and were used along the length of the rod for improved rigidity and to provide rotation correction (Figure 7.3). In 1988, they reported on 250 patients operated with this instrumentation, in which the mean Cobb angular correction (angle to determine scoliosis and scoliosis correction) was approximately 66% [Cotrel, Dubousset, and Guillaumat 1988]. Even though there were reported advantages on the use of this CD system, these were diminished by the difficulty of removing the system. In addition, the locking mechanism of the hooks was irreversible and only removable by destroying the hooks or cutting the rods [Houten 2005].

In 1986, Dr. Luque reported on his development of an interpeduncular segmental fixation (ISF), which he referred to as an evolution of his original segmental spine instrumentation (SSI) [Luque 1986]. This system was utilized for the

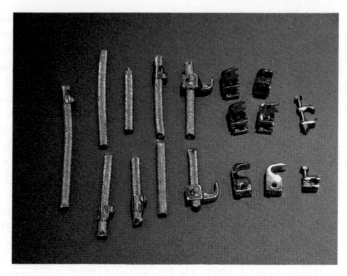

Fig. 7.3.
Cotrel-Duboussett (CD) instrumentation showing rods (cut for retrieval), hooks, and transverse rod connector retrieved after 8.3 years *in vivo*.

correction of lateral deviations, with the positioning of the ISF bar over the transverse processes to avoid rotational deformities and allow both flexion-extension and lateral deviation corrections. While only considered to be in a developmental stage, Dr. Luque reported on 50 patients, of which 20 had more than one year of follow-up. Due to the short follow-up period, no conclusions on the rate of pseudarthrosis were provided and no complications were reported. In a follow-up study published in 1988, Dr. Luque reported on 80 cases with an average follow-up of 18 months. In this series of patients, no pseudarthrosis was seen.

Following the development and use of the Harrington, Luque, and CD systems, other systems have been developed to treat scoliosis, including the Texas Scottish Rite System (TSRH, Medtronic Sofamor Danek, Memphis, TN) and the Isola and Moss-Miami implants (DePuy Spine, Raynham, MA) [An 1999; Bridwell 1997]. The TSRH system evolved as an adjunct to the Luque segmental instrumentation, providing a cross-link system similar to that used in the CD system, but with additional enhancements to facilitate removal during revision procedures. It differed from the CD system in the mode of attachment of the hooks to the rods, the surface characteristics of the rods, and the metallurgical properties of the implants [Benzel, Baldwin, and Ball 1995]. The cross link in this system was designed with the objective of preventing migration of the rod. The system also had pedicle screws available with variable or fixed angle options, and smooth rods [An 1999]. The method of hook fixation to the rod in this system utilizes a three-point shear clamp mechanism with an eyebolt/rod fixation method for all hooks, cross members, and screws. As such, this system requires that the rod fit into a groove in the hook, thus increasing the contact surface area between the hook and the rod due to the matching contours. This system has several types of hooks available, including offset hooks, laminar hooks, transverse process hooks, thoracic laminar hooks, and pedicle (facet) hooks [Benzel, Baldwin, and Ball 1995]. It has cross members available in various sizes to provide cross fixation of the two rods.

The Isola system (DePuy Spine, Raynham, MA) was designed by Dr. Mark Asher as an extension to the variable screw placement (VSP) system previously introduced by Dr. Steffee. This system includes anchors (hooks, screws, or wires) for attachment to rods [available in two sizes: 1/4 inch (6.35 mm) and 3/16 inch (4.76 mm)] and connectors (slotted, split, transverse, dual bypass, or tandem) [Flores, Rengachary, and Hitchon 1995]. The Isola system did not encourage the derotation maneuver as popularized with the CD system. The manner of application of this system involves initially securing the rod proximally and then with the application of cantilever bending and translational forces attaching the rod distally, where mainly pedicle screws are utilized [An 1999]. Isola systems come in both stainless steel and titanium alloy [Serhan et al. 2004].

The Moss-Miami system was designed by Drs. Schuffelbarger and Harms and includes low-profile 316LVM stainless steel rods (5-mm diameter) for applications on both the posterior and anterior spine. The insertion of this system follows sequential placement of pairs of screws and nut heads to be loaded, and provides the ability to use linkages between the rods [An 1999].

Of the systems previously mentioned, the TSHR and Isola tend to be bulky on thin patients, with the hooks and cross links being very prominent under the skin [Bridwell 1997]. The latest version of pedicle screws being used clinically are polyaxial in nature, thus facilitating rod placement in cases where pedicles are not physiologically well aligned [Mohan and Das 2003].

7.1.1.3 Applications for Spondylolisthesis

In 1959, Boucher reported his technique of using long screws posteriorly to fuse lumbar vertebrae to treat spondylolisthesis [Boucher 1959, 1997]. In a report of 49 operations, only four developed pseudarthrosis. One screw was fractured in a two-level fusion that appeared solid.

Following the introduction of the Harrington instrumentation for the treatment of scoliosis, Harrington and Tullos reported in 1971 the approach of utilizing posterior spinal instrumentation to also treat pediatric spondylolisthesis. They reported on the use of blunt hooks inserted into the lamina, two Moe hooks reversed and inserted into the sacral bars, and the use of 1/8-inch threaded rods with two hex nuts in place [Harrington and Tullos 1971]. With these rods in place, the proper distraction was induced to reduce the dislocation, and further incorporation of fusion (interbody and posterior) was included (Figure 7.4).

7.2 Anterior Instrumentation

In 1969, Dr. Dwyer presented an anterior (antero-lateral) approach to treat scoliosis by instrumenting the convex side of the curvature. The proposed implant system included titanium screws inserted in the convex side of each vertebral

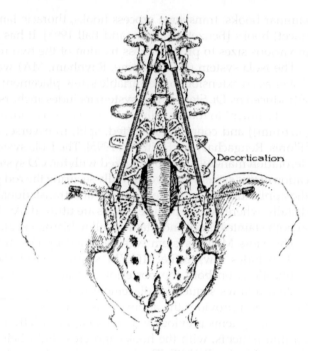

Decorlication

Fig. 7.4.

Harrington instrumentation to treat spondylolisthesis. (*Reproduced from Harrington et al. 1971 with permission from Lippincott, Williams & Wilkins.*)

body, with each screw holding down a titanium plate that hooked over the vertebral body ends. A titanium cable was threaded through the screw heads, and tension was applied between them to correct the curvature [Dwyer, Newton, and Sherwood 1969]. The eight case reports presented at the time indicated that the procedure allowed a considerable amount of corrective force on the scoliotic spine, while potentially allowing improved correction during growth. Dr. Dwyer further reported in 1974 a new set of 51 cases of scoliosis with follow-up periods from one to eight years. In this set of patients, the fusion rate was 96% with only two cases of pseudarthrosis. He claimed to provide a better correction for scoliosis with this method as compared to posterior fusion, citing the ability to provide a greater amount of tension with the tensioning device to pull the vertebral bodies together (given the vertebral body's increased size), and the increased mobility obtained from the complete removal of the intervertebral discs.

In 1978, Dr. Winter reported on the use of combined Dwyer and Harrington instrumentation for treating five adult idiopathic scoliosis patients. The two procedures were done two weeks apart, with the Dwyer implanted first and the Harrington second. In this series of patients he achieved the goal of obtaining two equal and balanced curves with no pseudarthrosis or complications reported.

The Zielke system was developed as an improvement to the Dwyer system, and included a compression rod with nuts allowing more de-rotation and thus greater correction of deformities [Cohen and McAfee 1995; Mohan and Das 2003]. The pseudarthrosis rate with the Zielke system was lower than with the Dwyer system. However, there were still reports of this system allowing kyphosis, and a higher rate of pseudarthrosis than the posterior systems [Bridwell 1997].

For the treatment of severe thoraco lumbar fractures, Dr. Dunn introduced an implant system to rigidly fix the spine anteriorly at a single level [Dunn 1984]. His design, which iterated through three versions, was finally implanted in patients as a configuration consisting of two rods rigidly linked by "vertebral body bridges" secured to each vertebra at two points: one posteriorly secured with a screw and the other more anteriorly secured with a staple. Dr. Dunn reported [1984] on surgeries done on 48 patients with successful bone union in 45.

The Kostuik-Harrington anterior distraction device was introduced for anterior fixation of thoracic and lumbar spine fractures [Kostuik 1984]. The technique recommended with this instrumentation highlighted the advantage of not needing posterior instrumentation. Dr. Kostuik presented a series of 49 patients treated anteriorly for bust injuries. In his series he indicated there were no cases of instrumentation failure or nonunion.

A bolt-plate fixation system was presented by Ryan et al. in 1986 for the fusion of the anterior thoraco lumbar and lumbar spine utilizing a lateral approach. The instrumentation presented consisted of two transverse bolts placed in the coronal plane and connected by a plate, all of which were made of titanium. The plate included a hole in the caudal portion and a slot in the cephalad portion. Only limited clinical experience of two patients were presented in this report, with fixation at the L4-L5 level and no reported complications.

Another plate proposed for anterior fixation of the thoraco lumbar spine was presented by Black et al. in 1986. The proposed design consisted of a 316LVM stainless steel low-profile contoured plate designed to fit closely on the lateral aspect of vertebral bodies by fixation via multiple screw holes, which allowed at least three screws per vertebral body and permitted bicortical purchase. Seven case studies were presented with encouraging early results.

To overcome incidences of pseudarthrosis, hardware failure, and loss of correction with the single-rod techniques [Mohan and Das 2003], Dr. Kaneda developed a titanium anterior fixation system that engaged on the vertebral bodies via vertebral body staples with two screws per vertebrae, and which are connected by two threaded longitudinal rods (Figure 7.5). He reported the use of his device in 1984 for the treatment of a thoraco lumbar burst fracture to achieve stabilization after the anterior decompression [Cohen and McAfee 1995]. This device allowed the reduction of kyphotic deformities by distracting the anterior column to compress across bone grafts intended for fusion [Ghanayem and Zdeblick 1997]. Reported rates of nonunion have been about 6% [Cohen and McAfee 1995]. This system was revolutionary in the area of anterior instrumentation, in that it allowed the surgical reduction of kyphotic deformities during the distraction of the anterior column while compressing the bone graft placed in the intervertebral space [Bridwell 1997].

Another implant system that was introduced following the Kaneda system was the Z-Plate (Medtronic Sofamor Danek, Memphis, TN), a titanium plate

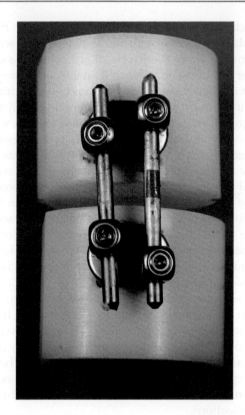

Fig. 7.5.
Kaneda anterior system showing two rods anchored on UHMWPE blocks with vertebral body staples, each attached with two screws.

with bolts and screws, having slots on the superior end and fixed holes at the inferior end. This implant system was introduced into the market on May of 1993 [Zdeblick 1995]. Among its features is included a radius of curvature similar to that of vertebral bodies so that it may adapt to kyphosis. The implantation involves placing a bolt and screws into the superior and inferior vertebral bodies, as well as screws into both vertebral bodies, with the bolt-plate interfaces being rigid and the screw-plate interfaces being semirigid [Zdeblick 1995]. The bolts can be used to provide distraction, thus reducing kyphotic deformities with their partial tightening. With the presence of the slots on the plate, compression can be placed on the bone graft before tightening.

7.3 Intervertebral Body Cages: Cervical and Lumbar

Prior to describing the introduction of intervertebral body cages, it is important to establish some historical perspective on the use of bone for intervertebral fusions. The use of ilium bone graft to promote fusion across the lumbar intervertebral body spaces was initially reported by Cloward in 1952. In his report, he indicated that he had been practicing this technique since 1943. The report also indicated the initial possibilities of using cadaveric bone (allograft) instead of the patient's own bone (autograft), and provided data for its safety and effectiveness. This application was the precursor to intervertebral body cages, which later became spacers used to promote fusion. Interbody cages have been utilized for anterior cervical and lumbar interbody fusions (ALIF), and have been utilized in posterior lumbar approaches. At times they have been used in conjunction with additional spinal instrumentation.

In 1984, Dr. Bagby presented to the orthopedics community the option of using his method for anterior cervical fusion. The method had been successful in horses, and reported previously [DeBowes et al. 1984] with the use of a hollow stainless steel implant (stainless steel basket, or SSB, or "Bagby basket") containing autogenous bone graft [Bagby 1988; Kuslich et al. 1998]. At the time, he indicated that it was not available for use in humans, but had the potential to be used with local autogenous bone in the human anterior cervical spine. Based on the concepts of the Bagby basket as a stepping-stone, along with certain material and design changes, the Bagby and Kuslich (BAK) implant evolved. It is a hollow, porous, threaded, and slightly tapered cylindrical titanium (Ti6Al4V) device that can be filled with bone graft to facilitate interbody lumbar spine fusion (Spine-Tech, Minneapolis, MN; now Zimmer Spine) [Kuslich et al. 1998]. The BAK was approved for clinical use by the Food and Drug Administration (FDA) on September 20, 1996 [FDA 1996]. A different version for the cervical spine (BAK-C) is utilized for anterior cervical interbody fusion and was approved in 2002 [Houten 2005; Matge 1998].

A multi-center study (19 centers and 42 surgeons) was carried out to evaluate the use of this implant for lumbar interbody stabilization to treat chronic discogenic low back pain secondary to degenerative disc disease. This study showed a rate of fusion of 91% at 24 months post surgery, with pain reduction in 84%. In this series, the rate of device-related re-operations was 4.4% [Kuslich et al. 1998]. For the cervical spine, a multi-center trial showed that successful fusion for one level procedures at one year was 97.9% for the BAK-C cage compared to 89.7% for the bone-only fusion group, and that symptom improvement was maintained at two years [Hacker et al. 2000].

Other cages that are used clinically include the Ray Threaded Fusion Cage (Stryker Spine, Allendale, NJ), the Harms titanium mesh cage (DePuy Spine, Raynham, MA), and the Brantigan cage (DePuy Spine, Raynam, MA) made out of carbon fiber. In 1991, Brantigan et al. presented a design for a carbon fiber reinforced polymer cage for posterior lumbar interbody fusion. The implant had ridges (or teeth) to resist pull-out, struts to support weight bearing, and a hollow center to allow autologous bone graft packing [Brantigan, Steffee, and Geiger 1991]. Mechanical testing done to characterize its performance indicated that the carbon fiber composite cage required a significantly greater pull-out force than a bone plug alone.

7.4 Cervical

Instrumentation for use in the cervical spine evolved for both the anterior and posterior approaches from basic inter-spinous wiring methods. This section first covers the history of posterior cervical instrumentation followed by that of anterior applications. Historically, internal stabilization of the cervical spine was carried initially only posteriorly with sublaminar or inter-spinous wiring. Anterior techniques have only evolved in the last four decades [Rengachary and Duke 1995].

7.4.1 Posterior Approaches: Grafts and Wiring

Cloward reported (1958) utilizing the same bone graft surgical technique as Robinson and Smith to treat ruptured cervical spine intervertebral discs. In this series he reported success (defined as pain relief) in 42 of 47 patients, and marked improvement in the remaining five by using bone from the patients or from a bone bank.

Wiring of the posterior cervical spine was first described by Rogers in 1942 for the treatment of fractures and dislocations of the cervical spine [An 1999]. It involved connecting several spinous processes together with wire and incorporating some bone graft to enhance the fusion [Slone et al. 1995]. Forsyth et al. further reported in 1959 the technique of posterior internal fixation in the cervical spine using 20-gauge stainless steel wire to wrap around the spinous processes and treat fracture-dislocations below the second cervical vertebra. They suggested the inclusion of bone graft against the base of the spinous processes, with additional graft added along the laminae and posterior articulations [Forsyth, Alexander, and Davis 1959].

Stabilization of the cervical spine following laminectomy by using wires through the articular processes and using ilium crest cortico-cancellous grafts was reported in the 1970s by Callahan et al. [1977]. In this series of 63 patients, 52 were followed for up to 17 years, of which 50 had a documented facet fusion at a mean follow-up period of 6.5 months [Callahan et al. 1977]. Even in the 1980s, Cahill et al. reported the bilateral approach at wiring the cervical spinous processes with the facets to stabilize facet fracture dislocations or subaxial flexion-compression injuries [Cahill, Bellegarrigue, and Ducker 1983].

7.4.2 Posterior Approaches: Instrumentation

In 1984, Holness et al. reported on the use of a stainless steel interlaminar clamp to treat cervical injuries by applying it to the adjoining laminae of the involved vertebrae. The indications were to treat cervical dislocations and subluxations with posterior instability, with minimal or no vertebral body involvement. A clinical study of 51 patients treated from 1972 to 1982 indicated that the long-term reports were largely satisfactory.

In the 1980s, Dr. Roy-Camille pioneered the use of posterior cervical stabilization by using screws on the lateral masses to stabilize the cervical spine [Roy-Camille, Saillant, and Mazel 1980]. His proposed stabilization technique induced spontaneous fusion of the bridged facets and therefore no complementary grafting was necessary. Clinical reports of the use of the Roy-Camille plate showed that successful fusion was achieved at three months, with only six patients showing loosening of short unicortical screws [Ebraheim et al. 1995]. These complications of loosening of screws led to the use of bicortical screws.

In 1989, Dr. Haid developed a posterior cervical plate (AME Haid Universal Bone Plate System, American Medical Electronics, Inc., Richardson, TX) made of titanium alloy to reduce artifacts in CT scanning [Traynelis and Haid 1995]. It had a slightly concave cross section to accommodate the anatomical shape of the articular pillars (lateral masses) [Slone et al. 1995]. One of the advantages of lateral mass plate fixation is that it is independent of posterior element integrity and can maintain the cervical lordosis. Reported fusion success rates were 98% [Traynelis and Haid 1995].

Halifax clamps (laminar clamps) were developed to engage on the lamina of the posterior cervical spine with a C-shaped hook that once tightened brought the two clamps together to produce compression [Slone et al. 1995]. Even though this device resisted flexion well, it did not provide enough stability against extension and rotation.

Lateral mass rods and screws were introduced to accommodate indications of spondylosis or trauma in the cervical spine [Omeis et al. 2004]. In addition, posterior instrumentation such as the CD rods used in the lumbar spine were also used in the cervical spine for applications requiring long-segment fusions [Slone et al. 1995]. Application of this instrumentation was more likely done when a fusion was necessary to include the thoracic spine. Examples of rod-screw systems that were developed to accommodate this include the CerviFix (Synthes, Paoli, PA), which is made out of titanium or titanium alloy; the Vertex (Medtronic Sofamor Danek, Memphis, TN); and the Summit system (DePuy Spine, Rayham, MA). Of these, the CerviFix and Summitt can also be utilized to include fixation to the occiput. Another rod application in the cervical spine was the O-ring or Luque rectangle, which were attached with wires or cables [Slone et al. 1995].

In 1994, Abumi et al. introduced the use of pedicle screws in the cervical spine for stabilizing subaxial traumatic instability. Biomechanical studies compared the pull-out force of pedicle screws to that of lateral masses, and showed that there was a significantly higher resistance to pull-out with this pedicle application [Jones et al. 1997].

7.4.3 Anterior Approaches: Plates

The original approach at fusing the spine anteriorly, known as the Smith-Robinson fusion, involved the removal of the disc and placement of a bone graft [Slone et al. 1995]. Cloward reported in 1958 on the anterior approach of removing ruptured cervical discs and fusion with iliac autograft or allografts in a series of 47 patients with a high success of pain relief. The term *Cloward fusion* has since been used when referring to a procedure that includes the removal of a portion of the vertebra [Slone et al. 1995].

Whereas the techniques presented previously were available to treat the cervical spine anteriorly, the use of anterior plates provided the capability to enhance stability with selective fusion of segments, while eliminating the need for external immobilization (i.e., halo, collar). A number of anterior cervical plates have been developed and utilized clinically over the years. In 2002, Haid et al. proposed a nomenclature for describing and *labeling* anterior cervical plates (ACPs) based on the biomechanical and graft-loading properties of these systems. The classification is presented in Figure 7.6 and the functionality and characteristics of most of these plates are described in this section, following a brief historical introduction of anterior cervical fusions.

Bohler is credited with the development of the first anterior cervical plate in 1964, which was the foundation of the plates available today [Bohler and Gaudernak 1980; Vaccaro and Balderston 1997]. In 1971, Orozco and Llovet reported their use of the plate made by the ASIF, which had an H-shape con-

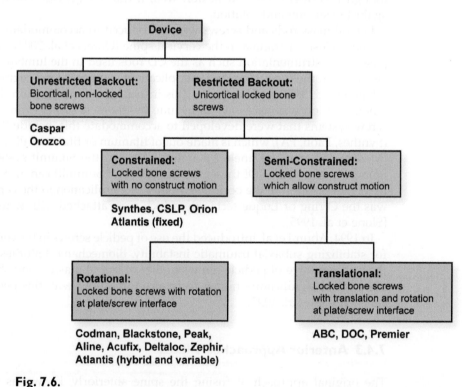

Fig. 7.6.

Proposed nomenclature presented by Haid et al. (2002) for classifying anterior cervical plates. (*Reproduced from Haid et al. 2002.*)

figuration, and later became known as the Orozco plate (Synthes, Padi, PA) [Moftakhar and Trost 2004; Slone et al. 1995; Vaccaro and Balderston 1997]. This plate was designed with a slight concavity to mate with the anterior vertebral body shape and to allow the edges to extend out at the screw sites, thus being known as having an H shape. Transcortical fixation with bicortical screws was utilized in this application [Slone et al. 1995].

The Caspar plate stabilization system for anterior cervical fusion was introduced in the late 1980s as manufactured by Aesculap, Inc. (South San Francisco, CA) [Caspar, Barbier, and Klara 1989; Traynelis and Ryken 1995]. The system was available for single- and multiple-level fixations in the lower cervical spine with a bicortical screw approach and the addition of bone graft, either from the iliac crest or autograft. The plate was made of either stainless steel or titanium and was wider at one end, shaped like a trapezoid with a slightly concave shape to accommodate the anterior vertebral body curvature [Slone et al. 1995; Traynelis and Ryken 1995]. The plate contained two rows of oval holes along its long axis. One of the reported advantages of this system was that it allowed immediate postoperative stability without external stabilization. In a report of the initial clinical cases, 60 patients with cervical trauma were treated with this system, and all patients obtained fusion with no unusual complications reported [Caspar, Barbier, and Klara 1989]. The incidence of screw loosening with this system has been reported to be 3.5%, with an overall fusion rate of 99% [Traynelis and Ryken 1995].

Both the Orozco and Caspar plates were considered nonrigid and nonlocking in that the screw angulation was determined at surgery and was not restricted by the plate geometry. These plates were designed with the inclusion of screws that engaged in bicortical purchase [Moftakhar and Trost 2004], the addition of which enhanced the stability of the system. Reported complications for both types of plates included screw loosening, screw migration [Rengachary and Duke 1995], back-out and fracture of the screws [Slone et al. 1995], and subsidence of the graft construct [Haid et al. 2002]. In the proposed classification of anterior cervical plates by Haid et al., these two plates were termed unrestricted back-out devices [Haid et al. 2002].

The Morscher cervical spine locking plate (CSLP, Synthes, Paoli, PA) was introduced, and included an expandable split screw that locks into the plate after the insertion of a small central screw [Moftakhar and Trost 2004; Morscher et al. 1986; Slone et al. 1995]. The plate and screws were made of titanium, and the screws included a tapped recess in the top to accept the small expansion screw (Figure 7.7). This dual screw mechanism works by allowing the head of the locking screw to expand and engage in the plate when the smaller screw is tightened, thereby reducing the risk of screw back-out [Slone et al. 1995]. With this mechanism in place, it utilized cancellous screws and as such did not require bicortical purchase. In addition, the caudal screw was oriented perpendicular and the cephalad screw was angled 12 degrees caudally for more screw purchase. Another feature of these screws was that they had multiple holes along the threaded portion, thereby allowing bone ingrowth for further anchoring in place. Improvements to this system have included lordotic precontouring [Haid et al. 2002].

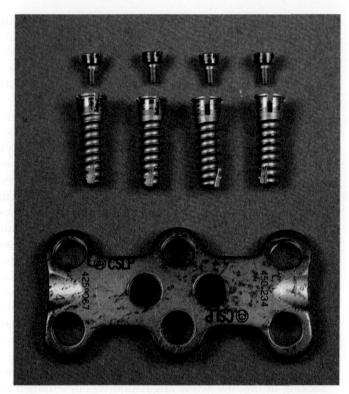

Fig. 7.7.
Cervical spine locking plate showing three-level plate with four unicortical screws and anchoring expanding screws. This implant was less than one year *in vivo* (0.9 years) and was removed due to progressive myelopathy and degeneration of the thecal sac.

The Orion anterior cervical plate system (Medtronic Sofamor Danek, Memphis, TN) was also developed in titanium alloy with a predetermined curved shape (lordosis) for use with unicortical screws or bicortical screws of variable lengths [Houten 2005; Lowery 1995]. The screw plate interface at both ends of the Orion plate (Figure 7.8) is secured by a single locking screw that covers both screw heads to prevent back-out. This plate has fixed screws that are oriented cephalad and caudal and also angled medially, which prevent cephalad or caudad motion of either the screw or the plate, thus providing stress shielding of the graft [Epstein 2001].

In the interest of reducing stress shielding of the bone graft in cervical spine fusions and preventing screw back-out, semiconstrained plates were designed next. The objective was to develop plates that would share the load with the graft and thus reduce some of the stress shielding [Houten 2005]. In contrast to constrained plates, the Atlantis system (Medtronic Sofamor Danek, Memphis, TN) is a semiconstrained plate that does not allow motion of the plate itself but has the option of variable angled screws that can toggle through an arch of 0 to 17 degrees in either direction. With this system, the amount of stress shield-

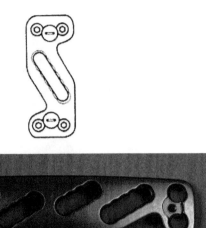

Fig. 7.8.
Orion Cervical Spine Plate in schematic form on the left for a two level intervention (reprinted with permission from Vaccaro et al. 1977 with permission from Lippincott, Williams & Wilkins) and for a multilevel corpectomy application on the right.

ing is reduced compared to the fixed screw designs. Even with these design options available, the Atlantis plate can also be used as a restricted constrained device if all screws are placed fixed and rigid [Haid et al. 2002]. Therefore, this system has the option of being fixed, hybrid (some fixed, some variable), or completely variable.

Another semiconstrained plate available is the Codman plate (Johnson and Johnson, Raynham, MA), which was designed to allow for variability in direction of all screws and prevent screw back-out with a built-in cam-locking system [Haid et al. 2002]. This plate allows for graft subsidence through a rotational mechanism via the rotation of all screws, thus providing an increased load on the graft and controlled subsidence.

In a continued effort to reduce the amount of stress shielding while still allowing compression of grafts in the cervical spine, dynamic plates were designed next. These plates perform this function due to the existence of slots that enable migration of the screws along the axial direction. Various dynamic plates have been introduced for use in the anterior cervical spine. A system that was designed for this purpose was the DOC Rod (DePuy Spine, Raynham, MA). This system allows for controlled vertical translation to permit settling of the graft (subsidence) by allowing the cephalad screws to slide along the rods, while maintaining anatomic alignment. Another example of a dynamic system is the ABC plate (Aesculap, Inc., Center Valley, PA), which has slots and variable angle screws to reduce stress shielding as much as possible (Figure 7.9). This system allows for translational motion of the screws and rotation at the screw-plate interface [Haid et al. 2002]. Epstein reports as much as 6 mm of migration of screws in the cephalad direction and 5 mm of caudad migration

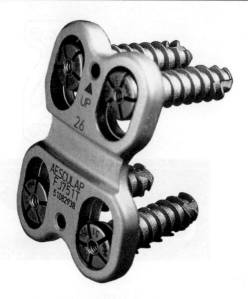

Fig. 7.9.
ABC dynamic plate, showing variable angles and cross-sectional view of screw anchoring mechanism. (*Image provided by Aesculap, Center Valley, PA.*)

with this system [Epstein 2001]. Other plates that have been introduced for anterior cervical application include the A-line (Codman, Johnson and Johnson) and the Premier (Medtronic Sofamor Danek, Memphis, TN), which were designed with the objective of maintaining load sharing between the graft and plate.

7.4.4 Clinical Performance of Anterior Cervical Plates

Retrospective studies have evaluated the risk of injury resulting from hardware failure (fracture or loosening) in a group of 133 patients who had constrained and unconstrained plates for anterior cervical spine reconstructions, with an average follow-up of 43 months [Lowery and McDonough 1998]. Plates evaluated included Orozco (unconstrained), CSLP, and Orion (constrained). In 38 patients (31%), there was some form of hardware failure, with 31 failures in unconstrained plates and 7 failures in constrained plates. Even though there was a significant difference in the failure rates between the constrained and unconstrained plates, neither posed a significant risk to patients. Of importance to note is that hardware would be a good indicator of nonunion, but immediate removal is rarely necessary.

Clinical reports indicate that surgeons have found benefits in using anterior cervical plates in cases of corpectomies and grafting to prevent extrusion of the graft [Vaccaro and Balderston 1997]. Biomechanically, anterior cervical plates function as a tension band when the neck is under extension, and as a buttress plate when the neck is in flexion. Animal models have been used to evaluate the additional rigidity and enhanced fusion rates with the use of anterior cervical plates [Vaccaro and Balderston 1997]. Even for the treatment of anterior corpectomies followed by fibular allograft with anterior plate reconstruction, acceptable fusions have been obtained using some of the plates mentioned previously (Caspar, CSLP, Orion, Codman) [Mayr et al. 2002]. No cases of plate fracture were reported, but fractured screws and screw pull-out were noted.

7.5 Summary

This chapter has traced the historical development of spine instrumentation in both the thoraco lumbar and cervical spine. It is clear that the development of spine instrumentation has increased the armamentarium of tools available to spine surgeons today as they treat patients with numerous pathologies with the goal of improving their quality of life. Even with more instrumentation choices available, success of their use in patients also depends on proper clinical evaluation of patient indications, as well as a thorough understanding of the biomechanical principles for their successful performance. A good understanding of the development of spinal instrumentation since the early 1900s lays the proper foundation for a better understanding of the clinical performance of these implants and of future developments.

7.6 Acknowledgments

I would like to thank Stephanie Teti for her incredible assistance collecting the literature for this chapter and to her and Sara Baxter for their review of this chapter.

7.7 References

Albertone, C. D., S. Naderi, and E. C. Benzel (2005). "History," in E. C. Benzel (ed.). *Spine Surgery Techniques, Complication Avoidance and Management* (2d ed.). Philadelphia: Elsevier.

An, H. S. (1999a). "Posterior Spinal Instrumentation of the Lower Cervical Spine," in H. S. An, and J. M. Cotler (eds.). *Spinal Instrumentation* (2d ed.). Philadelphia: Lippincott Williams & Wilkins.

An, H. S. (1999b). "Posterior Spinal Instrumentation of the Thoracolumbar Spine," in H. S. An, and J. M. Cotler (eds.). *Spinal Instrumentation* (2d ed.). Philadelphia: Lippincott Williams & Wilkins.

Bagby, G. W. (1988). "Arthrodesis by the Distraction-compression Method Using a Stainless Steel Implant," *Orthopedics* 11:931–934.

Bennett, G. J. (1995). "Cotrel-Dubousset Instrumentation for Thoracolumbar Instability," in P. W. Hitchon, V. C. Traynelis, and S. R. Rengachary (eds.). *Techniques in Spinal Fusion and Stabilization*. New York: Thieme Medical Publishers.

Benzel, E. C., N. G. Baldwin, and P. A. Ball (1995). "Texas Scottish Rite Hospital Hook-rod Spinal Fixation," in P. W. Hitchon, V. C. Traynelis, and S. R. Rengachary (eds.). *Techniques in Spinal Fusion and Stabilization*. New York: Thieme Medical Publishers.

Bohler, J., and T. Gaudernak (1980). "Anterior Plate Stabilization for Fracture-dislocations of the Lower Cervical Spine," *J. Trauma* 20:203–205.

Boucher, H. H. (1959). "A Method for Spinal Fusion," *J. Bone Joint Surg.* 41B:248–259.

Boucher, H. H. (1997). "Method of Spinal Fusion," *Clin. Orthop. Relat. Res.* 335:4–9.

Brantigan, J. W., A. D. Steffee, and J. M. Geiger (1991). "A Carbon Fiber Implant to Aid Interbody Lumbar Fusion: Mechanical Testing," *Spine* 16:S277–S282.

Bridwell, K. H. (1997). "Spinal Instrumentation in the Management of Adolescent Scoliosis," *Clin. Orthop.* 335:64–72.

Cahill, D. W., R. Bellegarrigue, and T. B. Ducker (1983). "Bilateral Facet to Spinous Process Fusion: A New Technique for Posterior Spinal Fusion After Trauma," *Neurosurgery* 13:1–4.

Callahan, R. A., R. M. Johnson, et al. (1977). "Cervical Facet Fusion for Control of Instability Following Laminectomy," *J. Bone Joint Surg Am.* 59:991–1002.

Caspar, W., D. D. Barbier, and P. M. Klara (1989). "Anterior Cervical Fusion and Caspar Plate Stabilization for Cervical Trauma," *Neurosurgery* 25:491–502.

Cohen, M. G., and P. McAfee (1995). "Kaneda Anterior Spinal Instrumentation," in P. W. Hitchon, V. C. Traynelis, and S. R. Rengachary (eds.). *Techniques in Spinal Fusion and Stabilization*. New York: Thieme Medical Publishers.

Cotrel, Y., and J. Dubousset (1984). "A New Technique for Segmental Spinal Osteosynthesis Using the Posterior Approach," *Rev. Chir. Orthop. Reparatrice Appar. Mot.* 70:489–494.

Cotrel, Y., J. Dubousset, and M. Guillaumat (1988). "New Universal Instrumentation in Spinal Surgery," *Clin. Orthop.* 227:10–23.

Curtis, R. S., J. H. Dickson, P. R. Harrington, and W. D. Erwin (1979). "Results of Harrington Instrumentation in the Treatment for Severe Scoliosis," *Clin. Orthop.* 144:128–134.

DeBowes, R. M., B. D. Grant, et al. (1984). "Cervical Vertebral Interbody Fusion in the Horse: A Comparative Study of Bovine Xenografts and Autografts Supported by Stainless Steel Baskets," *Am. J. Vet. Res.* 45:191–199.

Dickson, J. H., and P. R. Harrington (1973). "The Evolution of the Harrington Instrumentation Technique in Scoliosis," *J. Bone Joint Surg. Am.* 55:993–1002.

Dunn, H. K. (1984). "Anterior Stabilization of Thoracolumbar Injuries," *Clin. Orthop.* 55(5):993, 116–124.

Dwyer, A. F., N. C. Newton, and A. A. Sherwood (1969). "An Anterior Approach to Scoliosis. A Preliminary Report," *Clin. Orthop.* 62:192–202.

Ebraheim, N. A., R. E. Rupp, E. R. Savolaine, and J. A. Brown (1995). "Posterior Plating of the Cervical Spine," *J. Spinal Disord.* 8:111–115.

Epstein, N. (2001). "Anterior Approaches to Cervical Spondylosis and Ossification of the Posterior Longitudinal Ligament: Review of Operative Technique and Assessment of 65 Multilevel Circumferential Procedures," *Surg. Neurol.* 55:313–324.

FDA. (1996). "Summary of Safety and Effectiveness: BAK," *http://www.accessdata.fda.gov/scripts/cdrh/cfdocs/cfPMA/PMA.cfm?ID=12453.*

Flores, E., S. R. Rengachary, and P. W. Hitchon (1995). "ISOLA Instrumentation," in P. W. Hitchon, V. C. Traynelis, and S. R. Rengachary (eds.). *Techniques in Spinal Fusion and Stabilization*. New York: Thieme Medical Publishers.

Forsyth, H. F., E. Alexander, and C. Davis (1959). "The Advantages of Early Spine Fusion in the Treatment of Fracture Dislocations of the Cervical Spine," *J. Bone. Joint Surg.* 41-A:17–136.

Geremia, G. K., K. S. Kim, L. Cerullo, and L. Calenoff (1985). "Complications of Sublaminar Wiring," *Surg. Neurol.* 23:629–635.

Ghanayem, A. J., and T. A. Zdeblick (1997). "Anterior Instrumentation in the Management of Thoracolumbar Burst Fractures," *Clin. Orthop.* 335:89–100.

Hacker, R. J., J. C. Cauthen, T. J. Gilbert, and S. L. Griffith (2000). "A Prospective Randomized Multicenter Clinical Evaluation of an Anterior Cervical Fusion Cage," *Spine* 25:2646–2654; discussion 2655.

Hadra, B. (1891). "Wiring the Spinous Processes in Pott's Disease," *Trans. Am. Orthop. Assoc.* 4:206–210.

Haid, R. W., K. T. Foley, G. E. Rodts, and B. Barnes (2002). "The Cervical Spine Study Group Anterior Cervical Plate Nomenclature," *Neurosurg. Focus* 12:1–6.

Harrington, P. R. (1963). "The Management of Scoliosis by Spine Instrumentation: An Evaluation of More Than 200 Cases," *Southern Medical Journal* 56:1367–1377.

Harrington, P. R., and H. S. Tullos (1971). "Spondylolisthesis in Children: Observations and Surgical Treatment," *Clin. Orthop.* 79:75–84.

Hibbs, R. (1911). "An Operation for Progressive Spinal Deformities," *N.Y. Med. J.* 93: 1013–1016.

Hitchon, P. W., and K. A. Follett. (1995). "Luque Instrumentation for the Thoracic and Lumbar Spine," in P. W. Hitchon, V. C. Traynelis, and S. R. Rengachary (eds.). *Techniques in Spinal Fusion and Stabilization*. New York: Thieme Medical Publishers.

Holdsworth, F. W. (1970). "Fractures, Dislocations, and Fracture-dislocations of the Spine," *J. Bone Joint Surg. Am.* 52:1534–1551.

Holdsworth, F. W., and A. Hardy (1953). "Early Treatment of Paraplegia from Fractures of the Thoraco lumbar Spine," *J. Bone Joint Surg. Br.* 35-B:540–550.

Houten, J. K., and Errico, T. J. (2005). "History of Spinal Instrumentation: The Modern Era," in E. C. Benzel (ed.). *Spine Surgery Techniques, Complication Avoidance and Management* (2d ed.). Philadelphia: Elsevier.

Johnston, C. E. II, L. T. Happel Jr., et al. (1986). "Delayed Paraplegia Complicating Sublaminar Segmental Spinal Instrumentation," *J. Bone Joint Surg. Am.* 68:556–563.

Jones, E. L., J. G. Heller, D. H. Silcox, and W. C. Hutton (1997). "Cervical Pedicle Screws Versus Lateral Mass Screws: Anatomic Feasibility and Biomechanical Comparison," *Spine* 22:977–982.

King, D. (1948). "Internal Fixation for Lumbosacral Fusion," *J. Bone Joint Surg. Am.* 30A:560–565.

Kostuik, J. P. (1984). "Anterior Fixation for Fractures of the Thoracic and Lumbar Spine with or Without Neurologic Involvement," *Clin. Orthop. Relat. Res.* 189:103–115.

Kuslich, S. D., C. L. Ulstrom, et al. (1998). "The Bagby and Kuslich Method of Lumbar Interbody Fusion: History, Techniques, and 2-year Follow-up Results of a United States Prospective, Multicenter Trial," *Spine* 23:1267–1278; discussion 1279.

Lowery, G. L. (1995). "Anterior Cervical Osteosynthesis: Orion Anterior Cervical System," in P. W. Hitchon, V. C. Traynelis, and S. R. Rengachary (eds.). *Techniques in Spinal Fusion and Stabilization*. New York: Thieme Medical Publishers.

Lowery, G. L., and R. F. McDonough (1998). "The Significance of Hardware Failure in Anterior Cervical Plate Fixation: Patients with 2- to 7-year Follow-up," *Spine* 23:181–186; discussion 186–187.

Luque, E. R. (1982a). "The Anatomic Basis and Development of Segmental Spinal Instrumentation," *Spine* 7:256–259.

Luque, E. R. (1982b). "Segmental Spinal Instrumentation for Correction of Scoliosis," *Clin. Orthop. Relat. Res.* 163:192–198.

Luque, E. R. (1986a). "Interpeduncular Segmental Fixation," *Clin. Orthop.* 203:54–57.

Luque, E. R. (1986b). "Segmental Spinal Instrumentation of the Lumbar Spine," *Clin Orthop.* 203:126–134.

Luque, E. R., N. Cassis, and G. Ramirez-Wiella (1982). "Segmental Spinal Instrumentation in the Treatment of Fractures of the Thoracolumbar Spine," *Spine* 7:312–317.

Matge, G. (1998). "Anterior Interbody Fusion with the BAK-cage in Cervical Spondylosis," *Acta Neurochir (Wien)* 140:1–8.

Mayr, M., B. Subach, C. Comey, et al. (2002). "Cervical Spinal Stenosis: Outcome after Anterior Corpectomy, Allograft Reconstruction, and Instrumentation," *J. Neurosurg.* 96:10–16.

Moftakhar, R., and G. R. Trost (2004). "Anterior Cervical Plates: A Historical Perspective," *Neurosurg. Focus* 16:E8.

Mohan, A. L., and K. Das (2003). "History of Surgery for the Correction of Spinal Deformity," *Neurosurg. Focus* 14:e1.

Morscher, E., F. Sutter, H. Jenny, and S. Olerud (1986). "Anterior Plating of the Cervical Spine with the Hollow Screw-plate System of Titanium," *Chirurg.* 57:702–707.

Omeis, I., J. A. DeMattia, et al. (2004). "History of Instrumentation for Stabilization of the Subaxial Cervical Spine," *Neurosurg. Focus* 16:E10.

Rengachary, S. R., and D. A. Duke. (1995). "Stabilization of the Cervical Spine with the Locking Plate System," in P. W. Hitchon, V. C. Traynelis, and S. R. Rengachary (eds.). *Techniques in Spinal Fusion and Stabilization.* New York: Thieme Medical Publishers.

Roy-Camille, R., M. Roy-Camille, and C. Demeulenaere (1970). "Osteosynthesis of Dorsal, Lumbar, and Lumbosacral Spine with Metallic Plates Screwed into Vertebral Pedicles and Articular Apophyses," *Presse. Med.* 78:1447–1448.

Roy-Camille, R., G. Saillant, and C. Mazel (1980). "Internal Fixation of the Unstable Cervical Spine by a Posterior Osteosynthesis with Plates and Screws," in H. H. Sherk, E. J. Dunn, F. J. Eismont, J. W. Fielding, D. M. Long, K. Ong, L. Penning, and R. Raynor. *The Cervical Spine.* Lippincott, Williams and Wilkins Philadelphia.

Roy-Camille, R., G. Saillant, and C. Mazel (1986). "Internal Fixation of the Lumbar Spine with Pedicle Screw Plating," *Clin. Orthop.* 203:7–17.

Serhan, H., M. Slivka, T. Albert, and S. D. Kwak (2004). "Is Galvanic Corrosion Between Titanium Alloy and Stainless Steel Spinal Implants a Clinical Concern?," *Spine J.* 4:379–387.

Singh, H., S. Y. Rahimi, D. J. Yeh, and D. Floyd (2004). "History of Posterior Thoracic Instrumentation," *Neurosurg. Focus* 16:E11.

Slone, R. M., K. W. McEnery, K. H. Bridwell, and W. J. Montgomery (1995). "Fixation Techniques and Instrumentation Used in the Cervical Spine," *Radiol. Clin. North Am.* 33:213–232.

Stambough, J. L. (1997). "Posterior Instrumentation for Thoracolumbar Trauma," *Clin. Orthop. Relat. Res.* 335:73–88.

Steffee, A. D., R. S. Biscup, and D. J. Sitkowski (1986). "Segmental Spine Plates with Pedicle Screw Fixation: A New Internal Fixation Device for Disorders of the Lumbar and Thoracolumbar Spine," *Clin. Orthop. Relat. Res.* 203:45–53.

Sturz, H., J. Hinterberger, K. Matzen, and W. Plitz (1979). "Damage Analysis of the Harrington Rod Fracture After Scoliosis Operation," *Arch. Orthop. Trauma Surg.* 95:113–122.

Thomson, W., and E. Ralston (1949). "Pseudoarthrosis Following Spine Fusion," *J. Bone Joint Surg.* 31A:400–405.

Traynelis, V. C., and R. W. Haid (1995). "Posterior Cervical Plate Stabilization with the AME Haid Universal Bone Plate System," in P. W. Hitchon, V. C. Traynelis, and S. R. Rengachary (eds.). *Techniques in Spinal Fusion and Stabilization*. New York: Thieme Medical Publishers.

Traynelis, V. C., and T. C. Ryken (1995). "Caspar Plate Stabilization of the Cervical Spine," in P. W. Hitchon, V. C. Traynelis, and S. R. Rengachary (eds.). *Techniques in Spinal Fusion and Stabilization*. New York: Thieme Medical Publishers.

Vaccaro, A. R., and R. A. Balderston (1997). "Anterior Plate Instrumentation for Disorders of the Subaxial Cervical Spine," *Clin Orthop. Relat. Res.* 335:112–121.

Zdeblick, T. A. (1995). "Z-plate Anterior Thoracolumbar Instrumentation," in P. W. Hitchon, V. C. Traynelis, and S. R. Rengachary (eds.). *Techniques in Spinal Fusion and Stabilization*. New York: Thieme Medical Publishers.

Chapter 8

Clinical Performance of Rods, Plates, Screws, and Cages

Marta L. Villarraga, Ph.D.[1,2]
(1) Exponent, Inc. Philadelphia, PA
(2) Drexel University, Philadelphia, PA

The objective of this chapter is to evaluate the clinical performance of rods, plates, and cages used for spine stabilization and fusion. This chapter covers the common damage modes for spine implants, including corrosion, ion release, fatigue, and fracture.

8.1 Introduction

The number of choices of spinal instrumentation for treatment of various indications has increased dramatically over the last two decades. In addition to understanding indications and proper surgical techniques, clinicians and design engineers can also learn from the clinical performance of spine implants to design the next generation of implants. Successful procedures with positive patient outcomes not requiring re-operation are great examples from which to learn. In addition, damage modes or indications for retrieval can also provide valuable information for both the clinicians and design engineers as the next generation of implants continues to be developed.

Reasons for retrieval of spine instrumentation are not always indicative of instrumentation failure (e.g., fracture), but can also be patient or surgical related reasons. In contrast, instrumentation failure (e.g., fracture) may not always cause patient symptoms to manifest, and as such should be a signal that there can be other reasons leading to the failure, such as a pseudarthrosis (no fusion). Even

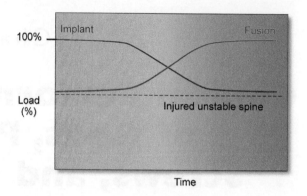

Fig. 8.1.

Perceived time rate of load sharing between spine instrumentation and fusion in bony segment. The relative time frames are not known with certainty and it is likely that the shape of the curves is not exact. *(Reproduced from White and Panjabi 1990.)*

with the identification of failed instrumentation, unless an appropriate source of the patient's symptoms is also identified, surgery to retrieve/revise the failed instrumentation will not always relieve any of the symptoms [Phillips 2004].

Spine implants are typically used to stabilize the spine while applying corrective forces (i.e., distraction, compression) as part of the treatment for a specific condition. For these applications, the goal is to achieve a bony fusion with the implants serving as a temporary load-bearing element while the bone achieves the fusion level sought and is able to bear the loads. Failure to achieve bony union will impose additional cyclic loading on the implants, which can ultimately result in fatigue failure, as implants are not made to support the loads indefinitely [Ashman et al. 1988]. Therefore, there is what appears to be a competition between the fusion mass that is forming as bone remodels and the implant that is fatiguing as it is being loaded. It is expected that as fusion progresses the loading on the implant is being reduced as it is being shared by the consolidated fusion mass (Figure 8.1) [Wang et al. 1979].

Spine implants are evaluated during the design process to determine if they meet performance criteria so that they can be considered for use in humans. The FDA issued a guidance document titled "Guidance for Industry and FDA Staff Spinal System 510(k)s" on May 3, 2004, which provides testing recommendations for spinal implant systems subject to 510(k) pre-market notification requirements [FDA 2004]. Industry standards issued by the American Society for Testing and Materials (ASTM) provide guidance for conducting mechanical and material evaluations for spine implant systems (Table 8.1). More details on the regulatory process for spine implants can be found in Chapter 15.

This chapter reviews the clinical performance of spine implants. First, anterior applications are discussed, including cervical and thoraco lumbar plates and rods. Then posterior applications are reviewed, including cervical and thoraco lumbar instrumentation. Finally, the performance of intervertebral cages is reviewed.

Table 8.1.

Relevant ASTM standards for materials used in spine implants or mechanical performance evaluation of spine implants.

Standard	Title	Scope
F543-02	Standard Specification and Test Methods for Metallic Medical Bone Screws	Performance considerations and standard test methods for measuring mechanical properties in torsion and axial pull-out for metallic medical bone screws
F1582-98 (2003)	Standard Terminology Relating to Spinal Implants	Basic terms & considerations for spinal implant devices & their mechanical analyses
F1717-04	Standard Test Methods for Spinal Implant Constructs in a Vertebrectomy Model	Materials & methods for static & fatigue testing of spinal implant assemblies, including cervical and lumbar for both anterior and posterior applications
F1798-97 (2003)	Standard Guide for Evaluating the Static and Fatigue Properties of Interconnection Mechanisms and Subassemblies Used in Spinal Arthrodesis Implants	Measurement of uniaxial static & fatigue strength, & resistance to component loosening
F2077-03	Test Methods for Intervertebral Body Fusion Devices	Materials & methods for static & dynamic testing of spinal implants designed to promote arthrodesis at a spinal motion segment
F2193-02	Standard Specifications and Test Methods for Components Used in the Surgical Fixation of the Spinal Skeletal System	Material, labeling, & handling requirements, & performance definitions for system components
F2267-04	Standard Test Method for Measuring Load Induced Subsidence of an Intervertebral Body Fusion Device Under Static Axial Compression	Materials & methods for the axial compressive subsidence testing of spinal implants designed to promote arthrodesis at a spinal motion segment

8.2 Anterior Applications

8.2.1 Cervical Spine

The use of anterior cervical plates (ACPs) to augment anterior cervical fusions has been reported to reduce the graft-related complications, maintain cervical alignment, allow immediate stabilization, and lead to higher success of fusion than grafting alone [Schultz et al. 2000]. In addition, there have been indications of improving rehabilitation following surgery and allowing a faster return to work [Geer and Papadopoulos 1999; Schultz et al. 2000]. Some earlier studies indicated that anterior cervical plating only added stability but did not increase the healing rate, promote rapid fusion, or reduce the frequency of graft-related complications [Zdeblick 1993]. The plethora of anterior cervical plate designs available has increased their use clinically, but their indication and success remains somewhat controversial [Grob et al. 1991; Wang et al. 1979; Zoega, Karrholm, and Lind 1998]. There appears to be a difference in success rates between their application for single-level versus two-level fusions [Yu and Tripuraneni 2004].

Despite this controversy, a number of anterior cervical plates have been developed and have been used clinically over the years. In 2002, Haid et al. proposed a nomenclature for describing and labeling anterior cervical plates (ACPs) based on the biomechanical and graft-loading properties of these systems. The classification is presented in Figure 7.6 and the functionality and characteristics of most of these plates are described in that section.

Examples of plates used for anterior fixation of the cervical spine include the Caspar anterior trapezoidal plate (Aesculap, San Francisco, CA), the cervical spine locking plate (CSLP, Synthes, Paoli, PA), the Orion anterior cervical plate (Medtronic Sofamor Danek, Memphis, TN), the Codman anterior cervical plate (Codman, Johnson & Johnson, Raynham, MA), the Atlantis system (Medtronic Sofamor Danek, Memphis, TN), the DOC rod (DePuy Spine, Raynham, MA), the ABC plate (Aesculap, Inc., Center Valley, PA), the A-line (Codman, Johnson & Johnson), and the Premier (Medtronic Sofamor Danek, Memphis, TN). Within these designs, new generations of plates have evolved to address the issues of minimizing graft dislodgement and reducing stress shielding of the graft in what has been termed a "dynamic plate."

Various studies have followed the outcomes of individual anterior cervical plates, whereas some have compared the performance of various implants. Among the common complications reported are indications of pseudarthrosis, screw fractures, screw pull-outs, screw or plate migration, malpositioned screws, and fractured plates [Connolly, Esses, and Kostuik 1996; Epstein 2001; Fogel et al. 2003; Grob et al. 1991; Healy and Ducheyne 1992; Heidecke, Rainov, and Burkert 1998; Lowery and McDonough 1998; Paramore, Dickman, and Sonntag 1996; Schultz et al. 2000; Zoega, Karrholm, and Lind 1998]. The importance of biomechanical evaluations of the various screw-plate constructs to gain a better understanding of each plate's physical characteristics and screw pull-out strength cannot be overestimated. This type of information is essential to allow clinicians to make a more educated decision based on biomechanical principles on what implants to utilize for different clinical indications.

In a study evaluating the effect of anterior plate fixation using the CSLP (Synthes, Paoli, PA) for one- and two-level anterior cervical discectomies and fusions, the use of this implant improved the outcome of two-level procedures compared to that of one-level uninstrumented fusions [Bolesta, Rechtine, and Chrin 2002]. On the contrary, a study following 43 patients treated with the Morscher titanium hollow screw-plate system indicated that the fusion rate of a one-level cervical fusion was not improved by the use of plate fixation and that the overall graft complication rate (pseudarthrosis plus delayed union and graft collapse) in multilevel fusions was decreased with the use of plate fixation [Connolly, Esses, and Kostuik 1996]. This study had two cases of screw lucencies on radiography, two malpositioned screws, one loose screw, and one fractured screw. These were plates that allowed no graft subsidence and thus created an environment with excessive stress shielding.

A clinical evaluation of the performance of the Codman anterior cervical plate (Codman, Johnson & Johnson, Raynham, MA) reported in 2003 based on patients at 10 centers with follow-up periods up to 24 months documented the load-sharing capabilities of this implant [Campbell et al. 1992]. Of the 190 patients followed, there was 93.7% fusion success, with 10.4% cases of hardware-related failure. These cases involved both screw fracture and partial or complete screw pull-outs and graft extrusions. There was evidence of load sharing between the plate and the bone graft as documented by the changes in the screw-plate angles over the first six months.

As part of a retrospective study in a single institution where 261 patients were followed after being treated with anterior plates following anterior corpectomy (removal of vertebral body) and allograft reconstruction, the success of fusion and related complications was reported [Mayr et al. 2002]. In this cohort, successful fusion was reported in 86.6% of the group, fibrous union in 12.6%, and unstable pseudarthrosis in 0.8% of the group. Successful fusion was defined as no motion upon review of dynamic radiographs (flexion/extension) and trabeculae present, bridging both ends of the graft. A fibrous union was defined as the absence of motion on flexion/extension views without the presence of trabeculae on either side of the graft. A pseudarthrosis was defined as the presence of motion on the dynamic radiograph and no evidence of trabeculae bridging the graft. This group had different types of implants utilized (Caspar, CSLP, Orion, and Codman), but the fusion rates were similar among the different types of instrumentation. Radiographic assessment of the patients was utilized to show that there had been hardware failure (screw fracture or pull-out) in 5.4% of the patients.

A follow-up study of 42 patients implanted with the dynamic ABC plate (Aesculap, Center Valley, PA) for single-level corpectomy documented the incidence and etiology of complications with an average follow-up of 34 months [Epstein 2001]. The reported design advantages of this slotted dynamic plate is that it allows up to 10 millimeters of cephalad and 10 millimeters of caudad migration, thus reducing stress shielding by intentionally allowing graft settling. Only four (9.5%) of the patients in this study showed evidence of plate-related failures, including one graft/plate extrusion, two indications of pseudarthrosis, and one delayed strut fracture. Of these patients, three were heavy smokers (>1 pack/day) and obese. Smoking has been noted as a factor affecting spine fusion [Bolesta, Rechtine, and Chrin 2002; Wang et al. 1979]. Despite the reported failures in this cohort, dynamic plates appear to provide a better biomechanical environment for load sharing and for minimizing stress shielding, both of which are qualities that will likely reduce pseudarthrosis.

In a prospective study evaluating the performance of the Orion locking plate (Medtronic Sofamor Danek, Memphis, TN), 96 patients were followed up for at least one year [Heidecke, Rainov, and Burkert 1998]. Only three cases (3%) of hardware failure were reported, all of which were attributed to both improper implantation technique and to osteoporosis. These cases involved screw fracture and screw and plate back-out. Despite these findings, all cases demonstrated a solid bony fusion, and thus the Orion plate was indicated as promoting a high rate of fusion.

Paramore et al. performed a retrospective clinical review of 49 patients evaluated one month postoperatively who had been implanted with the Caspar trapezoidal plate (Aesculap, Center Valley, PA) to analyze the failure mechanisms of this implant [Paramore, Dickman, and Sonntag 1996]. Of the cases reviewed, 11 displayed plate failure, five cases showed screw back-out, three had screw breakage, two had plate pull-out, and one case exhibited pseudarthrosis. Of importance to note was that the likelihood that construct failure was associated with both increased age and plate length. There was evidence of graft telescoping in 23 of the patients.

Lowery and McDonough followed 109 patients with anterior cervical fixation with an average follow-up period of 43 months and documented the incidence of hardware failure in this patient population [Lowery and McDonough 1998]. The type of instrumentation used in these patients included both constrained [CSLP (n = 22), Orion (n = 17)] and nonconstrained plates [Orozco (n = 70)]. In this group of patients, there were 38 patients (35%) with hardware failure, with 31 of these failures (44%) in nonconstrained plates and 7 failures (18%) in constrained implants. The study indicated that hardware failure was inconsequential if the patients were not symptomatic and if the hardware was not prominent. However, it was indicated that hardware failure should increase the surgeon's suspicion of nonunion, although immediate removal of the hardware is not necessary.

Hardware loosening (screws first and then followed by plates) may be the result of osteoporosis and thus insufficient bony purchase. As such, anterior cervical plating should be avoided in the osteporotic patient [An 1988]. Various bench-top cadaveric studies have shown that there is a significant correlation between screw insertion torque and bone mineral density, as well as a significant correlation between pull-out strength and bone mineral density, thereby making bone quality a great predictor of screw performance [Hitchon et al. 2003]. In addition, smoking has been associated with a higher nonunion rate and is not recommended following anterior cervical plating [Bolesta, Rechtine, and Chrin 2002; Wang et al. 1979].

Evaluation of these implant systems for their mechanical performance has been reported [Adams et al. 2001; Hitchon et al. 2003; Pitzen et al. 1999]. ASTM standard test methods (F1717) for evaluating the performance of anterior cervical plates have been established and are used extensively by engineers in the industry to assess the performance of these devices (Table 8.1). Additionally, evaluations of anterior cervical plates have been performed using cadaveric tissue to assess the biomechanical stability of various multilevel strut-graft cervical instrumentation systems in order to provide a better understanding of the load-sharing mechanics and the clinically observed instrumentation failure mechanisms [Di Angelo and Foley 2003].

8.2.2 Thoraco lumbar Anterior Plate/Rod Systems

Anterior fixation of the thoraco lumbar spine is typically done using a lateral approach with the instrumentation also being implanted on the lateral aspect of the vertebral bodies. Use of plates and/or rods via the anterior approach typically requires the use of a bone graft, a bone strut, or a cage to augment the anterior column. The use of anterior instrumentation offers the advantage of allowing the involvement of fewer segments than would be required in a posterior fixation approach. Failure modes of anterior instrumentation include implant loosening or subsidence of the strut or cage into the cancellous bone of the adjacent vertebral body, which can lead to failure of the fusion and additional unwanted deformity [Phillips 2004]. Additional reported failure modes include bending, axial slipping or fracture of rods (i.e., Dwyer system), or screw fracture (Kaneda instrumentation), with presence of pseudarthrosis or screw advancement into the spinal canal due to poor placement [Cohen and McAfee 1995]. In addition, presence of osteoporosis can also lead to instrumentation failure because the bone purchase of the screw is compromised due to the poor quality of the bone [Bayley, Yuan, and Fredrickson 1991].

Plates, such as the Roy-Camille plates, have also been utilized to stabilize the thoracic and lumbar spine posteriorly via pedicle-screws. A study reported an average follow-up of up to 19.5 months for 30 patients implanted with the Roy-Camille pedicular screw fixation system in the thoracic or lumbar spine, including their use for treating fractures, spondylolisthesis, metastatic disease, or degenerative disc disease [Simpson et al. 1993]. In this group, there was a 20% (n = 6) reported screw fracture rate, of which only one case had pseudarthrosis.

Biomechanical studies have also assisted clinicians in understanding the bone-screw interface fixation strength (pull-out) of anterior spinal instrumentation systems for scoliosis such as the Kaneda system in order to compare its fatigue performance to more traditional posterior systems used for treatment of scoliosis [Shimamoto et al. 2001]. Understanding the potential for screw loosening is an important factor to elucidate the potential loss of correction for these one-rod systems and how this loss of correction can compare to the two-rod systems. ASTM standards such as F543 and F1717 (Table 8.1) are utilized to evaluate pull-out strength of screws and to evaluate these types of implants, respectively.

8.3 Posterior Systems: Rods and Screws

8.3.1 Cervical Spine Systems

Posterior rod systems in the cervical spine are mainly used as part of longer fusions to include either the occiput or the thoracic spine. Examples of rod-screw systems that have been developed to accommodate this application in conjunction with fixation of the thoracic spine include the CerviFix (Synthes,

Paoli, PA), which is made out of titanium or titanium alloy; the Vertex (Medtronic Sofamor Danek, Memphis, TN); and the Summitt system (DePuy Spine, Rayham, MA). Of these, the CerviFix and Summitt can also be utilized to include fixation to the occiput. Another rod application for the cervical spine is the O-ring or Luque rectangle, which is attached with wires or cables [Slone et al. 1995]. These systems use screws or hooks as the mode of attachment to the lamina or pedicle.

Prospective studies evaluating the clinical performance of lateral mass screw-rod fixation systems in the cervical spine indicate that they offer advantages over plating systems [Deen et al. 2003]. Deen et al. followed 21 patients up to one year after surgery who were implanted with lateral mass screw-rod (polyaxial) constructs, and none of them showed any screw back-out or other implant related failures [Deen et al. 2003]. One of their conclusions was that screw placement is more precise because it is not constrained by the hole spacing of a plate and thus offers various advantages over plating techniques.

Posterior cervical plates have also been utilized by fixating with screws to the lateral masses for the management of cervical instability [Fehlings, Cooper, and Errico 1994]. Examples of implants that fit this category include the Roy-Camille plates and Haid posterior cervical plate (AME Haid Universal Bone Plate System, American Medical Electronics, Inc., Richardson, TX) (Figure 8.2). Reported hardware-related complications include screw loosening and subsequent pull-out related to faulty screw insertion [Fehlings, Cooper, and Errico 1994], as well as fractured plates and screws [Jones et al. 1997]. Insertion of screws at this location requires extreme caution due to the potential risk of injury to the cervical nerve roots. Removal of hardware (e.g., AO plates) from the cervicothoracic junction at the request of a patient in the hopes of reducing postoperative pain has also been reported [Chapman et al. 1996]. ASTM standards such as F1717 are utilized to evaluate the mechanical performance (static and fatigue behavior) of these types of devices (Table 8.1).

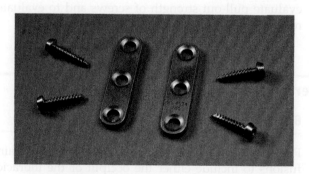

Fig. 8.2.
Haid plate and screws for lateral mass use in the cervical spine.

8.3.2 Thoraco lumbar Rods and Screws

In the thoraco lumbar and lumbar spine, posterior instrumentation consisting of rods is typically attached via pedicle-screws, hooks, or wires, with pedicle-screws being the most frequently used. The use of pedicle-screws for attachment of rods to the pedicles has been used extensively clinically over the last decade [Crawford and Esses 1994; Gertzbein et al. 1996]. Initially these screws were approved by the FDA only as bone screws and not for use in the pedicle for spinal fixation [Vaccaro and Balderston 1997], and were thus being used off-label when inserted in the spine via the pedicle. With the publication of a final rule (63 FR40025) on August 26, 1998—which classified and reclassified pedicle-screw systems—the classification of pedicle-screws was clarified [FDA 2004]. Pedicle-screw spinal systems are classified under 21 CFR Part 888, Subpart D, Section 3070 (Code of Federal Regulations) as either class II or class III devices, depending on their indication for use. The special controls these devices are subject to include compliance with material, mechanical testing, and biocompatibility standards. The recognized consensus standards that are applicable include ASTM F1717, F1798, and F1582 (Table 8.1). In addition, there are specific ASTM standards for each of the materials that can be utilized, such as 316L stainless steel, 316LVM stainless steel, 22Cr-13Ni-5Mn stainless steel, Ti-6Al-4V, and unalloyed titanium.

In the spine, the initial indications were for treatment of degenerative disorders of the lumbar spine, and then the indications were expanded to include adult lumbar scoliosis [Crawford and Esses 1994]. The variety of conditions for which they are being used clinically has expanded over the years. Pedicle-screws appear to have superior biomechanical fixation as compared with hooks, particularly in patients with good bone quality [Esses and Bednar 1989; Potter, Lehman, and Kuklo 2004]. Clinical studies have shown that despite there being a demonstrated improvement in fusion rate with transpedicular instrumentation [Zdeblick 1993], the clinical outcomes related to pain and increase in activity remain unchanged regardless of whether instrumentation is used or not [Fischgrund et al. 1997; France et al. 1999].

Failure of pedicle-screws by fracture of hardware has been reported extensively in the literature [Vaccaro and Balderston 1997]. Failure is likely to occur due to loosening or due to a loading situation that exceeds the load-bearing capacity of the implant. Likely scenarios for failure include (1) presence of pseudarthrosis that subjects the implants to continued fatigue loading until instrumentation failure occurs, (2) unstable or deficient anterior column due to the presence of tumors or unhealed fractures leading to excessive loading of posterior instrumentation [McLain, Sparling, and Benson 1993], (3) spinal deformities loading excessively the implants (kyphosis or spondylolisthesis) [Kramer, Rodgers, and Mansfield 1995], and (4) insufficient bone or poor bone quality for anchorage (osteoporosis) leading to loosening and pull-out [Phillips 2004]. Despite that pedicle-screw failures are typically only seen due to loosening and pedicle-screw fractures result mainly from pseudarthrosis, new instrumentation has evolved with more rigid and constrained connections between the screws and rods [Phillips 2004].

Pseudarthrosis as an indication of a failed fusion often cannot be made until about a year after surgery but can sometimes be identified by six months post-instrumentation [Govender 2004]. Comparisons of the incidence of pseud-arthrosis have often been done between treatment groups with instrumenta-tion against treatment groups without instrumentation. There is extensive literature on the higher incidence of pseudarthrosis in smokers versus non-smokers [Brown, Orme, and Richardson 1986; Govender 2004; Ransom, La Rocca, and Thalgott 1994; Rechtine et al. 1996; Schwab et al. 1995; Snider et al. 1999; Thalgott et al. 1997]. Despite pseudarthrosis being a likely scenario leading to hardware failure [Lagrone et al. 1988], there are reported cases where fracture of implants occurred even in the presence of a solid fusion that was confirmed during surgery [Lagrone et al. 1988] or confirmed with follow-up imaging at 18 to 37 months post-implantation [Kramer, Rodgers, and Mansfield 1995]. On the contrary, clinical study reports also exist in which despite the presence of pseudarthrosis there was no evidence of implant fracture in pedicle-screw/plate fixation of the lumbar and lumbo sacral spine [Bernhardt et al. 1992; Bohnen, Schaafsma, and Tonino 1997; Wood et al. 1995].

Failure of posterior instrumentation in the thoraco lumbar and lumbar spine typically involves loosening of the screws, or less commonly, fracture of the screws, rods, or plates (Figure 8.3) [Bailey et al. 1996; Bohnen, Schaafsman, and Tonino 1997; Enker and Steffee 1994; Esses and Bednar 1989; Gertzbein et al. 1996; Horowitch et al. 1989; Kramer, Rodgers, and Mansfield 1995; Marchesi and Aebi 1992; Ransom, La Rocca, and Thalgott 1994; Schwab et al. 1995; Weinstein, Rydevik, and Rauschning 1992; West, Bradford, and Ogilvie 1991]. These modes of fracture would typically be indicative of a failed fusion, loss of deformity correction, or excessive loading on the components beyond their fatigue strength. At times, instrumentation failure does not necessarily require surgical revision, but every case is different, and there are a number of clinical criteria that need to be considered in making that decision.

Whereas fracture of screws or rods is easily recognized in plane radiographs, screw loosening is not as obvious to detect. Evidence of screw loosening can typically be indicated by the presence of radiolucencies around the screw shafts, indicative of small motion and thus loosening and lack of fusion.

8.3.2.1 Clinical Studies

Numerous investigations have reported on the clinical performance of pedicle-screw instrumentation, all of which provide perspective to assess its short-term and long-term performance. This section reviews a few of these studies with the objective of providing the reader a brief overview of the various patient popu-lations, complications, and outcome measures identified in these studies.

Instrumentation for the thoracic spine attached via pedicle hook fixation has been reported to also utilize fixation screws passing through the interior facet into the pedicle to engage the superior end plate as an additional fixation means to prevent hook displacement [Cohen-Gadol et al. 2003]. In a study following 36 patients, there were reports of two revisions due to hook/end plate screw displacement (pull-out) and a case of end plate screw fracture.

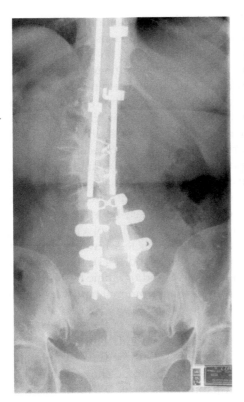
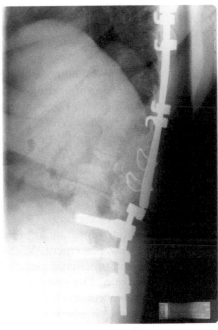

Fig. 8.3.
Radiographs of a fractured rod case with pseudoarthrosis; AP (left) and lateral (right). *(Personal spine retrieval collection.)*

In a clinical study, Wetzel et al. followed 74 patients for at least two years who underwent lumbar fusion with an unconstrained pedicle-screw system (AO/dynamic compression plate system, Synthes, Paoli, PA) and found that the overall fusion rate was 61% [Wetzel et al. 1999]. Of these patients, 22% (16) experienced hardware failure, and 12 of these had pseudarthrosis, with the failure typically occurring at the level of the pseudarthrosis. The hardware failure consisted of nine broken screws in eight patients, and 12 loose screws in the other eight patients.

Gertzbein et al. reported on a multi-center study evaluating the performance of semirigid pedicle-screw instrumentation (Moss-Miami) with circumferential (360-degree) fusion by incorporating anterior interbody fusion using allograft for patients for whom posterior fusion alone was not believed to be sufficient [Gertzbein et al. 1996]. The patient population included 82 patients with an average age of 44 years, with 54% males and 46% females, of whom 67 were followed up to two years. Complications related to instrumentation included two patients with fractured screws and one with a fractured rod, all of whom did not have the implants removed. However, two patients who complained of having painful hardware had the instrumentation removed. Despite these reported instrumentation complications, there was a 97% success rate in fusion at the two year follow-up.

In 1993, Esses et al. conducted a survey of members of the American Back Society's Committee on Surgery to focus on the type and frequency of pedicle-screw complications. As part of this survey, the respondents provided information on 617 patients and indicated that screw fracture occurred in 2.9% of their clinical cases, whereas screw loosening occurred in less than 1% (0.8%). Other complications reported were screw misplacement (5.2%), fracturing of the pedicle (2.3%), postoperative infection (4.2%) and nerve-related complications (2.4%). A comprehensive summary of pedicle-screw related complications (breakage, loosening, and misplacement) in the literature up to that date was presented with the results of this review (see Table 8.2).

In a long-term (10 years) follow-up evaluation of a group of 94 patients who underwent lumbar spine fusion with pedicle-screw instrumentation (variable screw placement, VSP, Acromed, Cleveland, OH), there were indications of good functional capacity, a low rate of radiographic failure, high patient satisfaction, a low rate of repeat surgery, and minimal hardware or surgical related complications [Glaser et al. 2003].

In a short-term (47 ± 14 months) follow-up of three groups of patients being evaluated to compare the performances of rigid, semirigid, and dynamic instrumentation, the findings indicated that all three types of implants maintained sagittal alignment of the lumbo sacral spine and showed similar improvements in pain and self-assessment [Korovessis et al. 2004]. Even though there was comparable performance among groups, there were still hardware failures reported in the dynamic group despite the lack of visible pseudarthrosis or loss of sagittal correction and asymptomatic radiolucencies present in a few patients with all three types of instrumentation.

Carson et al. reported on clinical implant failures of the Isola-VSP instrumentation (Acromed, Cleveland, OH) based on a multi-center retrospective study and their correlation to fatigue testing results in order to determine if the appropriate *in vitro* tests had been performed [Carson et al. 2003]. Five centers were surveyed to include a total of 2,499 mixed gender cases in the review. In total, there were 143 cases (5.7%) with 111 implant component failures, bone-implant interconnection failures, or complications possibly related to the instrumentation. In this set of cases, implant failure was frequently associated with a pseudarthrosis (37 confirmed) and thus indicative of an inappropriate load sharing with the anterior column of the spine. In the failures reported, 41 were screw failures (36.9%) and 57 were rod failures (51.4%). The authors indicated that the location of these failures corresponded to those observed during unilateral construct testing—namely at posterior locations, which are typically subject to higher flexion bending moments coupled with higher stresses within the component due to presence of a stress concentration and/or a surface alteration of the rod. Screw fractures were typically seen in the third (±1) cancellous thread from the integral nut, whereas rod fractures were typically seen adjacent to connectors. Both of these observations correlated well with locations identified during their *in vitro* tests. The third ranked clinical component failure

Table 8.2.

Complications associated with pedicle screws as reported by Esses et al. in 1993, to include breakdown of screw breakages (fracture), loosening, and misplacements. (*Reproduced from Esses* et al. *1993.*) See Esses et al. 1993 for references listed.

System	Authors	No. of Patients	Neurologic Complication	Screw	Infection Rate	Pseudo-arthrosis
Pedicle screw plates (Roy-Camille)	Roy-Camille et al.	227	12 (5%)	21 breakages (9%) 2 loosenings (1%) 10% of screws (in 84 patients) misplaced	13 (5.7%)	—
Pedicle screw plates (Roy-Camille)	Kinnard et al.	21	2 (10%)	5 breakages (24%)	—	—
Pedicle screw plates (modified)	Rene Louis	266	6 (2%)	8 breakages (3%) 6 loosenings (2%) 10 misplaced (4%)	3 (1%)	7 (2.6%)
VSP	Steffee et al.	120	2 (1.7%)	8 (7%)	7 (6%)	5 (4%)
VSP	Steffee et al.	14	1 (7%)	3 breakages (21.5%)	—	—
VSP (+PLIF)	Steffee et al.	36	2 (5.6%)	1 breakage (3%)	0	0
VSP	Zucherman et al.	77	—	19 breakages (25%)	4 (5%)	9 (12%)
VSP	Whitecloud et al.	40	9 (22.5%)	7 breakages (17.5%) 2 misplaced (5%)	3 (7.5%)	—
VSP	Matsuzaki et al.	57	4 (7%)	12 breakages (21%) 2 misplaced (3.5%)	—	—
Interpeduncular segmental fixation (ISF)	E. Luque	50	1 (2%)	0	1 (2%)	—
AO internal fixator	Dick	183	0	8 breakages (4%) 1 loosening (0.6%) 3 misplaced (2%)	2 (1%)	—
AO internal fixator	Aebi et al.	30	1 (3%)	2 loosening (6.7%)	0	—
AO internal fixator	Esses et al.	48	0	2 breakages (4%) 1 bent (2%) 1 loosening (2%) 2 misplaced (4%)	1 (2%)	—
AO internal fixator	Esses et al.	89	2 (2%)	3 breakages (3%) 8 misplaced (9%) 3 loosenings (3%)	4 (4.5%)	0

Continued

Table 8.2. *Continued*

System	Authors	No. of Patients	Neurologic Complication	Screw	Infection Rate	Pseudo-arthrosis
External spine fixator	Magerl	52	0	3 loosenings (6%)	4 (8%)	—
AO DCP plates	Thalgott et al.	46	3 (6.5%)	3 breakages (6.5%) 5 loosenings (11%) 3 misplaced (6.5%)	3 (6.5%)	8 (17%)
Wiltse (Longbeach)	Guyer et al.	170	5 (3%)	1 breakage (0.6%)	6 (3.5%)	—
Wiltse (Longbeach)	Horowitch et al.	99	4 (4%)	5 breakages (5%) 3 loosenings (3%)	4 (4%)	31.7%
Zielke	Hehne et al.	177	4 (2%)	4 (2%)	6 (3%)	0

observed was transverse connector failure (nine, or 8.1%), which was also observed in the *in vitro* tests when evaluating them with an H construct that produced reversed direction of lateral bending in the transverse member.

Screw misplacement leading to further complications (lateral wall intrusions, and so on) has also been reported as a complication in retrospective studies of posterior instrumentation [Bohnen, Schaafsma, and Tonino 1997; Lee et al. 2004]. Even when utilizing traditional or minimally invasive techniques, surgical complications are still reported that are sometimes attributed to screw placement [Boachie-Adjei et al. 2000]. Minimally invasive approaches for lumbar spine fusion are gaining more notoriety, but more long-term studies are still needed to assess if they truly minimize approach related morbidities [Haid et al. 2002].

Steffee et al. reported in 1993 on a prospective study in which 250 patients had been enrolled to evaluate the performance of the variable screw placement (VSP) spinal fixation system (Acromed, Cleveland, OH) for the treatment of spondylolisthesis, spinal stenosis, and postsurgical failed back syndrome and for whom there were two-year follow-up data on 73% of the patients. Of the patients followed up, there was evidence of screw fracture in 31 patients (33 screws), thus indicative of 2.5% of all screws implanted (1,314 screws total). Based on estimates obtained from other studies, the authors indicated that the fatigue life of VSP screws could vary from three days to 100 years, depending on the adequacy of load sharing in the anterior column, such that with a weak anterior column it would induce a higher bending moment and consequently an earlier fracture.

A high rate of hardware failure (fracture and disengagement) has been reported in pedicle-screw instrumentation used for short segment fusions (Figure 8.4) intended to treat fractures [Kramer, Rodgers, and Mansfield 1995; McKinley et al. 1999; McLain, Sparling, and Benson 1993; Sanderson et al. 1999].

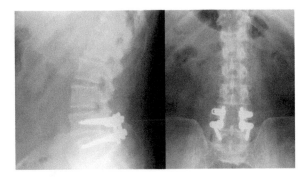

Fig. 8.4.
Example of lateral (left) and AP (right) radiographs showing a short-segment fusion. This includes levels L5-S1. *(Personal spine implant retrieval collection.)*

Screw loosening and screw breakage have also been reported in cases of short segment fixations intended for treating spondylolisthesis [Niu et al. 1996]. Kramer et al. reported on additional postoperative loss of fracture reduction at the intermediate level of the short segment fusion [Kramer, Rodgers, and Mansfield 1995]. Screw fractures were noted at the transition from 5 to 6 millimeters in diameter, but during retrieval there was no evidence of pseudarthrosis. In another study following 52 patients (mean age 29 years) treated with short-segment pedicle instrumentation (CD) for thoraco lumbar fractures, 10 patients had some sort of failure of the fixation within the early postoperative period (before six months) [McLain, Sparling, and Benson 1993]. These failures were manifested as (1) progressive kyphosis secondary to bending of the screws (Figure 8.5), (2) kyphosis resulting from osseous collapse or vertebral translation without hardware bending, and (3) segmental kyphosis after caudad screw failure. In this group of patients, there was a higher failure rate (bending) of the screws placed caudad to the fracture than cephalad (36% versus 29%) [McLain, Sparling, and Benson 1993]. This study indicated that pre-stressing of the screws through forced compression or due to *in situ* loading increased bending moments due to the short nature of the fusion and contributed to their early failure. In another retrospective study evaluating short segment posterior fixation used for patients with thoraco lumbar fractures without fusions (n = 28), there was a 14% failure rate of implants, manifested as screw fractures [Sanderson et al. 1999]. The implant failure rate for this study was comparable to that of others being treated with fusion.

8.3.2.2 Biomechanical Studies

Understanding the range of loads supported by spinal instrumentation has been evaluated biomechanically using various approaches. One approach that has been reported is via telemetrized load measurement, and another is with the use of computational models. Rohlmann et al. measured loads in internal spine fixation devices *in vivo* by implanting a telemetrized device in a patient

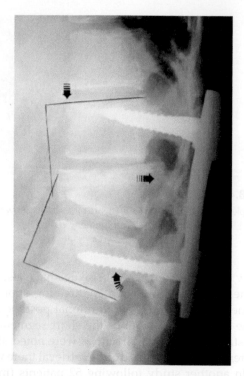

Fig. 8.5.
Progressive kyphosis secondary to bending of screws. *(Reprinted from McLain et al. 1993. The copyright is owned by* The Journal of Bone and Joint Surgery, *Inc.)*

at L2-L4 and following the patient through a variety of daily activities [Rohlmann et al. 1995]. This study indicated that while the patient was lying in a relaxed position the loads were small, but the highest loads were measured with the patient sitting, standing, and walking with a maximum of bending moments up to 5 to 8 Nm in these activities. The other way to get an understanding of the loads on spinal instrumentation is through finite element modeling of instrumented spine segments [Goel and Gilbertson 1995; Goel et al. 1988]. The approach of utilizing modeling as a tool has provided the means to gain insight into load sharing with spinal instrumentation and the stress levels imposed on spinal implants.

Various bench-top cadaveric studies have evaluated a number of important issues regarding the stability of posterior instrumentation, including the pedicle-screw system [Barber et al. 1998; Carlson et al. 1992; Ferrara et al. 2003; Fogel et al. 2003; Yamagata et al. 1992]. One set of these studies has shown that there is a significant correlation between screw insertion torque and bone mineral density, as well as a significant correlation between pull-out strength and bone mineral density, thereby making bone quality a great predictor of screw performance [Carlson et al. 1992; Fogel et al. 2003; Zdeblick 1993; Zdeblick et al. 1993]. Therefore, the presence of osteoporosis can also lead to posterior instrumentation failure because the bone purchase of the screw is compromised due to the poor quality of the bone.

Human spines are not typically able to withstand long-term loading because most donors are from an older age group and also due to long-term deterioration of the specimens. As such, only a few biomechanical studies exist that have evaluated the fatigue endurance of posterior instrumentation on tissue. Instead, calf spine models have been utilized [Wittenberg et al. 1992]. One such study compared the fatigue performance of Harrington rods, Luque plates, AO fixators, Steffee plates, and the Kluger fixation system on a calf spine model by subjecting these to compressive cyclic loading at 2 Hz over a range of 605 to 275 N after a compressive preload of 440 N and by limiting the loading cycles to a maximum of 100,000 [Wittenberg et al. 1992]. Of the implants evaluated, there were no fatigue failures in the Harrington rods or Luque plates, whereas the others had either screw or rod fatigue failures.

As an alternative, testing methodologies have been developed utilizing vertebral body surrogate models to evaluate the fatigue performance of various posterior implants [Cunningham et al. 1993]. The use of these UHMWPE cylinders representative of vertebral bodies has even been adopted in standardized testing methodologies utilized to evaluate implant performance as per ASTM F1717 (Table 8.1).

Various biomechanical bench-top studies have been performed to evaluate the failure mechanisms of pedicle-screws in short-segment fusions [Chiba et al. 1996; McKinley et al. 1999]. One of these has shown increased bending moments resulting from failure to insert screws to their full depth [McKinley et al. 1999]. The potential effect that the increased bending moment can have in reducing the cycles to failure of a pedicle-screw is important to consider especially when a fusion fails to consolidate. Some clinicians have protected pedicle-screw constructs to avoid screw bending failure by adding offset laminar hooks, increasing the length of the posterior instrumentation, or augmenting the posterior procedure with an anterior reconstruction [McKinley et al. 1999].

Although these approaches can provide assistance in reducing the bending moment, the benefits need to be considered as they will increase the number of interconnections available for micro-motion. An increased number of interconnections will provide more potential sites for fretting corrosion, increase the surgical burden on the patient (morbidity), and add to the cost of the procedure. Another biomechanical study showed the advantage of including supplemental offset hooks. These have been shown to increase construct stiffness when bending loads were applied without sacrificing the biomechanical principles of short-segment fixation [Chiba et al. 1996]. Of importance is that the reduction of the bending moments on the screws can prevent their early failure.

Other cadaveric studies have evaluated insertion techniques to determine optimal screw placement to evaluate the resistance to pull-out strength and to enhance fixation. One particular study found that there was an advantage to placing pedicle-screws in 30 degrees of convergence as compared to placing them in parallel to offer more resistance to axial pull-out [Barber et al. 1998].

Another study compared the biomechanical effects of short-term and long-term cyclic loading (180,000 cycles) on lumbar motion segments instrumented with either pedicle-screws or transfacet pedicle-screw systems [Ferrara et al. 2003]. The cadaveric model showed that the stability of both systems was not compromised after cyclic loading and that both appeared biomechanically equivalent as tested *in vitro*. The transfacet pedicle-screw fixation provides the opportunity of less dorsal destruction in the posterior elements.

In evaluating the pull-out behavior of pedicle-screws using cadaveric or animal models, another study has noted the importance of the contribution of the stress relaxation properties of bone and their effect on the pull-out behavior of pedicle-screws [Inceoglu et al. 2004]. The pull-out strength of pedicles augmented with carbonated apatite cement was shown to be greater than that of a control group (non-augmented) in human lumbar cadaveric testing designed to evaluate enhancement options for screw fixation [Lotz et al. 1997].

Pull-out strength testing of screws is described extensively in the literature and is outlined in ASTM standard F543 (Table 8.1). This testing guideline is easily implemented and most valuable to compare strength of various screw designs. Dawson et al. noted that despite the value of this comparative information, there are few clinical reports that actually cite screw loosening and pull-out as the failure mechanism [Dawson et al. 2003].

In addition, bench-top biomechanical studies evaluating numerous commonly used posterior polyaxial screw systems have also shown that the polyaxial screw head coupling is the first failure point and may be a protective feature of the pedicle-screw, thus preventing pedicle-screw and rod fracture [Fogel et al. 2003]. A comparison of the pull-out strength of conical and cylindrical pedicle-screws in a fully inserted setting and backed out 180 degrees was performed using a calf-spine model [Lill et al. 2000]. This study indicated that after cyclic loading, the conical screws had displaced significantly more than cylindrical ones, especially after being backed out by 180 degrees as compared to when they were fully inserted. Knowledge gained from bench-top biomechanical evaluations and computational modeling of spinal instrumentation can be a valuable resource of information for clinicians when choosing the most adequate instrumentation for a given clinical indication [Abumi, Panjabi, and Duranceau 1989; Ashman et al. 1988; Duffield et al. 1993; Farcy et al. 1987; Ferrara et al. 2003; Gaines et al. 1991; Law, Tencer, and Anderson 1993; McKinley et al. 1999].

In addition to rods, screws, and hooks, there is another component that is part of posterior instrumentation sets. Cross links or transverse connectors exist to connect two rods in order to increase torsional stiffness and to enhance stability of the construct [Dick et al. 1997]. The idea is that with a more rigid construct fusion will be enhanced. There are a number of different cross-link designs that have been made available by the different manufacturers of posterior instrumentation, all of which have the same ultimate goal of enhancing stability. Jensen et al. evaluated the relevance of interconnection strength as outlined in ASTM F1798-97 (Table 8.1) and the relevance to reported clinical complications [Jensen et al. 2003]. They concluded that the tests outlined in the standard do not adequately test for relevant clinical failures as reported in the literature, and as such that interconnection failure was not well documented *in vivo*.

8.3.2.3 Other Reasons for Removal: Prominence, Corrosion, or Operative Site Pain

Prominence of hardware [Deckey, Court, and Bradford 2000; Weinstein, Rydevik, and Rauschning 1992] and operative site pain have also been cited as a reason for removal of posterior thoraco lumbar spine instrumentation [Bohnen, Schaafsma, and Tonino 1997; Christensen et al. 1998; Cook et al. 2000; Gaine et al. 2001; Hume et al. 1996; Lagrone et al. 1988; Schwab et al. 1995; Senaran et al. 2004]. Although not very common, persistent low back pain can result from hardware irritation, and unsatisfactory outcomes have been documented as reasons for instrumentation removal [Gaine et al. 2001; Gertzbein et al. 1996; Hume et al. 1996; Lagrone et al. 1988]. This has also been termed late-onset discomfort or late operative site pain (LOSP) related to pseudarthrosis or to the presence of the implants in the spine [Cook et al. 2003]. Cook et al. have noted how regardless of implant type, LOSP of no apparent cause after instrumentation for treatment of scoliosis is relieved in most patients once the implants are removed [Asher, Cook, and Lai 2001; Cook et al. 2000, 2003].

Various studies have documented removal of hardware for these reasons. In a study following only the patients that required hardware removal (24% of original patients implanted with Wiltse pedicle-screw fixation), radiolucency was documented around the screws indicative of pseudarthrosis. In this study, hardware removal did not always offer a substantial improvement to the back pain noted earlier [Hume et al. 1996]. In another study, hardware removal led to loss of correction, pain, and further surgery due to new graft fracture or pseudarthrosis [Deckey, Court, and Bradford 2000]. In a retrospective study including 875 patients implanted with 4,790 pedicle-screws, 23% of the screws were associated with late-onset discomfort of the patient. These patients were those who necessitated removal of the instrumentation [Lagrone et al. 1988]. Only 20.7% of the patients that had the hardware removed had evidence of pseudarthrosis. In this same group of patients, only 0.5% of the screws were fractured.

In a study of six cases reporting removal of Isola instrumentation due to late operative site pain, symptoms were relieved immediately following implant removal [Gaine et al. 2001]. In these patients, the implants were removed 12 to 20 months after surgery and all showed a granulation tissue reaction with the presence of metallic debris that varied from very sparse to abundant due to the presence of fretting at the cross-connector junctions. Histological evaluations confirmed that there was infection at these sites along with clear evidence of fretting at the cross connectors. Cook et al. reported that the most frequent observation (9 of 14) noted in the group of patients that had the implants removed for LOSP was corrosion alone or corrosion with bursa formation, with the most frequent sites for corrosion being where upper compression and distraction hooks connected, or where open hooks and transverse connectors interfaced [Cook et al. 2000].

Metallic implants do corrode, and with corrosion there is release of metal ions into the surrounding environment. There are a number of reports documenting corrosion on spine implants [Aulisa et al. 1982; Vieweg et al. 1999]. Metal wear debris released due to fretting corrosion can occur due to the number of interconnecting surfaces present in spinal instrumentation and their resulting micro-motion [Aulisa et al. 1982; Bidez et al. 1987; Clark and Shufflebarger 1999; Hallab, Cunningham, and Jacobs 2003; Prikryl et al. 1989; Soultanis et al. 2003; Wang et al. 1979]. Even though stainless steel is more susceptible to fretting corrosion than titanium alloys, spinal instrumentation devices made from both materials have been reported to release metal debris [Vieweg et al. 1999; Villarraga et al. 2000; Wang et al. 1979] and have shown evidence of corrosion following *in vitro* testing [Serhan et al. 2004]. Corrosion findings have been reported in Harrington and Luque rods [Prikryl et al. 1989], and in TLS-Kluger instrumentation [Vieweg et al. 1999]. As such, corrosion of stainless steel components has been reported in previous retrieval studies of spinal implants [Prikryl et al. 1989; Simpson et al. 1993; Vieweg et al. 1999] to worsen the fatigue performance of orthopedic implants [Jacobs, Gilbert, and Urban 1998], and corrosion by-products are suspected of causing deleterious biologic tissue responses in the adjacent tissue surrounding the implant [Vieweg et al. 1999].

Cook et al. proposed a possible correlation between LOSP and fretting corrosion [Cook et al. 2003]. In his report, 27 cases of late operative site pain (LOSP) were clinically reported, and fretting corrosion was reported to exist in 14 of those cases. When evaluating the *in vitro* tests, there was a greater tendency for fretting corrosion within interconnections that had lower axial-torsional gripping. They noted that stronger cross linking (interconnection) appeared to correlate with a decreased incidence of LOSP in their biomechanical and clinical study.

Despite these findings from *in vitro* and *in vivo* reports, there are currently no corrosion standards to evaluate the performance of spine instrumentation. Kirkpatrick et al. performed a literature review to note the frequency of reporting of corrosion on retrieved spinal implants and combined this information with an evaluation of retrieved implants from 33 patients [Kirkpatrick et al. 2003]. In their retrieval evaluation, they noted that polished-finished stainless steel implants commonly exhibited fretting damage and corrosion at interconnection interfaces. In addition, the matte-finished stainless steel components had corrosion at more interconnections and more extensively than the polished-finished implants. In contrast, there was little evidence of corrosion on Ti6Al4V implants. They concluded that as more insight is gained into corrosion of spinal implants, with the advent of dynamic implants and intervertebral disc replacements, there should be consideration in the future as to whether standards to evaluate corrosion are necessary.

The identification of cellular responses to wear debris in periprosthetic tissue [Mody, Esses, and Heggeness 1994; Wang et al. 1979], serum, and hair have also been studied [Geremia et al. 1985; Kasai, Iida, and Uchida 2003]. In addition, other studies document the identification of elevated serum levels of nickel and chromium even after four years of follow-up of patients implanted with posterior instrumentation for the treatment of scoliosis [Geremia et al. 1985]. These studies had posterior implants with multiple connectors as potential sources for micro-motion and crevice corrosion.

Senaran et al. have reported on the ultrastructural analysis of metal debris as well as on the tissue reaction around stainless steel spinal implants in patients complaining of late operative site pain (LOSP). Analysis of the tissue around pedicle-screws revealed greater counts of macrophages as compared to tissue obtained from other locations. In contrast, the tissue around the transverse rod connectors revealed more abundance of particulate debris identified to be mostly iron and chromium. This study indicated the likelihood that this metal debris was the result of fretting corrosion of the stainless steel implants as evident by the metal debris identified.

In a retrieval program established locally, we evaluated posterior thoracolumbar rod implants retrieved from 57 patients, whose average age at implantation was 43.9 years to look for evidence of wear and corrosion. The time of implantation ranged from two months to 13.5 years. Wear was present in 75%, corrosion in 39%, and fractures in 7% of the retrieved implants. Wear and/or corrosion were more prevalent, with respect to the total number of implants retrieved, in implants that had been in service at least one year. There was no evidence of corrosion in any of the Ti implants, whereas corrosion was present (with wear) in 58% of the stainless steel (SS) implants. Implantation times were longer for SS implants than for Ti implants. Wear and corrosion (Figures 8.6 and 8.7) were more frequently observed in long rods than in short rods. Tissue retrieved at the time of implantation for the two stainless steel implants that remained *in vivo* the longest (up to 13.5 years) was analyzed for trace metal content (inductively coupled plasma) and found to contain noticeable amounts of Fe, Ni, and Cr (up to 3,580 ppm Ni, 480 ppm Fe, and 48 ppm of Cr), indicative of corrosion processes taking place.

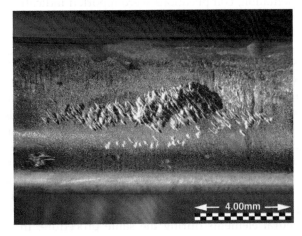

Fig. 8.6.

Evidence of wear on a retrieved rod. This implant was *in vivo* for 3.9 years. (*Personal spine implant retrieval collection.*)

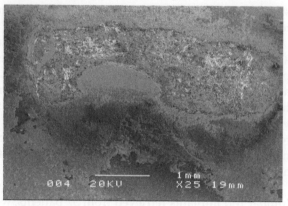

Fig. 8.7.

Evidence of corrosion on a retrieved rod at 25× magnification. This implant was *in vivo* for 1.4 years. *(Personal spine implant retrieval collection.)*

8.4 Intervertebral Body Devices: Cages

Intervertebral body devices are typically placed via anterior, posterior, or lateral approaches and can include implants that are impacted to interface with the vertebral body end plates or threaded implants. Each approach has its advantages and disadvantages from the perspectives of both the surgical technique and surgical outcome [Pavlov et al. 2000]. Each of these approaches is described with an acronym: PLIF for posterior lumbar interbody fusion, ALIF for anterior lumbar interbody fusion, and TLIF for transverse lumbar interbody fusion.

Despite early successes with the use of cages without any posterior instrumentation, complications were reported indicative of failed interbody devices [Cohen and McAfee 1995; Kuslich et al. 1998]. The indications for failure of these devices were more due to inadequate placing and improper sizing (inadequate operative approach), leading to inappropriate load sharing and failure of the intended fusion rather than to failure of the implants themselves [Cohen and McAfee 1995]. Typical failures of interbody devices include failure of the fusion to take place, cage loosening, subsidence and/or migration [Hacker et al. 2000], and inappropriately positioned cages leading to failure of fusion [Hacker et al. 2000; Phillips 2004]. Removal of these devices is difficult and not typical. Rather, supplemental intervention is done either anteriorly or posteriorly to stabilize the motion segments and to enhance the segment to promote stability and eventually fusion [Bozkus et al. 2004].

Posterior lumbar interbody fusion (PLIF) describes the surgical technique to fuse the spine from a posterior approach while allowing decompression of the neural elements during the same procedure. In doing so, PLIF dynamically decompresses the neural structures [Lin, Cautilli, and Joyce 1983]. This approach includes use of bone (autologous from the iliac crest or allograft from donors) or bone chips to promote fusion. Recently the use of interbody cages (carbon fiber or titanium mesh) have been used in addition to the bone to prevent graft subsidence. A clinical report of 60 patients with an average follow-up of up to 5.3 years operated with PLIF combined with posterolateral instrumentation indicates an 83% satisfaction [Freeman, Licina, and Mehdian 2000]. This approach, which can be described as a circumferential fusion, has been associated with superior outcomes despite an increase in the surgery time and costs. Circumferential (or 360 fusion), which can also include ALIF and posterior pedicle instrumentation, has also shown superior outcomes [Thalgott et al. 2000]. It appears that the addition of the instrumentation provides compression of the interbody space, likely reducing graft/cage migration.

Examples of cages that have been used clinically include the BAK (Centerpulse Spine Tech, Minneapolis, MN), the threaded interbody fusion device (TIFBD, Medtronic Sofamor Danek, Memphis, TN), the Harms titanium mesh cage (DePuy Spine, Raynham, MA), and the Brantigan rectangular and rounded cages (DePuy Spine, Raynham, MA) [Cohen and McAfee 1995].

A clinical study compared the performance of cages, bone dowel, and dowel-plate constructs in the cervical spine for anterior fusion [Hacker et al. 2000]. The cage being evaluated for this study was the BAK/C (Centerpulse Spine Tech, Minneapolis, MN). This study showed that out of 88 patients evaluated the cage group had the lowest graft requirement/risks, achieved similar patient outcomes, and fused at a higher rate than the bone dowel or bone-dowel plate groups.

A study reported on the clinical results and implant-related complications in anterior cervical fusion using titanium mesh (Figure 8.8) and anterior plates [Kanayama et al. 2003]. Of the 24 cases reported, 42% had indications of cage subsidence in the upper vertebrae (up to more than 3 mm) and 50% in the lower vertebrae (up to more than 3 mm). Displacement of the titanium mesh was another noted complication. Despite the elimination of the need for an iliac

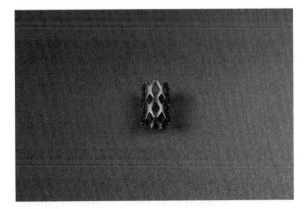

Fig. 8.8.
Titanium mesh.

autograft because of the use of local autograft packed in the titanium mesh, the fusions took longer to become solid as compared to iliac autografts.

Clinical studies evaluating the safety and efficacy of intervertebral body cages under FDA-sponsored approved protocols have documented outcome measures indicative of clinical success and fusion success as well as complications [Brantigan, Steffee, and Geiger 1991]. Brantigan et al. reported on the evaluation of a wedge-shaped carbon fiber reinforced polymer cage used in a posterior lumbar interbody fusion (PLIF) along with pedicle-screw fixation (VSP spine system, DePuy Acromed Corporation, Raynham, MA) in a group of 36 patients [Brantigan, Steffee, and Geiger 1991]. Despite the clinical and fusion success rates reported being higher than previously reported with a square cage, device-related complications of fractured screws were still reported (n = 2). The authors noted that the device-related complications were within the expected range for complex spinal reconstructive surgery.

In another clinical study by Brantigan et al., they reported on long-term follow-up on part of the patient group that had been enrolled in the original clinical study conducted prior to the approval of the carbon fiber reinforced polymer cage in 1999 [Brantigan, Steffee, and Geiger 1991]. At 10 years, the clinical success increased as compared to the two-year follow-up, with comparable patient satisfaction as originally reported. There were indications of adjacent segment degeneration in 61% of the patients and no difference in the clinical or fusion success between smokers and nonsmokers.

Subsidence through the vertebral end plates is one of the complications considered when designing intervertebral cages. Designs that induce increased stresses at the host implant area of contact have been associated with end plate failure and subsidence, and as such are not desirable [Burkus 2002]. Similarly, considering tapered cage designs and their benefits in maintaining the segmental lordosis when used anteriorly (ALIF) is of value because it provides anatomic restoration of the intervertebral disc space. This approach establishes a more biomechanically adequate sagittal alignment to the patients, which ultimately impacts their long-term outcome [Burkus et al. 2004].

Likewise, resorption of bone allograft cages has been cited as a reason for loss in disc space height and subsequent screw fracture in the adjoining posterior instrumentation [Brantigan, Steffee, and Geiger 1991]. Following the crushing of the graft and its resorption, the lack of fusion was evident due to the presence of a lucency at the end-plate/allograft boundary.

Biomechanical studies have also increased our understanding of the load sharing occurring in the presence of intervertebral body cages. Carson et al. [1990] presented a finite element analysis of load distribution and bending moments in an instrumented spine. This study concluded that the presence of anterior load sharing through an intact disc or an intervertebral body cage (like a carbon fiber cage) can improve the load sharing and thereby extend the fatigue life of the pedicle instrumentation used in conjunction with the interbody device [Carson et al. 1990]. In essence, the lack of load sharing in the anterior column (no cage) can lead to fatigue failures (fractures) of pedicle-screws. ASTM standard F2077 exists for evaluating these intervertebral body devices (Table 8.1).

8.5 Conclusions

As was reviewed in this chapter, successful clinical performance of spine instrumentation is the goal of the original clinical intervention. However, sometimes patient or surgical related factors place the implants in situations that lead to failure. The intended intervention is therefore considered unsuccessful. Proper training and use of implants in the hands of experienced surgeons can help minimize complications [Sidhu and Herkowitz 1997]. An additional complication due to the presence of implanted devices in the spine is the development of pathology at adjacent segments to the treated ones, which is also known as adjacent segment disease. This has been documented to take place in both the lumbar and cervical spine. Extensive reviews exist on this topic and as such were not covered here [Park et al. 2004].

Learning from analysis of retrievals and clinical indications accompanying those retrieved implants can provide valuable information to both improve implants and enhance clinical practices for the use of spinal instrumentation. Implant spine registries can also be a valuable source to track the clinical performance and failures of spine instrumentation in the patient population [Roder et al. 2002].

8.6 Acknowledgments

I would like to thank Stephanie Teti for her assistance collecting the literature for this chapter and also to her and Jill Heinly for their review of this chapter.

8.7 References

Abumi, K., M. M. Panjabi, and J. Duranceau (1989). "Biomechanical Evaluation of Spinal Fixation Devices. Part III. Stability Provided by Six Spinal Fixation Devices and Interbody Bone Graft," *Spine* 14:1249–1255.

Adams, M. S., N. R. Crawford, et al. (2001). "Biomechanical Comparison of Anterior Cervical Plating and Combined Anterior/Lateral Mass Plating," *Spine J.* 1:166–170.

An, H. S. (1988). "Anterior Instrumentation of the Cervical Spine," in H. S. An and L. H. Riley III (eds.). *An Atlas of Spine Surgery.* London: Martin-Dunitz.

Asher, M., S. Cook, and S. M. Lai (2001). "Late Operative Site Pain with Isola Posterior Instrumentation Requiring Implant Removal: Infection or Metal Reaction?," *Spine* 26:2516–2517.

Ashman, R. B., J. G. Birch, et al. (1988). "Mechanical Testing of Spinal Instrumentation," *Clin. Orthop.* 227:113–125.

Aulisa, L., A. di Benedetto, et al. (1982). "Corrosion of the Harrington's Instrumentation and Biological Behaviour of the Rod-human Spine System," *Biomaterials* 3:246–248.

Bailey, S. I., P. Bartolozzi, et al. (1996). "The BWM Spinal Fixator System: A Preliminary Report of a 2-year Prospective, International Multicenter Study in a Range of

Indications Requiring Surgical Intervention for Bone Grafting and Pedicle-Screw Fixation," *Spine* 21:2006–2015.

Barber, J. W., S. D. Boden, T. Ganey, and W. C. Hutton (1998). "Biomechanical Study of Lumbar Pedicle-Screws: Does Convergence Affect Axial Pullout Strength?," *J. Spinal Disord.* 11:215–220.

Bayley, J. C., H. A. Yuan, and B. E. Fredrickson (1991). "The Syracuse I-plate," *Spine* 16:S120–S124.

Bernhardt, M., D. E. Swartz, et al. (1992). "Posterolateral Lumbar and Lumbosacral Fusion with and Without Pedicle-Screw Internal Fixation," *Clin. Orthop. Relat. Res.* 284:109–115.

Bidez, M. W., L. C. Lucas, et al. (1987). "Biodegradation Phenomena Observed In Vivo and In Vitro Spinal Instrumentation Systems," *Spine* 12:605–608.

Boachie-Adjei, O., F. P. Girardi, M. Bansal, and B. A. Rawlins (2000). "Safety and Efficacy of Pedicle-Screw Placement for Adult Spinal Deformity with a Pedicle-probing Conventional Anatomic Technique," *J. Spinal Disord.* 13:496–500.

Bohnen, I. M., J. Schaafsma, and A. J. Tonino (1997). "Results and Complications After Posterior Lumbar Spondylodesis with the Variable Screw Placement Spinal Fixation System," *Acta Orthop. Belg.* 63:67–73.

Bolesta, M. J., G. R. Rechtine II, and A. M. Chrin (2002). "One- and Two-level Anterior Cervical Discectomy and Fusion: The Effect of Plate Fixation," *Spine J.* 2:197–203.

Bozkus, H., R. H. Chamberlain, et al. (2004). "Biomechanical Comparison of Anterolateral Plate, Lateral Plate, and Pedicle-Screws-rods for Enhancing Anterolateral Lumbar Interbody Cage Stabilization," *Spine* 29:635–641.

Brantigan, J. W., A. D. Steffee, and J. M. Geiger (1991). "A Carbon Fiber Implant to Aid Interbody Lumbar Fusion. Mechanical Testing," *Spine* 16:S277–S282.

Brown, C. W., T. J. Orme, and H. D. Richardson (1986). "The Rate of Pseudarthrosis (Surgical Nonunion) in Patients Who Are Smokers and Patients Who Are Nonsmokers: A Comparison Study," *Spine* 11:942–943.

Burkus, J. K. (2002). "Intervertebral Fixation: Clinical Results with Anterior Cages," *Orthop. Clin. North Am.* 33:349–357.

Burkus, J. K., T. C. Schuler, M. F. Gornet, and T. A. Zdeblick (2004). "Anterior Lumbar Interbody Fusion for the Management of Chronic Lower Back Pain: Current Strategies and Concepts," *Orthop. Clin. North Am.* 35:25–32.

Campbell, P., S. Nasser, N. Kossovsky, and H. C. Amstutz (1992). "Histopathological Effects of Ultrahigh-molecular-weight Polyethylene and Metal Wear Debris in Porous and Cemented Surface Replacements," in K. R. St. John (ed.). *Particulate Debris from Medical Implants: Mechanisms of Formation and Biological Consequences, ASTM STP 1144.* Philadelphia, PA: American Society for Testing and Materials.

Carlson, G. D., J. J. Abitbol, et al. (1992). "Screw Fixation in the Human Sacrum: An In Vitro Study of the Biomechanics of Fixation," *Spine* 17:S196–S203.

Carson, W., M. Asher, et al. (2003). "History of Isola-VSP Fatigue Testing Results with Correlation to Clinical Implant Failures," in M. L. Melkerson, S. L. Griffith, and J. S. Kirkpatrick (eds.). *Spinal Implants: Are We Evaluating Them Appropriately.* West Conshohocken, PA: ASTM International.

Carson, W. L., R. C. Duffield, et al. (1990). "Internal Forces and Moments in Transpedicular Spine Instrumentation: The Effect of Pedicle-Screw Angle and Transfixation—the 4R-4bar Linkage Concept," *Spine* 15:893–901.

Chapman, J. R., P. A. Anderson, et al. (1996). "Posterior Instrumentation of the Unstable Cervicothoracic Spine," *J. Neurosurg.* 84:552–558.

Chiba, M., R. F. McLain, et al. (1996). "Short-segment Pedicle Instrumentation: Biomechanical Analysis of Supplemental Hook Fixation," *Spine* 21:288–294.

Christensen, F. B., K. Thomsen, et al. (1998). "Functional Outcome After Posterolateral Spinal Fusion Using Pedicle-Screws: Comparison Between Primary and Salvage Procedure," *Eur. Spine J.* 7:321–327.

Clark, C. E., and H. L. Shufflebarger (1999). "Late-developing Infection in Instrumented Idiopathic Scoliosis," *Spine* 24:1909–1912.

Cohen, M. G., and P. McAfee (1995). "Kaneda Anterior Spinal Instrumentation," in P. W. Hitchon, V. C. Traynelis, and S. R. Rengachary (eds.). *Techniques in Spinal Fusion and Stabilization.* New York: Thieme Medical Publishers.

Cohen-Gadol, A. A., M. B. Dekutoski, et al. (2003). "Safety of Supplemental Endplate Screws in Thoracic Pedicle Hook Fixation," *J. Neurosurg. Spine* 98:31–35.

Connolly, P. J., S. I. Esses, and J. P. Kostuik (1996). "Anterior Cervical Fusion: Outcome Analysis of Patients Fused with and Without Anterior Cervical Plates," *J. Spinal Disord.* 9:202–206.

Cook, S., M. Asher, W. Carson, and S. M. Lai (2003). "Effect of Transverse Connector Design on Development of Late Operative Site Pain: Preliminary Clinical Findings," in M. L. Melkerson, S. L. Griffith, and J. S. Kirkpatrick (eds.). *Spinal Implants: Are We Evaluating Them Appropriately.* West Conshohocken, PA: ASTM International.

Cook, S., M. Asher, S. M. Lai, and J. Shobe (2000). "Reoperation After Primary Posterior Instrumentation and Fusion for Idiopathic Scoliosis: Toward Defining Late Operative Site Pain of Unknown Cause," *Spine* 25:463–468.

Crawford, M. J., and S. I. Esses (1994). "Indications for Pedicle Fixation: Results of NASS/SRS Faculty Questionnaire," North American Spine Society and Scoliosis Research Society. *Spine* 19:2584–2589.

Cunningham, B. W., J. C. Sefter, Y. Shono, and P. C. McAfee (1993). "Static and Cyclical Biomechanical Analysis of Pedicle-Screw Spinal Constructs," *Spine* 18:1677–1688.

Dawson, J. M., P. Boschert, M. M. Macenski, and N. Rand (2003). "Clinical Relevance of Pull-out Strenght Testing of Pedicle-Screws," in M. L. Melkerson, J. S. Kirkpatrick, and S. L. Griffith (eds.). *Spinal Implants: Are We Evaluating Them Appropriately?* West Conshohocken, PA: ASTM International.

Deckey, J. E., C. Court, and D. S. Bradford (2000). "Loss of Sagittal Plane Correction After Removal of Spinal Implants," *Spine* 25:2453–2460.

Deen, H. G., B. D. Birch, R. E. Wharen, and R. Reimer (2003). "Lateral Mass Screw-rod Fixation of the Cervical Spine: A Prospective Clinical Series with 1-year Follow-up," *Spine J.* 3:489–495.

Di Angelo, D. J., and K. T. Foley (2003). "An Improved Biomechanical Testing Protocol for Evaluating Multilevel Cervical Instrumentation in a Human Cadaveric Corpectomy Model," in M. L. Melkerson, J. S. Kirkpatrick, and S. L. Griffith (eds.). *Spinal Implants: Are We Evaluating Them Appropriately?* West Conshohocken, PA: ASTM International.

Dick, J. C., T. A. Zdeblick, B. D. Bartel, and D. N. Kunz (1997). "Mechanical Evaluation of Cross-link Designs in Rigid Pedicle-Screw Systems," *Spine* 22:370–375.

Duffield, R. C., W. L. Carson, L. Y. Chen, and B. Voth (1993). "Longitudinal Element Size Effect on Load Sharing, Internal Loads, and Fatigue Life of Tri-level Spinal Implant Constructs," *Spine* 18:1695–1703.

Enker, P., and A. D. Steffee (1994). "Interbody Fusion and Instrumentation," *Clin. Orthop. Relat. Res.* 300:90–101.

Epstein, N. (2001). "Anterior Approaches to Cervical Spondylosis and Ossification of the Posterior Longitudinal Ligament: Review of Operative Technique and Assessment of 65 Multilevel Circumferential Procedures," *Surg. Neurol.* 55:313–324.

Esses, S. I., and D. A. Bednar (1989). "The Spinal Pedicle-Screw: Techniques and Systems," *Orthop. Rev.* 18:676–682.

Farcy, J. P., M. Weidenbaum, et al. (1987). "A Comparative Biomechanical Study of Spinal Fixation Using Cotrel-Dubousset Instrumentation," *Spine* 12:877–881.

FDA (2004). "Guidance for Industry and FDA Staff Spinal Systems 510(k)s" Orthopedic Devices Branch; Division of General, Center for Device and Radiological Health.

Fehlings, M. G., P. R. Cooper, and T. J. Errico (1994). "Posterior Plates in the Management of Cervical Instability: Long-term Results in 44 Patients," *J. Neurosurg.* 81:341–349.

Ferrara, L. A., J. L. Secor, et al. (2003). "A Biomechanical Comparison of Facet Screw Fixation and Pedicle-Screw Fixation: Effects of Short-term and Long-term Repetitive Cycling," *Spine* 28:1226–1234.

Fischgrund, J. S., M. Mackay, et al. (1997). "1997 Volvo Award Winner in Clinical Studies: Degenerative Lumbar Spondylolisthesis with Spinal Stenosis: A Prospective, Randomized Study Comparing Decompressive Laminectomy and Arthrodesis with and Without Spinal Instrumentation," *Spine* 22:2807–2812.

Fogel, G. R., W. Liu, C. A. Reitman, and S. I. Esses (2003). "Cervical Plates: Comparison of Physical Characteristics and In Vitro Pushout Strength," *Spine J.* 3:118–124.

Fogel, G. R., C. A. Reitman, W. Liu, and S. I. Esses (2003). "Physical Characteristics of Polyaxial-headed Pedicle-Screws and Biomechanical Comparison of Load with Their Failure," *Spine* 28:470–473.

France, J. C., M. J. Yaszemski, et al. (1999). "A Randomized Prospective Study of Posterolateral Lumbar Fusion: Outcomes with and Without Pedicle-Screw Instrumentation," *Spine* 24:553–560.

Freeman, B. J., P. Licina, and S. H. Mehdian (2000). "Posterior Lumbar Interbody Fusion Combined with Instrumented Postero-lateral Fusion: 5-year Results in 60 Patients," *Eur. Spine J.* 9:42–46.

Gaine, W. J., S. M. Andrew, et al. (2001). "Late Operative Site Pain with Isola Posterior Instrumentation Requiring Implant Removal: Infection or Metal Reaction?," *Spine* 26:583–587.

Gaines, R. W. Jr., W. L. Carson, C. C. Satterlee, and G. I. Groh (1991). "Experimental Evaluation of Seven Different Spinal Fracture Internal Fixation Devices Using Non-failure Stability Testing: The Load-sharing and Unstable-mechanism Concepts," *Spine* 16:902–909.

Geer, C. P., and S. M. Papadopoulos (1999). "Instrumentation After Anterior Cervical Fusion," *Clinical Neurosurgery* 45:25–29.

Geremia, G. K., K. S. Kim, L. Cerullo, and L. Calenoff (1985). "Complications of Sub-laminar Wiring," *Surg. Neurol.* 23:629–635.

Gertzbein, S. D., R. Betz, et al. (1996). "Semirigid Instrumentation in the Management of Lumbar Spinal Conditions Combined with Circumferential Fusion: A Multi-center Study," *Spine* 21:1918–1925; discussion 1916–1925.

Glaser, J., M. Stanley, et al. (2003). "A 10-year Follow-up Evaluation of Lumbar Spine Fusion with Pedicle-Screw Fixation," *Spine* 28:1390–1395.

Goel, V. K., and L. G. Gilbertson (1995). "Applications of the Finite Element Method to Thoracolumbar Spinal Research: Past, Present, and Future," *Spine* 20:1719–1727.

Goel, V. K., Y. E. Kim, T. H. Lim, and J. N. Weinstein (1988). "An Analytical Investigation of the Mechanics of Spinal Instrumentation," *Spine* 13:1003–1011.

Govender, S. (2004). "Lumbar Pseudoarthrosis," in H. N. Herkowitz, M. Nordin, J. Dvorak, D. Grob, and G. R. Bell (eds.). *The Lumbar Spine* (3d ed.). Philadelphia: Lippincott Williams & Wilkins.

Grob, D., B. Jeanneret, M. Aebi, and T. M. Markwalder (1991). "Atlanto-axial Fusion with Transarticular Screw Fixation," *J. Bone Joint. Surg. Br.* 73:972–976.

Hacker, R. J., J. C. Cauthen, T. J. Gilbert, and S. L. Griffith (2000). "A Prospective Randomized Multicenter Clinical Evaluation of an Anterior Cervical Fusion Cage," *Spine* 25:2646–2654; discussion 2655.

Haid, R. W., K. T. Foley, G. E. Rodts, and B. Barnes (2002). "The Cervical Spine Study Group Anterior Cervical Palte Nomenclature," *Neurosurg. Focus* 12:1–6.

Hallab, N. J., B. W. Cunningham, and J. J. Jacobs (2003). "Spinal Implant Debris-induced Osteolysis," *Spine* 28:S125–S138.

Healy, K. E., and P. Ducheyne (1992). "The Mechanisms of Passive Dissolution of Titanium in a Model Physiological Environment," *J. Biomed. Mater. Res.* 26:319–338.

Heidecke, V., N. G. Rainov, and W. Burkert (1998). "Anterior Cervical Fusion with the Orion Locking Plate System," *Spine* 23:1796–1802; discussion 1803.

Hitchon, P. W., M. D. Brenton, et al. (2003). "Factors Affecting the Pullout Strength of Self-drilling and Self-tapping Anterior Cervical Screws," *Spine* 28:9–13.

Horowitch, A., R. D. Peek, et al. (1989). "The Wiltse Pedicle-Screw Fixation System: Early Clinical Results," *Spine* 14:461–467.

Hume, M., D. A. Capen, et al. (1996). "Outcome After Wiltse Pedicle-Screw Removal," *J. Spinal Disord.* 9:121–124.

Inceoglu, S., R. F. McLain, et al. (2004). "Stress Relaxation of Bone Significantly Affects the Pull-out Behavior of Pedicle-Screws," *J. Orthop. Res.* 22:1243–1247.

Jacobs, J. J., J. L. Gilbert, and R. M. Urban (1998). "Corrosion of Metal Orthopaedic Implants," *J. Bone Joint Surg. Am.* 80:268–282.

Jensen, L. M., S. S. Springer, S. F. Campbell, and E. Gray (2003). "Interconnection Strength Testing and Its Value in Evaluating Clinical Performance," in M. L. Melkerson, S. L. Griffith, and J. S. Kirkpatrick (eds.). *Spinal Implants: Are We Evaluating them Appropriately.* West Conshohocken, PA: ASTM International.

Jones, E. L., J. G. Heller, D. H. Silcox, and W. C. Hutton (1997). "Cervical Pedicle-Screws Versus Lateral Mass Screws: Anatomic Feasibility and Biomechanical Comparison," *Spine* 22:977–982.

Kanayama, M., T. Hashimoto, et al. (2003). "Pitfalls of Anterior Cervical Fusion Using Titanium Mesh and Local Autograft," *J. Spinal Disord. Tech.* 16:513–518.

Kasai, Y., R. Iida, and A. Uchida (2003). "Metal Concentrations in the Serum and Hair of Patients with Titanium Alloy Spinal Implants," *Spine* 28:1320–1326.

Kirkpatrick, J. S., R. Venugolopalan, et al. (2003). "Corrosion on Spinal Implant Constructs: Should Standards Be Revised?," in M. L. Melkerson, S. L. Griffith, and J. S. Kirkpatrick (eds.). *Spinal Implants: Are We Evaluating them Appropriately.* West Conshohocken, PA: ASTM International.

Korovessis, P., Z. Papazisis, G. Koureas, and E. Lambiris (2004). "Rigid, Semirigid Versus Dynamic Instrumentation for Degenerative Lumbar Spinal Stenosis: A Correlative Radiological and Clinical Analysis of Short-term Results," *Spine* 29:735–742.

Kramer, D. L., W. B. Rodgers, and F. L. Mansfield (1995). "Transpedicular Instrumentation and Short-segment Fusion of Thoracolumbar Fractures: A Prospective Study Using a Single Instrumentation System," *J. Orthop. Trauma* 9:499–506.

Kuslich, S. D., C. L. Ulstrom, et al. (1998). "The Bagby and Kuslich Method of Lumbar Interbody Fusion: History, Techniques, and 2-year Follow-up Results of a United States Prospective, Multicenter Trial," *Spine* 23:1267–1278; discussion 1279.

Lagrone, M. O., D. S. Bradford, et al. (1988). "Treatment of Symptomatic Flatback After Spinal Fusion," *J. Bone Joint Surg. Am.* 70:569–580.

Law, M., A. F. Tencer, and P. A. Anderson (1993). "Caudo-cephalad Loading of Pedicle-Screws: Mechanisms of Loosening and Methods of Augmentation," *Spine* 18:2438–2443.

Lee, S. H., W. G. Choi, et al. (2004). "Minimally Invasive Anterior Lumbar Interbody Fusion Followed by Percutaneous Pedicle-Screw Fixation for Isthmic Spondylolisthesis," *Spine J.* 4:644–649.

Lill, C. A., U. Schlegel, D. Wahl, and E. Schneider (2000). "Comparison of the In Vitro Holding Strengths of Conical and Cylindrical Pedicle-Screws in a Fully Inserted Setting and Backed Out 180 Degrees," *J. Spinal Disord.* 13:259–266.

Lin, P. M., R. A. Cautilli, and M. F. Joyce (1983). "Posterior Lumbar Interbody Fusion," *Clin. Orthop. Relat. Res.* 180:154–168.

Lotz, J. C., S. S. Hu, et al. (1997). "Carbonated Apatite Cement Augmentation of Pedicle-Screw Fixation in the Lumbar Spine," *Spine* 22:2716–2723.

Lowery, G. L., and R. F. McDonough (1998). "The Significance of Hardware Failure in Anterior Cervical Plate Fixation: Patients with 2- to 7-year Follow-up," *Spine* 23:181–186; discussion 186–187.

McKinley, T. O., R. F. McLain, et al. (1999). "Characteristics of Pedicle-Screw Loading: Effect of Surgical Technique on Intravertebral and Intrapedicular Bending Moments," *Spine* 24:18–24; discussion 25.

McLain, R. F., E. Sparling, and D. R. Benson (1993). "Early Failure of Short-segment Pedicle Instrumentation for Thoracolumbar Fractures: A Preliminary Report," *J. Bone Joint Surg. Am.* 75:162–167.

Marchesi, D. G., and M. Aebi (1992). "Pedicle Fixation Devices in the Treatment of Adult Lumbar Scoliosis," *Spine* 17:S304–S309.

Mayr, M., B. Subach, et al. (2002). "Cervical Spinal Stenosis: Outcome After Anterior Corpectomy, Allograft Reconstruction, and Instrumentation," *J. Neurosurg.* 96:10–16.

Mody, D. R., S. I. Esses, and M. H. Heggeness (1994). "A Histologic Study of Soft-tissue Reactions to Spinal Implants," *Spine* 19:1153–1156.

Niu, C. C., W. J. Chen, L. H. Chen, and C. H. Shih (1996). "Reduction-fixation Spinal System in Spondylolisthesis," *Am. J. Orthop.* 25:418–424.

Paramore, C. G., C. A. Dickman, and V. K. Sonntag (1996). "Radiographic and Clinical Follow-up Review of Caspar Plates in 49 Patients," *J. Neurosurg.* 84:957–961.

Park, P., H. J. Garton, et al. (2004). "Adjacent Segment Disease After Lumbar or Lumbosacral Fusion: Review of the Literature," *Spine* 29:1938–1944.

Pavlov, P. W., M. Spruit, et al. (2000). "Anterior Lumbar Interbody Fusion with Threaded Fusion Cages and Autologous Bone Grafts," *Eur. Spine J* 9:224–229.

Phillips, F. M. (2004). "Failed Surgery and Revision Surgery: Failed Instrumentation," in H. N. Herkowitz, J. Dvorak, G. R. Bell, M. Nordin, and D. Grob (eds.). *The Lumbar Spine* (3d ed.). Philadelphia: Lippincott Williams & Wilkins.

Pitzen, T., H. J. Wilke, et al. (1999), "Evaluation of a New Monocortical Screw for Anterior Cervical Fusion and Plating by a Combined Biomechanical and Clinical Study," *Eur. Spine J.* 8:382–387.

Potter, B. K., R. A. Lehman, and T. R. Kuklo (2004). "Anatomy and Biomechanics of Thoracic Pedicle-Screw Instrumentation," *Curr. Opin. Ortho.* 15:133–141.

Prikryl, M., S. C. Srivastava, et al. (1989). "Role of Corrosion in Harrington and Luque Rods Failure," *Biomaterials* 10:109–117.

Ransom, N., S. H. La Rocca, and J. Thalgott (1994). "The Case for Pedicle Fixation of the Lumbar Spine," *Spine* 19:2702–2706.

Rechtine, G. R., C. E. Sutterlin, et al. (1996). "The Efficacy of Pedicle-Screw/Plate Fixation on Lumbar/Lumbosacral Autogenous Bone Graft Fusion in Adult Patients with Degenerative Spondylolisthesis," *J. Spinal Disord.* 9:382–391.

Roder, C., A. El-Kerdi, D. Grob, and M. Aebi (2002). "A European Spine Registry," *Eur. Spine J.* 11:303–307.

Rohlmann, A., G. Bergmann, F. Graichen, and H. M. Mayer (1995). "Telemeterized Load Measurement Using Instrumented Spinal Internal Fixators in a Patient with Degenerative Instability," *Spine* 20:2683–2689.

Sanderson, P. L., R. D. Fraser, et al. (1999). "Short Segment Fixation of Thoracolumbar Burst Fractures Without Fusion," *Eur. Spine J.* 8:495–500.

Schultz, K. D. Jr., M. R. McLaughlin, et al. (2000). "Single-stage Anterior-posterior Decompression and Stabilization for Complex Cervical Spine Disorders," *J. Neurosurg. Spine* 93:214–221.

Schwab, F. J., D. G. Nazarian, F. Mahmud, and C. B. Michelsen (1995). "Effects of Spinal Instrumentation on Fusion of the Lumbosacral Spine," *Spine* 20:2023–2028.

Senaran, H., P. Atilla, et al. (2004). "Ultrastructural Analysis of Metallic Debris and Tissue Reaction Around Spinal Implants in Patients with Late Operative Site Pain," *Spine* 29:1618–1623; discussion 1623.

Serhan, H., M. Slivka, T. Albert, and S. D. Kwak (2004). "Is Galvanic Corrosion Between Titanium Alloy and Stainless Steel Spinal Implants a Clinical Concern?," *Spine J.* 4:379–387.

Shimamoto, N., Y. Kotani, et al. (2001). "Biomechanical Evaluation of Anterior Spinal Instrumentation Systems for Scoliosis: In Vitro Fatigue Simulation," *Spine* 26: 2701–2708.

Sidhu, K. S., and H. N. Herkowitz (1997). "Spinal Instrumentation in the Management of Degenerative Disorders of the Lumbar Spine," *Clin. Orthop. Relat. Res.* 335:39–53.

Simpson, J. M., N. A. Ebraheim, W. T. Jackson, and S. Chung (1993). "Internal Fixation of the Thoracic and Lumbar Spine Using Roy-Camille Plates," *Orthopedics* 16:663–672.

Slone, R. M., K. W. McEnery, K. H. Bridwell, and W. J. Montgomery (1995). "Fixation Techniques and Instrumentation Used in the Cervical Spine," *Radiol Clin. North Am.* 33:213–232.

Snider, R. K., N. K. Krumwiede, et al. (1999). "Factors Affecting Lumbar Spinal Fusion," *J. Spinal Disord.* 12:107–114.

Soultanis, K., G. Mantelos, A. Pagiatakis, and P. N. Soucacos (2003). "Late Infection in Patients with Scoliosis Treated with Spinal Instrumentation," *Clin. Orthop.* 411:116–123.

Thalgott, J. S., A. K. Chin, et al. (2000). "Minimally Invasive 360 Degrees Instrumented Lumbar Fusion," *Eur. Spine J.* 9 (Suppl. 1):S51–S56.

Thalgott, J. S., R. C. Sasso, et al. (1997). "Adult Spondylolisthesis Treated with Posterolateral Lumbar Fusion and Pedicular Instrumentation with AO DC Plates," *J. Spinal Disord.* 10:204–208.

Vaccaro, A. R., and R. A. Balderston (1997). "Anterior Plate Instrumentation for Disorders of the Subaxial Cervical Spine," *Clin. Orthop. Relat. Res.* 335:112–121.

Vieweg, U., D. van Roost, et al. (1999). "Corrosion on an Internal Spinal Fixator System," *Spine* 24:946–951.

Villarraga, M. L., R. C. Anderson, et al. (2000). "Mechanisms of Titanium Release from Posterior Cervical Spine Plates in a Canine Model Based on Computational and Biocompatibility Studies," in W. Soboyejo (ed.). *Functional Biomaterials.* Winterthur, Switzerland: Trans Tech Publications Ltd.

Wang, G. J., R. Whitehill, W. G. Stamp, and R. Rosenberger (1979). "The Treatment of Fracture Dislocations of the Thoracolumbar Spine with Halofemoral Traction and Harrington Rod Instrumentation," *Clin. Orthop. Relat. Res.* 142:168–175.

Weinstein, J. N., B. L. Rydevik, and W. Rauschning (1992). "Anatomic and Technical Considerations of Pedicle-Screw Fixation," *Clin. Orthop. Relat. Res.* 284:34–46.

West, J. L. III, D. S. Bradford, and J. W. Ogilvie (1991). "Results of Spinal Arthrodesis with Pedicle-Screw-plate Fixation," *J. Bone Joint Surg. Am.* 73:1179–1184.

Wetzel, F. T., M. Brustein, F. M. Phillips, and S. Trott (1999). "Hardware Failure in an Unconstrained Lumbar Pedicle-Screw System: A 2-year Follow-up Study," *Spine* 24:1138–1143.

Wittenberg, R. H., M. Shea, et al. (1992). "A Biomechanical Study of the Fatigue Characteristics of Thoracolumbar Fixation Implants in a Calf Spine Model," *Spine* 17:S121–S128.

Wood, G. W. II, R. J. Boyd, et al. (1995). "The Effect of Pedicle-Screw/Plate Fixation on Lumbar/Lumbosacral Autogenous Bone Graft Fusions in Patients with Degenerative Disc Disease," *Spine* 20:819–830.

Yamagata, M., H. Kitahara, et al. (1992). "Mechanical Stability of the Pedicle-Screw Fixation Systems for the Lumbar Spine," *Spine* 17:S51–S54.

Yu, W. D., and K. R. Tripuraneni (2004). "Cervical Interbody Cage Fusions," *Seminars in Spine Surgery* 16:2–8.

Zdeblick, T. A. (1993). "A Prospective, Randomized Study of Lumbar Fusion: Preliminary Results," *Spine* 18:983–991.

Zdeblick, T. A., D. N. Kunz, M. E. Cooke, and R. McCabe (1993). "Pedicle-Screw Pullout Strength: Correlation with Insertional Torque," *Spine* 18:1673–1676.

Zoega, B., J. Karrholm, and B. Lind (1998). "Plate Fixation Adds Stability to Two-level Anterior Fusion in the Cervical Spine: A Randomized Study Using Radiostereometry," *Eur. Spine J.* 7:302–307.

Chapter *9*

Biologics to Promote Spinal Fusion

Bill McKay, ME; Steve Peckham, Ph.D.;
and Jeff Scifert, Ph.D.
Medtronic Sofamor Danek, Memphis, TN

9.1 Introduction

Spinal fusion has become the standard of care for the treatment of back and leg pain due to spinal instability and deformity. Spinal instability and deformity result in excessive motion and compression of neural structures within and exiting the spinal canal. By decompressing the neural structures and limiting this abnormal motion through a spinal fusion, back and leg pain can often be reduced. Use of autogenous bone graft from the iliac crest has been the gold standard for conducting spinal fusions because of its ability to promote new bone formation and fusion. Fusion rates of approximately 85% have typically been reported with the use of autogenous bone, but ranges as large as 35 to 100% have been published. The reason for this large range in fusion rates is primarily due to surgeon technique differences and the quality and quantity of the autogenous bone used. The problems of harvesting autogenous bone are also well documented and include postoperative pain, infection, possible harvest site fracture, and limited quantity. The desire to avoid these harvest site complications and potentially improve on fusion rate consistency has led to the development of numerous commercial bone graft substitutes.

The flood of new bone graft substitutes on the market today has led to confusion in the surgical community about the differences among them. The lack of a consistent level of both pre-clinical and clinical data on many of them has only added to the confusion. This chapter attempts to review the various bone graft substitutes being used in spinal fusion and compare and contrast their relative efficacy.

Bone graft substitutes can be categorized into three major categories; osteoinductive, osteoconductive, and a new frequently utilized term osteopromotive. Osteoinductive bone graft materials have the inherent ability to induce new bone formation, and by definition can form bone in a non-bony site. Therefore, osteoinductivity is assessed by a materials ability to form *de novo* bone in a two- to four-week period in the standard rat ectopic model. The only osteoinductive materials known today are bone morphogenetic proteins (BMPs) and allograft demineralized bone matrix (DBM). The relative efficacy of these osteoinductive materials will be covered first, followed by the osteoconductive and osteopromotive bone graft materials. Osteoconductive materials do not have the inherent ability to induce new bone formation, but simply act as a scaffold on which new bone may form. The term *osteopromotive* has recently been used to describe those materials that play an active role in bone metabolism but are not inherently osteoinductive, such as platelet rich plasma and bone marrow. Comparison of the relative efficacy of bone graft substitute materials will guide how they should be used surgically, either as a true bone graft replacement for autogenous bone or as a bone graft extender that has to be used in combination with autograft bone to be effective. In the review of these various technologies, it is important to take note of the relative level and quality of the data available. The available level and quality of data will help establish whether a particular bone graft can be used as an autograft replacement or extender.

Prospective, randomized, level 1, clinical data provide the highest level of data possible, followed by nonhuman primate data, and finally lower-order animal data. Intertransverse spinous process spinal fusion is also typically more challenging that an intervertebral interbody spinal fusion, and provides a higher level of proof of a materials efficacy or ability to form bone. This is because an intertransverse process fusion has less bleeding bone in the area, more adjacent soft tissue, and is a much larger gap in which new bone must form to be successful. All of these variables should be considered when comparing and contrasting the efficacy of bone grafting substitutes. In general, as shown in Table 9.1, only recombinant bone morphogenetic proteins have been shown clinically to be effective autogenous bone graft replacements while all the other bone graft substitute materials should only be used as autograft extenders (i.e., DBM, bone marrow, ceramics).

9.2 Osteoinductive Bone Graft Substitutes

Iliac crest autograft has long been considered the "gold standard" for bone grafting in spinal fusion surgery. Host bone acts as a scaffold on which new bone can grow (osteoconductive), provides biochemical signals to produce new bone (osteoinductive), and contains the cells that can respond to the osteoinductive signal (osteogenic). It is against this standard that prospective bone grafting materials are measured. Although iliac crest autograft is considered an

Table 9.1.

Surgical use of bone graft substitutes based on published human clinical studies.

	Autograft Replacement	Autograft Extender
Osteoinductive		
Bone morphogenetic protein (BMP)	X	
Allograft demineralized bone (DBM)		X
Osteoconductive		
Ceramics		X
Ceramics/collagen composites		X
Osteopromotive		
Platelet-rich plasma (PRP)		?
Bone marrow		X

effective bone grafting material, its use does present several disadvantages. First, the amount of iliac crest bone graft that can be harvested is, by nature, limited. Also, many patients experience pain at the graft harvest site postoperatively with some patients reporting pain out to two years and beyond. Finally, serious complications such as graft site infection or fracture at the graft site do occur, although these complications are rare. For these reasons, there is tremendous interest in finding graft materials that offer the effectiveness of iliac crest autograft without the complications.

As described previously, purely osteoconductive bone grafting materials have limited utility in spinal applications. These are passive materials that provide a scaffold on which new bone may form. In spinal fusion surgery, the goal is to grow bone at sites where bone normally does not. Therefore, osteoinductive materials that are capable of producing de novo bone formation are the only materials that have any chance of acting as autograft substitutes in spinal bone grafting procedures. Osteoinductive materials are those that contain bone morphogenetic proteins, the only known biochemical compounds that can induce new bone formation.

9.3 Bone Morphogenetic Proteins

Bone morphogenetic proteins (BMPs) are naturally occurring proteins found in bone that are responsible for the ability of bone to regenerate itself. The concept that bone contains factors that stimulate new bone formation was advanced by Dr. Marshall Urist in 1965. In his early work, Urist demonstrated that new bone would form when demineralized bone was implanted intramuscularly in rats and rabbits. It was Urist who later used the term *bone morphogenetic protein* to describe the bone inducing factors present in bone matrix. Since that time, researchers have worked to try and harness the natural inductive capacity of bone for use in orthopedic bone grafting procedures.

Over the last forty years, much has been learned about BMPs. BMPs are members of the transforming growth factor β (TGF-β) superfamily of proteins. A number of different BMPs have been isolated and identified. Several of these have been shown to be osteoinductive, and the mechanisms by which BMPs induce new bone have been elucidated. The primary function for BMPs is to induce differentiation of mesenchymal stem cells or preosteoblasts into bone forming osteoblasts. These responding cells come from the surrounding tissue or from bleeding bone which occurs through decortication of host bone as part of the spinal fusion procedure. Some osteoinductive BMPs are also chemotactic. That is, certain cells respond to BMPs by migrating from areas of low BMP concentration to areas of higher BMP concentration. Also, BMPs have been shown to cause cell division or proliferation. It is through these chemotactic and mitogenic mechanisms that BMPs can increase the number of responding cells at the site of implantation.

There are two types of bone grafting materials available today that contain BMP and that can be considered to be osteoinductive. These are demineralized bone matrix (DBM) products and products containing recombinant human bone morphogenetic protein (rhBMP). Although both types of product are inductive and contain BMP, the level of osteoinductivity and the capacity to induce new bone formation are vastly different between the two material classes. For this reason, the clinical applications for these products in spinal surgery are generally different. DBM products are most often positioned as autograft extenders or enhancers, while rhBMP products are positioned as autograft replacements. This distinction is supported by the available literature as described in the next two sections of this chapter.

9.4 Demineralized Bone Matrix

Demineralized bone matrix (DBM) is produced by acid treatment of donor bone tissue to remove the mineral component of the bone. What remains after processing is primarily collagen. However, there are small amounts of growth factors including BMPs present in this matrix. Attempts to quantify the amount of BMP in bone have shown that a kilogram of bone contains only nanogram quantities of BMP [Jaw, Keesling, and Wironen 2001; Wozney 1993]. It is these BMPs that are responsible for whatever osteoinductive potential exists for DBM. Blum et al. [2004] extracted BMP from DBM and measured BMP-2 and BMP-4 levels. The samples were also tested in a rat ectopic model. The authors

Table 9.2.

Commercially available DBM products.

Company	Brand Name and Form(s)	Carrier
Medtronic Sofamor Danek/RTI, Inc.	OSTEOFIL DBM paste, ICM	Porcine gelatin
Osteotech	Grafton gel, putty, flex, matrix, crunch	Glycerol
	Grafton plus	Starch
Synthes/MTF	DBX paste, putty mix	Hyaluronic acid
Wright Medical/ Allosource	Allomatrix putty	Calcium sulfate and CMC
	Osteoset DBM pellets	Calcium sulfate
	Ignite ICS injectable mix	Calcium sulfate, CMC, and aspirated bone marrow
ISOTIS	DynaGraft gel, putty, Orthoblast	Reverse-phase polymer
	Accell DBM putty, total bone matrix	DBM derived
Stryker	Allocraft DBM putty	Acellular dermis
DePuy	Optium DBM gel, putty	Glycerol
EBI	Osteostim DBM putty	Human collagen derived from allograft tendon
Interpore Cross	InterGro DBM putty	Soy bean based lipid
Smith and Nephew	Viagraf DBM gel, putty, Flex crunch	Glycerol

found a strong correlation between the level of extractable BMP-2 and the amount of bone formation. For commercial purposes DBM powder is mixed with a carrier of some type to provide the desired handling properties. The most commonly used additives include glycerol, hyaluronic acid, carboxymethylcellulose, synthetic polymer, and gelatin. Some of the DBM products also have corticocancellous allograft chips added to the DBM to provide an osteoconductive scaffold for new bone formation. A list of currently marketed DBM products is provided in Table 9.2.

Although the basic premise is the same for all products in that they contain osteoinductive DBM combined with a carrier matrix, the final products may be very different. Each tissue bank has its own processing methods that may affect the degree of demineralization and ultimately the osteoinductivity of the final product. Even if the DBM were processed in the same way for each product and there were no variability in the osteoinductive potential of the DBM initially, there would still be differences among the available products. The effects of the various additives cannot be neglected since they will determine how well the material stays in place initially and the residence time of the material at the site of implantation. Some materials may be less cohesive than others and may tend to wash away very easily. On the other hand, a very cohesive material may not allow good cell penetration unless the carrier is removed relatively quickly by the body. Finally, some DBM products are terminally sterilized while others are aseptically processed which may affect osteoinductivity of the final product.

All of the previously cited differences would be present even if the starting DBM material were the same. Unfortunately, the issue is further complicated by the fact that all DBM is not the same. There are potential differences in osteoinductivity of the DBM based on processing techniques, donor age, and inherent variability in allograft tissue. Although processing techniques could be modified, donor variability is a fact, and each tissue bank has to decide how best to mitigate this variability. Some tissue banks may test DBM for osteoinductivity by implanting samples of DBM intramuscularly in athymic rats or nude mice and looking for de novo bone formation. Others may use cell based assays to test for inductivity. Still others may use donor age limits to increase the probability that the processed DBM is osteoinductive. Regardless, there is no standard by which one product may be compared to another and no requirement that products be tested for osteoinductivity. Ultimately, there is no guarantee to the surgeon that every lot of a particular DBM containing product will have the same osteoinductivity level.

Osteoinductivity testing of DBM products has been directed in two specific areas. These areas of research include studies to understand the variables that affect osteoinductivity and studies to compare various methods of assessing osteoinductivity to find methods that provide fast, accurate, and reproducible results for use in routine screening of DBM. Research on factors that affect osteoinductivity has given mixed results. Traianedes et al. [2004] tested DBM from 248 donors grouped by age up to 85 years. These authors found a small reduction in osteoinductivity with increasing donor age for male donors but not for female donors. They concluded that with proper processing DBM from donors up to age 85 could produce viable grafting material. The idea that processing is more important than donor variability in determining osteoinductivity of the final product is supported by Takikawa et al. [2003]. These authors tested multiple lots of two commercially available DBM products and found that one consistently produced more bone than the other. These results are contrasted by the work of Nyssen-Behets et al. [1996], who did find a trend toward decreasing osteoinductivity with increasing donor age.

In comparing different lots of DBM, Maddox et al. [2000] found wide variability in performance in the rat ectopic model for individual lots from the same tissue bank. Han et al. [2003] tested DBM from five established tissue banks and also found wide batch to batch variability both between samples from different tissue banks and also between lots from the same tissue bank. These results suggest a greater role of donor variability than processing method in determining osteoinductivity of DBM. With these differing results, it remains questionable whether consistent osteoinductivity can be assured by controlling processing methods or setting arbitrary age limits for donors.

The results of research on the osteoinductivity testing methods themselves have been less controversial and more consistent. Edwards et al. [1998] showed that the rat ectopic model was sensitive enough to distinguish between DBM samples with different osteoinductive potential. This was done by mixing inactivated DBM with normal DBM in different ratios and assessing the amount of bone formation. While this model is widely used and accepted, it is time consuming because the samples are generally collected at 28 days before being subjected to histological processing. Another option is in vitro testing in which alkaline phosphatase activity in cells is measured in response to exposure to DBM. Three separate studies have reported good correlation between results of *in vitro* testing and bone formation in the rat ectopic model [Edwards, Diegmann, and Scarborough 1998; Han, Tang, and Nimni 2003; Zhang, Powers, and Wolfinbarger 1997]. While osteoinductivity testing of some sort would seem like a logical step in the tissue preparation process, there are currently no requirements for any standardized testing for DBM products. Although both the *in vivo* and *in vitro* testing do give some information on the inherent osteoinductivity of the DBM component of a product, they do not give any information on the effectiveness of that particular product in any clinical application.

In order to better understand the potential efficacy of DBM in spinal surgery, a review of the published pre-clinical and clinical data on the use of DBM products in spinal surgery is provided here. Even though these products are often used in spinal fusion surgery, it should be understood that none of the available DBM products have an FDA cleared indication for use as an autograft replacement in spinal fusion surgery. In fact, until recently DBM products have been considered to be minimally manipulated human tissue which means that their marketing would not be regulated by FDA. With no requirements for large multi-center prospective randomized human clinical investigations prior to commercial release, available data are limited primarily to lower order animal spinal fusion studies or prospective and retrospective summaries of clinical experience in relatively small numbers of patients.

9.5 DBM: Pre-clinical Studies

Pre-clinical lower-order animal studies with DBM include rat, rabbit, and canine models. In the models, DBM products are used alone, combined with bone marrow or as an adjunct to autograft bone for either interbody or posterolateral fusion in the lumbar spine. Direct comparison between studies is often difficult because technique may vary from site to site, and the duration of the studies is not always consistent. Therefore, it is best to consider the body of evidence in order to draw general conclusions regarding the efficacy and utility of DBM products in these lower-order animal models.

Studies of DBM alone have been performed in rat posterolateral fusion models. Peterson et al. [2004] compared three commercial DBM products in an athymic rat posterolateral fusion model and found that Grafton (Osteotech,

Eatontown, NJ), DBX (Synthes, West Chester, PA), and Allomatrix (Wright Medical, Memphis, TN) produced fusion rates of 100, 50, and 0% (respectively) at eight weeks. The authors concluded that there were differences in the osteoinductive potential of these commercial DBM products. In a similar study it was found that Grafton yielded a fusion rate of 13% at three weeks and 39% at six weeks [Bomback et al. 2004]. Autograft was not tested in either of these studies. It is not known whether lot to lot variability could have contributed to the different results seen in this study. Additional testing of multiple lots could help determine whether this is the case.

Several studies have also been published using a canine posterior fusion model. In one of these studies Helm et al. [1997] showed no benefit of adding DBM to autograft and even suggested that the DBM may have had an inhibitory effect on bone formation. This study achieved a different result from that published by Frenkel [1993], where DBM added to autograft yielded more bone formation than autograft alone, suggesting a role for DBM as an autograft enhancer or extender. For his part, Cook [1995] found that neither DBM alone nor DBM added to allograft was able to achieve fusion in the canine model by 26 weeks. Once again these seemingly contradictory results may have been due to differences in DBM processing or handling or inherent osteoinductivity of the donor bone.

Finally, studies in the rabbit posterolateral fusion model have been performed with DBM products alone, in combination with iliac crest autograft and with the addition of bone marrow. In the rabbit posterior fusion model, Ragni showed that a combination of DBM and bone marrow gave a fusion rate of 83%. However, there was no testing of DBM alone so the effect of the addition of bone marrow could not be assessed [Ragni, Lindholm, and Lindholm 1987]. In a subsequent study, the same authors found that DBM with and without bone marrow gave equivalent results suggesting no added benefit of the bone marrow [Lindholm, Ragni, and Lindholm 1988]. A third study by these authors showed equivalence between DBM combined with a hyaluronic acid carrier and iliac crest autograft in a rabbit interbody fusion model [Ragni and Lindholm 1991]. Other authors using the rabbit posterolateral fusion model have found that various DBM products can act to enhance autograft, extend autograft, or replace autograft, depending on the formulation that was used. Yee et al. [2003] showed that adding DBM plus hyaluronan putty to autograft increases the fusion rate at eight weeks. Martin et al. [1999] demonstrated that Grafton flex and Grafton putty were effective as graft enhancers and graft extenders in the rabbit model. In fact, Grafton flex (100% fusion) and Grafton putty (83% fusion) both had higher fusion rates and more bone formation than autograft (33% fusion) in this model. In another rabbit study, Morone and Boden [1998] found that DBM was effective as a graft extender when used at up to a 3:1 ratio with iliac crest autograft.

With respect to use of DBM products in higher-order animals, the authors know of only one published study. In this study, Louis-Ugbo et al. [2004] examined Grafton flex and Grafton matrix added to iliac crest bone graft in a nonhuman primate model of lumbar posterolateral fusion. At 24 weeks postsurgery, two out of four animals treated with autograft plus Grafton flex and three out of four treated with autograft plus Grafton matrix were fused. The authors concluded the matrix formulation may work as a graft enhancer as well as a graft extender. To date, there are no published nonhuman primate studies demonstrating that DBM is equivalent to autograft or that DBM may be used as an autograft replacement.

When viewed as a whole, the amount of pre-clinical data on the use of DBM products in the spine are minimal in light of the number of products that are commercially available. There is only a single nonhuman primate spinal fusion study in the published literature. In particular, the lower-order pre-clinical studies demonstrate the difficulty of evaluating DBM products in terms of efficacy in spinal applications. Virtually all of the studies show that DBM products are capable of forming bone in the spine in these animal models. However, the ability of DBM products to produce spinal fusion in these models on a consistent basis may depend on a number of factors that are poorly understood. While there are a number of studies involving DBMs as a class of materials in spinal applications, for any particular DBM product or demineralization process there are at most a few studies. Even where there are multiple studies with the same product, the results with that product from study to study are not consistent. If a product does not give consistent results in a lower-order animal, it is unlikely to do so in higher-order animals where bone formation is more challenging or in clinical application where there are many new factors that may influence bone formation such as different disease states, lifestyle differences, and patient age.

9.6 DBM: Clinical Investigations

While pre-clinical data are important as supportive information and are often used as a stepping-stone toward clinical evaluation of a device, ultimately it is the clinical evaluation that is used to assess the efficacy of products. This is an area where data on individual DBM formulations are particularly lacking. There are no FDA regulated prospective randomized multi-center clinical investigations on the use of DBM products in spinal fusion. There are however several prospective and retrospective reports of clinical experience. These reports can provide important information, but they typically lack the level of control found in an FDA approved investigation. For example, the number of spinal levels treated, the indication that requires surgical intervention and types of instrumentation used in a patient may vary across the treatment group, making direct comparison between the DBM product and the control difficult. For the same reasons, it is difficult to compare results from different publications.

Most of the published clinical experience is with Grafton gel used as an extender for autograft. However, there is at least one example of Grafton being used with allograft as a replacement for iliac crest autograft. An et al. [1995] reported on 77 patients undergoing anterior cervical fusion who received iliac crest autograft or freeze-dried allograft augmented with Grafton. The fusion rate with autograft was 73.7% in this study compared to 53.8% for the allograft and DBM composite. Results were more promising when the DBM product was combined with local or iliac crest autograft. In a report of 108 patients undergoing posterolateral fusion, 60% of patients receiving local autograft mixed with Grafton had solid fusion while 56% of patients receiving iliac crest bone graft were fused [Sassard et al. 2000]. These results were supported by Cammisa et al. [2004] in a prospective single-level posterolateral fusion investigation with 81 patients. The patients in this investigation received iliac crest autograft on one side of the spine and Grafton gel mixed with iliac crest autograft in a 2 : 1 ratio on the opposite side. Fusion rates at 24 months were 54% and 52% for the autograft and Grafton gel plus autograft treated sides respectively.

In another investigation of posterolateral fusion, patients received either iliac crest autograft mixed with coralline hydroxyapatite or this same mixture with the addition of Grafton gel [Thalgott et al. 2001]. In this retrospective study, the Grafton did not lead to an improvement of fusion rate. In a subsequent report, the combination of coralline HA and Grafton gel used in an anterior interbody fusion procedure yielded a fusion rate of 96% [Thalgott et al. 2002]. With no controls in this study, the relative contribution of the DBM to the fusion results cannot be determined. Finally, Price et al. [2003] showed that bone marrow added to DBM powder gave equivalent fusion results to iliac crest autograft in an investigation of adolescent idiopathic scoliosis.

As discussed previously, the majority of the available clinical data describe the use of a single commercially available DBM product. At least two authors have indicated that it may be useful as an extender of autograft in posterolateral fusion application. Other authors have suggested that it has no added benefit over a purely osteoconductive material in the same application. It should also be noted that, with the differences between the various DBM products in terms of carriers, osteoinductivity testing, processing, and sterilization methods, results presented for a particular DBM formulation cannot be automatically assumed to apply to other materials. Overall, there are still many questions about the value of DBM products in spinal fusion. Prospective randomized and properly controlled clinical investigations would help surgeons to better understand where these products could most benefit their patients. However, it is recognized that these studies are very time consuming, expensive, difficult to accomplish, and unlikely to occur in the near future.

9.6.1 Recombinant Human Bone Morphogenetic Proteins (rhBMP)

With the recognition that bone contains osteoinductive factors capable of promoting new bone formation, it was a natural progression to attempt to isolate, purify, and identify the proteins responsible for this osteoinductive potential of bone matrix. While it is possible to purify bone morphogenetic proteins from bone, it is not a practical method for clinical application due to the very low concentrations of these proteins in bone. It was not until the 1980s that the genes for specific BMPs were identified and used for recombinant genetic production of pure, manufactured versions of the naturally occurring BMPs. With this advance, the goal of being able to make unlimited quantities of BMP for use in bone regeneration became a real possibility. A number of researchers began investigating these recombinant proteins for use in spinal fusion applications. This occurred first in some of the same lower-order animal models that have been used to study DBM products. Success in this area led to higher-order animal studies and eventually to FDA approved human clinical investigations.

The first of these products to become a commercial reality was recombinant human bone morphogenetic protein-2 (rhBMP-2) on an absorbable collagen sponge (ACS). Marketed under the name INFUSE® Bone Graft, this product was approved in July, 2002, for use with an LT-CAGE® lumbar tapered fusion device for single-level anterior lumbar interbody fusion (ALIF) in patients with single-level degenerative disc disease. Additional clinical investigations have been performed with INFUSE Bone Graft, with rhBMP-2 on other carriers, and other rhBMP products for a number of different clinical spinal indications. As this is an area for significant pre-clinical and clinical, investigation it is anticipated that more rhBMP products will reach the market within the next several years. The following sections of this chapter focus on the pre-clinical and clinical data supporting the use of rhBMPs in spinal fusion applications. Since rhBMP-2 and rhBMP-7 (rhOP-1) are the most often studied and the BMPs being targeted for commercial application, the review will focus on data for these two proteins. The body of data for each protein will be examined separately and will include information on lower-order animal, higher-order animal, and clinical data that have been published in the literature to date.

9.6.2 General Principles of rhBMP

A number of BMPs have been identified and all have some level of sequence homology that places them into the TGF-β superfamily of proteins. Not all of the BMPs have been shown to be osteoinductive. However, the BMPs being developed for use in spinal fusion (BMP-2 and BMP-7) are clearly osteoinductive. Both BMP-2 and BMP-7 work through the same mechanisms of chemotaxis, mitogenesis, and differentiation of cells toward the osteoblast lineage. Yet BMP-2 and BMP-7 seem to differ in the type of cells for which they can induce differentiation. One published study investigated the ability of 14 different BMPs to induce cell differentiation [Cheng et al. 2003]. The authors found that BMP-7 was capable of causing differentiation of preosteoblastic cells while BMP-2 caused differentiation of those cells as well as differentiation of mesenchymal cells. Therefore, BMPs should not be considered to be interchangeable in terms of their ability to produce bone in any particular model.

While the protein itself is competent to induce new bone formation, for practical use in bone grafting applications, they are used with a carrier matrix. This introduces another variable when trying to compare two rhBMP products. The carrier serves to maintain the rhBMP at the site of implantation and may act as a scaffold for new bone formation. The importance of the carrier should not be underestimated. Carriers for rhBMP should be appropriate for the desired application. For example, compression resistance may be important in a posterolateral application where muscle compression of the carrier may be a concern. This is less of a concern in interbody fusion application where the carrier is protected by the interbody device. While direct comparison between rhBMP products may be difficult, there are significant pre-clinical and clinical data on the use of these products in spinal applications to help the clinician assess their utility.

9.7 rhBMP-7 (rhOP-1): Preclinical Studies

Published literature on the use of rhBMP-7 in spinal applications consists of a combination of lower-order animal studies and clinical investigations. The rhBMP-7 is lyophilized onto a bovine collagen powder and mixed with carboxymethylcellulose (OP-1 putty). In general, the OP-1 product has been shown to be successful in lower-order animal spinal fusion application as compared to iliac crest autograft alone. In a rat posterolateral fusion model, doses of OP-1 as low as 10 µg resulted in a fusion rate of 100% [Salamon et al. 2003]. OP-1 has also been studied in at least two canine spinal fusion models. Cook et al. found that OP-1 induced posterior fusion in canines by 12 weeks as opposed to the 26 weeks that were required for iliac crest autograft [Cook et al. 1994]. In another study comparing iliac crest autograft, OP-1, and a combination of the two, it was shown that the fusion rate at 8 weeks was 22% for autograft, 66% for OP-1, and 88% for the combination [Cunningham et al. 2002]. Thus, OP-1 was more effective than autograft and it showed an additive benefit when combined with autograft.

In sheep fusion models, OP-1 was found to be equivalent to iliac crest autograft when placed inside an interbody fusion cage, when placed into an instrumented disc space without an interbody device, or when used in a challenging multilevel posterolateral fusion model [Cunningham et al. 1999; Magin and Delling 2001; Mermer et al. 2004]. In this multilevel posterolateral fusion model, none of the animals in either treatment group fused all three levels. The importance of the carrier is demonstrated in a study by Blattert et al. [2002]. When the OP-1 material was combined with a hydroxyapatite carrier in a sheep transpedicular interbody fusion model in sheep, it was found to be superior to autograft. In this study 10 out of 12 animals treated with the HA and OP-1 fused, while only 1 out of 10 autograft treated levels fused.

OP-1 fared better than autograft in all of the published reports using a rabbit posterolateral fusion model. The fusion rate for OP-1 was 100% at five weeks compared to a fusion rate of 63% for iliac crest autograft in one study [Grauer et al. 2001]. In a follow-up study, it was demonstrated that OP-1 still produced a 100% fusion rate in rabbits exposed to nicotine, while the autograft fusion rate dropped to 25% [Patel et al. 2001]. Similar results for OP-1 were shown by Jenis et al., where OP-1 produced a fusion rate of 100% [Jenis et al. 2002]. In this study, autograft did not produce any fusions. Finally, with the superiority of OP-1 to iliac crest autograft and the ability of OP-1 to overcome the negative effects of nicotine shown in the rabbit, Grauer et al. [2004] looked at the ability of OP-1 to heal a pseudarthrosis in the rabbit model. OP-1 was able to fuse 82% of pseudarthroses in this study compared to a fusion rate of 42% for autograft.

In summary, the lower-order animal spinal fusion data demonstrate that the OP-1 product is osteoinductive and able to form bone in a variety of different species. Depending on the model and the application, OP-1 was shown to be equivalent to or better than autograft in all cases. These data should be considered to be supporting information for clinical investigation of OP-1. As is the case with all animal models, they cannot be directly extrapolated to anticipated efficacy in human clinical use.

9.8 rhBMP-7 (rhOP-1): Clinical Investigations

The published human clinical experience with OP-1 in spinal fusion applications consists of two reports on a pilot study in which the OP-1 was used as an adjunct to autograft and several small case report studies from clinical practice in Europe where OP-1 is approved for use in treatment of tibial nonunions. The first of the published clinical experiences with OP-1 was a study in five patients with unstable thoraco lumbar burst fractures [Laursen et al. 1999]. One patient showed significant bone resorption at the site of implantation at three and six months. By 12 months new bone had started to fill in the resorbed area. OP-1 was unable to produce enough bone to get early structural support in any patient. In another small patient series, OP-1 was used in atlanto-axial posterior fusions in four patients [Jeppsson et al. 1999]. Only one of these patients went on to successful fusion. The final clinical series report was a randomized study of 20 patients comparing OP-1 to iliac crest autograft in noninstrumented posterolateral fusions [Johnsson, Stromqvist, and Aspenberg 2002]. Treatment with OP-1 resulted in bilateral fusion in 6 out of 10 patients, while autograft treatment led to fusion in 8 out of 10 patients. The authors concluded that there was no difference between the two treatment groups.

The final two published clinical reports relate to a twelve person multi-centered clinical FDA approved pilot investigation. In this study, patients underwent single level noninstrumented posterolateral fusion in which a combination of OP-1 and iliac crest autograft was placed across the decorticated transverse processes. The twelve-month results were published by Vaccaro et al. [2003]. In this study, 75% of patients were a clinical success based on a 20% improvement in their oswestry disability scores. With respect to radiographic success, 55% of the evaluable patients were determined to be fused according to the study criteria for fusion. Although no autograft control was used in this study, the authors concluded that the results were no different from a historic control in which 45% of patients receiving iliac crest alone had solid fusion. The same authors published a follow-up report with two-year data from this study [Vaccaro et al. 2005]. Clinical results were available for nine patients, and radiographic data were available for ten patients at two years post-op. Of these patients 89% were clinical successes while 50% were radiographic successes.

To date the promising data in lower-order animal models have not translated into successful demonstration of the superiority of OP-1 to iliac crest autograft in clinical spinal fusion applications. This underscores the danger of using lower-order animal models to predict clinical results. One thing that this study did demonstrate is that OP-1 did not lead to any adverse events, which will help support the notion that rhBMPs are safe for use in spinal surgery. Additional clinical investigations with OP-1 are currently underway. Results of these studies may further elucidate the proper role for this product in spinal fusion.

9.9 rhBMP-2 (INFUSE): Pre-clinical Studies

There is far more pre-clinical and clinical published literature on the use of rhBMP-2 in spinal applications than there is for any other osteoinductive biologic product. Lower-order animal models include multiple studies in canine, sheep, goat, and rabbit spinal fusion models. There are also at least six published studies in nonhuman primate interbody and posterolateral fusion models. Finally, there are currently 13 clinical publications in a variety of applications.

Canine fusion studies have been performed using collagen sponge and polylactic acid polymer carriers for rhBMP-2. In the earliest study, all canines that received rhBMP-2 on an open pore polylactic acid sponge in a posterior fusion model achieved fusion at three months, while none of the autograft animals were fused [Sandhu et al. 1995]. In a subsequent dosing study in the same model, all of the rhBMP-2 treated animals were fused using doses down to 58 μg of rhBMP-2 [Sandhu et al. 1996]. A final study in which fusion was performed with and without decortication of the transverse processes found that 100% of decorticated and 89% of undecorticated spines were fused at three months [Sandhu et al. 1997]. Another canine study performed by combining autograft with rhBMP-2 showed that rhBMP-2 significantly increased bone graft volume [Fishgrund 1997]. A canine fusion study comparing rib autograft to rhBMP-2 on either an absorbable collagen sponge (rhBMP-2/ACS) or polylactic acid polymer carrier also led to a 100% fusion rate for animals receiving rhBMP-2 compared to 33% fusion for the autograft group.

Positive results for rhBMP-2 have also been found in goat and sheep interbody fusion models. The goat model is typically used for cervical fusion studies while the sheep model is most often used for lumbar interbody fusion. In a three-level cervical fusion model in a goat, titanium cages filled with rhBMP-2/ACS fused 95% of the time while the same cages filled with autograft fused 48% of the time [Zdeblick et al. 1998]. Another three-level cervical study in goats yielded a 100% fusion rate for 50 μg rhBMP-2 on a porous hydroxyapatite carrier [Takahashi et al. 1999]. In this study, an order of magnitude lower dose of rhBMP-2 fused 50% of the time which was comparable to the results with the carrier alone. rhBMP-2 has also been shown to enhance bone ingrowth into porous tantalum implants and to enhance fusion relative to autograft when placed in a resorbable cage in the goat cervical fusion model [Lippman et al. 2004; Sidhu et al. 2001].

rhBMP-2 was also found to be superior to autograft in a sheep interbody fusion study. In this study, either rhBMP-2/ACS or iliac crest autograft was placed inside a cylindrical titanium interbody fusion device in a single-level interbody fusion model [Sandhu et al. 2002]. Once again all of the rhBMP-2/ACS treated levels fused compared to 33% of the autograft levels. In addition to the lower fusion rate, the autograft treated levels had 16 times more fibrous tissue inside the cages than the rhBMP-2/ACS levels.

The bulk of pre-clinical lower-order animal studies have been performed with the rabbit posterolateral fusion model. The fact that this is a validated model in which autograft does not lead to fusion all of the time and the relatively short duration of the study (five weeks) make this model a good option for screening rhBMP-2 carriers. One of the earliest studies was done using rhBMP-2 on a collagen sponge carrier [Schimandle, Boden, and Hutton 1995]. All of the rhBMP-2 treated animals were fused while only 42% of autograft treated levels fused. Fusions achieved with rhBMP-2 were also biomechanically stronger and stiffer than autograft fusions. A follow-up study showed rhBMP-2 induced fusions to have greater volume and higher contact area with the transverse processes than autograft fusions [Holliger et al. 1996]. The 100% efficacy of rhBMP-2/ACS in rabbit posterolateral fusion was then confirmed in a study designed to assess different surgical techniques [Boden et al. 1996]. A dosing study of rhBMP-2 and collagen in this model showed that a dose as low as 50 μg was sufficient to achieve a fusion rate of 100% [Itoh et al. 1999].

Other studies of rhBMP-2 on different carriers have demonstrated efficacy greater than iliac crest. One of these studies employed a bovine bone carrier infiltrated with collagen [Minamide et al. 1999]. Another study by the same authors suggested that the bovine bone/collagen carrier was superior to the collagen sponge carrier in terms of time to fusion and strength of fusion mass [Minamade et al. 2001]. This study contrasts the results summarized above where the collagen sheet led to 100% fusion even at relatively low protein doses. Additional work with hydroxyapatite/tricalcium phosphate (HA/TCP) granules, HA/TCP granules embedded in collagen sponges, or HA alone yielded the same 100% fusion rate for rhBMP-2 loaded carriers [Konishi et al. 2002; Suh et al. 2002]. Finally, other authors have examined alpha-tricalcium phosphate cement, nano-hydroxyapatite/collagen composite, and mineralized collagen plus polylactic acid and found these to be successful carriers for rhBMP-2 in the rabbit fusion model [Liao et al. 2003; Minamide 2004].

One thing that separates rhBMP-2 research from that of other osteoinductive bone graft materials is the amount of nonhuman primate data that exists. A total of six published studies covering both interbody and posterolateral applications and multiple carriers augment the lower-order animal data and support subsequent clinical investigations. In the interbody model, rhBMP-2/ACS was used to achieve 100% fusion when placed inside a threaded titanium interbody fusion cage or in a smooth walled allograft dowel [Boden et al. 1998; Hecht et al. 1999]. Boden et al. found that ACS alone led to fibrous tissue formation inside the cage, while Hecht et al. reported a 33% fusion rate for iliac crest autograft when placed inside the allograft bone dowel. In addition, rhBMP-2/ACS led to faster incorporation of the allograft tissue than that found for autograft.

The remaining nonhuman primate studies were performed in a single-level uninstrumented lumbar posterolateral fusion model. In the first of these studies, Martin et al. found that the rhBMP-2/ACS did not work well in the posterolateral fusion application unless it was protected from compression [Martin et al. 1999]. This example demonstrates the importance of higher-order animal data. The same product worked well in a similar application in rabbits and canines. Had a clinical investigation been initiated without benefit of these nonhuman primate data, patients could have been exposed to a potentially sub-optimal product for that application. This example also underscores the importance of matching the osteoinductive product and carrier to the proposed application. Subsequent work showed that 100% fusion could be achieved using compression resistant carriers or by adding a bulking agent to the rhBMP-2/ACS for compression resistance and space maintenance during bone formation. Boden et al. [1999] first used an HA/TCP block carrier combined with rhBMP-2 at doses ranging from 6 to 12mg per side of the spine. All of the rhBMP-2 treated levels fused compared to none of the iliac crest treated autograft levels. Suh et al. [2002] used an HA/TCP/collagen sponge as the carrier for rhBMP-2 and found that all of the levels treated with rhBMP-2 at a concentration of 2mg of protein per ml of carrier were fused. Animals treated with the same dose but a lower overall concentration did not fuse. This concentration was more than sufficient to achieve fusion on the same carrier in rabbits, highlighting once again the importance of identifying appropriate concentrations in nonhuman primate models. Finally, Akamuru et al. [2003] found that a lower dose of rhBMP-2 on ACS could be effective in the nonhuman primate posterolateral fusion model provided that it was used with an appropriate bulking agent. By wrapping the rhBMP-2/ACS around HA/TCP granules or allograft chips, 100% fusion was achieved in a study in which only one out of three iliac crest autograft treated levels fused.

9.10 rhBMP-2 (INFUSE): Clinical Investigations

A very significant volume of clinical data is also available for rhBMP-2. These data come in the form of both FDA approved prospective randomized multi-center controlled clinical investigations (level 1 data) and surgeon reports of clinical experience. The first clinical report of the use of rhBMP-2 in spinal fusion came from Boden et al. [2000]. In this small pilot study, all 11 patients who received rhBMP-2/ACS (at the same concentration shown to be effective in a nonhuman primate interbody study) inside a tapered threaded titanium fusion device were judged to be fused by independent radiologists at 6, 12, and 24 months postoperative. In contrast, 2 out of 3 control patients who received iliac crest inside the cage were fused. These data were used to support a larger pivotal clinical investigation in which 143 patients received rhBMP-2/ACS and 136 patients received autograft inside the same tapered threaded interbody device [Burkus et al. 2002]. At 24 months, the fusion rates based on strict FDA protocol definition (i.e., revision surgeries in patients with radiographic fusion count as fusion failures) were 94.5% and 88.7% for the investigational and control groups, respectively. Based solely on radiographic readings of independent radiologists, the fusion rates at 24 months were 100% and 95.7%. Clinical improvements were similar for both groups. These data were used to gain FDA approval of the INFUSE Bone Graft device for use with an LT-cage lumbar tapered fusion device in 2002. In addition to the pilot and pivotal studies described previously, the INFUSE Bone Graft and LT-cage lumbar tapered fusion device combination has also been used to replace autograft in a laproscopic ALIF technique as reported by Kleeman et al. [2001]. In a series of 22 patients at a single investigational site, all patients had improvement in back and leg pain, significant functional improvement, and solid fusion at the 6-month follow-up.

Additional FDA approved pilot clinical investigations of INFUSE Bone Graft have been performed using threaded allograft bone dowels in an ALIF surgery, allograft rings in an anterior cervical fusion procedure, and in threaded titanium cages in a posterior lumbar interbody fusion (PLIF) technique. In the ALIF study, 46 patients received either INFUSE Bone Graft or iliac crest autograft inside threaded cortical allograft dowels [Burkus et al. 2002]. All patients in the INFUSE Bone Graft group were fused at 12 months and remained fused at 24 months compared to fusion rates for the autograft group of 89.5% and 68.4% at 12 and 24 months, respectively. In addition to higher fusion rates, INFUSE treated patients had improved back and leg pain compared to the control. In the anterior cervical fusion study, 33 patients received a cortical allograft ring filled with either INFUSE Bone Graft or iliac crest autograft in a one- or two-level fusion procedure [Baskin et al. 2003]. Treated levels were stabilized with an anterior cervical plate. All patients in both groups were fused at 6, 12, and 24 months after surgery. The investigational group did have statistically greater improvement in neck disability and arm pain scores at 24 months. In the PLIF study, 67 patients underwent a single-level PLIF procedure with INFUSE Bone Graft or iliac crest autograft inside the interbody cage [Haid et al. 2004]. The fusion rates at 24 months were 92.3% and 77.8% for the investigational and control groups, respectively. Both groups experienced clinical improvement over time, but there was no statistically significant difference between the groups with the exception of superior improvement in back pain for the investigational group at 24 months.

The individual clinical investigations were designed to demonstrate equivalence to iliac crest autograft. Burkus et al. [2003] compiled data from multiple clinical studies including a total of 679 patients (277 received INFUSE Bone Graft, 402 received autograft), and performed an integrated analysis. This analysis showed that patients who received INFUSE Bone Graft had statistically superior length of surgery, blood loss, hospital stay, reoperation rate, median time to return to work, fusion rate, and oswestry scores at 6, 12, and 24 months as compared to control patients.

Since the approval of INFUSE Bone Graft, several clinical series have been reported in the literature using different fusion devices and surgical techniques. Mummaneni et al. [2004] reported on 40 patients who underwent a transforaminal lumbar interbody fusion (TLIF) procedure with either INFUSE Bone Graft or iliac crest autograft placed inside the cages. Patients also had either iliac crest autograft or local autograft placed posterior to the cage. At a mean follow-up of 9 months, there was one patient in each group who had a pseudarthrosis. The authors did report more rapid fusion when INFUSE Bone Graft was used inside the cage. In another TLIF study, Lanman and Hopkins [2004] described results from 43 patients who received INFUSE Bone Graft inside a resorbable polymer device. At the 6-month follow-up, 98% of the 41 patients who had radiographic data were fused. All 11 patients that had a 12-month CT were fused. The same authors [2004] also used INFUSE in a series of 20 patients undergoing anterior cervical fusion with resorbable polymer implants. All treated levels were fused at 3 months, based on radiographs and CT data.

As INFUSE Bone Graft is the only commercially available form of rhBMP-2, the vast majority of human clinical data has been generated with the rhBMP-2/ACS combination. As described in the pre-clinical summary of rhBMP-2, other carriers have been investigated in lower-order animal and nonhuman primate spinal fusion models. Results from an FDA-approved clinical investigation with one of these carriers have been published [Boden et al. 2002]. Patients underwent a single level posterolateral fusion in which they received one of three treatments: iliac crest autograft with posterior instrumentation, rhBMP-2 on an HA/TCP carrier (rhBMP-2/BCP) with posterior instrumentation, or rhBMP-2/BCP with no instrumentation. The radiographic fusion rate was 40% for the autograft control and 100% for the rhBMP-2/BCP groups with or without instrumentation. It was also suggested that patients who received rhBMP-2 had quicker clinical improvement than control patients.

The volume of published pre-clinical and clinical data supporting the use of rhBMP-2 in spinal fusion applications is far greater than that for any other osteoinductive biologic product. In virtually every pre-clinical study, from lower-order animals to nonhuman primates in interbody and posterolateral fusion applications, rhBMP-2 led to greater efficacy than the "gold standard" iliac crest. In a number of clinical investigations, both class I data and clinical practice reviews, rhBMP-2 was at least equivalent to if not better than autograft. Furthermore, the progression from lower-order animals to nonhuman primates to clinical investigations used in the development of rhBMP-2 provides a model for development of future osteoinductive biologic products.

9.10.1 Osteoconductive Bone Graft Substitutes

Osteoconductive graft materials are those that provide a scaffold or framework into which newly forming and remodeling bone can grow. These grafts provide no inherent growth functions to enhance the local environment for bone growth and act as substrates onto which osteoblasts can attach and proliferate. Osteoconductive materials require certain key characteristics (proper pore size, proper resorption rate locally (if bioresorbable), good affiliation with the local osteoblasts, etc.) in order to function properly as scaffolding. These materials are strictly passive in nature and therefore do not provide the capability by themselves to regrow or stimulate new bone production. However, they do act as scaffolding around which the newly forming bone can incorporate and also as a delivery vehicle for other agents that may act in a more osteopromotive or osteoinductive fashion, such as bone marrow or BMP, respectively.

There are many types of materials presently that function in an osteoconductive fashion, from naturally occurring materials such as processed human tissue (i.e., cortical-cancellous allograft chips) or animal tissue (i.e., bovine collagen) to pure synthetics such as ceramics containing hydroxyapatite (HA), tricalcium phosphate (TCP), calcium sulfate, or various blends of these materials.

9.10.2 Ceramics

Ceramics are formed through sintering nonmetallic mineral salts at high temperatures. They are generally crystalline in nature and are known to have good biocompatibility characteristics. Ceramics offer some advantages over processed tissue graft materials in that there is no possibility for disease transmission. Examples of ceramics typically used in bone grafting procedures of the spine include hydroxyapatite (HA), tricalcium phosphate (TCP), calcium sulfate, or various blends of these materials. Bone growth incorporation with these ceramic materials depends on a variety of factors, such as granule size, interconnection of pores in the ceramic structure, packing density of the ceramic, sintering temperature, and chemical structure and crystallinity. Consensus of research indicates that the requisite pore size for bone ingrowth into porous implants is 100 to 500 microns, and the interconnections must be larger than 100 microns. Kühne et al. [1994] demonstrated that average pore sizes of around 260 µm for implants showed the greatest ingrowth as compared to an empty defect. Kühne et al. further reported that propagation of osteoblasts is facilitated by the interaction of the primary osteons via the interconnections between the pores.

The FDA regulatory approval process of these osteoconductive substances is through a short three-month 510-K application to the FDA as a "bone void filler." They have to be able to demonstrate the ability to facilitate the healing of a small bone defect in animals. For this reason, on class I prospective, randomized clinical data exist for these bone void fillers demonstrating their efficacy in spine surgery.

9.11 Calcium Sulfate

Calcium sulfate ($CaSO_4$), also known as gypsum or plaster of Paris, was first used to fill bony defects in 1892 by Dressmann. The application of calcium sulfate as a bone void filler, and the use of calcium sulfate as a vector for antibiotic delivery, has been described by various studies [Armstrong et al. 2001; Beardmore et al. 2005; Benoit et al. 1997; Bohner et al. 1997; Doadrio et al. 2004; Mousset et al. 1993; Rogers-Foy et al. 1999]. Medical grade calcium sulfate is manufactured under controlled conditions and crystallized to produce regularly shaped crystals of similar morphology. It possesses a more predictable solubility and bioresorption (weeks).

Pre-clinical studies have demonstrated the use of calcium sulfate to treat bone defects and assist in bone regeneration as a scaffold. Hadjipavlou et al. [2000, 2001] demonstrated use of calcium sulfate in an ovine interbody spine fusion model and showed equivalency to autograft. Turner et al. [2001] showed that calcium sulfate compared favorably to autogenous bone in a canine humeral defect model. Histological results confirmed that the calcium sulfate resorbed as healing of the defects progressed.

Clinical studies have also demonstrated successful use of calcium sulfates *in vivo*. Using clinical and radiographic assessment, Kelly et al. [2001] described the use of calcium sulfate either alone (35% of patients) or combined with other materials (65% of patients) in a series of 109 patients with contained bone defects, primarily long bone defects of the femur, tibia, ilium, and humerus (73% of patients). Results showed that 88% of the defects demonstrated full trabecular bone healing. Kelly and Wilkins [2004] also described the use of an injectable calcium sulfate paste placed into bone voids created in place of previous benign space-occupying lesions in which 14 of 15 grafted defects showed complete incorporation of the graft material at an average of eight weeks. Alexander et al. [2001] showed in a small 40-patient study that calcium sulfate could successfully be used in lumbar spinal fusion in conjunction with locally harvested autogenous bone to act as an autogenous bone extender.

An example of a commercially available calcium sulfate is OsteoSet (Wright Medical Technology, Arlington, TN), which was approved by the FDA in 1996 as a bone void filler. OsteoSet comes in pellet form and dissolves *in vivo* within 30 to 60 days, depending on the volume and location. Its main advantages include the fact that it can be used in the presence of active infection and that it is relatively inexpensive. Since it is bioresorbable, it has inherent advantages over other non-resorbable antibiotic carriers, and it eliminates dead space and creates an acidic environment during its resorption. These qualities allow for OsteoSet to be an effective treatment for acute bony infections with bone loss. However, these qualities also make it less of an advantage in situations where longer-term scaffolding (i.e., six months and beyond) is required for bone growth. As a bone graft extender used with autogenous bone, it has been demonstrated to work in both canine spine and femoral defect models and in human lumbar spinal fusions clinically [Armstrong et al. 2001; Beardmore et al. 2005; Benoit et al. 1997; Bohner et al. 1997; Doadrio et al. 2004; Mousset et al. 1993; Rogers-Foy et al. 1999]. However, the long-term use as a bone graft replacement scaffolding for use alone or as a vehicle for delivery of osteoinductive or osteogenic factors is questionable due to its short resorption time. Glazer et al. [2001] performed posterolateral fusions using a rabbit lumbar fusion model to assess a calcium sulfate bone graft substitute in combination with electrical stimulation for spinal fusion. The authors used 36 adult New Zealand white female rabbits and divided them into three groups: group 1 had no electrical stimulator applied, group 2 received a 40-microA implantable electrical stimulator, and group 3 received a 100-microA implantable electrical stimulator. Each group underwent a single-level (L5-L6) fusion, receiving 3.0 cc calcium sulfate granules with bone marrow aspirate from the iliac crest. Survival was eight weeks, and the rabbit spines were subjected to radiographic assessment, manual palpation, and mechanical testing. Radiographic assessment demonstrated no fusions occurred at the adjacent nonoperated control levels (L4-L5). There were no fusions observed within group 1, containing the calcium sulfate and bone marrow aspirate alone, while the sites with the implantable stimulators showed a dose-dependent increase in fusion stiffness, although no fusion mass in group 2 or 3 was graded as bilaterally complete. The authors concluded that calcium sulfate as a bone graft substitute was unsuccessful in promoting spinal fusion in this rabbit model. They found radiographic evidence of rapid resorption of the calcium sulfate within four weeks after surgery. The use of electrical stimulation created a dose-dependent increase in mechanical competence of the bony mass, although the addition of direct current (DC) did not significantly alter fusion rates. Like any foreign material placed into the body, there exists the potential for inflammatory and/or allergic reactions. Three cases of inflammatory reactions and a single case of allergic reaction have been reported with OsteoSet [Robinson et al. 1999].

9.12 Hydroxyapatite

Hydroxyapatite is a family of calcium orthophosphate molecules. It is widely considered to be extremely biocompatible, and synthetic HAs are used as a bone graft substitute material in many forms. Hydroxyapatite is the major constituent of the inorganic component of bone. Although similar to natural bone in many respects, synthetic HAs vary from the natural bone in that they tend to contain larger and more uniform crystals with a more homogenous composition than those found in natural bone. Due to this more crystalline and organized structure and since hydroxyapatite is resorbed by foreign-body giant cells, which stop ingesting once 2 to 10 um of hydroxyapatite has been consumed, synthetic HAs tend to resorb extremely slowly in the body, often taking many decades to resorb fully.

Since the 1980s, coral and converted coralline hydroxyapatite have been used as bone grafts in lumbar and cervical spinal fusion, in tibial plateau and distal radius fractures in orthopedics, as bone void fillers in oncology procedures, and as orbital implants [Agrillo, Mastronardi, and Puzzilli 2002; Boden et al. 1999; Bozic et al. 1999; Bucholz, Carlton, and Holmes 1989; Dutton 1991; Fong and Choo 1997; Georgiadis, Terzidou, and Dimitriadis 1997; Georgiadis, Terzidou, and Dimitriadis 1999; Irwin, Bernhard, and Biddinger 2001; Jordan 2004; Jordan, Gilberg, and Bawazeer 2004; Karaismailouglu et al. 2002; Ladd and Pliam 1999; Thalgott 2002; Thalgott et al. 2002; White and Shors 1986; Wolfe et al. 1999; Ylinen et al. 1991]. Derived from certain species of marine corals, coral and converted coralline hydroxyapatites contain a pore structure of coralline calcium phosphate that is similar to human cancellous bone and contains interconnected pores, providing the capability for bone to form throughout the interstices of the material. The porous nature of the structure allows vascularization into the material to supply blood for new osteoid tissue, which is eventually mineralized and remodeled into mature bone. Bone graft materials derived from coral typically come in either block or granular forms, and the pore sizes vary.

An example of a commercially available fully sintered coralline hydroxyapatite product is Pro Osteon (Interpore Cross International Inc., Irvine, CA), which was approved by the FDA in 1998 as a bone void filler. Several preclinical and clinical studies have been done to look at this material for a variety of indications [Feifel 2000; Irwin, Bernhard, and Biddinger 2001; Jensen et al. 1996; Stubbs et al. 2004; Thalgott et al. 1999, 2001; Walsh et al. 2004]. A version of hybrid, partially sintered coralline product consisting of a calcium carbonate core layered by a 2- to 10-micron thickness layer of hydroxyapatite is also available (Pro Osteon 200-R and 500-R). The thickness of the hydroxyapatite layer is modified to alter the resorption rates.

9.13 Tricalcium Phosphates

Tricalcium phosphate (TCP) is typically more soluable and less crystalline than hydroxyapatite, and its cell-mediated bioresorption is 10 to 20 times faster (months). TCP is extremely biocompatible and acts as an osteoconductive scaffold. Due to its relative solubility, it has many of the same issues as the calcium sulfates regarding a relatively short residence time as a bone graft replacement scaffolding.

Tricalcium phosphate comes in two forms: alpha and beta TCP. The alpha-TCP is more soluble than beta-TCP and has a faster bioresorbable profile *in vivo*. It is typically available commercially in powder, block, or granule form. Beta-TCP is generally more available commercially and is sold in block or granule form. After 25 years of use, there are no known literature reports of significant unfavorable biologic responses to β-TCP implants. It is degraded by cell-mediated osteoclastic resorption.

An example of a commercially available beta-TCP is Vitoss (Orthovita, Malvern, PA), which was approved by the FDA in 2000 as a bone void filler. Vitoss has particles approximately 100 Nm in size, making up highly porous, 3D beta-TCP scaffolds (pores ranging from 1 to 1000 μm in size). It is available in either block or granular form.

TCP has been used in pre-clinical studies in pigs as a bone void filler and as a bone graft extender mixed with allograft and/or autogenous bone [Li et al. 2004; Li et al. 2004; Ohyama et al. 2002, 2004; Shima et al. 1979].

There have been two published clinical studies of using Vitoss in spinal fusion surgery. Linovitz and Peppers presented a retrospective review of seven patients who underwent anterior (ALIF) or posterior (PLIF) interbody fusion with pedicle screw fixation using only allograft plus a combination of Vitoss and venous blood as an extender with a total of 12 levels grafted with a 3- to 6-month follow-up. All 12 levels were solidly fused radiographically at the last follow-up [Linovitz and Peppers 2002]. Meadows et al. [2002] showed in a clinical study with 50 patients who received Vitoss bone void filler combined with autogenous bone graft in spinal posterolateral fusion procedures. Thirty-two patients were studied for at least 5 to 7 months postoperatively and all of these patients demonstrated good consolidation on follow-up radiographs. The use of iliac crest bone graft (ICBG) was avoided entirely in 7 (14%) of the 50 patients, and 30% less ICBG volume was required on average in others with use of the TCP [Meadows et al. 2002]. To date, no prospective randomized clinical evaluation to establish its efficacy in humans has been conducted with Vitoss. Muschik et al. [2001] demonstrated the use of TCP (chronOS, Mathys Medical, Ltd Battlach, Germany) combined with autograft in a posterolateral application for dorsal spondylodesis in adolescent idiopathic scoliosis (AIS) in 28 patients followed up for 13 +/− 8 months. Patients were evaluated by clinical examination, X-rays, and CT scans. Fusion involved 12 vertebrae on average and the segments were radiographically fused after approximately 6 months in both groups. Resorption of TCP was complete on the radiographs after 8 months on average. Based on the results of their small preliminary study, the authors determined that the use of TCP appears to be a valuable alternative to allografts as an extender to autogenous bone.

9.14 Biphasic Calcium Phosphate (BCP)

Biphasic calcium phosphate (BCP) is a composite consisting of HA and beta-TCP. The properties of the composite make it more rapidly bioresorbable compared to pure HA but slower resorbing than pure beta-TCP. An example of a commercially available BCP is MasterGraft (Medtronic Sofamor Danek, Memphis, TN) that was approved by the FDA in 2002 as a bone void filler. MasterGraft comes in granular form, and the chemical makeup is a 15% HA/ 85% TCP blend. It is designed to resorb through a cell-mediated osteoclastic resorptive process *in vivo* within six to nine months, depending on the volume and location.

There have been several pre-clinical studies evaluating the use of BCP materials both as an autogenous bone replacement and also as an extender. Emery et al. performed a study looking at various groups of materials, including BCP, in an anterior interbody fusion in the canine thoracic spine [Emery, Fuller, and Stevenson 1996]. Survival was eight weeks for all animals. Biomechanical and histological analyses were performed on all specimens after surgery. Biomechanical testing showed that spines from the autogenous tricortical iliac crest group were statistically significantly stiffer in all loading modes compared to the synthetic replacements studied. There were no differences in stiffnesses observed among the three ceramic groups. Histologically, the autogenous iliac crest graft performed best. The BCP and calcium carbonate demonstrated more consistent junction healing than the HA group. The authors concluded that ceramics in general are not suitable as replacement technologies in spinal fusion without a concurrent presence of autogenous bone. Toth et al. [1995] compared the efficacy of a 50/50 hydroxyapatite/beta-tricalcium phosphate BCP ceramic of varying porosity versus autograft in a goat cervical interbody spinal fusion model. The authors used radiographs, histology, dual energy X-ray absorptiometry analysis, and biomechanical testing to evaluate the ability of the materials studied to promote cervical interbody fusion. In contrast to the results from Emery et al. results showed that the ceramics performed equal to or better than the autograft.

BCP has been used in a variety of areas, from backfilling the iliac crest after autogenous bone harvesting to a bone graft extender mixed with autogenous bone for posterolateral fusions of the lumbar spine. Delacrin et al. [2000] reported on a series of 58 patients who underwent posterolateral spinal fusions using local bone grafts combined with either autogenous iliac bone (30 patients) or with porous biphasic calcium phosphate ceramic blocks (28 patients). Surgical results were assessed clinically and radiographically. Patient observation was a minimum of 24 months after surgery, with a mean postoperative observation time of 48 months. The results indicated that patients treated with BCP had a lower average blood loss than those in the iliac graft group and were free from secondary site pain at the iliac crest region as compared to the autogenous harvest group. Radiography demonstrated ceramic incorporation within one year and deformity correction was maintained similarly in both groups. Passuti et al. investigated the use of BCP for posterolateral spinal fusion in 12 adolecent patients with scoliosis for whom there was limited bone graft available [Passuti et al. 1989]. Assessment was done clinically and with roentgenogram assessment up to 24 months, and in two cases biopsies were obtained. Clinical and biologic assessments were normal, and the histologic and ultrastructural evaluation demonstrated the bioactivity and the osteoconduction of this material. There was demonstrated bioresorption of the BCP on histology. Fujibayashi et al. [2001] reported on a 32-patient study involving single-level posterolateral fusion with instrumentation where BCP was used as an extender to autogenous bone. The histologic findings of three biopsy specimens obtained during second operations for metallic implant removal showed excellent bone incorporation around the HA-TCP granules. All patients assessed were deemed fused. The authors concluded that combining BCP with autogenous bone for achieving spinal fusion was a "safe and effective procedure."

9.15 Calcium Phosphate/Collagen Composite Matrices

In an effort to improve the handling, surgical implantation, and bone healing response of granular ceramic bone void filler substances, ceramics have been combined with type I bovine collagen to form sponges and puttys (Chapman, Bucholz, and Cornell 1997; Cheng, Zhao, and Liu 1998; Cornell et al. 1991; Du et al. 1999; Feng, Cui, and Zhang 2002; Itoh et al. 2001, 2002, 2004, 2005; Kraiwattanapong et al. 2005; Liao and Cui 2004; Liao et al. 2003; Marouf, al-Khateeb, and Cataldo 1999; Mehlisch, Leider, and Roberts 1990; Porter et al. 2000; Suh and Lee 1995; Sun et al. 2004; Tay et al. 1998; Thomson et al. 1998; Walsh et al. 2000; Zhang et al. 1996, 2003; Zhang, Sucato, and Welch 2005].

Examples of commercial calcium phosphate/collagen composite matrices include MasterGraft Matrix (15% HA/85% TCP ceramic (75% by volume)/collagen sponge; Medtronic Sofamor Danek, Memphis, TN), Collagraft (65% HA/35% TCP ceramic/collagen; Zimmer Inc., Warsaw, IN), Healos (100% HA ceramic (1% by volume)/collagen; Depuy, Raynam, MA), and Vitoss Scaffold Foam (100% TCP ceramic/collagen; Orthovita, Malvern, PA).

Healos in combination with bone marrow aspirate was evaluated in a rabbit posterolateral spine fusion model by two investigators [Kraiwattanapong et al. 2005; Tay et al. 1998]. Conflicting results were obtained by the two investigators. Tay et al. [1998] aspirated bone marrow from all four of the long bones of rabbits and reported 0% and 100% fusion rates for Healos and Healos with bone marrow respectively based on plain radiographs. No manual palpation fusion assessment was reported. Biomechanically there was no statistical difference in the Healos alone and Healos with bone marrow study groups. In contrast, Kraiwattanapong et al. [2005], who aspirated bone marrow from the rabbits' iliac crest, reported a 0% fusion rate for Healos with bone marrow based on manual palpation, biomechanical testing, CT scans, and histology. A second arm in this study consisted of 1.5 mL of rhBMP-2 (0.43 mg/mL solution) on a type 1 collagen sponge (INFUSE Bone Graft, Medtronic Sofamor Danek, Memphis, TN) wrapped around an additional 1.5-mL collagen-ceramic (15% HA/85% TCP) sponge (MasterGraft matrix) as a bulking agent to provide 3 mL of graft on each side of the spine. 100% fusion rate was achieved with statistically stronger and stiffer fusion masses than the Healos with bone marrow group. To date, no prospective randomized clinical data have been published on either of these products. (See Table 9.3.)

Table 9.3.
Commercially available bone void filler products.

Company	Brand Name and Form(s)
Medtronic Sofamor Danek	MasterGraft resorbable ceramic granules
Medtronic Sofamor Danek	MasterGraft Matrix
Depuy	Healos bone graft material
Orthovita, Inc.	Vitoss scaffold foam
Orthovita, Inc.	Vitoss scaffold synthetic cancellous bone void filler
Interpore Cross International	Boneplast bone void filler
Wright Medical Technology, Inc.	Osteoset pellets
Interpore Cross International	Pro Osteon
EBI	Osteostim resorbable bone graft substitute
Zimmer, Inc.	Collagraft

9.15.1 Osteopromotive Bone Graft Substitutes

Osteopromotive substances are those natural biological compounds and cells that play a role in bone metabolism but are not inherently osteoinductive (i.e., platelet rich plasma and bone marrow). Researchers have been attempting to utilize them in bone grafting applications to increase spinal fusion rates. In order for osteopromotive substances to contribute meaningfully to the process of bony healing in the spine, they must be exposed to a local bony environment that contains the necessary differentiation signals and responding cells to ellicit a synergistic effect. Although use of these compounds has some merit, data on their effectiveness are limited, especially in controlled clinical studies.

9.15.2 Platelet-rich Plasma

Within the past several years, platelet concentrates or platelet rich plasmas (PRP) have undergone evaluation in spinal surgery as an adjunct material to either autologous bone graft and/or in conjunction with other graft extenders, such as ceramics and DBM materials. The thought behind such procedures is that, because platelets are a source of a myriad of growth factors (such as PDGF, TGF-beta, VEGF, etc.) that have some function in bone formation and the addition of platelets would provide a potential enhancement to the healing milieu. Also, the creation of a platelet gel tends to improve handling properties of the morselized autologous bone used surgically. There are several pre-clinical studies that demonstrate the potential benefits of PRP in a variety of areas from, including general orthopedic bone grafting, spinal and oral maxillofacial applications, and wound healing general orthopedic [Atri et al. 1990; Hudson-Goodman, Girard, and Jones 1990; Lowery, Kulkarni, and Pennisi 1999; Walsh et al. 2004; Whitman, Berry, and Green 1997].

A majority of the applications for PRP presented in the literature to date have been for soft tissue indications, with relatively little data to support its use in bone grafting applications outside of the oral maxillofacial arena. Recently, however, some clinical data have been published which cast doubt onto the efficacy of platelet concentrates for bone grafting applications in the spine. Hee et al. [2005], Weiner et al. [2004], Carreon et al. [2003], and Castro et al. [2003] have recently all published articles relating to the use of platelet concentrates in the spine. In general, the authors found reduction in spinal fusion rates and concluded that the efficacy of platelet concentrates for use in bone grafting applications in the spine was questionable at best, with several of the authors stating that the use of this technology in the area of spinal arthrodesis is not recommended for areas such as posterolateral fusion. Certainly, larger, prospective, randomized studies need to be accomplished before the efficacy of PRP technologies as an adjunct for bone grafting can be properly determined.

9.15.3 Bone Marrow Aspirate (BMA)

Bone marrow aspirate theoretically contains many of the necessary osteoprogenitor stem cells which can aid in bone regeneration. The use of BMA is an attractive concept. Because it is drawn through a simple needle aspiration in a minimally invasive fashion, use of BMA could potentially alleviate the need to harvest iliac crest bone, which is associated with donor site morbidity and other complications.

In order to be clinically useful for spinal fusion, BMA still requires a scaffolding in order to provide a matrix on which the new bone matrix and osteoblasts can proliferate. If the osteoprogenitor cell count from BMA is sufficiently high, the bony environment into which it is placed is sufficiently active in osteoinductive signaling to "activate" the pluripotent stem cells to cause them to become osteoblasts, and the BMA is contained on a highly osteoconductive scaffold, then BMA could well be an excellent component of the ideal graft agent.

Many pre-clinical studies have been performed to look at the potential for BMA in orthopedic fracture healing. Tiedeman et al. reported on the use of a BMA-DBM composite grafting technique in a series of 6-mm diaphyseal defects in canines [1991]. Healing of the defects was assessed radiographically, biomechanically, histologically, and biochemically. Results indicated that the combination of BMA with DBM created a synergistic response in the defect and that healing was better than with either material alone. Arinzeh et al. [2003] demonstrated that (over 3–4 weeks) culture-expanded *in vitro* allogeneic mesenchymal stem cells loaded onto an HA-TCP carrier could successfully enhance healing of critical-sized segmental femoral bone defects in canines at 16 weeks.

Connolly et al. have reported on the use of BMA in pre-clinical and clinical situations for general orthopedic applications. It appears to have some clinical merit, although larger, prospective randomized clinical trials have yet to be done in this arena [Connolly 1995; Connolly and Shindell 1986; Connolly et al. 1989, 1991; Strates and Connolly 1989; Tiedeman et al. 1991]. Connolly et al. reported on the first use of BMA injected percutaneously into an ununited tibia site as early as 1986. The fracture site healed clinically, and healing was confirmed by radiographic assessment six months after initial injection. In a subsequent report, Connolly et al. used percutaneous marrow injection rather than standard operative bone grafting on a series of 10 delayed tibial unions over a three-year period. Nine of the 10 fractures responded by forming callus in the area where the bone marrow was injected. The authors reported that this technique avoided potential problems associated with traditional operative grafting methods and encouraged early treatment of delayed healing fractures.

A report issued in 1995 summarized Connolly et al.'s experience with 100 patients for whom BMA was used as a treatment modality. The experience showed an 80% patient response to the BMA grafting technique used with standard fracture stabilization. Tiedeman et al. [1995] reported on the use of a BMA-DBM composite used clinically to treat tibial nonunions in a series of 48 patients, of which 39 were available for follow-up and review. Results demonstrated that healing of the nonunions was comparable to results achieved with standard iliac crest bone graft. The authors concluded that the results indicated that a DBM-BMA composite graft is a suitable alternative to autologous iliac crest bone graft for use in "certain clinical situations, such as bone defects in children, comminuted fractures with associated bone loss, ununited fractures, or to augment an intended arthrodesis site." Khanal et al. [2004] demonstrated in a prospective, randomized study on 40 patients injected with BMA into fresh closed tibial fractures that the mean union time was significantly reduced with the use of BMA as opposed to the control group in which there was no BMA utilized (all fractures using BMA healed in 3.65 +/– 0.49 months; 19/20 fractures treated conventionally united in 4.31 +/– 0.48 months (p = 0.0004). Price et al. [2003] reported on a series of patients treated for adolescent idiopathic scoliosis who achieved fusion results equivalent to the use of autologous iliac crest grafting using a composite graft of DBM and BMA.

Although there have been a variety of pre-clinical and clinical studies looking at the potential for bone marrow aspirate to facilitate healing in a variety of orthopedic applications, the use of BMA is not widespread clinically today for a variety of reasons [Chapman, Bucholz, and Cornell 1997; Connolly 1995; Connolly et al. 1986, 1989, 1991; Curylo et al. 1999; den Goer et al. 2003; Gebhart and Lane 1991; Jean, Wang, and Au 1997; Kai, Shao-qing, and Geng-ting 2003; Ragni, Ala-Mononen, and Lindholm 1993; Tay et al. 1998; Walsh et al. 2000]. There is significant variability in BMA draws due to patient factors and the difficulty in performing a proper draw technique. There is a relative scarcity of osteoprogenitor cells in a given bone marrow aspirate draw, with a majority of the cellular component of the aspirate containing blood components [Muschler et al. 2001]. Finally, the marrow is often placed on substandard carrier matrices which are potentially inappropriate for the surgical application. For all the aforementioned reasons, to date bone marrow aspirate has not demonstrated the capability to act as a bone graft replacement technology despite being able to demonstrate the potential to act as an osteopromotive agent given the proper environment.

In order to attempt to address the aforementioned limitations, researchers have begun to look into ways to concentrate bone marrow stem cells intra-operatively to reinfuse into the patient on matrix carriers. The early work on this idea of concentrating BMA was performed by Connolly et al. in which the authors looked at three methods of concentrating BMA using simple centrifugation, isopyknic centrifugation, and unit gravity segmentation. Although results indicated that the isopyknic preparation of marrow yielded the highest cell populations, the challenges this preparation presented for use in the OR made this preparation method impractical. Results indicated that improved healing of an orthotropically grafted rabbit delayed-union model was achieved using simply centrifuged marrow as compared to controls of whole marrow injections, although the difference was not significant. The authors also concluded that the lack of significant difference between data for centrifuged versus uncentrifuged marrow suggests that the concentration of marrow may be limited to benefiting areas clinically that are limited in volume and that for larger fracture sites, the benefits are outweighed by increased preparation time and chance of contamination.

A relatively new technique uses a filtration method to control the flow of BMA through particular matrices in order to "selectively retain" the cells of interest (i.e., osteoprogenitor cells such as stem cells and osteoblasts) in the matrix. This technique has the disadvantage of requiring aspiration of large quantities of bone marrow. Pre-clinical studies in canines using a demineral-

Table 9.4.

Commercially available osteopromotive products.

Company	Brand Name and Form(s)
Medtronic Sofamor Danek	Magellan autologous platelet separation system
Depuy	Cellect selective retention device
Depuy	Symphony II platelet concentrate system
Biomet, Inc.	GPS platelet concentrator
Harvest Technologies	SmartPReP platelet concentrate system
Interpore Cross International	AGF

ized cancellous bone (DBM) matrix have demonstrated the capability to generate spinal fusions comparable to that of autograft, and demonstrably better than whole marrow alone, DBM alone, or whole marrow plus DBM [Muschler et al. 2003, 2005]. While the pre-clinical results demonstrate the potential of concentrating bone marrow to deliver "enhanced" grafts for spinal fusions and other general orthopedic applications, there has been little evidence clinically that these grafts have the potential to obviate the need for autogenous bone and/or demineralized bone completely in all of these areas. Future studies looking into the potential and limitations of these grafts need to be accomplished before the clinical efficacy for these techniques in spinal fusion can be fully understood. (See Table 9.4.)

9.16 Conclusions

The spinal surgeon today has an extensive array of bone graft substitutes available to use clinically, but based on available published pre-clinical and clinical data, all of them (except for the rhBMPs) should only be used as autogenous bone graft extenders. Many of the commercially available bone graft substitutes are composed of materials that have been available for decades such as calcium phosphate ceramics, ceramic-collagen composites, calcium sulfates, demineralized bone, and bone marrow, which to date have only been demonstrated effective as bone graft extenders. Therefore, harvesting of autogenous bone is still required with these bone graft substitutes. Demineralized bone is the only osteoinductive (weakly) bone graft extender, which may allow for slightly less autogenous bone graft to be harvested.

Only recently have the recombinant human bone morphogenetic proteins become commercially available that can be used as bone graft replacements in spinal fusion procedures, eliminating the need to harvest autogenous bone.

INFUSE Bone Graft is currently the only product that has obtained FDA approval based on a prospective randomized clinical trial. Other BMPs for spinal fusion are still under clinical investigation.

9.17 References

Agrillo, U., L. Mastronardi, and F. Puzzilli (2002). "Anterior Cervical Fusion with Carbon Fiber Cage Containing Coralline Hydroxyapatite: Preliminary Observations in 45 Consecutive Cases of Soft-disc Herniation," *J. Neurosurg.* 96:273–276.

Akamaru, T., et al. (2003). "Simple Carrier Matrix Modifications Can Enhance Delivery of Recombinant Human Bone Morphogenetic Protein-2 for Posterolateral Spine Fusion." *Spine* 28:429–434.

Alexander, D. I., N. A. Manson, and M. J. Mitchell (2001). "Efficacy of Calcium Sulfate Plus Decompression Bone in Lumbar and Lumbosacral Spinal Fusion: Preliminary Results in 40 Patients," *Can. J. Surg.* 44:262–266.

An, H. S., et al. (1995). "Comparison Between Allograft Plus Demineralized Bone Matrix Versus Autograft in Anterior Cervical Fusion: A Prospective Multicenter Study," *Spine* 20:2211–2216.

Arinzeh, T. L., et al. (2003). "Allogeneic Mesenchymal Stem Cells Regenerate Bone in a Critical-sized Canine Segmental Defect," *J. Bone Joint Surg. Am.* 85A:1927–1935.

Armstrong, D. G., et al. (2001). "The Use of Absorbable Antibiotic-impregnated Calcium Sulphate Pellets in the Management of Diabetic Foot Infections," *Diabet. Med.* 18:942–943.

Atri, S. C., et al. (1990). "Use of Homologous Platelet Factors in Achieving Total Healing of Recalcitrant Skin Ulcers," *Surgery* 108:508–512.

Baskin, D. S., et al. (2003). "A Prospective, Randomized, Controlled Cervical Fusion Study Using Recombinant Human Bone Morphogenetic Protein-2 with the CORNERSTONE-SR Allograft Ring and the ATLANTIS Anterior Cervical Plate," *Spine* 28:1219–1225.

Beardmore, A. A., et al. (2005). "Effectiveness of Local Antibiotic Delivery with an Osteoinductive and Osteoconductive Bone-graft Substitute," *J. Bone Joint Surg. Am.* 87:107–112.

Benoit, M. A., et al. (1997). "Antibiotic-loaded Plaster of Paris Implants Coated with Poly Lactide-coglycolide as a Controlled Release Delivery System for the Treatment of Bone Infections," *Int. Orthop.* 21:403–408.

Blattert, T. R., et al. (2002). "Successful Transpedicular Lumbar Interbody Fusion by Means of a Composite of Osteogenic Protein-1 (rhBMP-7) and Hydroxyapatite Carrier: A Comparison with Autograft and Hydroxyapatite in the Sheep Spine," *Spine* 27:2697–2705.

Blum, B., et al. (2004). Measurement of Bone Morphogenetic Proteins and Other Growth Factors in Demineralized Bone Matrix," *Orthopedics* 27(Suppl. 1):S161–S165.

Boden, S. D., et al. (1996). "Video-assisted Lateral Intertransverse Process Arthrodesis: Validation of a New Minimally Invasive Lumbar Spinal Fusion Technique in the Rabbit and Nonhuman Primate (Rhesus) Models," *Spine* 21:2689–2697.

Boden, S. D., et al. (1998). "Laparoscopic Anterior Spinal Arthrodesis with rhBMP-2 in a Titanium Interbody Threaded Cage," *J. Spinal Disord.* 11:95–101.

Boden, S. D., et al. (1999). "Posterolateral Lumbar Intertransverse Process Spine Arthrodesis with Recombinant Human Bone Morphogenetic Protein 2/hydroxyapatite-tricalcium Phosphate After Laminectomy in the Nonhuman Primate," *Spine* 24: 1179–1185.

Boden, S. D., et al. (1999). "The Use of Coralline Hydroxyapatite with Bone Marrow, Autogenous Bone Graft, or Osteoinductive Bone Protein Extract for Posterolateral Lumbar Spine Fusion," *Spine* 24:320–327.

Boden, S. D., et al. (2000). "The Use of rhBMP-2 in Interbody Fusion Cages: Definitive Evidence of Osteoinduction in Humans, A Preliminary Report," *Spine* 25:376–381.

Boden, S. D., et al. (2002). "Use of Recombinant Human Bone Morphogenetic Protein-2 to Achieve Posterolateral Lumbar Spine Fusion in Humans: A Prospective, Randomized Clinical Pilot Trial," *Spine* 27:2662–2673.

Bohner, M., et al. (1997). "Gentamicin-loaded Hydraulic Calcium Phosphate Bone Cement as Antibiotic Delivery System," *J. Pharm. Sci.* 86:565–572.

Bomback, D. A., et al. (2004). "Comparison of Posterolateral Lumbar Fusion Rates of Grafton Putty and OP-1 Putty in an Athymic Rat Model," *Spine* 29:1612–1617.

Bozic, K. J., et al. (1999). "In Vivo Evaluation of Coralline Hydroxyapatite and Direct Current Electrical Stimulation in Lumbar Spinal Fusion," *Spine* 24:2127–2133.

Bucholz, R. W., A. Carlton, and R. Holmes (1989). "Interporous Hydroxyapatite as a Bone Graft Substitute in Tibial Plateau Fractures," *Clin. Orthop. Relat. Res.* 240:53–62.

Burkus, J. K., et al. (2003). "Is INFUSE Bone Graft Superior to Autograft Bone?: An Integrated Analysis of Clinical Trials Using the LT-CAGE Lumbar Tapered Fusion Device," *J. Spinal Disord. Tech.* 16:113–122.

Burkus, J. K., et al. (2002a). "Anterior Lumbar Interbody Fusion Using rhBMP-2 with Tapered Interbody Cages," *J. Spinal Disord. Tech.* 15:337–349.

Burkus, J. K., et al. (2002b). "Clinical and Radiographic Outcomes of Anterior Lumbar Interbody Fusion Using Recombinant Human Bone Morphogenetic Protein-2," *Spine* 27:2396–2408.

Cammisa, F. P. Jr., et al. (2004). "Two-year Fusion Rate Equivalency Between Grafton DBM Gel and Autograft in Posterolateral Spine Fusion: A Prospective Controlled Trial Employing a Side-by-side Comparison in the Same Patient," *Spine* 29:660–666.

Carreon, L. Y., et al. (2005). "Platelet Gel (AGF) Fails to Increase Fusion Rates in Instrumented Posterolateral Fusions," *Spine* 30:E243–E246; discussion E247.

Castro, F. P. Jr. (2004). "Role of Activated Growth Factors in Lumbar Spinal Fusions," *J. Spinal Disord. Tech.* 17:380–384.

Chapman, M. W., R. Bucholz, and C. Cornell (1997). "Treatment of Acute Fractures with a Collagen-calcium Phosphate Graft Material: A Randomized Clinical Trial," *J. Bone Joint Surg. Am.* 79:495–502.

Cheng, H., et al. (2003). "Osteogenic Activity of the Fourteen Types of Human Bone Morphogenetic Proteins (BMPs)," *J. Bone Joint Surg. Am.* 85A:1544–1552.

Cheng, Y., G. Zhao, and H. Liu (1998). "Histological Evaluation of Collagen-hydroxyapatite Composite as Osseous Implants in the Repair of Mandibular Defect," *Zhongguo Xiu Fu Chong Jian Wai Ke Za Zhi* 12:74–76.

Connolly, J. F. (1995). "Injectable Bone Marrow Preparations to Stimulate Osteogenic Repair," *Clin. Orthop. Relat. Res.* 313:8–18.

Connolly, J. F., and R. Shindell (1986). "Percutaneous Marrow Injection for an Ununited Tibia," *Nebr. Med. J.* 71:105–107.

Connolly, J. F., et al. (1989a). "Autologous Marrow Injection for Delayed Unions of the Tibia: A Preliminary Report," *J. Orthop. Trauma* 3:276–282.

Connolly, J., et al. (1989b). "Development of an Osteogenic Bone-marrow Preparation," *J. Bone Joint Surg. Am.* 71:684–691.

Connolly, J. F., et al. (1991). "Autologous Marrow Injection as a Substitute for Operative Grafting of Tibial Nonunions," *Clin. Orthop. Relat. Res.* 266:259–270.

Cook, S. D., et al. (1994). "In Vivo Evaluation of Recombinant Human Osteogenic Protein (rhOP-1) Implants as a Bone Graft Substitute for Spinal Fusions," *Spine* 19: 1655–1663.

Cook, S. D., et al. (1995). "In Vivo Evaluation of Demineralized Bone Matrix as a Bone Graft Substitute for Posterior Spinal Fusion," *Spine* 20:877–886.

Cornell, C. N., et al. (1991). "Multicenter Trial of Collagraft as Bone Graft Substitute," *J. Orthop. Trauma* 5:1–8.

Cunningham, B. W., et al. (1999). "Osteogenic Protein Versus Autologous Interbody Arthrodesis in the Sheep Thoracic Spine: A Comparative Endoscopic Study Using the Bagby and Kuslich Interbody Fusion Device," *Spine* 24:509.

Cunningham, B. W., et al. (2002). "Osseointegration of Autograft Versus Osteogenic Protein-1 in Posterolateral Spinal Arthrodesis: Emphasis on the Comparative Mechanisms of Bone Induction," *Spine J.* 2:11–24.

Curylo, L. J., et al. (1999). "Augmentation of Spinal Arthrodesis with Autologous Bone Marrow in a Rabbit Posterolateral Spine Fusion Model," *Spine* 24:434–438; discussion 438–439.

Delecrin, J., et al. (2000). "A Synthetic Porous Ceramic as a Bone Graft Substitute in the Surgical Management of Scoliosis: A Prospective, Randomized Study," *Spine* 25:563–569.

den Boer, F. C., et al. (2003). "Healing of Segmental Bone Defects with Granular Porous Hydroxyapatite Augmented with Recombinant Human Osteogenic Protein-1 or Autologous Bone Marrow," *J. Orthop. Res.* 21:521–528.

Doadrio, J. C., et al. (2004). "Calcium Sulphate-based Cements Containing Cephalexin," *Biomaterials* 25:2629–2635.

Dreesmann, H. (1892). "Ueber Knochenplombierung," *Beitr. Klin. Chir.* 9:804–810.

Du, C., et al. (1999). "Three-dimensional Nano-HAp/collagen Matrix Loading with Osteogenic Cells in Organ Culture," *J. Biomed. Mater. Res.* 44:407–415.

Dutton, J. J. (1991). "Coralline Hydroxyapatite as an Ocular Implant," *Ophthalmology* 98:370–377.

Edwards, J. T., M. H. Diegmann, and N. L. Scarborough (1998). "Osteoinduction of Human Demineralized Bone: Characterization in a Rat Model," *Clin. Orthop. Relat. Res.* 357:219–228.

Emery, S. E., D. A. Fuller, and S. Stevenson (1996). "Ceramic Anterior Spinal Fusion: Biologic and Biomechanical Comparison in a Canine Model," *Spine* 21:2713–2719.

Feifel, H. (2000). "Bone Regeneration in Pro Osteon 500 Alone and in Combination with Colloss in the Patellar Gliding Model of the Rabbit," *Mund Kiefer Gesichtschir* 4(Suppl. 2):S527–S530.

Feng, Q. L., F. Z. Cui, and W. Zhang (2002). "Nano-hydroxyapatite/collagen Composite for Bone Repair," *Zhongguo Yi Xue Ke Xue Yuan Xue Bao* 24:124–128.

Fischgrund, J. S., et al. (1997). "Augmentation of Autograft Using rhBMP-2 and Different Carrier Media in the Canine Spinal Fusion Model," *J. Spinal Disord.* 10:467.

Fong, K. S. and C. T. Choo (1997). "Hydroxyapatite Orbital Implants: Our Local Experience," *Ann. Acad. Med. Singapore* 26:405–408.

Frenkel, S. R., et al. (1993). "Demineralized Bone Matrix: Enhancement of Spinal Fusion," *Spine* 18:1634–1639.

Fujibayashi, S., et al. (2001). "Lumbar Posterolateral Fusion with Biphasic Calcium Phosphate Ceramic," *J. Spinal Disord.* 14:214–221.

Gebhart, M. and J. Lane (1991). "A Radiographical and Biomechanical Study of Demineralized Bone Matrix Implanted into a Bone Defect of Rat Femurs with and Without Bone Marrow," *Acta Orthop. Belg.* 57:130–143.

Georgiadis, N. S., C. D. Terzidou, and A. S. Dimitriadis (1998). "Restoration of the Anophthalmic Socket with Secondary Implantation of a Coralline Hydroxyapatite Sphere," *Ophthalmic Surg. Lasers* 29:808–814.

Georgiadis, N. S., C. D. Terzidou, and A. S. Dimitriadis (1999). "Coralline Hydroxyapatite Sphere in Orbit Restoration," *Eur. J. Ophthalmol.* 9:302–308.

Glazer, P. A., et al. (2001). "In Vivo Evaluation of Calcium Sulfate as a Bone Graft Substitute for Lumbar Spinal Fusion," *Spine J.* 1:395–401.

Grauer, J. N., et al. (2001). "Evaluation of OP-l as a Graft Substitute for Intertransverse Process Lumbar Fusion," *Spine* 26:127–133.

Grauer, J. N., et al. (2004). "Development of a New Zealand White Rabbit Model of Spinal Pseudarthrosis Repair and Evaluation of the Potential Role of OP-1 to Overcome Pseudarthrosis," *Spine* 29:1405–1412.

Hadjipavlou, A. G., et al. (2000). "Plaster of Paris as an Osteoconductive Material for Interbody Vertebral Fusion in Mature Sheep," *Spine* 25:10–15; discussion 16.

Hadjipavlou, A. G., et al. (2001). "Plaster of Paris as Bone Substitute in Spinal Surgery," *Eur. Spine J.* 10(Suppl. 2):S189–S196.

Haid, R. W. Jr., et al. (2004). "Posterior Lumbar Interbody Fusion Using Recombinant Human Bone Morphogenetic Protein Type 2 with Cylindrical Interbody Cages," *Spine J.* 4:527–538; discussion 538–539.

Han, B., B. Tang, and M. E. Nimni (2003). "Quantitative and Sensitive In Vitro Assay for Osteoinductive Activity of Demineralized Bone Matrix," *J. Orthop. Res.* 21:648–654.

Hecht, B. P., et al. (1999). "The Use of Recombinant Human Bone Morphogenetic Protein 2 (rhBMP-2) to Promote Spinal Fusion in a Nonhuman Primate Anterior Interbody Fusion Model," *Spine* 24:629–636.

Hee, H. T., et al. (2003). "Do Autologous Growth Factors Enhance Transforaminal Lumbar Interbody Fusion?," *Eur. Spine J.* 12:400–407.

Helm, G. A., et al. (1997). "Utilization of Type I Collagen Gel, Demineralized Bone Matrix, and Bone Morphogenetic Protein-2 to Enhance Autologous Bone Lumbar Spinal Fusion," *J. Neurosurg.* 86:93–100.

Holliger, E. H., et al. (1996). "Morphology of the Lumbar Intertransverse Process Fusion Mass in the Rabbit Model: A Comparison Between Two Bone Graft Materials: rhBMP-2 and Autograft," *J. Spinal Disord.* 9:125–128.

Hudson-Goodman, P., N. Girard, and M. B. Jones (1990). "Wound Repair and the Potential Use of Growth Factors," *Heart Lung* 19:379–384.

Irwin, R. B., M. Bernhard, and A. Biddinger (2001). "Coralline Hydroxyapatite as Bone Substitute in Orthopedic Oncology," *Am. J. Orthop.* 30:544–550.

Itoh, H., et al. (1999). "Experimental Spinal Fusion with Use of Recombinant Human Bone Morphogenetic Protein 2," *Spine* 24:1402.

Itoh, S., et al., (2001). "The Biocompatibility and Osteoconductive Activity of a Novel Hydroxyapatite/collagen Composite Biomaterial, and Its Function as a Carrier of rhBMP-2," *J. Biomed. Mater. Res.* 54:445–453.

Itoh, S., et al. (2002a). "Development of an Artificial Vertebral Body Using a Novel Biomaterial, Hydroxyapatite/collagen Composite," *Biomaterials* 23:3919–3926.

Itoh, S., et al. (2002b). "Implantation Study of a Novel Hydroxyapatite/collagen (HAp/col) Composite into Weight-bearing Sites of Dogs," *J. Biomed. Mater. Res.* 63:507–515.

Itoh, S., et al. (2004). "Development of a Hydroxyapatite/collagen Nanocomposite as a Medical Device," *Cell Transplant* 13:451–461.

Itoh, S., et al. (2005). "Development of a Novel Biomaterial, Hydroxyapatite/collagen (HAp/Col) Composite for Medical Use," *Biomed. Mater. Eng.* 15:29–41.

Jaw, R. Y. Y., J. Keesling, and J. F. Wironen (2001). "The Level of BMP-2/4 Extracted from Human Bone Correlates with the Osteoinductive Potential of That Bone In Vivo," 25th Annual Meeting, American Association of Tissue Banks. Washington DC.

Jean, J. L., S. J. Wang, and M. K. Au (1997). "Treatment of a Large Segmental Bone Defect with Allograft and Autogenous Bone Marrow Graft," *J. Formos. Med. Assoc.* 96: 553–557.

Jenis, L. G., et al. (2002). "The Effect of Osteogenic Protein-1 in Instrumented and Non-instrumented Posterolateral Fusion in Rabbits," *Spine J.* 2:173–178.

Jensen, S. S., et al. (1996). "Tissue Reaction and Material Characteristics of Four Bone Substitutes," *Int. J. Oral Maxillofac Implants* 11:55–66.

Jeppsson, C., et al. (1999). "OP-1 for Cervical Spine Fusion: Bridging Bone in Only 1 of 4 Rheumatoid Patients But Prednisolone Did Not Inhibit Bone Induction in Rats," *Acta Orthop. Scand.* 70:559–563.

Johnsson, R., B. Stromqvist, and P. Aspenberg (2002). "Randomized Radiostereometric Study Comparing Osteogenic Protein-1 (BMP-7) and Autograft Bone in Human Noninstrumented Posterolateral Lumbar Fusion," *Spine* 27:2654–2661.

Jordan, D. R. (2004). "Problems After Evisceration Surgery with Porous Orbital Implants: Experience with 86 Patients," *Ophthal. Plast. Reconstr. Surg.* 20:374–380.

Jordan, D. R., S. Gilberg, and A. Bawazeer (2004). "Coralline Hydroxyapatite Orbital Implant (Bio-eye): Experience with 158 Patients," *Ophthal. Plast. Reconstr. Surg.* 20:69–74.

Kai, T., G. Shao-qing, and D. Geng-ting (2003). "In Vivo Evaluation of Bone Marrow Stromal-derived Osteoblasts-porous Calcium Phosphate Ceramic Composites as Bone Graft Substitute for Lumbar Intervertebral Spinal Fusion," *Spine* 28: 1653–1658.

Karaismailoglu, T. N., et al. (2002). "Comparison of Autograft, Coralline Graft, and Xenograft in Promoting Posterior Spinal Fusion," *Acta Orthop. Traumatol. Turc.* 36:147–154.

Kelly, C. M., and R. M. Wilkins (2004). "Treatment of Benign Bone Lesions with an Injectable Calcium Sulfate-based Bone Graft Substitute," *Orthopedics* 27:S131–S135.

Kelly, C. M., et al. (2001). "The Use of a Surgical Grade Calcium Sulfate as a Bone Graft Substitute: Results of a Multicenter Trial," *Clin. Orthop. Relat. Res.* 382:42–50.

Khanal, G. P., M. Garg, and G. K. Singh (2004). "A Prospective Randomized Trial of Percutaneous Marrow Injection in a Series of Closed Fresh Tibial Fractures," *Int. Orthop.* 28:167–170.

Kleeman, T. J., U. M. Ahn, and A. Talbot-Kleeman (2001). "Laparoscopic Anterior Lumbar Interbody Fusion with rhBMP-2: A Prospective Study of Clinical and Radiographic Outcomes," *Spine* 26:2751–2756.

Konishi, S., et al. (2002). "Hydroxyapatite Granule Graft Combined with Recombinant Human Bone Morphogenic Protein-2 for Solid Lumbar Fusion," *J. Spinal Disord. Tech.* 15:237–244.

Kraiwattanapong, C., et al. (2005). "Comparison of Healos/bone Marrow to INFUSE(rhBMP-2/ACS) with a Collagen-ceramic Sponge Bulking Agent as Graft Substitutes for Lumbar Spine Fusion. *Spine* 30:1001–1007; discussion 1007.

Kuhne, J. H., et al. (1994). "Bone Formation in Coralline Hydroxyapatite: Effects of Pore Size Studied in Rabbits," *Acta Orthop. Scand.* 65:246–252.

Ladd, A. L., and N. B. Pliam (1999). "Use of Bone-graft Substitutes in Distal Radius Fractures," *J. Am. Acad. Orthop. Surg.* 7:279–290.

Lanman, T. H., and T. J. Hopkins (2004a). "Early Findings in a Pilot Study of Anterior Cervical Interbody Fusion in Which Recombinant Human Bone Morphogenetic Protein-2 Was Used with Poly(L-lactide-co-D,L-lactide) Bioabsorbable Implants," *Neurosurg. Focus* 16:E6.

Lanman, T. H., and T. J. Hopkins (2004b). "Lumbar Interbody Fusion After Treatment with Recombinant Human Bone Morphogenetic Protein-2 Added to Poly(L-lactide-co-D,L-lactide) Bioresorbable Implants," *Neurosurg. Focus* 16:E9.

Laursen, M., et al. (1999). "Recombinant Bone Morphogenetic Protein-7 as an Intracorporal Bone Growth Stimulator in Unstable Thoracolumbar Burst Fractures in Humans: Preliminary Results," *Eur. Spine J.* 8:485–490.

Li, H., et al. (2004a). "Anterior Lumbar Interbody Fusion with Carbon Fiber Cage Loaded with Bioceramics and Platelet-rich Plasma: An Experimental Study on Pigs," *Eur. Spine J.* 13:354–358.

Li, H., et al. (2004b). "Effects of Autogenous Bone Graft Impaction and Tricalcium Phosphate on Anterior Interbody Fusion in the Porcine Lumbar Spine," *Acta Orthop. Scand.* 75:456–463.

Liao, S. S., et al. (2003). "Lumbar Spinal Fusion with a Mineralized Collagen Matrix and rhBMP-2 in a Rabbit Model," *Spine* 28:1954–1960.

Liao, S. S., and F. Z. Cui (2004). "In Vitro and In Vivo Degradation of Mineralized Collagen-based Composite Scaffold: Nanohydroxyapatite/collagen/poly(L-lactide)," *Tissue Eng.* 10:73–80.

Lindholm, T. S., P. Ragni, and T. C. Lindholm (1988). "Response of Bone Marrow Stroma Cells to Demineralized Cortical Bone Matrix in Experimental Spinal Fusion in Rabbits," *Clin. Orthop. Relat. Res.* 230:296–302.

Linovitz, R. J., and T. A. Peppers (2002). "Use of an Advanced Formulation of Beta-tricalcium Phosphate as a Bone Extender in Interbody Lumbar Fusion," *Orthopedics* 25:S585–S589.

Lippman, C. R., et al. (2004). "Cervical Spine Fusion with Bioabsorbable Cages," *Neurosurg. Focus* 16:E4.

Louis-Ugbo, J., et al. (2004). "Evidence of Osteoinduction by Grafton Demineralized Bone Matrix in Nonhuman Primate Spinal Fusion," *Spine* 29:360–366; discussion Z1.

Lowery, G. L., S. Kulkarni, and A. E. Pennisi (1999). "Use of Autologous Growth Factors in Lumbar Spinal Fusion," *Bone* 25:47S–50S.

Maddox, E., et al. (2000). "Optimizing Human Demineralized Bone Matrix for Clinical Application," *Tissue Eng.* 6:441–448.

Magin, M. N., and G. Delling (2001). "Improved Lumbar Vertebral Interbody Fusion Using rhOP-1: A Comparison of Autogenous Bone Graft, Bovine Hydroxylapatite (Bio-Oss), and BMP-7 (rhOP-1) in Sheep," *Spine* 26:469–478.

Marouf, H. A., T. L. al-Khateeb, and E. Cataldo (1999). "Enhancement of Bone Ingrowth into Collagen/HA Composite Implants Using e-PTFE Membranes," *J. Ir. Dent. Assoc.* 45:52–57.

Martin, G. J. Jr., et al. (1999a). "New Formulations of Demineralized Bone Matrix as a More Effective Graft Alternative in Experimental Posterolateral Lumbar Spine Arthrodesis," *Spine* 24:637–645.

Martin, G. J. Jr., et al. (1999b). "Posterolateral Intertransverse Process Spinal Arthrodesis with rhBMP-2 in a Nonhuman Primate: Important Lessons Learned Regarding Dose, Carrier, and Safety," *J. Spinal Disord.* 12:179–186.

Meadows, G. R. (2002). "Adjunctive Use of Ultraporous Beta-tricalcium Phosphate Bone Void Filler in Spinal Arthrodesis," *Orthopedics* 25:S579–S584.

Mehlisch, D. R., A. S. Leider, and W. E. Roberts (1990). "Histologic Evaluation of the Bone/graft Interface After Mandibular Augmentation with Hydroxylapatite/

purified Fibrillar Collagen Composite Implants," *Oral Surg. Oral Med. Oral Pathol.* 70:685–692.

Mermer, M. J., et al. (2004). "Efficacy of Osteogenic Protein-1 in a Challenging Multilevel Fusion Model," *Spine* 29:249–256.

Minamide, A., et al. (1999). "Experimental Spinal Fusion Using Sintered Bovine Bone Coated with Type I Collagen and Recombinant Human Bone Morphogenetic Protein-2," *Spine* 24:1863–1870; discussion 1871–1872.

Minamide, A., et al. (2001). "Evaluation of Carriers of Bone Morphogenetic Protein for Spinal Fusion," *Spine* 26:933–939.

Minamide, A., et al. (2004). "Experimental Study of Carriers of Bone Morphogenetic Protein Used for Spinal Fusion," *J. Orthop. Sci.* 9:142-151.

Morone, M. A., and S. D. Boden (1998). "Experimental Posterolateral Lumbar Spinal Fusion with a Demineralized Bone Matrix Gel," *Spine* 23:159–167.

Mousset, B., et al. (1993). "Plaster of Paris: A Carrier for Antibiotics in the Treatment of Bone Infections," *Acta Orthop. Belg.* 59:239–248.

Mousset, B., et al. (1995). "Biodegradable Implants for Potential Use in Bone Infection: An In Vitro Study of Antibiotic-loaded Calcium Sulphate," *Int. Orthop.* 19:157–161.

Mummaneni, P. V., et al. (2004). "Contribution of Recombinant Human Bone Morphogenetic Protein-2 to the Rapid Creation of Interbody Fusion When Used in Transforaminal Lumbar Interbody Fusion: A Preliminary Report," Invited submission from the Joint Section Meeting on Disorders of the Spine and Peripheral Nerves, March 2004. *J. Neurosurg. Spine* 1:19–23.

Muschik, M., et al. (2001). "Beta-tricalcium Phosphate as a Bone Substitute for Dorsal Spinal Fusion in Adolescent Idiopathic Scoliosis: Preliminary Results of a Prospective Clinical Study," *Eur. Spine J.* 10(Suppl. 2):S178–S184.

Muschler, G. F., et al. (2001). "Age- and Gender-related Changes in the Cellularity of Human Bone Marrow and the Prevalence of Osteoblastic Progenitors," *J. Orthop. Res.* 19:117–125.

Muschler, G. F., et al. (2003). "Spine Fusion Using Cell Matrix Composites Enriched in Bone Marrow-derived Cells," *Clin. Orthop. Relat. Res.* 407:102–118.

Muschler, G. F., et al. (2005). "Selective Retention of Bone Marrow-derived Cells to Enhance Spinal Fusion," *Clin. Orthop. Relat. Res.* 432:242–251.

Nyssen-Behets, C., et al. (1996). "Aging Effect on Inductive Capacity of Human Demineralized Bone Matrix," *Arch. Orthop. Trauma Surg.* 115:303–306.

Ohyama, T., et al. (2002). "Beta-tricalcium Phosphate as a Substitute for Autograft in Interbody Fusion Cages in the Canine Lumbar Spine," *J. Neurosurg.* 97:350–354.

Ohyama, T., et al. (2004). "Beta-tricalcium Phosphate Combined with Recombinant Human Bone Morphogenetic Protein-2: A Substitute for Autograft, Used for Packing Interbody Fusion Cages in the Canine Lumbar Spine," *Neurol. Med. Chir.* (Tokyo) 44:234–240; discussion 241.

Passuti, N., et al. (1989). "Macroporous Calcium Phosphate Ceramic Performance in Human Spine Fusion," *Clin. Orthop. Relat. Res.* 248:169–176.

Patel, T. C., et al. (2001). "Osteogenic Protein-1 Overcomes the Inhibitory Effect of Nicotine on Posterolateral Lumbar Fusion," *Spine* 26:1656–1661.

Peterson, B., et al. (2004). "Osteoinductivity of Commercially Available Demineralized Bone Matrix. Preparations in a Spine Fusion Model," *J. Bone. Joint Surg. Am.* 86-A:2243–2250.

Porter, B. D., et al. (2000). "Mechanical Properties of a Biodegradable Bone Regeneration Scaffold," *J. Biomech. Eng.* 122:286–288.

Price, C. T., et al. (2003). "Comparison of Bone Grafts for Posterior Spinal Fusion in Adolescent Idiopathic Scoliosis," *Spine* 28:793–798.

Ragni, P., and T. S. Lindholm (1991). "Interaction of Allogeneic Demineralized Bone Matrix and Porous Hydroxyapatite Bioceramics in Lumbar Interbody Fusion in Rabbits," *Clin. Orthop. Relat. Res.* 272:292–299.

Ragni, P., P. Ala-Mononen, and T. S. Lindholm (1993). "Spinal Fusion Induced by Porous Hydroxyapatite Blocks (HA): Experimental Comparative Study with HA, Demineralized Bone Matrix and Autogenous Bone Marrow," *Ital. J. Orthop. Traumatol.* 19:133–144.

Ragni, P., T. S. Lindholm, and T. C. Lindholm (1987). "Vertebral Fusion Dynamics in the Thoracic and Lumbar Spine Induced by Allogenic Demineralized Bone Matrix Combined with Autogenous Bone Marrow: An Experimental Study in Rabbits," *Ital. J. Orthop. Traumatol.* 13:241–251.

Robinson, D., et al. (1999). "Inflammatory Reactions Associated with a Calcium Sulfate Bone Substitute," *Ann. Transplant* 4:91–97.

Rogers-Foy, J. M., et al. (1999). "Hydroxyapatite Composites Designed for Antibiotic Drug Delivery and Bone Reconstruction: A Caprine Model," *J. Invest. Surg.* 12:263–275.

Salamon, M. L., et al. (2003). "The Effects of BMP-7 in a Rat Posterolateral Intertransverse Process Fusion Model," *J. Spinal Disord. Tech.* 16:90–95.

Sandhu, H. S., et al. (1995). "Evaluation of rhBMP-2 with an OPLA Carrier in a Canine Posterolateral (Transverse Process) Spinal Fusion Model," *Spine* 20:2669–2682.

Sandhu, H. S., et al. (1996). "Effective Doses of Recombinant Human Bone Morphogenetic Protein-2 in Experimental Spinal Fusion," *Spine* 21:2115–2122.

Sandhu, H. S., et al. (1997). "Experimental Spinal Fusion with Recombinant Human Bone Morphogenetic Protein-2 Without Decortication of Osseous Elements," *Spine* 22:1171–1180.

Sandhu, H. S., et al. (2002). "Histologic Evaluation of the Efficacy of rhBMP-2 Compared with Autograft Bone in Sheep Spinal Anterior Interbody Fusion," *Spine* 27:567–575.

Sassard, W. R., et al. (2000). "Augmenting Local Bone with Grafton Demineralized Bone Matrix for Posterolateral Lumbar Spine Fusion: Avoiding Second Site Autologous Bone Harvest," *Orthopedics* 23:1059–1064; discussion 1064–1065.

Schimandle, J. H., S. D. Boden, and W. C. Hutton (1995). "Experimental Spinal Fusion with Recombinant Human Bone Morphogenetic Protein-2," *Spine* 20:1326–1337.

Shima, T., et al. (1979). "Anterior Cervical Discectomy and Interbody Fusion: An Experimental Study Using a Synthetic Tricalcium Phosphate," *J. Neurosurg.* 51:533–538.

Sidhu, K. S., et al. (2001). "Anterior Cervical Interbody Fusion with rhBMP-2 and Tantalum in a Goat Model," *Spine J.* 1:331–340.

Stubbs, D., et al. (2004). "In Vivo Evaluation of Resorbable Bone Graft Substitutes in a Rabbit Tibial Defect Model," *Biomaterials* 25:5037–5044.

Strates, B. S., and J. F. Connolly (1989). "Osteogenesis in Cranial Defects and Diffusion Chambers: Comparison in Rabbits of Bone Matrix, Marrow, and Collagen Implants," *Acta Orthop. Scand.* 60:200–203.

Suh, H., and C. Lee (1995). "Biodegradable Ceramic-collagen Composite Implanted in Rabbit Tibiae," *Asaio J.* 41:M652–M656.

Suh, D. Y., et al. (2002). "Delivery of Recombinant Human Bone Morphogenetic Protein-2 Using a Compression-resistant Matrix in Posterolateral Spine Fusion in the Rabbit and in the Non-human Primate," *Spine* 27:353–360.

Sun, T. S., et al. (2004). "Effect of Nano-hydroxyapatite/collagen Composite and Bone Morphogenetic Protein-2 on Lumbar Intertransverse Fusion in Rabbits," *Chin. J. Traumatol.* 7:18–24.

Takahashi, T., et al. (1999). "Use of Porous Hydroxyapatite Graft Containing Recombinant Human Bone Morphogenetic Protein-2 for Cervical Fusion in a Caprine Model," *J. Neurosurg.* 90:224–230.

Takikawa, S., et al. (2003). "Comparative Evaluation of the Osteoinductivity of Two Formulations of Human Demineralized Bone Matrix," *J. Biomed. Mater. Res.* A65:37–42.

Tay, B. K., et al. (1998). "Use of a Collagen-hydroxyapatite Matrix in Spinal Fusion: A Rabbit Model," *Spine* 23:2276–2281.

Thalgott, J. S., et al. (1999). "Anterior Interbody Fusion of the Cervical Spine with Coralline Hydroxyapatite," *Spine* 24:1295–1299.

Thalgott, J. S., et al. (2001). "Instrumented Posterolateral Lumbar Fusion Using Coralline Hydroxyapatite with or Without Demineralized Bone Matrix, as an Adjunct to Autologous Bone," *Spine J.* 1:131–137.

Thalgott, J. S., et al. (2002a). "Anterior Lumbar Interbody Fusion with Processed Sea Coral (Coralline Hydroxyapatite) as Part of a Circumferential Fusion," *Spine* 27:E518–E525; discussion E526–E527.

Thalgott, J. S., et al. (2002b). "Anterior Lumbar Interbody Fusion with Titanium Mesh Cages, Coralline Hydroxyapatite, and Demineralized Bone Matrix as Part of a Circumferential Fusion," *Spine J.* 2:63–69.

Thomson, R. C., et al. (1998). "Hydroxyapatite Fiber Reinforced Poly(alpha-hydroxy ester) Foams for Bone Regeneration," *Biomaterials* 19:1935–1943.

Tiedeman, J. J., et al. (1991a). "Healing of a Large Nonossifying Fibroma After Grafting with Bone Matrix and Marrow: A Case Report. *Clin. Orthop. Relat. Res.* 265:302–305.

Tiedeman, J. J., et al. (1991b). "Treatment of Nonunion by Percutaneous Injection of Bone Marrow and Demineralized Bone Matrix: An Experimental Study in Dogs," *Clin. Orthop. Relat. Res.* 268:294–302.

Tiedeman, J. J., et al. (1995). "The Role of a Composite, Demineralized Bone Matrix and Bone Marrow in the Treatment of Osseous Defects," *Orthopedics* 18:1153–1158.

Toth, J. M., et al. (1995). "Evaluation of Porous Biphasic Calcium Phosphate Ceramics for Anterior Cervical Interbody Fusion in a Caprine Model," *Spine* 20:2203–2210.

Turner, T. M., et al. (2001). "Radiographic and Histologic Assessment of Calcium Sulfate in Experimental Animal Models and Clinical Use as a Resorbable Bone-graft Substitute, a Bone-graft Expander, and a Method for Local Antibiotic Delivery: One Institution's Experience," *J. Bone Joint Surg. Am.* 83A:8–18.

Traianedes, K., et al. (2004). "Donor Age and Gender Effects on Osteoinductivity of Demineralized Bone Matrix," *J. Biomed. Mater. Res.* 70B:21–29.

Urist, M. R. (1965). "Bone: Formation by Autoinduction," *Science* 150:893–899.

Vaccaro, A. R., et al. (2003). "A Pilot Safety and Efficacy Study of OP-1 Putty (rhBMP-7) as an Adjunct to Iliac Crest Autograft in Posterolateral Lumbar Fusions," *Eur. Spine J.* 12:495–500.

Vaccaro, A. R., et al. (2005). "A 2-year Follow-up Pilot Study Evaluating the Safety and Efficacy of Op-1 Putty (rhbmp-7) as an Adjunct to Iliac Crest Autograft in Posterolateral Lumbar Fusions," *Eur. Spine J.* 14:623–629.

Walsh, W. R., et al. (2000). "Mechanical and Histologic Evaluation of Collagraft in an Ovine Lumbar Fusion Model," *Clin. Orthop. Relat. Res.* 375:258–266.

Walsh, W. R., et al. (2004). "Spinal Fusion Using an Autologous Growth Factor Gel and a Porous Resorbable Ceramic," *Eur. Spine J.* 13:359–366.

Weiner, B. K., and M. Walker (2003). "Efficacy of Autologous Growth Factors in Lumbar Intertransverse Fusions," *Spine* 28:1968–1970; discussion 1971.

White, E., and E. C. Shors (1986). "Biomaterial Aspects of Interpore-200 Porous Hydroxyapatite," *Dent. Clin. North Am.* 30:49–67.

Whitman, D. H., R. L. Berry, and D. M. Green (1997). "Platelet Gel: An Autologous Alternative to Fibrin Glue with Applications in Oral and Maxillofacial Surgery," *J. Oral Maxillofac. Surg.* 55:1294–1299.

Wolfe, S. W., et al. (1999). "Augmentation of Distal Radius Fracture Fixation with Coralline Hydroxyapatite Bone Graft Substitute," *J. Hand Surg. Am.* 24:816–827.

Wozney, J. M. (1993). "Bone Morphogenetic Proteins and Their Gene Expression," in M. Noda (ed.). *Cellular and Molecular Biology of Bone.* San Diego: Academic Press.

Yee, A. J., et al. (2003). "Augmentation of Rabbit Posterolateral Spondylodesis Using a Novel Demineralized Bone Matrix-hyaluronan Putty," *Spine* 28:2435–2440.

Ylinen, P., et al. (1991). "Lumbar Spine Interbody Fusion with Reinforced Hydroxyapatite Implants," *Arch. Orthop. Trauma Surg.* 110:250–256.

Zdeblick, T. A., et al. (1998). "Cervical Interbody Fusion Cages: An Animal Model with and Without Bone Morphogenetic Protein," *Spine* 23:758–765; discussion 766.

Zhang, H., D. J. Sucato, and R. D. Welch (2005). "Recombinant Human Bone Morphogenic Protein-2-enhanced Anterior Spine Fusion Without Bone Encroachment into the Spinal Canal: A Histomorphometric Study in a Thoracoscopically Instrumented Porcine Model," *Spine* 30:512–518.

Zhang, M., R. M. Powers Jr., and L. Wolfinbarger Jr. (1997). "A Quantitative Assessment of Osteoinductivity of Human Demineralized Bone Matrix," *J. Periodontol.* 68: 1076–1084.

Zhang, Q. Q., et al. (1996). "Porous Hydroxyapatite Reinforced with Collagen Protein," *Artif. Cells Blood Substit. Immobil. Biotechnol.* 24:693–702.

Zhang, S. M., et al. (2003). "Synthesis and Biocompatibility of Porous Nano-hydroxyapatite/collagen/alginate Composite," *J. Mater. Sci. Mater. Med.* 14: 641–645.

Chapter *10*

Nucleus Replacement of the Intervertebral Disc

Michele S. Marcolongo, Ph.D.[1];
Marco Cannella, Ph.D.[1]; *and*
Christopher J. Massey, M.S.[2]

(1) Department of Materials Science and Engineering
(2) Department of Mechanical Engineering and
Mechanics, Drexel University, Philadelphia, PA

10.1 Introduction

Nucleus replacement was first performed by David Cleveland [Frost & Sullivan 2004] in 1955, when he injected methyl acrylic into 14 patients after discectomies. In more recent years, the first commercialized (in Europe) nucleus replacement device was realized in the Raymedica PDN. Currently, there is much interest in the orthopedic community in the fundamental premise, and patient diagnosis or disc degenerative state that would realize benefit from this procedure. In the beginning of this new millennium, there are numerous corporate activities that are investigating nucleus replacement as well as a few academic groups that are researching these concepts. This chapter will serve to summarize the disease state, principles that are important in the state of disc degeneration, and nucleus replacement design concepts that have been put forth.

10.2 Intervertebral Disc

The mechanical function of the spine allows motion and load transmission [Borenstein and Weisel 1989; Hardy 1982; White and Panjabi 1990]. The spine motion segment is the smallest structural unit allowing motion and load transmission. This consists of two vertebrae, an intervertebral disc, two zygapophyseal joints and capsules, and the associated ligaments and muscles. Within the motion segment, the intervertebral disc is the primary load-bearing dynamic element providing passive motion restraint. This is accomplished by transferring loads from one intervertebral body to the next and by maintaining a deformable space to accommodate the normal spine movement.

The intervertebral discs comprise approximately 20 to 30% of spine length [Borenstein and Weisel 1989]. They are composed of three tissue structures. The central nucleus pulposus tissue is contained at the vertebral end plates by end plate cartilage and circumferentially by the annulus fibrosus tissue. On gross inspection the nucleus pulposus tissue is an amorphous mucoid structure [White and Panjabi 1990]. The annulus fibrosus consists of highly ordered collagen fibers. The collagen fibers of the annulus fibrosus are oriented at a 60-degree angle to the longitudinal axis of the disc and arranged in 10 to 20 lamellae with alternating angulation [White and Panjabi 1990]. This crisscross arrangement of collagen fibers within the annulus fibrosus enables it to withstand torsional and bending loads. The disc end plates are composed of hyaline and fibro cartilage in the central portion of the vertebrae. The inner third of the annulus fibrosus attaches directly to this cartilage.

The normal disc mechanics are such that the hydrated nucleus exerts a hydro-static pressure (called intradiscal pressure) on the internal surface of the annulus, placing the annular fibers into tension. For the same reason that a rope can take more load when pulled than pushed, the annulus fibers operate more efficiently in tension, and are able to effectively transfer loads between the adjacent vertebral bodies. Loads sustained for all normal motions of the disc are limited by tension within the fibers of the annulus fibrosus and maintenance of pressure within the nucleus pulposus. Compressive and tensile loading of the disc provides the most uniform distribution of forces within the annulus fibrosus fibers, whereas torsional and translational loading provides the least uniform loading of fibers.

10.3 Degenerative Disc Disease: Etiology

At the level of the motion of the segment, degenerative spine disease is synonymous with degenerative disc disease although the degenerative process involves not only the discs but the other articulating soft tissues. The etiology of the degenerative process is not fully understood but is thought to involve aging, genetic, and environmental factors. Both the nucleus pulposus and annulus fibrosus undergo a change with aging [Beard and Stevens 1980; Gower and Pedrini 1969; Sylven et al. 1951]. With aging, the concentration of proteoglycans within the nucleus pulposus decreases and the proteoglycans have reduced molecular weights [Adams and Muir 1976; Bushell et al. 1977; Comper and Preston 1974; Urban and Maroudas 1980]. In addition, the ratio of keratin sulfate to chondrotin sulfate increases [Adams, Eyre, and Muir 1977; Gower and Pedrini 1969; Naylor 1976; Naylor and Shental 1976; Urban and Maroudas 1980]. There is an increase in the collagen content as well as collagen-proteoglycan binding [Adams and Muir 1976; Hirsch et al. 1953]. The nucleus pulposus becomes less hydrophilic with age [Adams and Muir 1976; Hirsch et al. 1953]. The loss of hydration is not only due to change in ratio of the keratin sulfate to chondrotin sulfate but also due to changes in the collagen and collagen-proteoglycan binding [Comper and Preston 1974; Hirsch et al. 1953]. Whether or not these changes are due to change in phenotypic expression, to change in percentage of cell type, to alteration of the disc metabolism, or to mechanical stimulation is not fully appreciated.

The biochemical changes that take place with loss of hydration and increased collagen-proteoglycan binding render the nucleus pulposus more fibrous and less resilient. The mechanical consequence of the dehydration is a reduction in intradiscal pressure resulting in greater deformation of the disc under load. Annular radial expansion (disc bulging) and loss of disc height result, and these herald early degenerative disc disease. With increasing disc deformation, the annulus lamellae become increasingly fibrillated and may develop clefts and fissures [Harris and MacNab 1954; Pritzker 1977; Vernon-Roberts and Pirie 1977].

Ultimately, with the reduced intradiscal pressure the fibers of the annulus are no longer loaded in tension. The loads between vertebral bodies are then transferred by the annulus fibers in compression and the disc is now operating as the proverbial flat tire. Structural weaknesses in the annulus fibrosus, fissures, or tears may result in focal concentrations in annular loading and a decreased ability of the disc to handle normal physiologic loads. Consequential overloading may tear the annulus fibrosus and repeated micro trauma may hasten propagation of fissures and cracks. If a complete radial tear in the annulus fibrosus develops, there can be expulsion of the nucleus pulposus material, disc herniation. This may further increase stress within the annulus fibrosus.

Throughout the degenerative process tissue injury evokes an injury response. The ability of the disc to heal is limited, and healing does not restore normal physiologic function. In summary, loss of disc mechanical integrity with nucleus pulposus dehydration and fibrosis results in a cascade of loss of normal disc mechanical function, tissue injury, and injury response. The time course of the injury and injury response determines the clinical manifestation of degenerative disc disease.

10.4 Current Treatments for Degenerative Disc Disease

Current treatment for degenerative disc disease focuses primarily on relieving back and leg pain. The inflammatory response secondary to tissue injury and nerve root impingement are frequently observed in association with degenerative disc changes and are thought to mediate a pain response. Although the exact mechanism of pain generation is debated, more than 75% of low back pain is associated with degenerative disc disease [Schaaf 1998]. Moreover, sciatica has an even stronger association with disc herniation and nerve root impingement. In the absence of neurological impairment, treatment begins with conservative care, activity modification, and anti-inflammatory medication. Under this regimen, 85 to 90% of patients are treated successfully in three months [Ahn 2002; Bush et al. 1992]. However, the remaining 10 to 15% result in over 75% of the treatment costs, often requiring highly invasive surgical interventions. The most common surgical treatments, discectomy and spinal fusion, are performed to reduce pain, and not to restore disc function. Discectomy is employed when the disc has herniated and is impinging on nerve roots causing patient pain, but when the annulus degeneration is not severe. In this surgery, the impinging region of the annulus fibrosus and nucleus pulposus is excised, hence alleviating pressure on the nerves and eliminating pain. Pain is eliminated in 90 to 95% of cases [Kambin and Savitz 2000]. However, as previously noted, this approach does nothing to restore normal biomechanics of the vertebral segment [Weber 1983]. The nucleus pulposus is still dehydrated and the annulus fibers are still likely operating in compression. Therefore, the patient may continue along the path of disc degeneration over ensuing years.

Surgical fusion, inducing bone growth across the functional spinal unit to eliminate disc loading and motion, is reserved for patients with chronic severely disabling pain. Generally, discs treated with fusion are farther along the path of degeneration. Without delineating the specific indications for fusion of the functional spinal unit (which are varied dependant on the signs and symptoms of the degenerative disease), suffice here to say that approximately 150,000 spinal fusions are performed per year in the United States alone. The numbers are growing exponentially. Regardless of the extent to which this procedure is performed, the results of spine fusion vary extensively [Lee et al. 1991]. More perplexing is the clinical outcome, which may not improve with increased rates of fusion. There are significant long-term limitations associated with a spine fusion. Spinal fusion does nothing to restore the normal biomechanics of the vertebral segment. In fact, the lack of motion within the segment can lead to further degeneration of the adjacent intervertebral discs [Leong et al. 1983]. Lehman et al. [1987] pursued a long-term follow-up of lumbar fusions in patients from 21 to 52 years of age, and found that 44% of the patients were currently still experiencing low back pain, 50% had back pain within the previous year, 53% were on medications, 5% had late sequelae secondary to surgery, and 15% had repeat lumbar surgery. This suggests the need for alternatives to fusion.

In the past three years, the spine industry has changed dramatically. The recent success of nonfusion technologies in markets outside the United States has increased the research and development activities into nonfusion and motion-preservation approaches. Only recently (October of 2004), the FDA approved the first nonfusional device to enter the U.S. market. Over the past four years, more than 50,000 patients worldwide have received nonfusional spinal implants and only recently more than 3,000 U.S. patients have been treated in FDA-approved Investigation Device Exemption (IDE) studies of nonfusional products [Viscogliosi 2005]. The nonfusion device can be divided into two main categories: total disc replacement (TDR) and nucleus disc replacement (NDR).

10.5 Total Disc Replacement

A nonfusion surgical approach to the treatment of degenerative disc disease is to remove the diseased disc in its entirety and replace it with a synthetic implant. Disc replacement may serve to eliminate pain while restoring physiological motion. This approach for total knee and hip replacement has been highly successful. More than 56 reports on mechanical replacement have been described [McMillin and Steffee 1994], most from the standpoint of design concept with very few clinical reports, until the recent commercialization of the Charité LINK (the first commercialized total disc replacement in the United States) and the Prodisc (commercialized in Europe at the time of this writing). These promising devices are aimed at replacing the intervertebral disc of patients that have severely degenerated discs (grade III or IV) at this time. The question remains if there could be an earlier surgical intervention that would slow or prevent the severe pain associated with end-stage disc disease. This requires some further understanding of the degenerative path of the disc to examine points at which an intervention might make sense.

10.6 Nucleus Pulposus Replacement

Rather than replacing the entire disc, several investigators have attempted to replace the nucleus pulposus alone. This would result in a surgical technique that would offer a less invasive approach to pain relief while potentially restoring the functional biomechanics to the system. This approach could be most effective in patients with early diagnosis of disc disease, before the annulus has suffered significant degeneration. The concept of nucleus replacement was investigated by several scientists and doctors in the late 1950s. Originally, the aim was to prevent disc collapse, but later it was to mimic the mechanical properties of the nucleus. Nachemson, in the early 1960s, injected a self-curing silicone into the disc space in cadavers [Nachemson 1962]. Further research into silicone replacement of the nucleus continued into the early part of the nineties [Ashida, Yolurnvaniva, and Okumulu 1990; Bost 1982; Fassie and Ginestle 1978; Roy-Camille, Saillant, and Lavaste 1978; Schneider and Oven 1974]. The silicone prostheses have been promising as far as mechanical properties and ease of insertion into the nucleus. However, silicone synovitis and its associated complications may play a significant role in limiting the clinical success of this material as it has in other orthopedic joints [Chan et al. 1998]. More recently, Gan et al. [2000] have investigated nucleus tissue engineering as a way of regenerating the degenerated tissue. While the cells clearly adhered to the glass substrate and primarily held their phenotype after three weeks *in vitro*, it was not clear that the matrix was that of a healthy nucleus pulposus. This approach is reasonable in an era of tissue engineering solutions, but cell and molecular biologists are still struggling to determine the nature of the nucleus pulposus cell, and so setting and meeting the requirements of regenerating the tissue, while promising, has many challenges to overcome before adaptation as a clinical treatment.

10.6.1 What Is the Goal of Nucleus Replacement?

This might be the trickiest question of all. We as a research and clinical community are good at solving problems, but the definition of the problem is the most significant issue in disc degeneration. What causes lower back pain? How can we diagnose the structural and biochemical changes associated with lower back pain? If we can answer these questions, we can then develop a barrage of treatment modalities that would help to relieve this severely debilitating condition. At least at present, we have some insights into the disc features that are associated with pain. We know that there is lumbar nerve impingement that leads to sciatica and we know that there is a mechanical pain associated with different pressures exerted by the disc (for example, with specific motions). The root cause of the pain, however, is not always clear. Therefore, the goal of nucleus replacement is not clear. Should the nucleus replacement restore disc height? Will this relieve pain? Should the nucleus replacement restore intradiscal pressure and will this relieve pain? The crucial answers to these questions are difficult to anticipate, but with some good clinical feedback we can better define this problem and then better solve it. Nucleus replacement may be a viable treatment alternative to patients with early degenerative disc disease, but the efficacy of the treatment will likely evolve as our clinical understanding of pain becomes more clear.

10.6.2 Who Are the Surgical Candidates for Nucleus Replacement?

Clearly, there are different treatment approaches to lower back pain according to the state of degeneration of the intervertebral disc. For patients whose conservative treatment has failed, it may be that discectomy is an option if the annulus fibrosus is not significantly compromised. While discectomy is helpful in eliminating pain, it does not restore normal biomechanics or disc height. This has been shown to lead to further degeneration and pain in some cases [Bao and Yuan 2002]. Because the restoration of biomechanics has proven to be so important for other implant systems, an assumption that biomechanics would play an important role in the treatment of degenerative disc disease in relieving pain and restoring function of the structure is reasonable. Therefore, for patients who have a severely compromised annulus it is unlikely that replacing or regenerating the nucleus will have any lasting biomechanical benefit, unless the annulus can be regenerated or repaired synthetically. In addition, since replacing the nucleus is an inside-out type of procedure, the success of the procedure relies on an intact annulus to constrain the device, at least in part. However, if one could replace the nucleus of a patient earlier on in the degenerative process—where there has been a loss of hydration of the nucleus but a relatively intact annulus—the chance of repressurizing or tensioning the annulus fibrosus may limit or eliminate the mechanical consequences that may be responsible for further degeneration of the annulus. It is for this large group of patients that nucleus replacement may add a great benefit.

10.6.3 Fundamental Concepts of Nucleus Replacement

There have been two approaches to replacing the nucleus pulposus of the intervertebral disc using synthetic biomaterials. The first approach holds the premise that by removing the nucleus pulposus and implanting a replacement device one would restore the height of the disc thereby relieving pressure on the nerves on which the disc is impinging and alleviating lower back pain. This approach was investigated using vitalium spheres [Harmon 1959] and stainless steel balls [Fernstrom 1965]. More recently, this approach is being used by Raymedica (polyethene fiber encased polyacrylonitrile spacers), Replication New Brunswilcle, NJ (polyacylonitrile) and Biomet Warsaw, IN (pyrolytic carbon spacer). The height restoration approach does not intend to mimic the biomechanical function of the nucleus to pressurize the annulus fibrosus, but does in some way tension the annulus by distraction of the nuclear cavity. Outcomes of this approach will depend, in part, on the restored disc height and the method proposed to determine this height. Some details of the results of the height restoration approach follow in the text.

There has been clinical evidence that the restoration of disc height with a nucleus replacement will provide normal ranges of motion for the anterior column unit; for example, for the Raymedica PDN [Wilke et al. 2001]. Risks to this type of approach and the use of devices that are of a significantly higher modulus (and hardness) than the nucleus tissue is that there could be migration of the device into the end plate (a process that could significantly alter disc mechanics and potentially exacerbate pain). In addition, by implanting a relatively large solid device into the nuclear space by incision through the annulus the result could be expulsion of the implant through the implantation site (or another weakened area of the annulus fibrosus). Indeed, the height restoring PDN has suffered from an unacceptable incidence of expulsion (12% worldwide results) [Shim et al. 2003].

The second approach to nucleus replacement is to restore biomechanics by mimicking the biomechanical function of the nucleus pulposus, which is to pressurize the annulus fibrosus in a hydrostatic manner and hence tension the collagen fibers of the annulus so that they can more efficiently transfer stress between vertebral bodies. Devices that are intended to mimic this function utilize softer materials that can utilize the Poisson effect [Joshi et al. 2005] to provide a radial stress on the inner annulus fibers to tension them in much the same way that the water-containing nucleus pulposus tissue tensions the fibers. This approach has also resulted in restoration of biomechanics of the anterior column unit [Joshi et al. 2006]. While the second approach mimics the biomechanical function of the nucleus, it does not preclude the restoration of disc height. The volume of material used to fill the nuclear space may be more important in the restoration of biomechanics than the modulus of the material used within a certain range. Therefore, overfilling or underfilling of the cavity in this approach may prove to be clinically relevant [Joshi et al. 2005]. The Zimmar Newcleus (Warsaw, IN) and Stryker Howmedica Osteonics Acquarelle (Mahwah, NJ) are examples of designs of this approach.

10.6.4 Minimally Invasive Implantation and Expulsion

Implantation of the nucleus replacements has been through the annulus fibrosus either in an open anterior approach or in a posterior-lateral or lateral approach. In any case, the annulus fibrosus is incised and instrumentation is incorporated to remove the nucleus pulposus. The amount of nucleus removed will depend on the device. Subsequently, the nucleus device is inserted into the cavity.

One issue associated with the device implantation is the retention of the device in the disc space. Raymedica showed a 12% device migration after six months in their clinical study [Shim et al. 2003]. The Aquarelle nucleus replacement expulsed in 20% of cases in a primate model (n = 5) *in vivo* [Allen et al. 2004]. Recognizing this challenging situation of filling a large (approximately 16-mm diameter by 10-mm height) nucleus cavity with an implant that should be placed through the smallest possible incision site presents some challenges. Some approaches to this issue have been very clever including exploiting the shape memory properties of hydrogels and polyurethanes. Hydrogels exhibit a shape memory with hydration level so that a dehydrated material would hold its shape when rehydrated *in situ* in the disc space, for instance. The dehydrated material, losing approximately 40 to 90% of its mass, would result in a volumetric reduction. Upon the introduction to an aqueous solution, the material would theoretically swell to a much larger volume with water uptake. This principle is used in the Raymedica PDN. Another interesting application of this technique is via the Replication device, which is engineered to preferentially hydrate longitudinally, intending in this way to restore disc height but to allow for a minimal incision site in the annulus. Sulzer's Newcleus is a polyurethane ribbon formed in a spiral. For implantation, the device is uncoiled and straightened, thus reducing the cross-sectional area needed to allow implantation. As the device is inserted, the shape memory of the polyurethane is exploited and the material will coil *in situ* to fill the nuclear cavity.

The trade-off between providing a cavity filling implant with the smallest possible incision is intended to limit the rate of expulsion of the device from the disc. The severe loading of the spine puts tremendous pressure on the device with significant off-axis loading. A bending, twisting, compression condition is known to produce herniations *in vitro*. This same motion might be important in the expulsion tendency of the nucleus replacement, although the clinical motions and loads responsible for nucleus implant expulsion have not been well defined. For this reason, injectable biomaterials have been considered for nucleus replacement. Bao et al. have worked on injectable polyurethane/protein polymers to discover an injectable material system that would allow for a minimally invasive replacement of the nucleus pulposus where the limitation to the incision site would then be limited by the size needed to remove the nucleus pulposus tissue [Ahrens et al. 2005]. The complication to this injectable approach is that the polyurethane polymerized *in situ*, which may result in residual unreacted agents that could lead to biocompatibility concerns.

10.6.5 Mechanical Requirements

The mechanical requirements of the nucleus replacements fall into two categories: (1) the mechanical requirements of the implant itself and (2) the biomechanical performance of the implanted device with the surrounding tissues. For the first category, the implant itself must exhibit a repeatable, reliable mechanical behavior. The compressive modulus and strength as well as shear modulus and strength should be well understood. The implant should be able to survive the repeated loading cycles of the spine in compression, bending, and shear. Appropriate methods for testing in fatigue are still in discussion [Joshi et al.]. The implant could be tested in a constrained [Bao et al. 1996] or unconstrained [Thomas et al. 2003] fashion to determine the device interaction with the annulus fibrosus or the material property, respectively.

Some issues arise with the feasibility of truly unconstrained injectable nucleus replacements. In addition, the viscoelastic behavior of the nucleus replacement (applicable for protein solutions and for polymeric materials) should match the viscoelastic behavior of the disc (as described in Chapter 3). There should be full recovery and no permanent set of the material over time of implantation that might result in a loss of disc height. Bain et al. measured the creep behavior of the PDN-implanted disc and found that the PDN-implanted creep behavior and the recovery behavior closely tied with that of the intervertebral disc itself [Bain et al. 2000].

Biomechanical performance of the implanted disc should mimic that of the normal intact disc. Meakin et al. [2001] used the sheep discs to assess the effect of nucleus implant on bulging direction of the Anulus Fibrosus fibers, in pure compression. They observed that a nucleus implant with a modulus in the range of 0.2 to 40 MPa prevented the inward bulging of the AF, seen in the case of the denucleated specimen. However, their numerical modeling [Meakin, Reid, and Hukins 2001] showed that the stresses were restored to those of the intact Functional Spinal Unit only with an implant in the modulus range of 3 to 5 MPa. Further reports of the compressive behavior of different moduli materials for nucleus replacement showed that the modulus over a range from 150 to 1,500 kPa did not show a difference in compressive stiffness in human lumbar cadaveric anterior column units. However, the volumetric fill of the cavity did have an effect with an undersized fill of the cavity (resulting in a significant reduction of compressive ACU stiffness, especially at high strain levels), whereas an overfilled cavity resulted in a significant increase of ACU stiffness regardless of implant modulus tested [Joshi et al. 2005]. Work reported by Butterman et al. showed that the PDN was able to restore the range of motion of the implanted ACUs to the level of the intact of the same segment in bending and torsion [Buttermann and Beaubien 2004]. A more recent abstract by Ahrens et al. [2005] showed that the motion was restored with a polyurethane injectable system. For space-filling designs, mimicking the exact intradiscal stress of the nucleus pulposus may not be as critical to the biomechanics as the fill of the cavity in providing stability to the system. For the PDN, the space filling does not seem to be as critical. Here, the modulus may play a more dominant role.

10.6.6 Biocompatibility Requirements

Biocompatibility is an obvious yet essential component to a successful nucleus replacement. In addition to the required ISO standard battery of testing, some considerations need to be made as to the specific location and function of the device. While these requirements have yet to be formalized in a standard, one might consider some important biological interactions. The first is the tissue response to the implant in the physiological implantation site (i.e., the nucleus cavity). This harsh, osmotically dynamic environment is unique in the body, and thus a biomaterial response to this environment is essential for understanding the impact of the material on the surrounding tissue pathology. For this type of safety analysis, animal models would be best employed with direct implantation in the nucleus. The specific animal model has not yet been agreed on by the community and to date a major challenge in developing these devices has been the creation of an animal model for safety, much less efficacy. In an ideal design, one might be able to induce disc degeneration, subsequently repair the disc using the nucleus replacement technology, and allow the animal to load the device according to a loading pattern that is similar (although scaled for geometrical considerations) to the human. In reality, although animal models have been considered from the empire penguin to the kangaroo even primates do not serve as adequate biomechanical models for nucleus replacement. It is often challenging to scale a device to the size of smaller mammals and so the sheep has been put forth as a model that provides the implantation site (nucleus) environment, but that does not adequately replicate the biomechanical environment. At best, to date, one can propose an animal model that will test the safety but not the efficacy of a nucleus replacement *in vivo*.

Further considerations for biocompatibility include the potential inflammatory response to particulate debris that may be created through wear of the device. The long-standing body of experience and literature on polyethylene wear debris from hip and knee arthroplasty give good reason to consider this biological response. In addition, because of the proximity to sensitive neurological tissues some consideration of their response to particulates may be warranted. Certainly, the inflammatory nature of the materials chosen could be considered in a standard model, such as the rat pouch model. The tests to determine the inflammatory nature of potential particulates will be affected by the number, size, and shape of the particulates. Generation of these particulates *in vitro* is challenging (especially for soft elastomers and hydrogels) when it is not known how the material will wear *in vivo*, leaving the option of using ranges of particle sizes and doses to best determine the potential inflammatory nature of the particulates of the implant material.

10.7 Historical Design Perspective

The earliest description of spinal column disorders was discovered in an Egyptian papyrus scroll, dated to approximately 1550 BCE. It describes two spinal cord injuries involving fracture or dislocation of the neck vertebrae accompanied by paralysis. The first scientific description of a spinal condition may have been done by Hippocrates (460–377 BCE), but no treatment options were reported for spinal cord injuries that resulted in paralysis. In about 200 CE, the Roman physician Galen introduced the concept of the central nervous system and he suggested that the spinal cord was an extension of the brain that carried sensation to the limbs and back. This observation moved Paulus of Aegina, in the seventh century CE, to suggest surgery as a treatment for spinal column injury by removing bone fragments that he was convinced caused paralysis. Only in the late nineteenth century, with the use of antiseptics and sterilization in surgical procedures, could a spinal surgery be done without severe risk of infection. In 1909, Oppenheim and Kruse performed the first surgery for disc herniation. More recently, the use of X-rays in the 1920s definitely improved surgeons' skills in locating the spine injury and making a diagnosis and a prediction of the outcome [Chedid and Chedid 2003].

Spinal fusion, the most popular surgical treatment for degenerative disc disease causing instability and back pain, has been used by Albee and Hibbs since 1911. They believed that these painful symptoms could be relieved by elimination of unstable spinal motion segments by fusing adjacent vertebral bodies together. They developed, almost simultaneously but independently, autograph and allograph procedures in order to (1) provide immediate stability, (2) induce osteogenic regeneration, and (3) restore disc height. However, the nonphysiological nature of interbody fusion affects the stress on the adjacent discs and this may accelerate their degeneration. The issue becomes trying to stabilize the joint without greatly altering the biomechanical stiffness of the disc joint [Bao and Yuan 2002]. Prosthetic disc replacement is considered a solution to degenerative disc disease, but the design of a device that mimics the multicomponent structure and the multifunction of the intervertebral disc is extremely complicated. As of 2005, most designs have been able to mimic some of the properties of the normal disc, but one that mimics all of its functions still eludes us. Moreover, it is unlikely that disc replacement will be suitable for every patient, particularly in early-stage disc degeneration. In these cases, most of the annulus is left intact and it may be feasible to restore the normal stiffness using a nucleus prosthesis rather than using a total disc prosthesis [Bao and Yuan 2002].

Although it is not clear who developed the first nucleus disc prosthesis, in the 1950s several researchers attempted disc replacement in order to prevent disc collapse after discectomy. These first attempts can be considered as either disc or nucleus prostheses because their main goal is to restore the disc height by mimicking some of the nucleus functions.

One of the first attempts to prevent disc collapse was made by Hamby and Cleveland in 1955 by injecting methyl-acrylic into the disc space during discectomy [Carl et al. 2004; Sagi, Bao, and Yuan 2003, 2004]. The main function of the methyl-acrylic injection was to restore disc height and to provide stability by fusion of the two adjacent vertebrae. Of the more than 200 patients treated with methyl methacrylate fusion, no major complications had been reported and none of the patients required re-operation at the same level. Later, in 1959, Harmon inserted Vitalium unknow source spheres (which were commercialized for a short time), but his results were never reported [Frost & Sullivan 2004].

The first real attempt to mimic the mechanical properties of the nucleus was done on cadavers by Nachemson in 1962 using silicone as a nucleus replacement. The silicone prostheses have been promising as far as mechanical properties and ease of insertion into the nucleus. However, silicone synovitis and its associated complications may play a significant role in limiting the clinical success of this material.

Fernström, in 1965, used a solid stainless steel ball with a diameter of 10 to 16 mm, which was designed to serve as a spacer allowing movement between the adjacent vertebrae. This is generally considered the first human nucleus prosthesis. The prosthesis was able to restore original disc height and did not limit the range of motion of the vertebral segment. However, it was stiff in compression and very compliant in rotation. The device did not restore the normal load distribution and was discarded because of basic problems such as implant migration within the cavity and its tendency to subside into the vertebral end plates and bodies [Bao and Yuan 2002; Sagi, Bao, and Yuan 2003]. Nevertheless, McKenzie presented good long-term results [Carl et al. 2004] and recently (1995) this approach has been used by Cook, Salkeld, and Wang in designing other nucleus replacements (EBI Regain). A pilot clinical trial of this nucleus replacement (EBI, Parsippany, NJ) has been initiated on the encouraging results obtained in a primate model.

In 1973, Stubstad and his team developed the first multicoil or spiraled implant. They describe a spiral implant with elastic memory which after introduction wraps into a disc-shaped prosthesis [Szpalski, Gunzburg, and Mayer 2002]. In the same year, Urbaniak published a clinical study on the insertion of a silicone-Dacron composite device in chimpanzee discs. He reported bone resorption and reactive bone formation and he suggested the idea of a pre-formed or contained implant [Sagi, Bao, and Yuan 2003]. But it was Froning, in 1975, who patented a plastic device with a central collapsible bladder, which is filled with a fluid or plastic under adjustable pressure. The prosthesis was anchored to the two adjacent vertebrae by studs that set in place once the disc is inflated.

In 1977, Roy-Camille proposed to contain medical grade silicone in a latex bag during insertion into a human cadaver disc. After the silicone was polymerized, a 200-hour fatigue test was performed and no deterioration of the disc was observed. Several researchers contributed to the clinical study and in the improvement of the silicone rubber nucleus design: Fassio and Ginestie (1978), Horst (1982), and Ashida (1991) [Bao et al. 1996]. In 1994, Hou implanted a preformed silicon nucleus of horseshoe shape into over 30 patients. This may be the first human clinical study using silicone rubber for nucleus replacement [Hou et al. 1991; Sagi, Bao, and Yuan 2003]. Unfortunately, however, the results have not yet been published.

In 1981, Edeland first suggested the idea of a device that would mimic both the mechanical and the biological characteristics of the nucleus pulposus. He proposed to develop a material that under loading would allow the influx and efflux of water molecules because of its hydrophilic nature. He suggested the implantation of this device before the degeneration progress affects the facet joints. Unfortunately, he was not able to find the appropriate material for his device [Bao et al. 1996; Carl et al. 2004; Sagi, Bao, and Yuan 2003; Szpalski, Gunzburg, and Mayer 2002].

Based on the principles of Edeland and Froning, in 1988 Ray and Corbin developed a dual disc cylinder device, each one made by a bioresorbable material (polyglicolic acid PGA) that attracts tissue ingrowth. The core of each cylinder was filled by a hygroscopic thixotropic gel (i.e., hyalutropic acid) that exhibited swelling pressures intended to be similar to the natural nucleus pulposus. The cylinders were implanted in a deflated state after nucleotomy and then inflated by the injection of the thixotropic gel [Bao et al. 1996; Sagi, Bao, and Yuan 2003]. Later, in the mid 1990s, Ray proposed a different implant positioned in the medial-lateral position rather than anterior-posterior like the previous one [Carl et al. 2004; Sagi, Bao, and Yuan 2003]. The implants were made of a polyacrylonitrile (PAN) hydrogel surrounded by a flexible but inelastic polyethylene fiber. This device was the first to fully pursue commercialization in Europe and in the United States and is known as the Raymedica PDN. The PDN ushered in the modern era of nucleus replacement.

10.8 Recent Design Concepts

Of the several devices that have been designed as nucleus disc replacements, few are used in clinical practice outside the United States, and many are waiting for FDA approval in order to be sold in the United States. The following highlights the published results from numerous current efforts in nucleus replacement.

10.8.1 Raymedica Prosthetic Disc Nucleus (PDN)

In 1995, Ray et al. developed and internationally commercialized a polyacrylonitrile hydrogel nucleus replacement covered with a polyethylene fiber jacket, called the PDN. It is made by a hydrogel core (which replaces the function of the failed intervertebral disc) and a flexible polyethylene jacket surrounding the hydrogel, which maintains the size of the hydrogel and permits its expansion and contraction. The hydrogel core is intended to imbibe and expel fluids in response to different loads placed on the spinal unit. The polyethylene jacket is porous to allow fluids to pass to and from the hydrogel core. Its function is critical because it keeps the hydrogel height, which in turn controls the disc height and tensioning of the annulus fibers.

This device is intended to improve disc height, restore motion, and relieve pain due to disc herniation [Bertagnoli and Schanmayr 2002]. Initially, it was made into two separate units: a tapered anterior unit and a rectangular posterior unit, achieving a surgical success rate of 88% (1999 through 2001), with the primary failure being dislocation of the implant from the nucleus. The open procedure through the annulus can allow the devices (which are implanted in the hydrated state) to exit through the incision site. While the surgical technique is still evolving to the level of having a truly satisfactory procedure, patient pain in this short-term follow-up study was reduced 86% (oswestry and visual analog scale pain levels) and spinal flexibility increased 67%. During the first human trial period, it was discovered that an excessive end plate remodeling also occurred [Shim et al. 2003].

The design was improved and today the implant is available only as a single device (SOLO). The PDN device is implanted in a dehydrated low profile and has the ability to restore disc height as it expands with hydration. Three different surgical approaches have been used: the posterior approach, the Para spinal approach, and the anterolateral transpsoatic approach. Each of these approaches requires a discectomy (to remove the nucleus) in order to create enough room for the PDN device.

A minimum disc height of 5mm is required to implant the device. The annulus must be without calcification, excessive fissures, or delamination. The implant can be used also in patients with disc herniation. This device is indicated for the treatment of adult patients suffering from disc degenerative disease of the lumbar spine, represented by low back pain (with or without leg pain) that is discogenic in origin and unresponsive to nonsurgical treatment.

Since 1996, the PDN has been implanted in 423 patients with a 90% success rate. The remaining 10% of the patients have been converted to other surgical methods [Klara and Ray 2002]. From November of 1997 to February of 1999, 10 patients were implanted with the PDN device, after unilateral discectomy, at Sentara Leigh Memorial Hospital in Norfolk, Virginia. Intraoperative fluoroscopy verified correct positioning. The mean operative time was 91 minutes. Postoperative mobility was permitted the day after surgery, with restricted flexion. Complications related to the surgical procedure were limited to two device displacements without accompanying motor neurological deficit, and one patient with unresolved pain at the operative level. One patient reported pain following a motor vehicle accident after device implantation. These patients were converted to fusion [Klara and Ray 2002]. In 2001, Canada's therapeutic Directorate has given approval to begin clinical trials for this device and in 2002 the FDA approved a second U.S. clinical evaluation of the PDN prosthetic disc nucleus device.

10.8.2 Newcleus

Newcleus is a spinal nuclear replacement device constructed with a polycarbonate urethane elastomer (SULENE PCU). The material is biocompatible and has been used in cardiovascular application. Newcleus is manufactured in a manner that takes the form of a memory coiling spiral. The device has a rectilinear shape before the application and will roll automatically into a spire shape during the implantation in the disc cavity with no fixed mechanical axis. Once implanted, the device absorbs water to approximately 35% of its net weight. Functionally, it acts as a spacer with some shock-absorbing capabilities. The device is implanted using the same approach as for microdiscectomy.

This device has two main applications: single-level radiculalgia without back pain due to disc herniation and single-level radiculalgia with predominal leg pain and some back pain, due to disc herniation and degenerative disc disease. In order for the Newcleus to be used, the patient must be between the ages of 18 and 65, have posterior disc height at the affected level of >= 5 mm, and be a candidate for one-level discectomy from L2 to S1 [Korge et al. 2002]. The exclusion criteria include previous spine surgery, end plate lesions, significant spinal stenosis, degenerated facet joints, and severe osteoporosis [Korge et al. 2002].

Until 2002, five patients (two female and three male in the age range 24 to 52) had been treated with this implant. In all the patients, disc surgery, and implantation had been performed without complication and all the patients were satisfied with the result. In the first patient, after two years, the facet joints maintained completely their function. No implant migration occurred.

Biomechanical tests have demonstrated that this device compensates for the loss of disc height, decreases the compression of the facet joints, and restores the kinematics of the spinal segment, without deformation of the vertebral end plates or migration. The device is currently under clinical investigation [Korge et al. 2002].

10.8.3 Aquarelle

Bao and Higham [1993], in 1991, approached nucleus replacement with a hydrogel polymer, called the Aquarelle. This material selection has resulted in an implant that has similar mechanical properties to those of the nucleus as well as similar physiological properties, maintaining about 70% water content under physiological loading conditions. The particular hydrogel employed by this group is comprised of semicrystalline polyvinyl alcohol (PVA) [Bao and Higham 1993]. PVA has the ability to absorb water or physiological fluid and survive mechanical loading as would exist in the nucleus region of the intervertebral disc. However, PVA is not entirely stable within the physiological environment of the body, showing degradation through the melting out of small crystallites over time that can result in a reduction of mechanical properties and leaching of molecules into the physiological environment [Peppas 1977]. Biomechanically, the Aquarelle device has performed well in fatigue testing up to 40 million cycles [DiMartino et al. 2005].

Aquarelle is inserted through a 4- to 5-mm tapered cannula that enters the disc space via a small opening in the annulus. The interspace may be accessed via a lateral or posterior route. Once injected inside the annulus, the viscoelastic material exerts a uniform pressure across the end plates. However, a recent baboon study [Allen et al. 2004] shows a high expulsion rate (33%) using an anterior approach, and even when the surgical approach was modified to anterolateral positioning there remained a 20% expulsion rate for the devices. In the discs where the device remained, the PVA was generally well tolerated and considered biocompatible with no systemic effects. Additionally, particulates of the PVA were generated in a few discs. The biological response to the particulates was an inflammatory response, typical of other types of particulate debris (polyethylene and silicone) in other sites. Finally, microscopic evidence of end plate damage was seen in 22.59% of the animals used for this study, even in the controls with nucleotomy but with no implant. The authors attribute the end plate degeneration to damage caused by removal of the nucleus tissue and not a direct consequence of the implantation itself. The Aquarelle implant is currently in human trials in Europe [Dupont.com 2002].

10.8.4 NeuDisc

The NeuDisc (Replication Medical New Brunswick, NJ) is a prosthetic device that is composed of two parallel soft layers of an elastic deformable hydrogel, with at least one rigid layer. The rigid layer has less compressibility than the soft layer. The number of soft layers is usually one more than the number of rigid layers. Before implantation, the device is in a dehydrated state and rolled up "like a burrito." It is inserted in the annulus after discectomy through a cannula. Once inside the annulus, the device will unfurl and assume a flat shape in which it can start swelling in a predominantly axial direction (U.S. pat. 6726721). No studies describing the mechanical characteristic of this implant have been found in the literature. In 2003, the company was completing pre-clinical testing and is working toward a clinical evaluation of the device.

10.8.5 Regain

Regain (EBI, Parsippany, NJ) is a pyrocarbon nucleus prosthesis. It has a high level of compressive strength and is resistant to wear. The implant can have one of three different geometric profiles: lordotic, spherical, and anatomic [Salkeld et al. 2004]. An *in vivo* study on baboons (n = 6) showed no expulsion and the ability of the implant to restore normal range of motion. Based on these results, the company is starting a clinical evaluation in Europe. Unfortunately, no data have been published in the scientific literature to date.

10.8.6 Intervertebral Prosthetic Disc (IPD)

The intervertebral prosthetic disc (IPD) is a mechanical device composed of an elastic component (metallic springs) that is connected to one or two intervertebral bodies through a fixation component (plate). The elastic component consists of four cobalt chrome springs connected to a metallic plate [Buttermann and Beaubien 2004].

The main benefit of this device is that the annulus fibrosus is preserved during implantation. The implantation is by means of one or two cavities made in the vertebrae adjacent to the disc, through which the nucleus and the end plates are extracted.

A biomechanical testing on lumbar calf spines has been published [Buttermann and Beaubien 2004], which evaluated the effects of springs with different stiffness values on the device performance. Unfortunately, none of the springs tested has been able to restore the biomechanical properties of the intact disc in axial compression.

10.8.7 DASCOR

DASCOR (Disc Dynamics, Eden Prarie, MN) is an *in situ* curable polyurethane that is injected into a polyurethane balloon. The device is already under experimentation and development. A recent publication reports the DASCOR implant was able to restore stiffness and range of motion to nearly intact levels in a study of 12 human lumbar functional spinal units.

10.8.8 BioDisc

This implant is a protein-base hydrogel in which protein and water are "cross linked" to one another. The implant is composed by two parts: a bovine serum albumin (protein) and a cross linker (glutaraldehyde). The two parts are injected through a hypodermic needle in the void created after discectomy [Frost & Sullivan 2004]. No biomechanical studies of this approach have been found in the literature to date. The company claims to have completed the *in vivo* animal studies in 2000 and in 2005 declared to have treated its first patients with the BioDisc ((Cryolife, Kennesaw, GA) Atlanta).

10.8.9 NuCore

The NuCore (Spine Wave, Shelton, CT) injectable nucleus is an injectable, *in situ* curing protein polymer with physical properties specifically designed to mimic that of the natural nucleus. The polymer is a hydrogel composed of synthetic silk-elastin copolymer created through DNA bacterial synthesis fermentation.

These polymers are initially water soluble and can be injected through a needle: a chemical cross-linking agent is also injected into the disc along with the polymer. The mixture cures into an adhesive hydrogel, which fills and seals the void inside the disc space. The company claims that this hydrogel has the same properties as those of the nucleus pulposus [Frost and Sullivan 2004]. Currently, this device is an investigational device only—limited to clinical investigation. No studies on this device have been found in the literature. (See Table 10.1 for a summary of nucleus replacement devices under investigation.)

10.8.10 co.don Chondrotransplant Disc

The autologous disc-derived chondrocyte transplantation (ADTC) replaces the tissue lacking due to the disc herniation and the disc operation. Disc chondrocytes were harvested, expanded in culture, and then returned to the disc in a minimally invasive procedure. Transplanted disc chondrocytes remain viable after transplantation and produce an extracellular matrix that displays composition similar to normal intervertebral disc tissue. Therefore, the function of the disc can be restored and further degeneration can be prevented [co.don 2005].

As early as 1996, the first ADCTs were performed and in 1999 a pilot study for controlled clinical use was started. In a canine model, this technique was able to repair disc damage and retard disc degeneration. In 2002, co.don AG Teltow, Germany started a clinical program to show the efficacy and safety of this product on 104 patients. The follow-up data of these patients showed very good results over a period of more than five years. In 2004, they launched the co.don chondrotransplant DISC as the first biological method to treat disc degeneration [co.don 2005].

10.9 Future Directions

The next five to 10 years of nucleus replacement will be very telling. With the continuation and expansion of clinical trials, real patient data will be determined that will prove or disprove the concept that nucleus replacement can relieve pain and maybe even prevent or postpone the continuation of disc degeneration. More clinical data will help to fine-tune the patient population for which this treatment may be effective. Certainly, the clinical insights will help in refining the pre-clinical testing protocol and understanding of the potential limitations associated with the device.

More and different design concepts may be put forth, and indeed at the time of this writing are already underway in numerous companies and laboratories across the country. The concepts of cellular therapies and tissue engineered constructs to regenerate the nucleus may also be better understood. The one certainty in the next five to 10 years is that the prevalence of lower back pain will not be reduced. Real debilitation exists today and will continue to exist until better treatment options are developed for the patients who suffer from degenerative disc disease.

Table 10.1.

Summary of nucleus replacement devices currently under investigation.

Company	Device	Technology	Studies	Results
Raymedica, Inc., Bloomington, MN	Prosthetic disc nucleus solo (PDN)	Hydrogel core in a polyethylene jacket	Already implanted in more than 300 patients	Moderate to severe end plate change (about 83%). Due either to an inflammatory response or changes in load distribution. Extrusion rate 12%.
Stryker Howmedica Osteonics, Allendale, NJ	Aquarelle	Semihydrated poly vinyl alcohol hydrogel	Preclinical, including baboon study *in vivo*	High rates of expulsion have been reported (20 to 33%), depending on the approach used to implant the device (posterolateral or anterior). PVA appeared biocompatible. Currently in human trials in Europe.
Replication Medical, Inc., New Brunswick, NJ	NeuDisc	Modified hydrolyzed polyacrylonitrile polymer	Pre-clinical testing	No results of mechanical testing are available.
Sulzer	NewCleus	Polycarbonated urethane elastomer curled into a preformed spiral	Implanted in 5 patients	No implant migration was observed.
EBI, Parsippany, NJ	Regain	Polycarbon	Starting clinical trials in Europe	Implanted *in vivo* in baboon (n = 6).
Dynamic Spine, Nahtomedi, MN	IPD	Four cobalt chrome springs	Device feasibility	Incapable of restoring original disc mechanics.
Disc Dynamics, Inc., Eden Prairie, MN	DASCOR	Curable polyurethane	Pre-clinical testing	Able to nearly restore quasi-static biomechanics of the disc.
Cryolife, Kennesaw, GA	BioDisc	Protein base hydrogels (Bioglue)	First implantation in human	No results have been published.
Spine Wave, Shelton, CT	NuCore IDN	Hydrogel composed of synthetic silk-elastin	Undergoing experimentation *in vivo*	No results on the *in vitro* test have been published.

10.10 References

Adams, P., and H. Muir (1976). "Qualitative Changes with Age of Proteoglycans of Human Lumbar Discs," *Annals of the Rheumatic Diseases* 35:289–296.

Adams, P., D. R. Eyre, and H. Muir (1977). "Biochemical Aspects of Development and Ageing of Human Lumbar Intervertebral Discs," *Rheumatology and Rehabilitation* 16:22–29.

Ahn, S. H. (2002). "Comparison of Clinical Outcomes and Natural Morphologic Changes Between Sequestered and Large Central Extruded Disc Herniations," *Yonsei Medical Journal* 43:283–290.

Ahrens, M., N. Ordway, et al. (2005). "Nucleus Replacement with an *In Situ* Curable Balloon Contained Polymer and Restoration of Segmental Kinematics," *European Cells and Materials* 10:46.

Allen, M. J., J. E. Schoonmaker, et al. (2004). "Preclinical Evaluation of a Poly (Vinyl Alcohol) Hydrogel Implant as a Replacement for the Nucleus Pulposus," [miscellaneous article]. *Spine* 29:515–523.

Ashida, H., K. Yolurnvaniva, and A. Okumulu (1990). "An Attempt to Develop Artificial Nuclei Pulposi in Lumbar Intervertebral Discs," *Journal of the Japanese Orthopaedic Association* 64:S947.

Bain, A. C., T. Sherman, B. K. Norton, and W. C. Hutton (2000). *A Comparison of the Viscolelastic Behavior of the Lumbar Intervertebral Disc Before and After Implantation of a Prosthetic Disc Nucleus*. Advances in Bioengineering ASME 2000. Orlando, FL 5, 192, 326.

Bao, Q. B., and P. A. Higham (1993). Hydrogel Intervertebral Disc Nucleus. United States Patant 5, 192, 326.

Bao, Q.-B. P., and H. A. M. D. Yuan (2002a). "New Technologies in Spine: Nucleus Replacement." *Spine* 27:1245–1247.

Bao, Q.-B. P., and H. A. M. D. Yuan. (2002b). "Prosthetic Disc Replacement: The Future?" [Report]. *Clinical Orthopaedics & Related Research* 394:139–145.

Bao, Q.-B., G. M. Mccullen, et al. 1996. "The Artificial Disc: Theory, Design and Materials." *Biomaterials* 17:1157–1167.

Beard, H. K., and R. L. Stevens (1980). "Biochemical Changes in the Intervertebral Disc," in M. I. Jayson (ed.). *The Lumbar Spine and Backache* (2d ed.). London: Pitman.

Bertagnoli, R., and R. Schanmayr (2002). "Surgical and Clinical Results with the PDN Prosthetic Disc-nucleus Device," *European Spine Journal* 11:S143–S148.

Borenstein, D. G., and S. W. Weisel (1989). *Low Back Pain: Medical Diagnosis and Comprehensive Management*. Philadelphia: W. B. Saunders.

Bost, M. (1982). "Mechanical Loading of the Vertebral Body Cover Plate: Measurement of the Direct Stress Distribution at the Interface Between Intervertebral Disc and Intervertebral Body, "in H. Junulanns (ed.). *Die Wirbelsuule in Forschung and Praxis*. Stuttgart: Hippokrates.

Bush, K., N. Cowan, D. E. Katz, and P. Gishen (1992). "The Natural History of Sciatica Associated with Disc Pathology," *Spine* 17:1205–1212.

Bushell, G. R., P. Ghosh, T. F. Taylor, and W. H. Akeson (1977). "Proteoglycan Chemistry of the Intervertebral Disks," *Clinical Orthopaedics & Related Research* 129:115–123.

Buttermann, G. R., and B. P. Beaubien (2004). "Stiffness of Prosthetic Nucleus Determines Stiffness of Reconstructed Lumbar Calf Disc," *The Spine Journal* 4:265–274.

Carl, A., E. Ledet, H. Yuan, and A. Sharan. (2004). "New Developments in Nucleus Pulposus Replacement Technology," *The Spine Journal* 4:S325–S329.

Chan, M., P. Chowchuen, et al. (1998). "Silicone Synovitis: MR Imaging in Five Patients," *Skeletal Radiology* 27:13–17.

Chedid, K. J., and M. K. Chedid (2003). "The 'Tract' of History in the Treatment of Lumbar Degenerative Disc Disease," *Neurosurgical Focus* 16:1–4.

co.don (2005). *http://www.codon.de/_/index.php.*

Comper, W. D., and B. N. Preston (1974). "Model Connective-tissue Systems: A Study of Polyion-mobile Ion and of Excluded-volume Interactions of Proteoglycans," *Biochemical Journal* 143:1–9.

DiMartino, A., A. Vaccaro, et al. (2005). "Nucleus Pulposus Replacement: Basic Science and Indications for Clinical Use," *Spine* 30:S16–S22.

Dupont.com (2002). "Tyvek® Protects New Stryker® Howmedica Osteonics Implant That Could Revolutionize Lower Back Surgery," *http://medicalpackaging.dupont.com/en/applications/pdf/case_histories/lidstock/new_stryker.pdf.*

Fassie, B., and J. F. Ginestle (1978). "Disc Prosthesis Made of Silicone: Experimental Study and First Clinical Cases," *Nouvelle Presse Medical* 21:207.

Froning, E. C. (1975). "Intervertebral Disc Prosthesis and Instruments for Locating Same: United States," Patent No 3875595.

Frost and Sullivan (2004). *U.S. and Asia Markets for Non-Fusion Technologies in Spine Procedures.* Raymedica, Inc. *http://www.raymedica.com/images/pdn.jpg.*

Gan, J. C., P. Ducheyne, E. Vresilovic, and I. M. Shapiro (2000). "Bioactive Glass Serves as a Substrate for Maintenance of Phenotype of Nucleus Pulposus Cells of the Intervertebral Disc," *Journal of Biomedical Materials Research* 51:596–604.

Gower, W. E., and V. Pedrini (1969). "Age-related Variations in Protein-polysaccharides from Human Nucleus Pulposus, Annulus Fibrosus, and Costal Cartilage," *Journal of Bone and Joint Surgery* 51A:1154–1162.

Hardy, R. W. (1982). *Lumbar Disc Disease.* New York: Raven Press.

Harris, R. I., and I. MacNab (1954). "Structural Changes in the Lumbar Intervertebral Discs: Their Relationship to Low Back Pain and Sciatica," *Journal of Bone and Joint Surgery* 36B:304–322.

Hirsch, C., S. Paulson, B. Sylven, and O. Snellman (1953). "Biophysical and Physiological Investigations on Cartilage and Other Mesenchymal Tissues. VI. Characteristics of Human Nuclei Pulposi During Aging," *Acta Orthopaedica Scandinavica* 22:175–183.

Hou, T. S., K. Y. Tu, et al. (1991). "Lumbar Intervertebral Disc Prosthesis: An Experimental Study," *Chinese Medical Journal* 104:381–386.

Joshi, A., G. Fussell, et al. (2006). "Functional Compressive Mechanics of a PVA/PVP Nucleus Pulposus Replacement," *Biomaterials* 27:176–184.

Joshi, A., S. Mehta, et al. (2005). "Nucleus Implant Parameters Significantly Change the Compressive Stiffness of the Human Lumbar Intervertebral Disc," *Transactions of the ASME* 127:536–540.

Kambin, P., and M. H. Savitz (2000). "Arthroscopic Microdiscectomy: An Alternative to Open Disc Surgery," *The Mount Sinai Journal of Medicine* 67:283–287.

Klara, P. M., and C. D. Ray (2002). "Artificial Nucleus Replacement: Clinical Experience," *Spine* 27:1374–1377.

Korge, A., T. Nydegger, et al. (2002). "A Spiral Implant as Nucleus Prosthesis in the Lumbar Spine," *European Spine Journal* 11:S149–S153.

Lee, C., N. Langrana, J. Parsons, and M. Zimmerman (1991). "Development of a Prosthetic Intervertebral Disc," *Spine* 16:S253–S255.

Lehmann, T., K. Spratt, et al. (1987). Long Term Follow-up of Lower Lumbar Fusion Patients" *Spine* 12:97–104.

Leong, J., S. Chun, W. Grange, and D. Fang (1983). "Long Term Results of Lumbar Intervertebral Disc Prolapse," *Spine* 8:793–799.

McMillin, C., and A. Steffee (1994). "Artificial Spinal Disc with up to Five Years Follow-up," *Transcript of the 20th Annual Society for Biomaterials* 89.

Meakin, J. R., J. E. Reid, and D. W. Hukins (2001). "Replacing the Nucleus Pulposus of the Intervertebral Disc," *Clinical Biomechanics* 16:560–565.

Nachemson, A. (1962). "Some Mechanical Properties of the Lumbar Intervertebral Discs," *Bulletin of the Hospital for Joint Diseases* 23:130–143.

Naylor, A. (1976). "Intervertebral Disc Prolapse and Degeneration: The Biochemical and Biophysical Approach," *Spine* 1:108–114.

Naylor, A., and R. Shental (1976). "Biochemical Aspects of Intervertebral Discs in Aging and Disease," in M. I. Jayson (ed.). *The Lumbar Spine and Backache*. New York: Grune & Stratton.

Nikolaos, A., and E. W. M. Peppas (1977). "Development of Semicrystalline Poly(vinyl alcohol) Hydrogels for Biomedical Applications," *Journal of Biomedical Materials Research* 11:423–434.

Pritzker, K. P. (1977). "Aging and Degeneration in the Lumbar Intervertebral Disc," *Orthopedic Clinics of North America* 8:66–77.

Raymedica (2005). *http://www.raymedica.com/images/pdn.jpg*.

Roy-Camille, R., G. Saillant, and F. Lavaste (1978). "Experimental Study of Lumbar Disc Replacement," *Revue de Chirurgie Orthopédique et réparatrice de l'appareil Moteur* 64:106–107.

Sagi, H. C., Q. B. Bao, and H. A. Yuan (2003). "Nuclear Replacement Strategies," *Orthopedic Clinics of North America* 34:263–267.

Salkeld, S. L., K. C. Bailey, et al. (2004). *Partial Disc Replacement in the Lumbar Spine, Poster.* Washington, D.C.: National Academy of Sciences.

Schaaf, T. A. (1998). "Spinal Implants: Accelerating growth, increasing competition," *MedPro Month* VIII.

Schneider, P. G., and R. Oven. (1974a). "Intervertebral Disc Replacement: Experimental Studies, Clinical Consequences," *Zeitschrift für Orthopädie und ihre Grenzebiete* 112:791–792.

Schneider, P. G., and R. Oven. (1974b). "Plastic Surgery on Intervertebral Disc. Part 1: Intervertebral Disc Replacement in the Lumbar Region with Silicone Rubber. Theoretical and Experimental Studies," *Zeitschrift für Orthopädie und ihre Grenzebiete* 112:1078–1086.

Shim, C. S., S. H. Lee, et al. (2003). "Partial Disc Replacement with the PDN Prosthetic Disc Nucleus Device: Early Clinical Results," *Journal of Spinal Disorders & Techniques* 16:324–330.

Sylven, B., S. Paulson, C. Hirsch, and O. Snellman (1951). "Biophysical and Physiological Investigations on Cartilage and Other Mesenchymal Tissues," *Journal of Bone and Joint Surgery* 33A:320–333.

Szpalski, M., R. Gunzburg, and M. Mayer (2002). "Spine Arthroplasty: A Historical Review," *European Spine Journal* 11:S65–S84.

Thomas, J., A. Shuen, A. Lowman, and M. Marcolongo (2003). *The Effect of Fatigue on Associating Hydrogels for Nucleus Pulposus Replacement.* Proceedings of the 29th Annual Society for Biomaterials. Reno, NV.

Urban, J., and A. Maroudas (1980). "The Chemistry of the Intervertebral Disc in Relation to Its Physiological Function," *Clinics in Rheumatological Diseases* 6:51–57.

Vernon-Roberts, B., and C. J. Pirie (1977). "Degenerative Changes in the Intervertebral Discs of the Lumbar Spine and Their Sequelae," *Rheumatology and Rehabilitation* 16:13–21.

Viscogliosi, M. R. (2005). "Building a New Model for Spine Care," *http://www.devicelink.com/mx/archive/05/01/viscogliosi.html*.

Weber, H. (1983). "Lumbar Disc Herniation: A Controlled Perspective Study with Ten Years of Observation," *Spine* 8:131–140.

White, A. A., and M. M. Panjabi (1990). *Clinical Biomechanics of the Spine*. Philadelphia: J. P. Lippincott.

Wilke, H.-J., S. Kavanagh, et al. (2001). "Effect of a Prosthetic Disc Nucleus on the Mobility and Disc Height of the L4–5 Intervertebral Disc Postnucleotomy," *Journal of Neurosurgery (Spine)* 95:208–214.

Chapter *11*

Total Disc Arthroplasty

Steven Kurtz, Ph.D.

Exponent, Inc. Drexel University, Philadelphia, PA

11.1 Introduction

Total disc replacement (TDR) surgery is a promising treatment for advanced degenerative disc disease. Unlike nuclear replacements, which are targeted for patients with early disc degeneration, disc arthroplasty is primarily intended for patients in whom the annulus and nucleus are no longer biomechanically competent. The central aims of disc arthroplasty are to restore the pain free motion, as well as the load-carrying capacity of a diseased functional spinal unit. Therefore, disc replacement occupies a unique and important position in the treatment continuum spanning early degenerative disc disease, at one end of the pathological spectrum, and with spinal fusion at the other.

Today, the task of identifying patients who will benefit the most from total disc replacements—as opposed to some other spine technology such as fusion—represents a diagnostic challenge. The indications for disc arthroplasty vary somewhat, depending on the implant design, and whether the implant is to be implanted in the lumbar or cervical region. In the lumbar spine, disc replacement is specifically indicated for patients with disc-related ("discogenic") back pain, whereas in the cervical spine a broader range of indications can be addressed, including myelopathy and radiculopathy [McAfee 2004]. However, not all patients with a painful disc should receive a total disc replacement surgery because of the formidable list of contraindications, especially in the lumbar region. Central or lateral recess stenosis, facet arthrosis, spondylolisthesis or spondylolysis, herniated nucleus pulposus (HNP) with neural compression, scoliosis, osteoporosis, and any deficiency of the posterior elements are currently considered to be contraindications for lumbar total disc replacement. Indeed, among a consecutive series of 100 contemporary fusion and nonfusion lumbar spine surgery candidates Huang et al. [2004] found that only 5% of the patients would meet the strict inclusion/exclusion criteria for a total disc replacement. Thus, only a fraction of patients with lower back pain may be suitable candidates for total disc replacement surgery. Furthermore, because 100% of fusion patients in Huang's study had at least one contraindication for disc arthroplasty it is considered highly unlikely that disc replacements are going to eliminate the need for fusion surgeries in the foreseeable future.

Nevertheless, as we shall see subsequently in this chapter, one of the historical driving factors for the development of disc replacements has been growing dissatisfaction with fusion as a long-term treatment, especially for younger patients. Immobilization of a functional spinal unit by fusion can result in degenerative changes at adjacent levels, which is referred to as "adjacent segment disease" by some clinicians. However, based on the current state of knowledge it is still not clear whether long-term degenerative changes adjacent to a fused segment are causally related to the fusion itself, or merely represent the natural progression of spine disease [Hilibrand and Robbins 2004]. Proponents of total disc replacement have hypothesized that by maintaining the mobility of the treated disc long-term adjacent segment degeneration may be forestalled or possibly averted.

Therefore, disc replacement is currently considered by many clinicians to be a promising technology for discogenic back pain for a carefully selected patient population [Anderson et al. 2004; Bertagnoli et al. 2005; Errico 2005; Gamradt and Wang 2005; Huang and Sandhu 2004; Mathews et al. 2004; Phillips and Garfin 2005; Traynelis 2005]. The goals of total disc replacement are to restore intervertebral motion of the natural disc. In the short term, clinical data from multiple studies indicates that disc replacement patients may recover from surgery faster than during a fusion procedure [Blumenthal et al. 2005; McAfee et al. 2005]. Clinical data further documents that disc replacements preserve flexibility and range of motion at the treated level [Bertagnoli et al. 2005; Blumenthal et al. 2005; Delamarter, Bae, and Pradhan 2005; Huang et al. 2005; Le Huec et al. 2005; Lemaire et al. 2005; McAfee et al. 2005; Tropiano et al. 2005]. Additional long-term benefits of disc replacement have yet to be proven in randomized clinical trials, but are predicted to include a reduced incidence of adjacent level degeneration.

The state of knowledge in total disc replacements is evolving rapidly. In this field, the majority of published papers are either clinical studies or review articles. A much smaller percentage of publications are dedicated to the science and technology of total disc arthroplasty for an engineering audience. In this chapter, we review the past and current technologies used clinically in total disc replacements. Several previous review articles have focused heavily on describing the patent art. No such treatment is provided here, because of the glaring discrepancy between the number of inventions and the mere handful of designs that have survived the gauntlet of pre-clinical testing, animal testing, and human clinical trials. Therefore, our goal is to critically examine the previous (and soon to be realized) published technologies behind total disc arthroplasty from a bioengineering perspective. This chapter begins with a summary of early total disc replacement designs and summarizes current cervical and lumbar disc replacements. The information in this chapter is intended to provide a bioengineer with the foundation to understand current designs as well as to develop new implants for the future.

11.2 Pioneers of Total Disc Arthroplasty

Total disc arthroplasty can trace its clinical history back to the early 1960s, when Fernström first implanted stainless steel spheres to replace the intervertebral disc [Fernström 1966]. From these modest beginnings, developments in total disc replacement technology have progressed at a slow but exponentially increasing pace. The plethora of patents described by Szpalski et al. [2002] attest to engineering creativity over the past 40 years [Szpalski, Gunzburg, and Mayer 2002]. However, only a small fraction of the innovations described in the body of patent literature has been validated by biomechanical and animal testing, and an even shorter list of implant designs have ever been used clinically in humans.

   In this section, we focus on three historical disc replacement designs that were evaluated in patients: Fernström spheres, the AcroFlex artificial disc, and the Charité artificial disc. Neither Fernström's spheres from the 1960s nor the AcroFlex artificial disc, which evolved starting in the 1980s, were ever widely adopted by clinicians. In contrast, a third historical design, the Charité artificial disc (which also evolved in the 1980s), continues in clinical use to this day. Whether clinically accepted or not, the *in vivo* performance of these pioneering disc arthroplasties provides important insight into the complex and demanding environment in which disc replacement technologies must function.

11.2.1 Metallic Spheres

Paul Harmon is considered to have first implanted metallic spheres in the spine, starting in 1957, to stabilize and augment anterior fusion procedures [McKenzie 1995]. Apparently these Vitallium implants were commercialized [Szpalski, Gunzburg, and Mayer 2002]. However, very limited primary data on the extent of these fusion procedures is available in the literature. Vitallium is the trade name for a cobalt chromium alloy, which was proprietary to Howmedica (today, Stryker Orthopedics, Mahwah, NJ).

   In the early 1960s, Dr. Ulf Fernström implanted stainless steel ball bearings in the cervical and lumbar spines of 250 patients [Szpalski, Gunzburg, and Mayer 2002], and the outcomes of a subset of these patients were reported with some detail in 1966 [Fernström 1966]. In contrast with Harmon's spheres, which were intended as interbody fusion devices, Fernström referred to his implants as "another type of arthroplasty." Fernström further distinguished his prosthesis from the injection of polymethyl methacrylate and silicone polymeric materials into the degenerated disc. Today, we would classify Fernström's prosthesis as the forerunner of modern total disc replacement, as opposed to the polymeric nuclear replacements, which were also being experimented with at the time. The reader is referred to Chapter 10 for an overview of disc augmentation and nucleus replacement technologies.

11.2.1.1 Design and Outcomes of Fernström's Prosthesis

Fernström describes his implant as "an oxygen-resistant and stainless steel ball, supplied by The Swedish Ball Bearing Factory (SKF)" [Fernström 1966]. The grade of stainless steel used in these implants is not recorded. An example of a retrieved Fernström prosthesis is shown in Figure 11.1. The implant diameters were 10 to 16 mm for the lumbar spine, and 6 to 10 mm for the cervical spine. Fernström sized the implants 1 mm larger than the disc space. Between 1962 and 1964, Fernström inserted 191 spheres into the lumbar spines of 125 patients, and 13 spheres into the cervical spines of eight patients. Figure 11.2 shows radiographs of a Fernström prosthesis implanted at L5-S1.

In 1966, Fernström provided clinical data on 105 patients with follow-up ranging between six months and 2.5 years [Fernström 1966]. He found the best results, in terms of pain relief, when the implant was installed after complete evacuation of the disc. In these cases, the incidence of pain relief was compa-

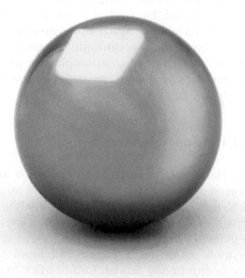

Fig. 11.1.
Photograph of a retrieved Fernström prosthesis.

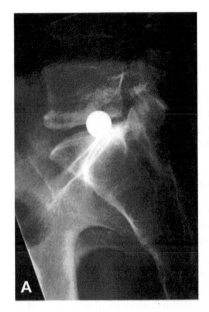
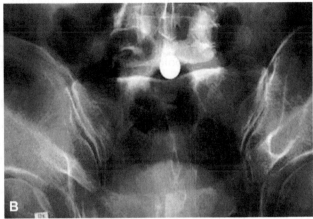

Fig. 11.2.
(A) Lateral and (B) anterior-posterior radiographs of a patient implanted with Fernström stainless steel interverte-bral arthroplasty, adapted from Szpalski et al. [2002]. Note the penetration of the ball into the superior end plate in A. *(Reproduced with kind permission of Springer Science and Business Media.)*

rable to fusion. The complication rates for the procedure were low. In one patient (0.7%), the sphere migrated posteriorly into the spinal canal. After three months the implant was removed and the segment was treated by fusion. In a second patient (0.7%), temporary paresis of the peroneus occurred. However, the clinical performance of the spheres was not entirely satisfactory. Radiographic examination, as well as examination upon retrieval of the devices, demonstrated subsidence into the end plates by 1 to 3mm (Figure 11.2).

Fernström's paper contains limited data regarding the performance of the implants themselves [Fernström 1966]. Retrieved implants from six patients reportedly showed "no signs of corrosion," but the methodology used for such an analysis was not provided. The tissues surrounding the implant also reportedly showed no evidence of a foreign body reaction, but again the methodology used for this assessment was not described.

No long-term results of Fernström's original series are available in the literature. However, some indication of the durability of the procedure is available from a cohort of patients who have been followed for up to 20 years [McKenzie 1995]. In 1969, Alvin McKenzie, a Canadian surgeon, visited Fernström's clinic in Sweden and learned Fernström's procedure [McKenzie 1995]. After returning to Canada, McKenzie performed disc arthroplasties in 103 patients using "acid-resistant coated steel balls ranging in size from 3/8 inch [9.5mm] to 3/4 inch [19mm] in diameter" [McKenzie 1995]. McKenzie states that "the steel ball itself has been shown to be innocuous when properly sized and properly placed in a suitably prepared intervertebral disc space." However, no further details about the implants themselves are reported in McKenzie's study.

Sixty-seven patients (65%) were followed by McKenzie for between 10 and 20 years (on average, 17 years). Excellent or good clinical results were reported in 75 to 83% of the 67 patients who were available for evaluation. Because no information is available on 35% of the patients who were lost to long-term follow-up, the generally positive results of McKenzie's long-term series must be interpreted with some caution. Nevertheless, McKenzie's study demonstrates the potential durability of Fernström's disc arthroplasty procedure.

11.2.1.2 Legacy of Fernström's Disc Arthroplasty

Recent historical reviews of disc arthroplasty have adopted a somewhat negative view of Fernström's prosthesis [Bono and Garfin 2004; Szpalski, Gunzburg, and Mayer 2002]. From a modern perspective, the subsidence of the spherical implants into the end plates is the greatest perceived drawback of Fernström's spherical implant design—and in and of itself limits its acceptance by surgeons today. According to the review by Bono and Garfin [2004], the intervertebral height was lost after four to seven years of implantation in about 88% of the cases due to subsidence [Bono and Garfin 2004]. In retrospect, it is hardly surprising for a bioengineer to conceive that the comparatively rigid spherical implant would act as a local stress concentration, thus producing local failure of the end plates and the underlying cancellous bone.

However, from a historical and implant design perspective Fernström was the first pioneer of disc arthroplasty. His work introduced the notion that a motion-preserving interbody prosthesis might possibly avoid undesirable complications of spine fusion procedures. Fernström's work also provides some evidence, albeit extremely limited, that metallic disc replacement components were biocompatible when implanted as bearing materials in the intervertebral disc space to articulate against the end plates. Ultimately, if not the implant design then certainly the motion preserving philosophy introduced by Fernström would inspire many other surgeons and inventors to develop alternate designs for disc arthroplasty.

11.2.2 The AcroFlex Artificial Disc

The AcroFlex artificial disc, developed starting in the 1970s by Arthur Steffee, M.D., represents a major evolutionary step in the conceptual design of total disc arthroplasties, especially when juxtaposed against the much simpler design of the Fernström sphere. The AcroFlex design basically consists of two porous coated metallic end plates fused to a hyperelastic polymer disc (Figure 11.3). In the AcroFlex design, the vertebral bone is intended to grow into the titanium end plates, providing long-term implant fixation, whereas the hyperelastic disc is intended to restore the flexibility and motion to the functional spinal unit [Steffee 1992]. Therefore, the AcroFlex design is an example of a non-sliding artificial disc.

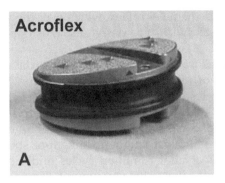
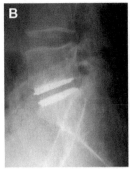
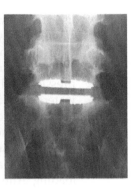

Fig. 11.3.
AcroFlex artificial disc. (A) Photograph of a third-generation AcroFlex; (B) anteroposterior and lateral radiographs of the third-generation AcroFlex implanted in the lumbosacral spine. *(Reproduced from Fraser et al. [2004] with permission from Elsevier.)*

Over time, there have been three generations of the design. All of these implant variations survived the standard mechanical testing protocols of their day, only to exhibit short-term failure modes in four series of limited human clinical trials [Fraser et al. 2004; Steffee 1992]. At each iteration of the design, failure of the AcroFlex was related to the mechanical performance of the hyperelastic polymer disc material. As a result, the AcroFlex was never widely used clinically, but details about the design and the clinical studies have been published in the scientific literature, so that the spine community can benefit from understanding the AcroFlex experience [Fraser et al. 2004]. Consequently, it is highly instructive to review the development of the AcroFlex, as it provides an example of a measured, responsible strategy for evaluating new spine technologies and sharing the results with the spine implant community.

11.2.2.1 Early Beginnings and the First-generation AcroFlex Design

Starting in 1976, Steffee's earliest artificial disc design, developed in collaboration with Thomas Hoogland, M.D., involved cemented components fabricated from CoCr alloy and "high density" polyethylene, which were to be implanted via an anterior approach [Steffee 1992]. This experimental design was mechanically tested in cadaveric spines and the results were published in 1978 at the Orthopedic Research Society Meeting [Hoogland et al. 1978]. However, concerns about bone-cement interface precluded human clinical trials, and the development of a cemented artificial disc design was subsequently abandoned.

The first cementless design evolved in the 1980s, using Ti end plates with two layers of sintered 250-μm-diameter beads for long-term fixation [Steffee 1992]. In this iteration of the design, each end plate also had four prominent tapered pegs for short-term fixation. The synthetic disc was fabricated from Hexsyn, which was a polyolefin rubber developed by Goodyear for fatigue-resistant biomedical applications such as artificial heart components [McMillin 1987; Steffee 1992]. Hexsyn was licensed to AcroMed Corporation (Akron, OH) for use in spine applications under the trade name AcroFlex, which over the years came to be synonymous with rubber sandwich-type design itself, as opposed to just the polymeric biomaterial.

In accordance with recommendations from the FDA at the time, axial compression and 45-degree shear testing of implants was performed in a 37°C water bath [Steffee 1992]. Discs were tested in each loading mode. Fatigue testing was conducted with a load of 100 lbs. (448 N) and 2 Hz. Tests of this type are now standardized for total disc replacements, as discussed in Chapter 13. The device survived 11.5 million cycles in axial fatigue loading, but showed evidence of a small nonpropagating tear after 4 million cycles under shear loading. After 11.5 million cycles, a small anterior hole was found. Despite evidence of local material failure, these tests were judged to be successful at the time [Steffee 1992].

At this early stage, animal testing of the AcroFlex design was not conducted. According to Steffee, they made "many futile attempts" to obtain permission to implant these artificial discs in kangaroos [Steffee 1992]. By 1992, animal testing had yet to be performed. Based on the *in vitro* testing results, which included biocompatibility of the implant materials, the decision was made to proceed to human clinical trials. Steffee later wrote that "there was some concern about implanting the prosthesis in a patient without the benefit of scientific data from animal studies. After further discussion with the patient, it was decided that the patient's need far outweighed the value of additional information to be gleaned from such studies" [Steffee 1992].

The first-generation AcroFlex device was implanted in six patients between October of 1988 and August of 1989 [Steffee 1992]. In four of these patients, the disc was implanted in patients with previous fusions above the existing fusion level. However, in 1990 the FDA withdrew approval for the use of Hexsyn as an implant material, due to concern about the potential carcinogenicity of 2-mercaptobenzothiazole, a compound used in the vulcanization process [Steffee 1992]. Further enrollment in the AcroFlex clinical trial was suspended.

After three years of follow-up, the outcome was good, excellent, or fair in 4/6 patients (66%) but poor in two patients (33%) [Enker et al. 1993]. In one case, involving a patient with multilevel fusions, the disc failed after one year of implantation, requiring removal. The failure mode was fracture of the rubber core, and appeared to originate where two pieces of the implant had been vulcanized together. Interestingly, the end plates were osseointegrated and required an osteotomy for removal. In a second case with a poor result, involving a patient with no prior surgery, the patient obtained no relief of pain from the procedure for reasons that were not clear, despite "satisfactory radiographic appearance."

11.2.2.2 Second-generation AcroFlex Design

In a second-generation design, the Hexsyn material was replaced with a silicone elastomer, and a clinical trial in eight patients was conducted between 1993 and 1994. Little information about this design iteration, or its clinical results, is available in the literature. Fraser reports that "one mechanical failure of the artificial disc occurred 6 months later in a patient with a prior fusion at an adjacent level" [Fraser et al. 2004]. However, silicone elastomers were a highly controversial choice for biomaterial in the 1990s due to the use of this polymer, both as a rubber and as a gel in breast implants. In light of the class action litigation against silicone implant manufacturers, such as Dow Corning in the mid 1990s, it is hardly surprising that the outcomes of the silicone AcroFlex were not widely published at the time.

11.2.2.3 Third-generation AcroFlex Designs

Details of the third-generation AcroFlex designs, which evolved in the late 1990s, were published by Fraser et al. [2004]. This design used, once again, a hexene-based polyolefin rubber core. However, the geometry of the end plates was reshaped, to include a lower overall profile to reduce the amount of overdistraction necessary for implantation, as well as to optimize bone ingrowth. Specifically, the redesigned end plates were machined from Ti alloy (Ti-6 Al-4 V ELI alloy), but the porous coated beads were commercially pure Ti [Fraser et al. 2004].

Static and dynamic axial compression and compressive shear tests were conducted of the third-generation AcroFlex by the manufacturer in accordance with draft ASTM standards [Serhan 2005]. The manufacturer considered that 3,400 N was the maximum load to be likely subjected to the implant. Testing demonstrated that the AcroFlex did not "catastrophically fail or significantly permanently deform" under these conditions [Serhan 2005]. Testing at higher loads (up to 7,000 N) demonstrated that the device was stronger than the underlying vertebral bodies. The manufacturer also conducted dynamic compression testing between the physiologic loads of 700 N (average daily living load) and 3,400 N (worst-case activity of bending while lifting a 20-kg weight with the back bent and knees straight) [Serhan 2005]. Disc height measurements indicated that less than 0.5% permanent deformation would be expected under compression fatigue loading conditions. Static compressive shear testing was also carried out by the manufacturer, and verified that the maximum shear strength of the AcroFlex Disc exceeded 351 to 653 N [Serhan 2005]. Because there were no articulating surfaces, wear debris testing was not performed [Serhan 2005].

Animal studies were conducted using the third-generation AcroFlex with 20 baboons. The goal of these studies was to evaluate segmental motion and the extent of bony ingrowth into the porous coating after 6 and 12 months of implantation [Cunningham et al. 2002]. In one baboon, failure of the core occurred after 12 months, and was attributed to insufficient curing of the polymer. In that animal, there was evidence of black wear particles and a localized histocytic foreign body reaction. However, there was no evidence of an inflammatory response around the end plates of the other baboons. Overall, there was strong evidence of osteointegration into the porous coating after 6 months, which remained unchanged after 12 months.

Two pilot human clinical studies were conducted using the third-generation AcroFlex, with subtle differences in end plate design [Fraser et al. 2004]. In the first pilot study—conducted with 11 patients in Adelaide, Australia, between 1998 and 1999—the end plates were relatively flat and there was a single ridge for short-term fixation. In a second pilot study, also conducted in Adelaide, with 17 patients between February and December of 2000, the end plates were slightly domed to encourage the apposition to the concave end plates, and four to six small fins were included for short-term fixation.

In the pilot human clinical trials, there were 16 complications in the 28 patients involved in the two studies mentioned previously [Fraser et al. 2004]. Patients in both pilot studies were found to have evidence of tears or failure of the polyolefin cores on CT imaging studies. Ultimately, 8/28 patients required revision surgery. One patient was revised after one year, and the remaining seven patients were revised between two to four years of implantation. The one-year revision was due to severe pain. Upon removal of the implant, it was found not to have osseointegrated. Three patients had extensive anterior disruptions of rubber or anterior tears, as well as a local granulomatous reaction to the particulate rubber debris. In two of the three patients, there was evidence of osteolysis and loosening at the bone-implant interface. In four patients with rubber tears, posterior fusions were performed for stabilization. Fraser reported that it was the intention of the investigators to initiate a prospective randomized trial of the AcroFlex following the completion of the two pilot studies [Fraser et al. 2004]. However, such a trial was not initiated, for reasons that were not illuminated in Fraser's paper.

11.2.2.4 Legacy of the AcroFlex Artificial Disc

Consequently, after nearly three decades of development the AcroFlex design did not reach fruition. The concept of a one-piece nonarticulating artificial disc replacement is attractive, as it would mimic the structure and function of the natural disc. However, neither the AcroFlex design nor any other design based on this premise has yet proven to be successful for the demanding loading environment of the lumbar spine. As we shall see, the current state-of-the-art disc replacement technologies achieve motion by articulating surfaces, by borrowing bearing concepts from hip and knee arthroplasty. Indeed, if we consider the successful aspects of the AcroFlex design—namely, the achievement of rapid osseointegration of the end plates—these were attributed to porous coating technology, which was already widely used in the 1980s for metal-backed hip replacements. Therefore, the first lesson of the AcroFlex is to incorporate historically successful fixation techniques whenever possible into a new implant design.

The second lesson from the AcroFlex would be to avoid employing novel, unproven biomaterials in a prosthesis design for long-term implantation, if a historically proven biomaterial can be employed instead. This lesson may be unglamorous, and it flies in the face of what a pioneering design is hoped to accomplish. However, bioengineers who ignore this lesson do so at their own peril. The AcroFlex clearly illustrates the risks associated with introducing a new biomaterial into a harsh, long-term loading environment that is not yet fully understood or well characterized. Fraser suggested that the standard mechanical test protocols did not incorporate coupled multiaxial motion, only uniaxial compression or shear [Fraser et al. 2004]. Perhaps the ultimate failure of the AcroFlex design may be attributed, more specifically, to the inability of bioengineers and implant designers of the day to identify a suitable polymeric biomaterial that could survive the multiaxial loading conditions of the lumbar spine. Ultimately, the AcroFlex is the story of an artificial disc design in search of a more durable biomaterial. Ironically, the design that would surpass the elegant philosophy of the AcroFlex to become the successful paradigm of modern total disc arthroplasty was not inspired by the structure of the natural disc, but by the principles of total hip replacement, established during the 1960s.

11.2.3 The Charité Artificial Disc

The history of the Charité differs dramatically from the AcroFlex, in that the designers sought to replicate the kinematics, but not the structure, of a vertebral disc. The Charité design, formally known as the SB Charité artificial disc by its inventors, basically consists of two metallic end plates fixed to the adjacent vertebral bodies, which articulate against a central core fabricated from ultrahigh molecular weight polyethylene (UHMWPE) (Figure 11.4). This artificial disc was invented by Kurt Shellnack, M.D., and Karin Büttner-Janz, M.D., Ph.D., who were at the time affiliated with the Charité Center for Musculoskeletal Surgery at the Medical University of Berlin (Universitätsmedizin Berlin, *http://www.charite.de*) [Büttner-Janz 2003].

In the Charité design, the polyethylene core has two domed (convex) surfaces, which articulate against the concave metallic end plates. In full flexion or extension, the core is (theoretically) free to translate and rotate, so that the polyethylene rim contacts the metallic rims of the end plates (Figure 11.5). This artificial disc is implanted by an anterior approach. An excellent summary of the design can be found in a recent monograph [Büttner-Janz, Hochschuler, and McAfee 2003].

The Charité has gone through four distinct phases in its design history. In this part of the chapter we review the details about the major phases of its design, and explain how the Charité helped to launch the field of modern total disc arthroplasty. In addition to the historical significance of this design, we also highlight some of the controversies surrounding its continued use today.

11.2.3.1 SB Charité I and II

The first two iterations of the design (i.e., the SB Charité I and II) occurred between 1984 and 1985 at the Charité hospital. In this phase of its history, the implants were not commercially available, and were implanted in a total of 49 patients [Büttner-Janz 2003]. The smooth end plates were fashioned from non-forged stainless steel, and only fixed to the vertebral end plates by a number of protruding teeth. A circumferential radiographic wire marker was also

Charité Disc Prototypes

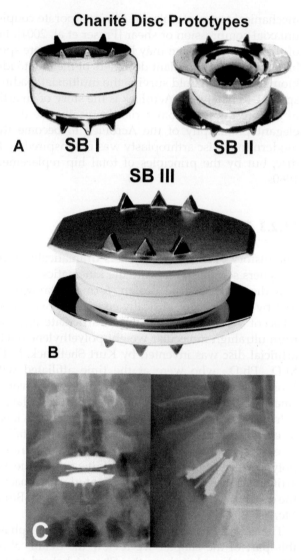

A   SB I   **SB II**

SB III

B

C

Fig. 11.4.
Charité artificial disc. (A) Photograph of the SB I and SB II Charité; (B) photograph of the SB III Charité with uncoated end plates; (C) anteroposterior and lateral radiographs of the SB III Charité implanted in the lumbosacral spine. *(Reproduced with permission from DePuy Spine, Rayhnam, MA.)*

included in the polyethylene core. In the SB I design, the end plates were circular and shaped like bottle caps. In the SB II design, the end plates were expanded with lateral wings to provide more coverage of the vertebral end plates (Figure 11.4a).

The Charité's designers adopted the "low-friction principle" of polymer-on-metal articulation, employed by Sir John Charnley when creating the first

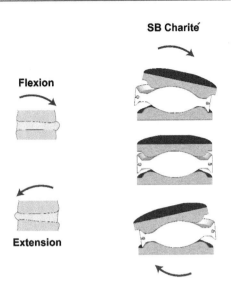

Fig. 11.5.

Kinematics of the Charité artificial disc. The metallic end plates are designed to contact the rim of the UHMWPE core in flexion and extension. In neutral alignment, load is transferred through the central domed portion of UHMWPE core.

successful hip replacement design [Charnley 1979]. Starting in the 1960s, Charnley's hip design evolved to become the dominant joint replacement technology in orthopedics during the 1970s, due largely to the outstanding frictional and fatigue properties of the polymeric bearing material, UHMWPE. In the 1980s (and still today), articulations with UHMWPE are the standard of care for degenerative joint disease [Kurtz 2004]. Specifically, the UHMWPE was CHIRULEN (Ticona), which is a trade name referring to a compression molded GUR 412 resin. The UHMWPE sheets were fabricated in Oberhausen, Germany. All of the implants were gamma sterilized in air. The complete details of UHMWPE materials of that era have been published [Kurtz 2004].

Only retrospective clinical data are available regarding the SB Charité I and II designs [Büttner-Janz, Hochschuler, and McAfee 2003; Putzier et al. 2005]. McAfee evaluated the early "suboptimal" results of the type I and II designs, which he attributed to suboptimal surgical technique (e.g., undersizing, malpositioning) rather than to deficiencies in the design [McAfee 2003]. Most recently, investigators from the Charité hospital have reviewed the performance of 15 patients with the type I design and 22 patients with the type II design after an average follow-up of 18.2 and 17.5 years for the two groups, respectively [Putzier et al. 2005] (Table 11.1). Fair to excellent results were found in 87% of patients with type I implants and in 68% of patients with SB II implants. The higher incidence of poorer results with the type II was due to stainless steel end plate fractures, which occurred in 7/22 patients. No end plate fractures were reported by the authors in the SB I design. Other long-term complications included subsidence, dislocation, and persisting pain (Table 11.1). Interestingly,

Table 11.1.

Long-term clinical performance of the SB Charité (I, II, and III), adapted from Putzier et al. [2005]. No significant difference in long-term clinical performance was noted between the three Charité designs.

Charité Design Type	Treatment Period (Year)	Average Follow-up (Years)	Number of Patients	Number of TDRs Implanted	Average Age	Fair to Excellent Patient Outcome (%)	Segmental Fusion for Subsidence	Segmental Fusion for Dislocation	Segmental Fusion for Persisting Pain	Arthrodesis or Spontaneous Fusion
SB I	1984–1985	18.2	15	16	44	13/15 (87%)	2/15	0/15	1/15	12/15 (80%)
SB II	1985–1987	17.5	22	25	45	15/22 (68%)	1/22	0/22	0/22	11/22 (50%)
SB III	1987–1989	16.1	16	22	43	12/16 (75%)	0/16	1/16	0/16	9/16 (56%)
Total	1984–1989		53	63		40/53 (75%)	3/53	1/53	1/53	32/53 (60%)

Putzier et al. reported that heterotopic ossification, leading to spontaneous fusion of the treated level, occurred in 12/15 (80%) of type I patients and 11/22 (50%) of type II patients [Putzier et al. 2005].

Static and dynamic biomechanical testing of the early (SB Charité I and II) designs was conducted by the inventors [Büttner-Janz, Schellnack, and Zippel 1989]. The devices were statically loaded in servohydraulic test frames for two to five cycles at loads ranging from 4.2 to 10.5 kN, at which point the height of the UHMWPE core was reduced by 10%. The artificial disc components were tested in a fixture intended to rock the prosthesis by ±10 degrees at 5 to 10 Hz under a compressive load. The loading ranged between 0.7 and 8.0 kN with intermediate load steps of unspecified duration and magnitude. The component was rocked for 20 million cycles, which they considered to be equivalent to 20 years of use. The authors report only "slight track marks" as a result of the fatigue testing.

The inventors further reported that "no macroscopic wear was found, and little would be expected because of the relatively slight movement of the intervertebral segments." [Büttner-Janz, Schellnack, and Zippel 1989]. Similar sentiments regarding the improbability of wear and surface damage are also reflected in the (much later) monograph [Büttner-Janz, Hochschuler, and McAfee 2003]. In retrospect, the lack of wear damage is consistent with the unidirectionality of the wear testing (flexion-extension rocking), which we know today produces orders of magnitude less wear debris in UHMWPE than multidirectional motion [Wang et al. 1998]. As we shall see, the inventors' *in vitro* observations have not been borne out by recent retrieval studies [Kurtz et al. 2005].

The inventors also conducted cadaver testing in 13 lumbar segments to evaluate subsidence and migration [Büttner-Janz, Schellnack, and Zippel 1989]. The donors' ages ranged between 27 and 62 years. Subsidence of the implants was observed at peak loads of 4.5 to 8.5 kN for the SB Charité I and between 10.7 and 11.6 kN for the SB Charité II. The publication provides no details about the bone quality of the lumbar segment donors, nor are details provided about the sizing and alignment of components during testing.

11.2.3.2 SB Charité III

The Charité artificial disc was commercialized by Waldemar Link GmbH & Co in 1987, resulting in the SB Charité III (i.e., third iteration design) [Büttner-Janz, Hochschuler, and McAfee 2003]. As an orthopedic implant manufacturer, Waldemar Link made major changes in the design of the metallic end plates, including changing the material from stainless steel to CoCr alloy. Specifically, Link employed a proprietary CoCr alloy, VACUCAST (0.20 to 0.25% C, 28.0 to 30.0% Cr, 5.5 to 6.5% Mo, max. 0.5% Ni, max. 0.5% Fe, 0.4 to 1.0% Si, 0.4 to 1.0% Mn, with the remainder 57.1 to 69% Co) [Link and Keller 2003]. The backside of the CoCr was "satin finished" by corundum blasting, and fixation was achieved with six sharp teeth [Link and Keller 2003]. Since the redesign of the end plates by Link, there have been no further reports of component fractures [Büttner-Janz, Hochschuler, and McAfee 2003; Putzier et al.

2005]. The geometry and properties of the UHMWPE core remained essentially unchanged by Link at that time. Unlike previous iterations of the design, which were only used at the inventors' institution, this version was launched internationally beginning with France and the Netherlands in 1989 and the United Kingdom in 1990.

The clinical performance of the Charité has been documented in a number of published studies, the majority of which pertain to the type III design (Table 11.2). Taken together, these studies demonstrate that in at least some patients the Charité TDR has the potential to preserve motion, result in good to excellent clinical outcomes, and survive long-term implantation in the human body. However, these largely retrospective cohort studies also demonstrate broad variations in their complication rates and clinical success rates, raising concerns about the repeatability and reproducibility of the procedure. The largest and most comprehensive body of clinical data about the Charité was collected for the prospective, randomized trial undertaken for the FDA's IDE study in the United States (Table 11.2). However, as shall be discussed in a subsequent section, both the retrospective studies as well as the randomized IDE study have generated considerable controversy due to questions about the risks and effectiveness of the Charité relative to instrumented fusions.

Link sponsored a number of promotional studies of the Charité, intended primarily for the FDA [Link 2002; Link and Keller 2003]. Static, dynamic, and wear testing of the UHMWPE core were conducted. Mechanical testing of the CoCr alloy end plates was not performed, because according to Link, mechanical failure had not been clinically reported. Static testing of the UHMWPE was conducted to a maximum load of 4.5 kN based on requirements of the FDA to obtain pre-market approval. The compressive testing was performed statically and dynamically at rates of 0.001 to 0.5 Hz at 37°C in Ringers' solution. At least five specimens from two different sizes (7.5 and 9.5 mm, size 2 cores) were tested. It was estimated based on the tests that 0.4 to 0.7 mm of permanent deformation would be expected after 10 years of implantation. Link concluded that "cold flow is not a major factor with the SB Charité III prosthesis" [Link and Keller 2003].

Promotional wear testing of an unspecified number of size 2, 9.5-mm cores was conducted using a single-station tester [Link and Keller 2003]. Sinusoidal loading was applied at 1 Hz with a range of 0.5 to 2.5 kN for 10 million cycles in 25% bovine serum, diluted with deionized water, at 37°C. The ranges of motion were +4°/−2° in flexion-extension, ±1° in axial rotation, and ±2° in lateral bending. No abrasive wear was found on either the UHMWPE or CoCr end plates under these conditions. Link concluded optimistically that "the implants exhibited very favorable tribologic properties" [Link and Keller 2003].

Subsequent testing by Serhan et al. [2005] was performed for 10 million cycles, at loads ranging between 0.9 and 1.85 kN. This testing used slightly different kinematics based on the existing draft ASTM disc wear standard at the time, rather than what had been previously used by Link. Two duty cycles were investigated: the first involved ±7.5° in flexion-extension with ±1.5° in axial rotation; the second involved ±7.5° in lateral bending with ±1.5° in axial rotation. The testing was performed in bovine serum at 37°C. In contrast with Link,

Table 11.2.

Clinical details of primary peer-reviewed studies involving the SB Charité (I, II, and III), adapted and expanded from de Kleuver, Oner, and Jacobs [2003].

	Büttner-Janz et al. (Büttner-Janz et al. 1988)	Wittig et al. (Wittig, Muller, and Staudte 1989)	David (David 1993)	Griffith et al. (Griffith et al. 1994)	Cinotti et al. (Cinotti, David, and Postacchini 1996)	Zeegers et al. (Zeegers et al. 1999)	Sott and Harrison (Sott and Harrison 2000)	Lemaire et al. (Lemaire et al. 2005)	Putzier et al. (Putzier et al. 2005)	FDA IDE Study (Blumenthal et al. 2005; McAfee et al. 2005)
Study type	Hcoh	Hcoh	Hcoh	Hcoh	Hcoh	Pcoh	Hcoh	Hcoh	Hcoh	RCT
Type of prosthesis	SB I, II, III	SB III	SB III	SB I, II, III	SB III	SB III	SB III	SB III	SB I, II, III	SB III
Average age	43		37	43	36	43	48	40	44	40
Age range	26–59	30–54	27–50	25–59	27–44	24–59	31–61	24–51	30–59	19–60
No. of patients	62	13	22	93	46	50	14	100	53	205
No. of arthroplasties	76	14	29	139	56	75	15	147	63	205
Follow-up in months	15	9	19	11.9	38	24	48	136	208	24
Range in follow-up	?–36	3–18	12–37	1–37	24–60		18–68	120–161	174–230	
Good or excellent	81%	NA	15/22	?	63%	70%	10/14	90%	75%	57.1%**

Continued

Table 11.2. *Continued*

	Büttner-Janz et al. (Büttner-Janz et al. 1988)	Wittig et al. (Wittig, Muller, and Staudte 1989)	David (David 1993)	Griffith et al. (Griffith et al. 1994)	Cinotti et al. (Cinotti, David, and Postacchini 1996)	Zeegers et al. (Zeegers et al. 1999)	Sott and Harrison (Sott and Harrison 2000)	Lemaire et al. (Lemaire et al. 2005)	Putzier et al. (Putzier et al. 2005)	FDA IDE Study (Blumenthal et al. 2005; McAfee et al. 2005)
Secondary surgery		6/13				17/50	1/14	5/100	12/53	11/205
Arthrodesis or spontaneous fusion		2/15	3/30					2/100	32/53	2/205
Complications	29/76	1?	1?	55/139	8/46	3/50	2/15	21/100	44/53	68/205
Motion on flexion-extension radiographs in degrees (range)										
Average	5	—	7.1*	?	12.2	9 (2–17)	?	10.3 (0–16)	?	7.1 (6.6–7.7)
L3/L4			2		—			12.0 (10–16)		
L4/L5			9.4		16			9.6 (0–15)		
L5/S1			6.4		9			9.2 (0–14)		

Hcoh (historical cohort study); Pcoh (prospective cohort study); RCT (randomized controlled trial).

*Average mobility was calculated from the reported data (de Kleuver, Oner, and Jacobs 2003).

**Overall clinical success was defined as patients having ≥25% improvement in ODI score at 24 months compared with the preoperative score, no device failure, no major complications, and no neurological deterioration [Blumenthal et al. 2005].

who found no measurable wear, Serhan et al. measured 0.11 mg of wear per million cycles. The median wear particle diameter was 0.2 microns, and they ranged between 0.08 and 16.3 microns. Serhan et al. concluded that "the long history of the Charité disc indicates that wear debris is clinically irrelevant" [Serhan et al. 2005].

However, the extremely low magnitudes of wear produced by these simulators should be interpreted with some caution. Hip and knee simulator studies have demonstrated that the wear rate of UHMWPE is sensitive to the lubrication conditions, as well as the extent of cross-shear motion at the articulating surfaces [Wang et al. 1998]. In particular, curvilinear motion can produce orders of magnitude less wear rates for UHMWPE, as compared with cross-shear motion [Wang et al. 1998]. Wear testing methods for total disc have only recently been standardized. For example, the ASTM Standard Test Guide for the Functional, Kinematic, and Wear Assessment of Total Disc Prostheses has only recently been approved (as of November of 2005), and no standard number is available as of yet. From a scientific perspective, until the spine simulators can be shown to produce comparable clinically relevant wear mechanisms and wear rates, the early promotional wear studies performed by Link must be viewed as unvalidated and irrelevant.

Thus far, only isolated case studies of retrieved Charité prostheses have been published in the peer-reviewed scientific literature [David 2005; Kurtz et al. 2005]. More recently, observations of wear from a large collection of clinical retrievals have also been reported at national conferences [Kurtz et al. 2005]. In an ongoing study, Kurtz et al. have analyzed 16 Charité retrievals from 14 patients undergoing TDR revision surgery after 2.9 to 16.0 years of implantation [Kurtz et al. 2005]. Revisions were performed between 2003 and 2005 due to intractable pain and facet degeneration (in all cases). The following complications were noted: subsidence (n = 6), anterior migration (n = 3), lateral subluxation (n = 1), wear with wire marker fracture (n = 1), end plate loosening (n = 2), and osteolysis (n = 1). The retrieved implants showed evidence of adhesive/abrasive wear mechanisms in the central domed region of the implants. In addition, there was also evidence of macroscopic rim damage, including radial cracking, plastic deformation, and third-body damage. The retrieved TDRs displayed surface damage observed previously in both hip and knee replacements. The results from large retrieval analyses will be useful for further development of the *in vitro* test methods that will be utilized to evaluate total disc replacements in the pre-clinical stage.

11.2.3.3 Recent Generations of the Charité Artificial Disc

There have been a number of changes in the Charité made by Link, in the late 1990s, and more recently by DePuy Spine in 2004. All of these changes have been made on a rolling basis, and it is therefore difficult to appreciate at the present time what effect these will have on the long-term clinical performance.

For example, in 1997 Link changed its packaging of the UHMWPE core, which was initially air permeable ("gamma air"), to two polymeric pouches in a nitrogen/vacuum process (N-VAC) (Figure 11.6) [Serhan 2005]. The

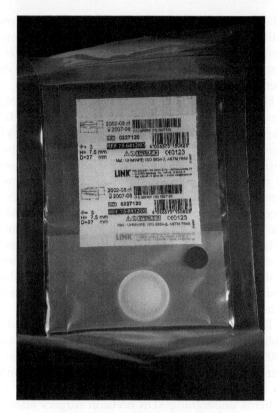

Fig. 11.6.
First-generation polymeric barrier packaging of the Charité UHMWPE core by Link, employed between 1998 and 2004.

UHMWPE material used in the cores was changed to compression molded GUR 1020, converted by Poly Hi Solidur (Fort Wayne, IN). At the FDA Panel meeting in 2004, it was revealed that the polymeric packaging was also air permeable, resulting in measurable oxidation of the UHMWPE during shelf storage [Currier 2004]. Therefore, it is currently unknown what benefit, if any, was achieved by this packaging change. All of the UHMWPE cores used in the U.S. IDE trial were sterilized in N-VAC packaging.

Link completed the fourth major design change to the Charité in 1998 with the introduction of textured, coated end plates [Link and Keller 2003]. The end plates are coated in a three-step process. In the first step, the CoCr alloy is coated with a thin layer of commercially pure (CP) Ti. In the second step, a plasma spray of CP Ti is applied to the initial bond coat, achieving a textured surface with surface features ranging between 75 and 300 μm for bone ongrowth. In the third step, the textured Ti surface is coated with calcium phosphate (CaP) in an electrochemical process (Figure 11.7). These end plates have been shown in primate studies to provide excellent bone ongrowth [Cunningham et al. 2003], thereby providing resistance for implant migration.

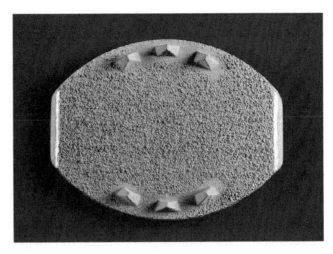

Fig. 11.7.
Textured CaP-Ti coated end plates (of the Charité), produced by Link starting in 1997.

However, they are currently unavailable for use in the United States (as of January of 2006) because textured end plates were not included in the clinical trial that was approved by the FDA.

The current manufacturer of the Charité (DePuy Spine, Raynhnam, MA) has made few changes to Link's design for the SB Charité III. Most notably, DePuy Spine has changed the packaging of the UHMWPE to a foil pouch (GVF). This most recent packaging change was initially implemented in April of 2004 and launched worldwide in October of 2004 [Serhan 2005]. Traceable retrieval studies will be necessary to establish the natural history of Charité polyethylene components stored within first-generation (N-VAC) and second-generation (GVF) barrier packaging.

In addition, coated end plates are expected to be clinically introduced for the Charité in the United States during 2006 (they continue to be available in Europe since 1998). Because of the strong scientific data [Cunningham 2004] supporting the advantages of coated end plate technology, both for the Charité and for previous artificial disc designs such as the AcroFlex, the use of smooth end plates will be most likely be discontinued in the future.

11.2.3.4 Bioengineering Studies of the Charité

Although most of the literature about the Charité is related to clinical outcomes, there are an increasing number of studies related to the bioengineering aspects of total disc replacement that have been published recently [Cunningham 2004; Cunningham et al. 2003; David 2005; Kurtz et al. 2005; O'Leary et al. 2005]. Among these, the work of Cunningham is perhaps the best known, as the data was made available to the FDA during the IDE study and has been published in the peer-reviewed scientific literature [Cunningham 2004; Cunningham et al. 2003]. Cunningham's research, therefore, is highly instructive as to the scope and quality of biomechanical testing that are needed to address questions by regulatory bodies, such as the FDA, for the evaluation of total disc replacement technologies. More recently, O'Leary et al. have also published biomechanical data, collected with *in vitro* cadaveric models, that characterize the motion patterns for the Charité [O'Leary et al. 2005]. In addition to *in vitro* biomechanical and animal studies, retrieval analyses of the Charité have started to appear in the literature [David 2005; Kurtz et al. 2005], as noted previously. For the remainder of this section, we focus on the test methods employed by Cunningham's group and O'Leary et al. in their evaluations of the Charité.

Cunningham's work has been summarized in a recent review article [Cunningham 2004], and includes both *in vitro* cadaveric spine testing and animal studies. Cunningham's research analyzes the biomechanics, osseointegration, and biocompatibility of wear debris for the Charité. For the *in vitro* biomechanical studies, Cunningham studied control (untreated) lumbar spines, as well as lumbar spines implanted with the Charité artificial disc as compared to the BAK cage and the AcroFlex artificial disc [Cunningham 2004; Cunningham et al. 2003]. The lumbar spines were tested with the application of pure moments [±8 Nm] in flexion-extension, lateral bending, and axial rotation. It is noteworthy that Cunningham's tests did not include axial preload, and thus quantify the maximum theoretical flexibility of an unloaded spine. Motion was characterized using an OptoTrak 3020 motion system (Northern Digital, Inc., Waterloo, Canada) as well as lateral plain radiographs. Under the applied moments, the Charité exhibited significantly greater axial rotation, but less lateral bending compared to the intact spine (Figure 11.8). In absolute terms, the average axial rotation of the intact spine was measured to be 2.4 degrees as opposed to 3.9 degrees after treatment with the Charité (Figure 11.8) [Cunningham et al. 2003]. There was no significant difference between the intact spine and the Charité in flexion/extension (Figure 11.8). Interestingly, the AcroFlex provided significantly less motion than the Charité and the intact spine in both flexion/extension and lateral bending (Figure 11.8).

Osseointegration of the coated end plates was evaluated in a baboon study (n = 27) with six months of follow-up [Cunningham 2004]. No radiolucencies were noted around the end plates using radiographs. Microradiographs of sections through the implants were used to evaluate bone apposition to the implant (Figure 11.9). Because the Ti/CaP coating of the Charité end plates does not contain subsurface pores that are connected with the surface, adjacent bone growth is more appropriately characterized as "ongrowth," as opposed to "ingrowth," which typically occurs with implant coatings that have subsurface porosity that is accessible for bone growth from the surface. The extent of ongrowth with the coated end plates was 48% ± 9% [Cunningham 2004]. Histochemical assays were used to look for local or systemic reactions to wear debris, but no evidence of such reactions was found. Although Cunningham's paper provides a bioengineering foundation for the use of coated end plate technology with the Charité, no data are provided about biological response to uncoated end plates, which are currently used clinically in the United States.

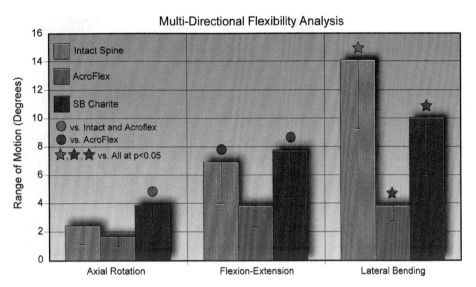

Fig. 11.8.
Summary of *in vitro* biomechanical range of motion tests for the Charité artificial disc, AcroFlex artificial disc, and the intact lumbar spine. All were tested with ±8 Nm of pure moments, but no axial preload, as reported by Cunningham [2004].

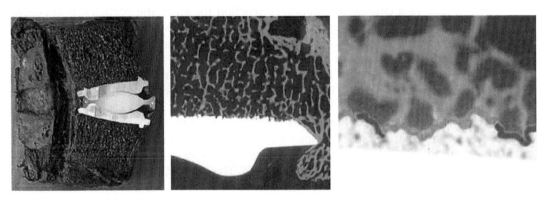

Fig. 11.9.
Sectioning technique and microradiographs used to evaluate bone ongrowth for coated textured Charité end plates by Cunningham [2004]. *(Reproduced with permission from Lippincott, Williams & Wilkins.)*

Neural tissue response to wear debris was evaluated by applying 4 mg of particles onto the epidura of New Zealand white rabbits (n = 50, total). Five groups of rabbits were tested (n = 10, each): (1) sham operation (control), (2) stainless steel 316LVM, (3) titanium alloy (Ti-6Al-4V), (4) CoCr alloy, and (5) UHMWPE. The particle sizes ranged between 0.5 and 10 microns in diameter, and were verified to be endotoxin free prior to implantation. Animals were

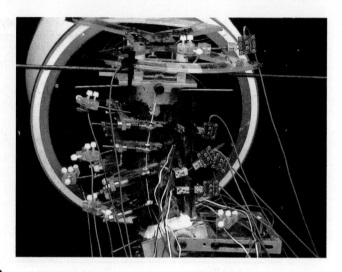

Fig. 11.10.

In vitro biomechanical testing apparatus of the lumbar spine, incorporating a follower preload for evaluation of motion patterns in total disc replacement. *(Reproduced from O'Leary et al. [2005] with permission from Elsevier.)*

sacrificed at three and six months postoperatively. Even though there was evidence of a chronic inflammatory reaction for all of the particles, it appeared localized within the epidural tissue. CoCr particles, in particular, were shown to diffuse from the epidural layers into the cerebrospinal fluid, and into spinal cord itself. Although this study provides some insight into the biological response following a massive particle load delivered directly to the epidural layer of the cord, the likelihood of this scenario occurring in the clinical situation is not clear.

O'Leary et al. [O'Leary et al. 2005] have recently studied the motion patterns of the Charité using an elegant *in vitro* biomechanical testing system that can simultaneously apply pure moments (up to 8 Nm in flexion and 6 Nm in extension) along with a 400-N axial preload. The preload is also referred to as a "follower load," because the orientation of the force is such that by means of cables it follows the curvature of the spine during flexion-extension testing (Figure 11.10). Motion was characterized using an OptoTrak 3020 motion system (Northern Digital, Inc., Waterloo, Canada) and bi-axial motion sensors. Motion of the UHMWPE core was tracked during flexion-extension using digital video fluoroscopy. Five lumbar spines were used in the testing from patients ranging in age from 39 to 60. Four distinct motion patterns were observed for the UHMWPE core when tested under compressive preload. With motion pattern 1, relative angular motion occurred predominantly between the superior end plate and the core, with little or no core translation (Figure 11.11a). In motion pattern 2, lift-off occurred by either the superior end plate from the core, or by the core from the inferior end plate (Figure 11.11b). In motion pattern 3, the UHMWPE core "locked" in plane, resulting in entrapment over a portion of

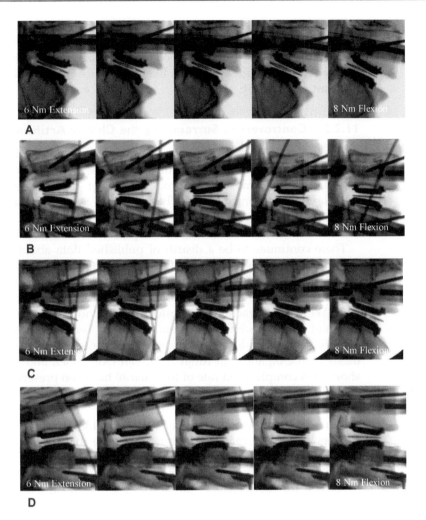

Fig. 11.11.
Four motion patterns of the UHMWPE core in the Charité total disc replacement observed during *in vitro* biomechanical testing. (A) With motion pattern 1, relative angular motion occurred predominantly between the superior end plate and the core, with little or no core translation. (B) In motion pattern 2, lift-off occurred by either the superior end plate from the core, or by the core from the inferior end plate. (C) In motion pattern 3, the UHMWPE core "locked" in plane, resulting in entrapment over a portion of the flexion-extension range. (D) In motion pattern 4, angular motion occurred between the core and both the superior and inferior end plates. *(Reproduced from O'Leary et al. [2005] with permission from Elsevier.)*

the flexion-extension range (Figure 11.11c). In motion pattern 4, angular motion occurred between the core and both the superior and inferior end plates (Figure 11.11d). O'Leary et al. concluded that "Charité TDR restored near normal quantity of flexion-extension range of motion under a constant physiologic preload; however, the quality of segmental motion differed from the intact case over the flexion-extension range " [O'Leary et al. 2005]. Because some of the implants in this study may have been undersized or not optimally placed, the authors further concluded that positioning, changes in lordosis, and the magnitude of the preload would also likely influence the kinematics of the Charité [O'Leary et al. 2005].

11.2.3.5 Controversies Surrounding the Charité Artificial Disc

The complete history of the Charité spans two decades and numerous iterations in design (1984 to 2004). During this time period, it has been implanted in 9,000 patients, mostly in Europe. However, the long-term success of the Charité remains controversial. The broad range of outcomes for the Charité reported in the literature (Tables 11.1 and 11.2) raises questions about the probability of long-term success of motion preservation with this implant.

There continues to be a dearth of published data about the complications with this implant system outside of the United States [van Ooij, Oner, and Verbout 2003]. There have been reported incidences of migration, subsidence, ejection of the core (either anteriorly or posteriorly), radiographic wire fracture, UHMWPE wear, fracture, and osteolysis [David 2005; Kurtz et al. 2005; van Ooij and van Rhijn 2005; van Ooij, Oner, and Verbout 2003]. Potential clinical complications include facet degeneration, spontaneous fusion, and spondylisthesis [van Ooij and van Rhijn 2005; van Ooij, Oner, and Verbout 2003]. The short-term complication rate of the Charité has been presented at international meetings [McAfee et al. 2005]. However, the long-term prevalence of complications with the Charité remains unknown.

In a systematic review of the artificial disc literature published in 2003, the authors concluded that "there is no evidence that disc arthroplasty reliably, reproducibly, and over longer periods of time fulfills the three primary aims of clinical efficacy, continued motion, and few adjacent segment degeneration problems" [de Kleuver, Oner, and Jacobs 2003]. Putzier, writing in 2005 from the Charité hospital in Berlin, where the implant was first used clinically, stated that "the long-term follow-up study demonstrates dissatisfying results after artificial disc replacement in the majority of the evaluated cases. . . . the Charité artificial disc replacement cannot guarantee long-term near to normal function of spinal motion segment in patients with moderate to severe [degenerative disc disease]" [Putzier et al. 2005]. As a result, the long-term prognosis for patients with a Charité total disc replacement remains uncertain.

The most comprehensive clinical trial of the Charité was the prospective randomized study performed for the FDA [Blumenthal et al. 2005; McAfee et al. 2005; Mirza 2005; Zindrick, Lorenz, and Bunch 2005]. In this study, the investigators successfully demonstrated that the Charité was not inferior to a historical anterior fusion procedure employing a BAK cage. The Charité was subsequently cleared by the FDA in October of 2004, and it remains at the beginning of 2006 to be the only commercially available artificial disc in the United States. Only two-year follow-up of this series has been reported, which is sufficient to demonstrate short-term safety and efficacy for the FDA, but inadequate to document long-term outcomes and complication rates.

Consequently, the adoption of the Charité in the United States in 2005 was much slower than initially expected. In addition to the paucity of long-term performance data, the IDE trial did not demonstrate, in the short-term, a clear superiority of the Charité over an anterior lumbar interbody fusion with a standalone cage, which is currently considered in the spine community to be of "dubious efficacy" [Mirza 2005]. Furthermore, there exists limited data demonstrating clinical superiority or cost effectiveness of the Charité over more contemporary fusion technologies (i.e., instrumented fusions augmented with biologics, which are described in Chapters 7 through 9).

As a result, many insurance companies, as well as Medicare and Medicaid, have authorized only very limited or no reimbursement at all for performing the procedure in the United States during 2005. On October 1, 2005, the Center for Medicare Services (CMS) denied the manufacturer's request for new technology add-on payments with the following justification: "Our medical officers could not find sufficient evidence to support a finding that this device meets the criteria for being a substantial clinical improvement. Specifically, we are concerned about the lack of comparative data beyond 24 months in the materials that were submitted for review. While the clinical studies above cited by the manufacturer suggest positive outcomes with the device for up to 24 months, other studies cast doubt on both its short-term and long-term performance, and raise troubling questions regarding longer term adverse outcomes. . . . Therefore, due to the lack of good evidence of long-term clinical benefit and safety, and because of the degree of controversy surrounding the device within the orthopedic and spine surgery community, we do not believe it meets the criterion for substantial clinical improvement and we are denying the application for new technology add-on payments for FY 2006" [cms.hhs.gov 2005]. Based on this ruling, difficulties in reimbursement for artificial disc replacement in the United States are expected to persist throughout 2006.

11.2.3.6 The Legacy of the Charité Artificial Disc

Despite the current controversies and reimbursement difficulties surrounding the Charité, it is nonetheless the icon for contemporary total disc arthroplasty. Other artificial disc designs are currently in clinical use in Europe, and may become available in the United States within the next one to two years. However, these newer designs build upon the design philosophy established by the Charité, which adapted the successful bearing concepts from hip and knee replacements for total disc replacement. As we have seen in the previous section describing the AcroFlex design, an alternative design philosophy—in which the designers sought to replicate both the structure and the function of the natural disc—has thus far failed to reach clinical fruition, at least for the lumbar spine. In contrast, the Charité artificial disc is the first design to establish a history of clinical use spanning two decades, with 10-year outcomes available in, albeit limited, retrospective studies. The Charité is a pioneering design for this reason.

Like any pioneering technology, the story of the Charité highlights a number of unexpected developments, especially with regard to reimbursement, that have complicated its smooth transition into the U.S. market. It is unclear how this unintended legacy of the Charité will influence the adoption of newer artificial disc designs as they are granted clearance by the FDA in the next one to two years. The current reimbursement difficulties for the Charité provide a sobering lesson for bioengineers about the importance of health care economics for the successful introduction of new spine implant technologies. With health care resources being increasingly limited in the future, new artificial disc technologies will need to demonstrate not only effectiveness but cost effectiveness with respect to established spine procedures. The reader is referred to Chapter 16, which reviews the concepts underlying medical device economics and cost effectiveness in greater detail.

11.3 Contemporary Lumbar Disc Replacements

As summarized in Table 11.3, there are four contemporary total disc replacement designs in clinical trials today: Charité, ProDisc, Maverick, and FlexiCore. In the previous section, we reviewed the clinical history and bioengineering studies related to the Charité. The three newer designs differ markedly from the Charité in many respects, such as the number of individual components to be installed by the surgeon, the number and type of biomaterials used for the articulating surfaces, the amount of constraint in the bearing, the incorporation of keels into the end plates, and the design of the bone-implant interfaces (Table 11.3).

The amount and quality of available clinical data also vary among the designs (Table 11.3). Although intermediate and long-term data are available for the ProDisc and the Charité, respectively, the reader should be aware that these studies are limited to retrospective evaluations [Putzier et al. 2005; Tropiano et al. 2005]. Intermediate-term prospective, randomized trial data are not available for any design, and long-term randomized data for all four artificial discs will not to be available for at least another decade.

In this section, we summarize the design theory and available literature for the ProDisc, Maverick, and FlexiCore artificial discs. Like the Charité, the three newer lumbar disc designs are based on well-established bearing and bone-implant fixation technologies used for hip and knee replacements. Furthermore, these devices are similarly implanted by an anterior approach, albeit with device-specific instrumentation of varying sophistication.

The newer designs represent significant departures from the unconstrained mobile bearing philosophy embodied by the Charité. The three designs incorporate varying degrees of constraint, ranging from a ball-and-socket design of the ProDisc and Maverick to the captured ball-and-socket design with stops of the FlexiCore. The increased constraint is intended to prevent hypermobility and overloading of the facets, which could lead to pain, degeneration, and spontaneous fusions. Two of the newer designs (Maverick and FlexiCore) also incorporate metal-on-metal articulations using CoCr alloys, to reduce wear and the risk of long-term osteolysis. Consequently, it is hoped that these newer

Table 11.3.
Summary of contemporary lumbar artificial disc designs.

Design	Charité	ProDisc	Maverick	FlexiCore
Current manufacturer	DePuy spine (Raynham, MA, USA; http://www.charitedisc.com/)	Synthes (Paoli, PA; http://www.synthes.com/)	Medtronic Sofamor Danek (Memphis, TN; http://www.sofamordanek.com/)	Stryker Spine (Allendale, NJ; http://www.strykerspine.com)
Number of components for surgeon assembly	Three	Three	Two	One*
Number of articulating surfaces	Two	One	One	One
Bearing design	Mobile bearing	Ball-and-socket	Ball-and-socket	Ball-and-socket w/stops
Articulating biomaterials	CoCr/UHMWPE	CoCr/UHMWPE	CoCr/CoCr	CoCr/CoCr
Constraint	Unconstrained	Semi-constrained	Semi-constrained	Constrained
Bone/implant fixation	teeth (USA only**); teeth and CaP/Ti coating (outside USA)	Keel and Ti textured coating	Keel and textured CoCr with hydroxyapatite	Spikes and plasma-sprayed Ti surface coating
Keel	No	Yes	Yes	No
Published clinical studies	Yes (see Table 11.2)	Yes (see Table 11.4)	Yes	No
Longest published average follow-up	18.2 years (Putzier et al. 2005)	8.7 years (Tropiano et al. 2005)	2 years (Le Huec et al. 2005)	None
2-year FDA randomized controlled trial	Completed and published (Blumenthal et al. 2005; McAfee et al. 2005)	In process	In process	In process
Control procedure in FDA randomized trial	Anterior interbody fusion with BAK cage	360-degree fusion	Anterior LT cage with INFUSE bone graft	360-degree fusion

*The FlexiCore consists of four components (a superior and inferior end plate, a captured ball, and a shield) preassembled by the manufacturer.
**Only smooth end plates, with no ongrowth surface, are currently available in the United States.

designs will be able to overcome some of the long-term complications and controversies, including facet degeneration and wear, that have been identified in recent studies of the Charité.

11.3.1 ProDisc

Conceived in 1989 by Thierry Marnay, M.D., from Montpellier in France, the ProDisc consists of two metallic end plates and a UHMWPE core (Figure 11.12) [Delamarter, Bae, and Pradhan]. Unlike the Charité, the UHMWPE core in the ProDisc is firmly attached to the flat, inferior end plate by a locking mechanism (Figure 11.13). The domed (convex) surface of the core articulates against the concave, superior metallic end plate. There have been two versions of the ProDisc (I and II), but only the more recent version of the design (ProDisc II) has been commercially available. The ProDisc II was originally produced by Aesculap AG & Co. (Tuttlingen, Germany) [Tropiano et al. 2005], and then commercialized by Spinal Solutions. Today it is manufactured by Synthes (Paoli, PA).

Besides the Charité, the ProDisc has the second-longest clinical follow-up of any currently available artificial disc design [Tropiano et al. 2005]. Marnay implanted 93 first-generation ProDisc I artificial discs in 64 patients between March of 1990 and September of 1993 [Huang et al. 2005; Tropiano et al. 2005]. The end plates of the ProDisc I were fabricated from Ti alloy (Figure 11.14). Each end plate featured two short, parallel keels for short-term fixation, and the back surfaces were plasma sprayed with titanium for bone ongrowth.

The intermediate-term clinical results of the ProDisc I patients were published in 2005 [Tropiano et al. 2005]. The mean follow-up of this study, which included 55 (86%) patients from Marnay's original cohort, was 8.7 years.

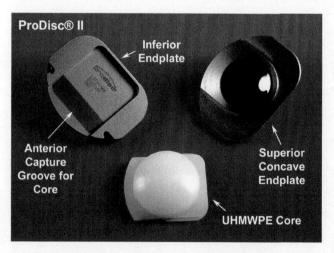

Fig. 11.12.
Two CoCr alloy end plates and UHMWPE core of the ProDisc II design.

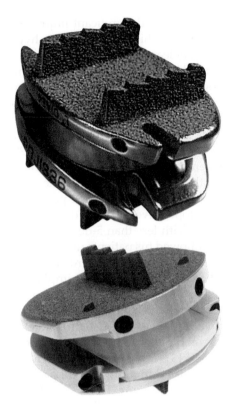

Fig. 11.13.
(A) Two titanium alloy end plates and UHMWPE core of the ProDisc I design. (B) Two CoCr alloy end plates and UHMWPE core of the ProDisc II design. *(Reprinted with permission from Synthes Spine, LP.)*

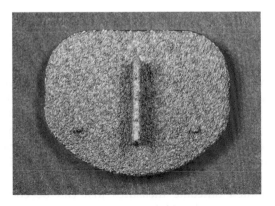

Fig. 11.14.
Textured titanium plasma spray backing and keel of the ProDisc II.

Marnay demonstrated significant improvement using non-validated outcome scoring methods, which confirmed his hypothesis that the ProDisc I was safe and effective, at least in his hands (Table 11.4). Procedure-related complications were observed in five cases (deep venous thrombosis, iliac vein laceration, transient retrograde ejaculation, and two incisional hernias), but none were implant related. The investigators were not able to detect any measurable UHMWPE wear when comparing the core height immediately after surgery with the core height at the longest follow-up. Subsequent analysis of the range in clinical performance for this cohort by Huang et al. [2005] revealed an intriguing correlation between patient outcomes and the range of motion of the operated levels. Patients with more than 5 degrees of flexion-extension range of motion had significantly less postoperative back pain and better clinical outcomes (as measured by postoperative oswestry disability index and Stauffer-Coventry scores) than patients with less than 5-degree range of motion.

Marnay followed his patients until 1998 before making further modifications, which resulted in the current ProDisc II design. Since 1999, more than 5,000 ProDisc II components have been implanted worldwide [Delamarter, Bae, and Pradhan 2005]. In the second-generation design, the end plates are fabricated from CoCr alloy, which has improved tribological properties as compared with Ti alloy. In addition, a single, slightly taller keel is used. The textured back surfaces of the end plates are plasma sprayed with titanium (Figure 11.14).

The UHMWPE core is machined from compression molded GUR 1020, and is gamma sterilized in nitrogen. Foil packaging is currently used for its oxygen barrier properties (Figure 11.15). The ProDisc II has a unique locking detail which engages the UHMWPE core with the inferior end plate. The capture mechanism for the core consists of a sliding, tongue-in-groove along the left and right (laterally), with a raised, triangular-profiled ridge on the inferior surface of the UHMWPE. During implantation, the surgeon slides the tongues on the core backward into the grooved capture mechanism of the inferior end plate until the anterior raised ridge of the UHMWPE snaps into a mating slot in the end plate, thereby preventing anterior ejection of the core (Figure 11.13).

The reports of generally positive clinical outcomes of the ProDisc II are limited to short-term studies (on average, 17 to 31 months of follow-up), which are summarized in Table 11.4. In addition, published prospective clinical data for the ProDisc II provide some evidence that the short-term outcomes of multilevel implantation are comparable to single-level disc replacement [Bertagnoli et al. 2005]. In general, the available clinical data for the ProDisc are stronger, scientifically speaking, than that for the Charité, which has historically been documented by mostly retrospective studies in Europe (Table 11.2). With the exception of the FDA trial, none of the Charité studies included validated outcome measures, such as the oswestry disability index. In contrast, the majority of available studies for the ProDisc II are prospective, and employ validated outcome measures that can be compared with alternative spine procedures (Table 11.4).

The prospective, randomized clinical trial for the ProDisc II, with both single-level and double-level arms, began in the United States in October of 2001 and completed its target enrollment by the end of 2003. The reference procedure

Table 11.4.

Clinical details of primary, peer-reviewed studies involving the ProDisc I and II.

	Tropiano et al. (Huang et al. 2005, Tropiano et al. 2005)	Mayer et al. (Mayer et al. 2002)	Tropiano et al. (Tropiano et al. 2003)	Zigler (Zigler 2004)	Bertagnoli et al. (Bertagnoli et al. 2005)	Bertagnoli et al. (Bertagnoli et al. 2005)	Delamarter et al. (Delamarter, Bae, and Pradhan 2005)
Study type	Hcoh	Pcoh	Pcoh	RCT	Pcoh	Pcoh	RCT
Type of prosthesis	ProDisc I	ProDisc II	ProDisc II	ProDisc II	ProDisc II	ProDisc II	ProDisc II
Average age	46	44	45	38	48 (median)	51 (median)	40
Age range	25–65	25–65	28–67		24–45	30–60	19–59
No. of patients	55	34	53	28	104	25	56
No. of arthroplasties	78	37	68		104	60	91
Follow-up in months	104	12	17	12	31 (median)	31 (median)	18
Range in follow-up	85–128		12–24		24–45	25–41	
Good or excellent	75%						
Initial Oswestry score (%). Average ± SD	N/A	19 ± 7	56 ± 8		54	65 (42–92)	31
Owestry score (%) at longest follow-up, average ± SD	18 ± 16	7.2 ± 9.6	14 ± 7	Decreased	29	22 (0–48)	20
Secondary surgery	3/55	0/34	3/53		1/104	1/25	
Arthrodesis or spontaneous fusion	1/55	0/34	0/53		0/104	0/25	
Complications	10/55	3/34	5/53		5/104	4/25	
Motion on flexion-extension radiographs in degrees (range)							
Average	4.0 (0–18)		9 (2–18)		7		
L4/L5			10 (8–18)				10
L5/S1			8 (2–12)				8

Hcoh (historical cohort study); Pcoh (prospective cohort study); RCT (randomized controlled trial).

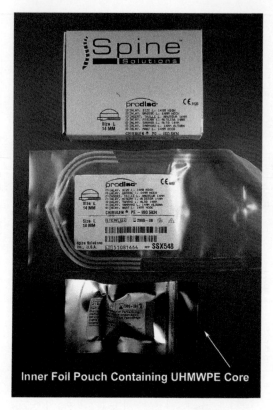

Inner Foil Pouch Containing UHMWPE Core

Fig. 11.15.
Outer polymeric pouch and inner foil barrier packaging of the ProDisc II UHMWPE core developed by Spine Solutions and currently employed by Synthes Spine.

was an anterior-posterior (360-degree) fusion: the control patients first underwent an anterior fusion procedure, involving a femoral ring allograft. The patients were then flipped, and a posterior fusion was performed, consisting of bilateral intertransverse fixation with pedicle screws [Zigler 2003]. Although by no means obsolete, a 360-degree procedure represents a highly conservative fusion strategy and arguably a "worst-case" scenario with which to compare with disc replacement. Two of the 19 clinical sites involved in the pivotal trial have published interim results, with follow-up periods of up to 18 months (Table 11.4) [Delamarter, Bae, and Pradhan 2005; Delamarter et al. 2003; Zigler 2003, 2004]. There was a major difference in the complexity, and hence the operative time between the disc replacement and the 360-degree fusion (on average, 75.4 versus 218.2 minutes, respectively) [Zigler 2003]. Although disc replacements patients recovered faster than controls, the longest-term available data suggest that the final outcomes of a 360-degree fusion and the ProDisc, as measured by VAS and oswestry disability scores, are not significantly different [Delamarter, Bae, and Pradhan 2005; Zigler 2004]. The aggregate clinical data from the U.S. IDE study, including all 19 centers from the randomized clinical

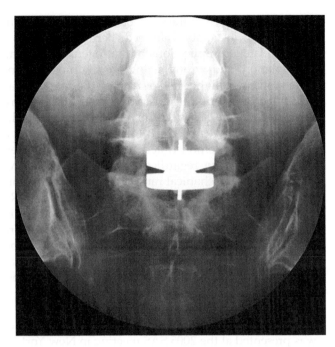

Fig. 11.16.
AP radiograph of a Maverick total disc replacement. *(Reprinted with permission from Medtronic Sofamor Danek.)*

trial, have not yet been published. Synthes has not received clearance by the FDA for marketing the ProDisc II in the United States. However, it is currently anticipated that the artificial disc will be commercially available to U.S. surgeons during 2006.

Even though little information about complications with the ProDisc II has appeared in the literature thus far [Bertagnoli et al. 2005; Shim et al. 2005], more extensive complication data have recently been presented at national meetings. At the 2005 North American Spine Society meeting, for example, Bertagnoli reported an overall complication rate for the ProDisc at 3.0% (15/522 patients) [Bertagnoli 2005]. Although relatively few in number [7/522, 1.4%], many of the complications reported for the ProDisc II—such as wound infections, retrograde ejaculation, and epidural or retroperitonial hematoma—appear related to the anterior approach itself [Bertagnoli 2005]. Device-related complications have been reported in 8/522 cases [1.6%], and include partial subsidence of the end plates, anterior migration or partial ejection of the UHMWPE core, and L5 root/motion deficit [Bertagnoli 2005]. Two cases of vertebral split fractures associated with the ProDisc have also been reported in the literature [Shim et al. 2005]. In both cases, the split fractures were caused by the surgeons when chiseling of the bone grooves to accommodate the keels. Thus, the vertebral split fractures, as well as the majority of the complications reported by Bertagnoli, are likely related to surgical technique. The cases of core ejection may be technique related, particularly if the surgeon fails to properly engage the capture mechanism during installation. Indeed, Bertagnoli opines that "more than 90% of device-related complications are iatrogenic. Poor patient selection, improper implantation, and wrong sizing are the most common examples of surgical errors causing a higher risk of failure" [Bertagnoli et al. 2005].

Limited test data, related to shock absorption, have been reported for the ProDisc II in the scientific literature [LeHuec et al. 2003]. Dynamic testing at frequency ranges between 0 and 100 Hz, as well as "shock loading" with 0.1 s durations, demonstrated that the ProDisc II exhibits negligible shock-absorption capacity, regardless of the fact that a UHMWPE core is included in the design. Biomechanical range-of-motion evaluations for the ProDisc II were presented at the 2003 meeting of the Orthopedic Research Society [Lipman et al. 2003]. Lipman et al. tested six lumbar spines, with and without a ProDisc II. The specimens were mounted in a 6-degree-of-freedom spine testing apparatus, attached to a bi-axial MTS load frame. The specimens were tested with ±10 Nm flexion/extension, lateral bending, and axial torsion, under applied compressive preloads of 600 N and 1,200 N. The investigators found no significant difference in the range of motion of the natural and treated lumbar spine when testing under these conditions.

Wear testing for 5 million cycles of the ProDisc II in comparison to the Charité was presented at the 2005 SAS meeting in New York [Bushelow, Aberman, and Kaddick 2005]. Two different types of duty cycle were employed. In one set of simulations, a curvilinear motion of the end plates was prescribed in flexion/extension and axial rotation. In a second set of simulations, crossing path motion was prescribed in flexion/extension, lateral bending, and axial rotation. The load magnitude varied between 350 and 1,750 N. However, no further details about the test conditions (e.g., test temperature and fluid) were provided in the abstract. Simulator kinematics had a significant effect on wear rates, with crossing path motion producing a higher wear rate as compared with curvilinear motion. The wear rates of the ProDisc II and Charité artificial discs were found to be similar under both sets of simulator conditions.

In summary, there is a growing body of literature supporting the clinical safety and effectiveness for the ProDisc II. However, many aspects of the clinical evaluation, in particular complication rates and *in vivo* wear rates, remain yet to be fully explored. The two-year results of the prospective randomized trial are not publicly available, but are expected within the coming year. Despite its clinical use since 1999, there currently exist no published retrieval studies for the ProDisc II, and thus the early clinical performance of the implant components remains unknown. Finally, biomechanical characterization of the ProDisc remains in its early stages, with the majority of test studies appearing at conferences, rather than in peer-reviewed journal publications.

11.3.2 Maverick

The Maverick total disc replacement device was developed in 2001 by an engineering team at Medtronic Sofamor Danek (Memphis, TN), working in close

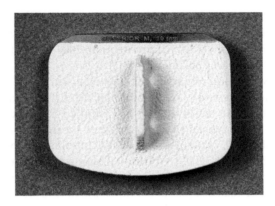

Fig. 11.17.
Hydroxyapatite-coated backing and keel of the Maverick.

collaboration with spine surgeons. Although early experimental prototypes were initially fabricated from alumina ceramic, the commercially available Maverick is a two-piece, metal-on-metal design consisting of superior and inferior CoCr alloy end plates (Figure 11.16). The ball-and-socket articulation is shifted posteriorly with respect to the geometric center of the end plates to more closely approximate the anatomic center of rotation for the intact motion segment. The bearing surfaces are CoCr alloy, similar to metal-on-metal hip replacements, because of the ultralow wear rates that have been achieved in hip replacements with this technology [Clarke et al. 2000]. The original end plates were designed with an 11-mm high, doubly fenestrated keel. The latest version has a reduced keel height of 6.5 mm. The entire keel and backside of the end plates are roughened and coated with hydroxyapatite to promote bone ongrowth (Figure 11.17).

Clinical use of the Maverick began in January of 2002 [Mathews et al. 2004]. Two-year prospective results have been reported by Le Huec for a cohort of 64 patients implanted with a single-level Maverick [Le Huec et al. 2005]. The mean age of the patients was 44 ± 7 years. The oswestry disability index (ODI) for the patients improved significantly from 43.8 preoperatively, to 23.1 at two years. Using a 25% improvement in ODI as the criteria for success (similar to the FDA study for the Charité), clinical success was achieved in 75% of the patients. The range of motion in flexion and extension was 7.9 degrees at L5-S1, 9.4 degrees at L4-L5, and 7.4 degrees at L3-L4. The few reported complications for the Maverick have been technique related, including a ureter tear, an injury to the common iliac vein, and a posterior wall fracture. There were no device related complications or revisions in this series. Additional, prospective analysis of sagittal balance in a series of 35 patients with no history of lumbosacral imbalance demonstrated that implantation of the Maverick had no significant effect on pelvic tilt, sacral tilt, or lordosis [Le Huec et al. 2005].

The prospective randomized trial for the FDA IDE study began in April of 2003. In contrast with other prospective trials, which employed conservative or obsolete control procedures, the control procedure for the Maverick is a state-of-the-art fusion procedure; namely, anterior fusion using an LT-cage filled with INFUSE bone graft [Mathews et al. 2004]. Data from the randomized trial have not yet been published.

A few preliminary biomechanical studies of the Maverick have been published in peer-reviewed journal articles [Hitchon et al. 2005; LeHuec et al. 2003; Mathews et al. 2004]. Le Huec studied the shock absorption characteristics of the Maverick and concluded that the metal-on-metal design, similar to the ProDisc II, provides negligible attenuation of dynamic or shock loading [LeHuec et al. 2003]. Additional biomechanical testing of the Maverick has been summarized by Mathews et al. [2004]. Compressive fatigue testing with a peak load of 10,000 N (2.3 to 3.2 times the failure strength of the vertebral body) produced no mechanical damage after 10 million cycles. Mathews further reports that wear testing was performed with the Maverick for 10 million cycles, and produced a total 12 to 14 mm^3 of debris by the end of the testing, but no details about the testing (aside from a 2-Hz rate and 60-day test duration) are provided. Mathews suggests that the testing is equivalent to 31.5 years of *in vivo* use, based on simplified theoretical estimates of the number of "significant bends" a patient might be expected to make during a year. However, in the absence of validation of the spine simulator it is not possible to state whether the wear debris in this study was generated in a clinically relevant manner. Hence, it is not at all clear how many years of *in vivo* use may be attributed to the wear testing reported by Mathews and co-workers [Mathews et al. 2004].

In vitro cadaveric testing of the Maverick revealed no significant difference between the intact and reconstructed spine [Hitchon et al. 2005]. These tests were performed with seven fresh-frozen lumbar spines under applied pure moments of ±6 Nm in flexion/extension, lateral bending, and axial rotation. Although the authors report performing the experiments on a "biomechanical testing frame," insufficient details were provided of the set up so that the testing could be repeated by another investigator. In particular, this testing was performed without a compressive follower load, and therefore assesses the theoretical maximum flexibility of the natural and treated spine in the absence of compression.

At the 2005 meeting for the Spine Arthroplasty Society, Chan and co-workers presented wear test results for the Maverick under unidirectional motion, which is one of the methods currently recommended in the recently approved "ASTM Standard Test Guide for the Functional, Kinematic, and Wear Assessment of Total Disc Prostheses" (no standard number is yet available for this standard) [Chan et al. 2005]. In this study, the surface morphology of wear tested implants were compared with a retrieved component that had been implanted for one year in a 43-year-old female patient, but was revised for nerve root impingement (Figure 11.18). Wear testing was performed for four million cycles under a constant load of 1,200 N with ±10 degrees of flexion/extension at 2 Hz in a spine simulator. The lubricant was bovine serum diluted to 25% concentration. In general, the articulating surfaces of the *in vitro*-tested implants exhibited (without magnification) directional scratching in the F/E direction, evident of abrasive wear mechanisms. In contrast, the retrieved

Wear-Tested Maverick

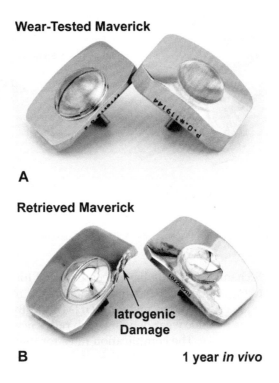

A

Retrieved Maverick

**Iatrogenic
Damage**

B   **1 year *in vivo***

Fig. 11.18.
(A) Wear-tested Maverick, evaluated under ASTM unidirectional test conditions; (B) retrieved component that was implanted for one year. Prior to revision, the posterior corner of the implant was abraded by the surgeon using a Dremel tool (iatrogenic damage), in an effort to relieve nerve root compression.

component exhibited highly polished articulated surfaces, with microabrasive wear mechanisms only visible under the SEM. These remarkable differences between the simulator-tested implants and the explant strongly suggest that the unidirectional testing specified as one of the options in the ASTM standard is an inappropriate analogue to the clinical scenario.

A second-generation Maverick, referred to as the A-Mav, was developed for the European market starting in 2005. With the A-Mav, the keel height was lowered by 4.5 mm to increase the keel-to-keel separation when multilevel disc replacements were employed. Reducing the keel height was thought not to affect the initial stability of the device, but could slightly improve its revisability, because the osteotomy that would be required to remove the taller keel would be reduced. In addition to changing the keel height, a number of slight changes in the edge chamfer and instrumentation holes were made, as summarized in Figure 11.19. This particular design is not being evaluated for clinical use in the United States.

In summary, the Maverick is a promising alternative to metal-on-polyethylene disc replacements. Prospective two-year clinical data and preliminary

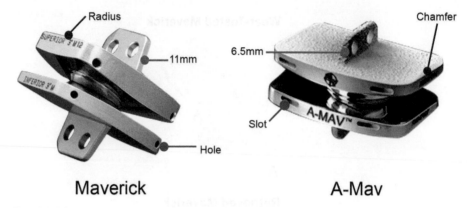

Maverick   **A-Mav**

Fig. 11.19.
Comparison of the Maverick and A-Mav total disc replacement designs.

biomechanical test data have been reported for the Maverick, but many unanswered questions still remain. Although the metal-on-metal articulation provides lower wear than metal-on-UHMWPE, the articulation of CoCr surfaces produces metallic wear debris, which raises new questions about the long-term biological risks. The complication rates for this design remain unknown. Clinical and biomechanical studies of the Maverick are ongoing and will be reported in the future.

11.3.3 FlexiCore

The FlexiCore lumbar artificial disc (Stryker Spine, Allendale, NJ) is the most constrained of the contemporary, lumbar artificial disc designs. The FlexiCore consists of four CoCr components, including a superior and inferior baseplate, a captured spherical head that attaches to the superior end plate, and a shield [Valdevit and Errico 2004]. These four components are preassembled by the manufacturer, so that the surgeon implants a one-piece device (Figure 11.20). The CoCr ball-and-socket bearing surface for the device is centrally located with respect to the end plates. Because the spherical head is captured beneath the shield, the device is capable of supporting tensile loads. The device also includes mechanical stops to limit flexion/extension and lateral bending motion. However, these stops are set beyond the normal ranges of motion for the lumbar spine. Short-term fixation of the implant is achieved with four spikes on each end plate, and a titanium plasma spray coating is applied to the end plates for bone ongrowth.

Static and dynamic fatigue testing, in tension, compression, and shear have been conducted [Valdevit and Errico 2004]. These tests demonstrated successful mechanical device performance, with strength limits exceeding the load limits for vertebral bodies. In addition, wear testing with up to 10 million loading cycles have been performed. According to the authors, "minimal or no damage resulting from wear was seen" [Valdevit and Errico 2004].

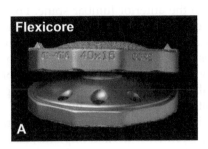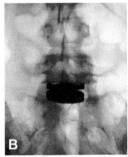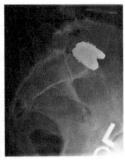

Fig. 11.20.
The FlexiCore total disc replacement. (A) Photograph of a FlexiCore; (B) anteroposterior and lateral radiographs of the FlexiCore implanted in the lumbosacral spine. *(Reproduced from Errico et al. [2005] with permission from Lippincott, Williams & Wilkins.)*

A prospective randomized trial for the FlexiCore is currently underway, but results are not expected for several years. The trial, which started in August of 2003, is designed to evaluate treatment of single-level disc degeneration with either a FlexiCore or a 360-degree fusion [Errico 2005], which, as noted previously, is the most conservative fusion procedure currently available. No clinical data for the FlexiCore have yet been published. In summary, it remains to be seen how the FlexiCore will perform clinically, and there is a paucity of hard data concerning this design in the literature.

11.4 Cervical TDRs

In several key aspects, total disc arthroplasty is a more attractive technology for the cervical spine than for the lumbar spine. First, the biomechanical demands on a cervical prosthesis, which must support the weight of the head and the neck above it, are about an order of magnitude less stringent than in the lumbar region, which must support the weight of the entire upper torso. The lower loads of the cervical spine also permit a much broader range of design and biomaterial options, which would not otherwise be feasible in the lumbar spine.

Second, the indications for cervical disc replacement, which include myelopathy and radiculopathy, are broader and more prevalent than for lumbar disc replacement. That is, more of the patients undergoing cervical fusions today may be candidates for disc arthroplasty, provided certain other contraindications are not met, such as non-intact posterior elements and osteoporosis. In contrast, the list of contraindications in lumbar disc replacement is currently so extensive that it effectively precludes the vast majority of lumbar fusion candidates from receiving an arthroplasty.

Third, the surgical access to the anterior cervical spine is easier and less risky for the patient than the access to the anterior lumbar spine. Furthermore, the ease of access for cervical disc replacements is preserved during revision, whereas in the lumbar spine, scar tissue, and adherent vessels greatly complicate the anterior revision process. For these main reasons, cervical disc arthroplasty appears to be a less risky proposition than lumbar arthroplasty, both in terms of the feasibility of available technology options for the implants as well as in terms of the risk to the patient from the procedure.

Currently, the clinical experience with cervical disc replacements is less mature than for lumbar disc replacements. Certain implants, such as the Prestige, have gone through several design iterations, and as a result the newest versions of the design have not yet been followed for prolonged periods of time. Regardless, very little clinical data about any of these designs are currently available, with the exception of pilot studies that helped to confirm the design concept of early prototypes. In particular, only one prospective randomized trial data for any cervical disc has yet been published in the peer-reviewed scientific literature [Porchet and Metcalf 2004], and no manufacturer has yet been given clearance for marketing any cervical disc in the United States. Therefore, cervical discs are all considered investigational devices in the United States.

As summarized previously, Fernström's stainless steel sphere was the first cervical disc arthroplasty implanted in the early 1960s [Fernström 1966]. Although Fernström's 1966 publication acknowledges his use of the spherical prosthesis in the cervical spine, two South African surgeons, Hjalmar Reitz and Mauritius Joubert, are credited with publishing the first paper on cervical disc arthroplasty two years earlier [Reitz and Joubert 1964]. Reitz and Joubert visited with Fernström in Sweden, and were "favourably impressed by his results" [Reitz and Joubert 1964]. After returning home, they implanted 75 spherical cervical disc replacements in 32 patients who suffered from severe headaches and neck-related arm pain. The surgeons reported generally positive outcomes for their patients who were followed for less than a year. However, Reitz and Joubert were optimistic that Fernström's prosthesis "preserves the mobility of the intervertebral joints, thus obviating the inherent disadvantages of all fusion procedures" [Reitz and Joubert 1964]. The surgeons acknowledged that longer-term follow-up would be necessary to confirm the viability of their technique. As we have seen earlier in the chapter, Fernström's spherical implant design is no longer widely used today as a disc replacement, because of hypermobility and subsidence. However, Fernström's pioneering design, along with the experience of Reitz and Joubert, would provide inspiration for future generations of cervical disc replacement technologies.

In this section, we summarize the design features, bearing technologies, and available literature for contemporary cervical artificial discs. Many cervical disc replacements have been proposed over the years, but today four contemporary designs have been documented in the peer-reviewed literature and are currently in clinical trials in the United States: Bryan, Prestige, ProDisc-C, and PCM (Table 11.5). As detailed in the following, these four designs differ markedly from each other in the number of individual components, the biomaterials employed, as well as in the philosophy and constraint in the bearing

Table 11.5.
Summary of contemporary cervical artificial disc designs.

Design	Bryan	Prestige	ProDisc-C	PCM
Manufacturer	Medtronic Sofamor Danek (Memphis, TN; http://www.sofamordanek.com/)	Medtronic Sofamor Danek (Memphis, TN; http://www.sofamordanek.com/)	Synthes (Paoli, PA; http://www.synthes.com)	Cervitech (Rockaway, NJ; http://www.cervitech.com/)
Number of components for surgeon assembly	One	Two	Two	Two
Number of articulating surfaces	Two	One	One	One
Bearing design	Elastomeric ball-and-socket	Ball-in-trough	Ball-and-socket	Surface replacement
Articulating biomaterials	Ti/PU	Stainless steel (ST design); Ti ceramic composite (LP design)	UHMWPE/CoCr	UHMWPE/CoCr
Constraint	Semi-constrained	Semi-constrained	Semi-constrained	"Minimally" constrained
Bone/implant fixation	Precision milled bone interface*; Ti textured coating	Keels and Ti textured coating (LP design only)	Keel and Ti textured coating	CaP/Ti coating
Keel	No	Yes	Yes	No
Published clinical studies	Yes	Yes	Yes	No

*Prior to implantation, the surgeon mills a recess into the superior and inferior vertebral bodies to accept the Ti end plates of the Bryan prosthesis.

(Table 11.5). Two designs, namely the ProDisc-C and PCM, are based on technologies and design principles already covered in detail for lumbar discs, which preceded them. In these cases, the overview of these designs makes reference to their lumbar predecessors. The Bryan and Prestige, on the other hand, have a number of unique designs and biomaterial technologies that differ from lumbar disc replacements, and therefore warrant additional attention.

11.4.1 Prestige

Based on the principles of metal-on-metal total joint arthroplasty, the Prestige has the longest clinical track record of contemporary cervical discs. Starting in 1989, the design was conceived by Brian Cummins, a neurosurgeon from the Frenchay Hospital in Bristol, England [Cummins, Robertson, and Gill 1998]. The original design has been given many names in the literature, including the Cummins Artificial Cervical Joint (ACJ), the Bristol Disc, and the Bristol/Cummins Disc. However, these various names all refer to the same historical design, which included two stainless steel end plates incorporating a ball-and-socket articulation. The end plates also featured anterior flanges for screw fixation. The Bristol/Cummins disc was first implanted in 1991, and then followed clinically for up to five years to evaluate its *in vivo* performance [Cummins, Robertson, and Gill 1998]. In 1998, the Bristol/Cummins design was modified by Medtronic Sofamor Danek (Memphis, TN) and renamed to Prestige [Traynelis 2004]. It has since undergone four additional design iterations (the most recent in 2004), as well as a change in biomaterials, in an effort to decrease its anterior profile, improve the joint kinematics, and improve its MRI compatibility [Traynelis 2005]. The clinical and design history of the Prestige is summarized in Figure 11.21, and is explored in greater detail in the following sections.

11.4.1.1 Bristol/Cummins Disc

In developing his cervical disc replacement, Cummins was motivated to provide a solution for the adjacent level degeneration he witnessed when treating many of his cervical fusion patients [Cummins, Robertson, and Gill 1998]. Familiar with the clinical history of the stainless steel Fernström prosthesis in the cervical spine [Fernström 1966; Reitz and Joubert 1964], and concerned about the problems associated with UHMWPE wear, Cummins chose to make his prosthesis from type 316 surgical stainless steel [Cummins, Robertson, and Gill 1998]. The ball-and-socket design was intended to provide rotation with "slight translation," because the diameter of the inferior concave component was slightly larger than the diameter of the convex superior end plate. The implant prototypes, all produced with a single size, were designed and manufactured in collaboration with engineering staff from the Department of Medical Engineering at Frenchay Hospital (Figure 11.21).

Starting in 1991, the Bristol/Cummins disc was implanted in 20 patients, the vast majority of which (19/20, 95%) had an adjacent preexisting cervical fusion. Eighteen patients were examined in 1996, with up to five years follow-up. By

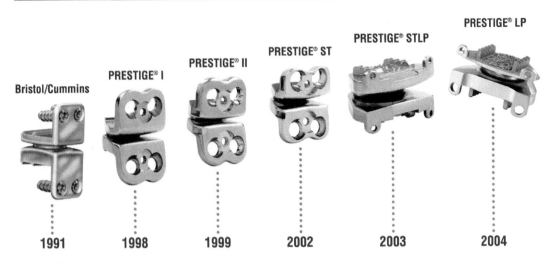

PRESTIGE® LP

PRESTIGE® STLP

PRESTIGE® ST

PRESTIGE® II

PRESTIGE® I

Bristol/Cummins

1991   1998   1999   2002   2003   2004

Fig. 11.21.
The clinical history of the Prestige cervical artificial disc. *(Reproduced with permission from Medtronic Sofamor Danek, Memphis, TN.)*

then one patient had died, for reasons unrelated to the implant, and the other patient could only be interviewed telephonically. Motion was detected radiographically in the prosthesis for 16/18 examined patients [Cummins, Robertson, and Gill 1998], with an average of 5 degrees of motion in flexion and extension. In the two patients without prosthesis motion, it was noted that the intervertebral space had been overdistracted during the operation. One patient sustained a drill-related injury to the cord during surgery, resulting in deltoid muscle paresis, and three patients found their pain symptoms unchanged or worsened by the surgery. In 2003, 16 of the patients were again examined, and the prostheses were found to be still functioning after up to 12 years *in vivo* [Porchet and Metcalf 2004].

A large number of implant-related complications were noted with these disc replacements. In the first five cases, the flange only had one screw hole to accommodate a stainless steel screw for fixation of the end plates in the superior and inferior vertebral bodies [Cummins, Robertson, and Gill 1998]. In this group, three of the screws backed out partially, one screw fractured, and one implant subluxed, causing the patient difficulty in swallowing. For the subsequent 15 patients, the anterior flanges of the implants were modified with an additional screw hole, and fenestrated titanium self-locking screws (14 mm) were used. One of these Ti screws was observed radiographically to have fractured, and two screws partially backed out. Due to the size of the anterior flanges, 3/15 patients experienced persistent difficulty with swallowing.

In addition, one implant became loose and persistently painful, due to an interference fit of the ball and socket, which was later confirmed to be a manufacturing error. The implantation time of this prosthesis was not reported. Cummins states that "no wear debris of metal was found in the surrounding soft tissue" [Cummins, Robertson, and Gill 1998], but the author provides no details of how the tissue was examined. Subsequent authors have noted that the retrieval "showed virtually no wear" [Porchet and Metcalf 2004], but again, the details of the retrieval examination were not published.

Technologically speaking, the Bristol/Cummins disc was far from a totally ideal implant prototype. These implants were all manufactured in a single size by a hospital machine shop, and the size chosen was invariably too large for several of the patients [Cummins, Robertson, and Gill 1998; Porchet and Metcalf 2004]. Although a total of four patients (20%) had significant persistent swallowing complications (as noted previously), all of the patients in this series reported at least some difficulty with swallowing due to size of the anterior profile of the implant [Cummins, Robertson, and Gill 1998]. Despite these notable limitations, the Bristol/Cummins disc did demonstrate the long-term feasibility of metal-on-metal arthroplasty using stainless steel bearing surfaces in the cervical spine, albeit in a demanding patient population with a history of previous, adjacent fusions. In this light, the Bristol/Cummins disc represents a significant historical advancement in cervical motion preservation technology, in comparison with the Fernström prosthesis, and provided the motivation for many alternative cervical total disc replacement designs, including the Prestige, that would follow.

11.4.1.2 Screw-fixation Designs: Prestige I, Prestige II, Prestige ST

Encouraged by the promising evidence of long-term motion preservation, the Bristol/Cummins disc was subsequently optimized, in collaboration with a spine implant manufacturer (Medtronic Sofamor Danek, Memphis, TN) and renamed to Prestige. Developed between 1998 and 2002, the Prestige I, II, and ST designs are metal-on-metal artificial discs fabricated from 316 stainless steel with anterior screw fixation, like the Bristol/Cummins disc (Figure 11.21) [Traynelis 2005]. However, there are a number of important design improvements in these three artificial disc designs that distinguish them from their historical predecessor. In the Prestige I implant (also referred to in the literature as the Frenchay artificial cervical joint), the bearing surface of the inferior end plate was changed from a spherical bowl to an ellipsoidal dish, with the long axis of the ellipsoid oriented parallel to the anterior-posterior axis to provide 2 mm of anterior translation (both sliding and rolling) during flexion/extension rotation of the cervical spine [Wigfield et al. 2002]. The anterior profile was reduced, customized stainless steel screws were developed, and a locking screw was introduced to prevent the fixation screws from backing out (Figure 11.21). In the Prestige II design, the bearing surface was unchanged, but modifications were made to further reduce the anterior profile (Figure 11.21). The backside of the end plates were also roughened with the Prestige II design to promote bone ongrowth [Porchet and Metcalf 2004]. In the Prestige ST design, the height of the anterior flange was reduced by an additional 2 mm (as compared with the Prestige II), and the backside of the end plates were roughened by grit blasting (Figure 11.22) [Traynelis]. Because the materials and bearing geometry are the same for the Prestige I, II, and ST, these designs are biomechanically and tribologically identical.

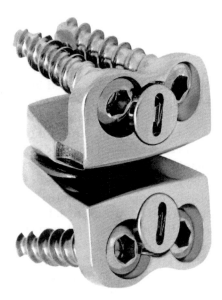

Fig. 11.22.
The Prestige ST cervical disc replacement. *(Reproduced with permission from Medtronic Sofamor Danek, Memphis, TN.)*

A small pilot study was conducted with 15 patients, to evaluate the clinical outcomes (in particular safety and efficacy) associated with the Prestige I [Robertson and Metcalf 2004; Wigfield et al. 2002]. Like the clinical study of the Bristol/Cummins disc, the pilot study for the Prestige I targeted patients at high risk of adjacent level degeneration, including patients with previous multilevel cervical fusions. The average Neck Disability Index improved from 43 (measured preoperatively) and stabilized at 30 after two and four years postoperatively, but the difference in the outcomes was not significant because the number of patients enrolled in the study was too small [Robertson and Metcalf 2004; Wigfield et al. 2002]. The cervical prosthesis was found to effectively preserve motion at the treated level. Measurable intervertebral motion was detected in all cases during flexion and extension, with a mean angular rotation of 6.5 degrees (range: 1 to 15 degrees), and with a maximum of 2 mm of anteroposterior translation [Wigfield et al. 2002]. Two of the fixation screws fractured in one patient at six months, but these were not related to clinical outcome [Wigfield et al. 2002]. None of the screws backed out, confirming the effectiveness of the locking screw in each end plate. Four patients reported neck pain during extension, which was unrelated to the implant (as confirmed by CT myelogram studies). One Prestige I implant was revised at 12 months due to persisting pain that did not resolve after the implant was removed and the treated level was fused. Analysis performed on the tissue surrounding the explanted device revealed "no histologic evidence of inflammation or infection and no significant wear debris" [Wigfield et al. 2002]. After four years of follow-up, none of the patients had developed adjacent level disease [Robertson and Metcalf 2004].

An international two-year prospective, randomized clinical trial (RCT) was conducted with the Prestige II, as compared with a "gold standard" anterior cervical decompression and fusion (ACDF) procedure using iliac crest autograft [Porchet and Metcalf 2004]. A total of 55 patients (27 patients with the Prestige II, 28 control patients) were enrolled in the study from four centers located in the United Kingdom, Belgium, Switzerland, and Australia. At the time of publication, 37 patients had been followed for 12 months, and nine patients had been followed for 24 months. No significant difference was noted in the number of adverse events between the two procedures. There was one technique-related complication related to the artificial disc (malpositioning) that required revision, device removal, and fusion at four months. However, there were no device related complications reported for the Prestige II series. For both the investigational and control groups, the Neck Disability Index (NDI) improved significantly after treatment, but remained essentially unchanged thereafter. There was no significant difference in NDI between ACDF and the Prestige II patients. The Prestige II patients maintained segmental mobility, with an average of 5.9 degrees of angular motion at 12 months, whereas no significant motion was observed in the ACDF group after the same time interval. Overall, the RCT data suggested that the Prestige II appeared as safe as ACDF, and was effective at maintaining the mobility of the treated level [Porchet and Metcalf 2004].

"Worst-case" static and fatigue testing was performed in which Prestige I components were installed with a 1 mm gap between the end plates and UHMWPE blocks, to induce accelerated bending failures [Wigfield et al. 2002]. Both 12- and 14-mm-diameter components were evaluated. Static axial loads of 1,300 N to 6,200 N produced 1 to 5 mm of displacement, but did not result in permanent deformation or failure. During fatigue conditions, cyclic loads of 150 to 225 N produced no evidence of failure up to 10 million cycles. Cyclic loading of greater than 500 N (up to 3,000 N) produced localized crack initiation near the anterior screw holes, but these cracks did not propagate to produce catastrophic failure of the implants. No details about the testing rate or environment were provided in this study. A similar battery of static and fatigue tests was repeated for the Prestige II design [Porchet and Metcalf 2004].

The *in vitro* biomechanics of the Prestige II were investigated in four cervical spines (C2-C7) by testing them sequentially in the intact state, following disc arthroplasty, and then after single-level anterior fusion using the Orion cervical plating system (Medtronic Sofamor Danek, Memphis, TN) [DiAngelo et al. 2003]. The investigators developed a custom-built load frame attached to a servo-motor load actuator (International Device Corp., Novato, CA) with a robotic controller (Adept, Inc., San Jose, CA) in line with a load cell. Custom fixtures were then used to drive the cervical spine in displacement control to produce flexion/extension, lateral bending, or axial rotation. They found no significant difference in the flexibility of the intact spines and the disc replacement. However, significantly less motion was detected between the intact spine and the fused condition. The authors concluded that the Prestige II design did not alter the kinematics of the operated site or the adjacent segments.

Wear testing results for the Prestige ST have been described by Anderson et al. [2004]. These tests were conducted for 10 million cycles in flexion/extension (±9.7 degrees ROM, with 148 N loading at 2 Hz), followed by five million cycles of coupled lateral bending (±4.7 degrees ROM, with 49 N loading at 2 Hz) and axial rotation (±3.8 degrees ROM, with 49 N loading at 2 Hz). Tests were performed at body temperature in bovine calf serum. After a total of 20 million cycles, the average wear rate was $0.2\,mm^3$/million cycles.

Anderson's study is also noteworthy as it is the only published paper that describes the wear assessment of retrieved Prestige discs (presumably of the ST design, implanted for 18 and 39 months) [Anderson et al. 2004]. Two discs were revised because of infection and malpositioning, respectively. Metallic wear debris was "observed ubiquitously" in histological sections of the retrieved tissues surrounding the two implants, but without an associated inflammatory response. Anderson and colleagues also compared the extent of wear observed in SEM images, taken from the 39-month retrieval, and components from a wear simulator. Overall, the retrieved component exhibited less wear than the wear-tested component. Anderson's paper also mentions fretting and/or crevice corrosion at the head of the screws in one of the retrieved implants.

The Prestige ST became commercially available in Europe in 2002. Medtronic Sofamor Danek has initiated a prospective randomized trial for the Prestige ST in the United States. No peer-reviewed data from this trial have yet been published.

11.4.1.3 Low-profile Designs (Prestige STLP, Prestige LP)

Starting in 2002, the Prestige was further redesigned to provide primary fixation without the use of bone screws and an anterior profile, resulting in the Prestige STLP (the LP stands for "low profile") [Traynelis 2004, 2005]. With the Prestige STLP, primary fixation is achieved using two parallel rails on each component (Figure 11.21) [Traynelis 2005]. The back surface was roughened to provide secondary fixation. The bearing geometry and the implant material (316 stainless steel) were not changed from the previous Prestige ST design. Clinical implantations of the Prestige STLP began in Europe in 2003.

Stainless steel is not MRI compatible, making it impossible to evaluate the soft tissues adjacent to the treated cervical level using this modality. Although titanium and titanium alloys are generally more MRI compatible than stainless steel, the wear properties of these materials are generally inferior. To overcome this limitation, the manufacturer developed a novel metal matrix composite with better wear properties than Ti alloy, but which retains its MRI compatibility. The composite chosen for cervical disc applications uses Ti6Al4V alloy as the metal matrix. The Ti alloy is hardened using a dispersed phase of titanium carbide (TiC). The carbide phase increases the stiffness of the material, thereby improving its wear resistance.

In addition to the use of a unique bearing material, the back surface of the Prestige LP is titanium plasma sprayed for bone ingrowth (Figure 11.23) [Traynelis 2005]. The Prestige LP was clinically used in Europe starting in 2004. The prospective randomized IDE trial for the FDA is currently underway.

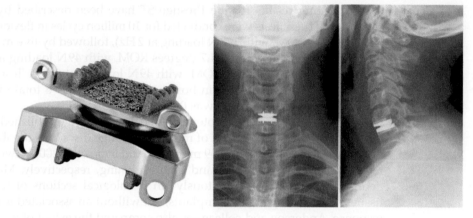

Fig. 11.23.
The Prestige LP cervical disc replacement. (A) Implant photograph; (B) AP and lateral radiographs of the Prestige LP implanted in the cervical spine. *(Reproduced with permission from Medtronic Sofamor Danek, Memphis, TN.)*

11.4.2 Bryan Artificial Disc

With over 10,000 patients having been implanted worldwide, the Bryan artificial disc has the distinction of being the most widely used cervical disc replacement in clinical use today [Rouleau 2005]. Invented by Vincent Bryan, Jr., in the early 1990s, and clinically implanted starting in 2000, the Bryan disc employs a unique mobile bi-convex hyperelastic core that articulates against dual concave titanium alloy shells (Figure 11.24). The following sections summarize the design, materials, clinical literature, and biomechanical test data for the Bryan artificial disc.

11.4.2.1 Design and Materials of the Bryan Artificial Disc

The design of the Bryan disc has remained essentially unchanged since its clinical introduction. In addition to preservation of normal disc motion, a unique design criterion for the Bryan artificial disc was that it should have axial compliance, similar to a natural disc [Rouleau 2005]. Bryan was acutely aware that historical orthopedic biomaterials, such as UHMWPE and metallic alloys, have negligible axial compliance and shock absorption as compared with the natural disc [Le Huec et al. 2003]. In this respect, the Bryan artificial disc embodies a biomimetic design philosophy, similar to the AcroFlex (detailed earlier in this chapter). Unlike the AcroFlex, however, the Bryan disc incorporates a deformable load-bearing polymeric nucleus that articulates against concave metallic shells. In this respect, the Bryan design incorporates total joint replacement technologies, albeit with novel nontraditional bearing materials.

Because of its design objectives of motion preservation and axial compliance, the Bryan disc is necessarily more complex that other artificial discs, as it

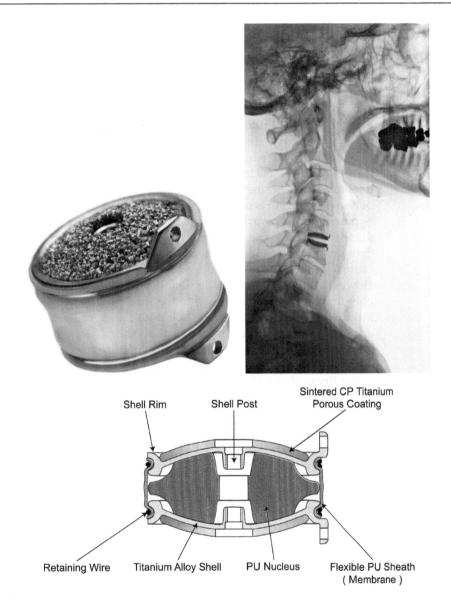

Fig. 11.24.
The Bryan cervical disc replacement. (A) Implant photograph; (B) design schematic; (C) lateral radiograph of the Bryan disc implanted in the cervical spine. *(Reproduced with permission from Medtronic Sofamor Danek, Memphis, TN.)*

includes two end plates or shells, a polymer core, a polymer sheath, and metallic centralizing pins (Figure 11.24a). The hyperelastic core is contained in a flexible polymeric sheath (also referred to as a membrane) that is filled with saline solution intraoperatively. The polymeric outer sheath was designed to prevent soft-tissue encroachment of the bearing surfaces, as well as to provide a controlled fluid lubrication environment for the articulations between the core and the end plate shells. Although the sheath prevents soft tissues and biological macromolecules from entering the artificial disc, it is permeable to water. Therefore, the nucleus is intended to remain hydrated *in vivo* and to articulate against the Ti alloy shells in an aqueous saline environment. Because the sheath is fixed to the shell, it is capable of supporting tensile stresses, and thus functions biomechanically as a soft "stop" or limit to flexion/extension motion.

To achieve its objective of axial compliance, Bryan's design employs polyurethane biomaterials that are available with varying durometers (hardness). The sheath and the core of the artificial disc are fabricated from two different types (or resins) of polyurethane. Specifically, a low-durometer (softer) polyurethane resin is used for the membranous sheath, whereas the central core is fabricated from a higher-durometer (stiffer) resin. Extremely tough and ductile, polyurethanes encompass a broad family of polymeric biomaterials that have an extensive clinical track record, especially in cardiovascular applications [Stokes, McVenes, and Anderson 1995; Zdrahala and Zdrahala 1999]. However, a well-established limitation with the use of certain polyether-based polyurethanes has been related to their biostability, which can result in chemical degradation *in vivo* [Stokes, McVenes, and Anderson 1995; Zdrahala and Zdrahala 1999]. The precise specifications and physical properties of the unique polyurethanes used in the Bryan artificial disc have not yet been published [Rouleau 2005]. However, to evaluate the susceptibility of the proprietary resins in the Bryan disc to biodegradation the molecular weight and chemical composition has been characterized using gel permeation chromatography (GPC) and Fourier transform infrared spectroscopy (FTIR), respectively, both before and after implantation [Anderson et al. 2004]. Although the sheath has a higher molecular weight than the core (170 ± 15 kD versus 116 ± 2 kD), no significant difference was detected between control and retrieved artificial discs [Anderson et al. 2004]. Consequently, the published GPC and FTIR analyses suggest that the two polyurethane resins used in the Bryan artificial disc are stable in a biological environment, but these data are only based on analysis of retrievals with up to 10 months of implantation.

The metal shells of the Bryan are fabricated from forged Ti-6Al-4V ELI alloy because of its MRI compatibility [Rouleau 2005]. The outer surfaces of Ti alloy shells are coated by sintering irregular shards of CP Ti, thereby forming an interconnected 3D porous network on the exterior of the prosthesis. Because of its porosity, this exterior surface has the potential for bone ingrowth, which has been verified in animal and retrieval studies, as will be further discussed later in this section [Jensen et al. 2005]. The inner articulating surfaces of the metal shells are highly polished.

11.4.2.2 Clinical Studies of the Bryan Artificial Disc

The Bryan disc is implanted using a typical ACDF approach, but the preparation of the disc space to accommodate the prosthesis is more complex than a fusion procedure [Wang, Leung, and Casey 2005]. Specifically, the circumferential edges of the metal shells in the Bryan disc are intended to be implanted

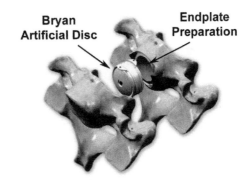

Fig. 11.25.

Implantation technique of the Bryan cervical disc, by milling the vertebral end plates to accommodate the domed outer surfaces of the prosthesis. *(Reproduced with permission from Medtronic Sofamor Danek, Memphis, TN.)*

flush with the rim of the vertebral end plates. Consequently, during the implantation procedure the vertebral end plates are precisely machined with specialized instrumentation, creating countersunk spherical mating concavities that accommodate the domed shells of the prosthesis (Figure 11.25).

The Bryan disc received clinical approval for implantation in Europe starting in January of 2000 [Goffin et al. 2003]. Consequently, only short-term clinical data, with two years of follow-up or less, have been published. The published clinical outcomes for the Bryan artificial disc are summarized in Table 11.6. The largest and most complete body of clinical data currently available has been published by a multi-center European consortium of spine surgeons, in what is referred to as the "Bryan Disc Study" [Goffin et al. 2002, 2003; Leung et al. 2005]. This prospective observational cohort study is being conducted by seven centers in six countries (Belgium, England, France, Germany, Italy, and Sweden). The Bryan Disc Study was established using SF-36, as opposed to the Oswestry Neck Disability Index, as a validated clinical outcome measure [Leung et al. 2005]. Overall, the Bryan Disc Study, as well as other prospective studies, have thus far reported encouraging short-term clinical success rates (Table 11.6). These studies, in particular the recent study by Pickett et al. [Pickett, Rouleau, and Duggal 2005], demonstrate that the Bryan disc also preserves intervertebral motion at the treated level (Table 11.6).

Procedure-related complications (e.g., hematomas, unresolved neck and arm pain, and cerebrospinal fluid leakage during posterior decompresssion) have been reported in the clinical literature (Table 11.6). Recently, heterotopic ossification (HO) has been reported as a rare complication in studies of the Bryan disc [Leung et al. 2005; Sekhon 2004]. In the Bryan Disc Study, the incidence of HO has been reported as high as 18% [Leung et al. 2005]. However, sufficient bone growth spanning the intervertebral spaces to limit movement of the treated level was only observed in 6/90 (7%) patients. The authors theorize that residual bone dust, produced during milling of the vertebral end plates, may stimulate HO, and they advocated copious irrigation as well as nonsteroidal

Table 11.6.
Clinical details of primary peer-reviewed studies involving the Bryan cervical artificial disc.

	Bryan (Bryan 2002)	Goffin et al. (Goffin et al. 2002, 2003; Leung et al. 2005)	Sekhon et al. (Sekhon 2003, 2004)	Pickett et al. (Pickett, Rouleau, and Duggal 2005)	Papadopoulos (Papadopoulos 2005)
Study type	Pcoh	Pcoh	Pcoh	Pcoh	RCT
Type of prosthesis	Bryan	Bryan	Bryan	Bryan	Bryan
Average age			44		
Age range	26–79	26–79	31–55		
No. of patients	97	146	11	20	56
No. of arthroplasties	97	189	15	24	56
Average follow-up in months			18.4	24	
Range in follow-up in months	0–24	6–24	10–32		12–24
Good or excellent	87–89% (n = 8–40)	90–96% (n = 25–49)	91%		
Initial NDI score, Average ± SD			54 ± 17		47
NDI score at longest follow-up, average ± SD			13 ± 12		7
Secondary surgery	1/97 (1%)	7/146 (5%)	0/11		N/A
Heterotopic ossificiation	0/97	16/90 (18%)	1/11		N/A
Complications	5/97 (5%)	11/146 (8%)	2/11		N/A
Average range of motion (± SD)	11° ± 5°	9° ± 5°	N/A	9°	7°

Pcoh (prospective cohort study); RCT (randomized controlled trial); NDI (Neck Disability Index); N/A (not available).

anti-inflammatory drugs as potential prophylactic countermeasures [Leung et al. 2005].

Although the Bryan disc has been widely used clinically, very few revisions have been reported requiring device removal. In a recent review article, Anderson indicated that 10 Bryan disc revisions had thus far been performed worldwide [Anderson et al. 2004]. Four revisions were reportedly due to infection, and the remaining six were caused by "incomplete neural decompression" [Anderson et al. 2004]. Thus far, none of the complications reported in clinical studies nor any of the reported worldwide revisions have been related to malfunctioning or failure of the Bryan prosthesis itself.

11.4.2.3 Biomechanical and Tribological Testing of the Bryan Artificial Disc

Because the Bryan disc employs not only an innovative design but also two novel polyurethane biomaterials—with no preexisting clinical history as long-term orthopedic bearing materials—the availability of detailed, pre-clinical test data for peer-reviewed scrutiny is an essential prerequisite to establish viability of the new design and biomaterial technologies for the clinical community. Currently, a body of biomechanical and tribological test data has already been published for the Bryan artificial disc in the peer-reviewed scientific literature [Anderson et al. 2003, 2004; Jensen et al. 2005]. Overall, the published studies demonstrate the wear resistance of the Bryan artificial disc design and confirm the biocompatibility of the wear debris and the porous coating.

Wear testing of the Bryan disc was performed using a cervical spine simulator, under sinusoidal peak loading of 130N [Anderson et al. 2003]. The duty cycle consisted of ±4.9 degrees flexion/extension and ±3.8 degrees axial/rotation. These two degrees of freedom were synchronized in phase (with both peaks occurring simultaneously) at a rate of 4Hz. Within 72 hours of the start of the test, the nuclei of the prostheses were hydrated with saline, but the assembled prostheses were then immersed in bovine serum at body temperature for the duration of the test. Six implants were wear tested to 10 million cycles, with three devices serving as load-soak controls. All of the prostheses survived the test protocol, with no externally detectable damage to the outer sheath. Pressure testing confirmed that the sheath was intact following the test. When the implants were disassembled and the nuclei measured following 10 million cycles of testing, a 1.8% mass loss and a 0.8% height reduction in the core were determined with respect to the load-soak controls. Absolute mass and height measurements were not reported for the nucleus. Wear particle characterization was performed in accordance with ASTM F1877-98. The overall size of the particles, characterized by the equivalent circle diameter, ranged between 1 and 315µm (3µm on average).

A second series of wear tests was performed without a membrane so that the height and weight of the nucleus could be routinely monitored throughout the test [Anderson et al. 2003]. The testing was performed in a saline environment, which is what would be expected to be lubricating the nucleus when the membrane was intact. Testing was conducted until end plate impingement occurred due to height loss (wear) of the nucleus, which occurred between 37.7 and 40 million cycles. Over that time, progressive wear was associated with a height loss of 0.02mm per million cycles.

Animal studies were conducted using both higher primate and caprine models [Anderson et al. 2003]. The Bryan disc was implanted in the cervical spines of two adult male chimpanzees [Anderson et al. 2003]. The devices were revised along with periprosthetic tissue biopsies after three months, and the primates received a fusion. Standard H&E-stained sections were analyzed, along with periodic acid-Schiff (PAS)-stained sections. Polymeric wear debris was detected in the tissues from one of the two chimpanzees, but no local inflammatory reaction was observed.

A series of 10 nubian goats were also implanted with the Bryan disc [Anderson et al. 2003]. After 3, 6, and 12 months, the animals were euthanized and both the periprosthetic tissue, as well as the lymph nodes, liver, spleen, and cervical spinal cord were examined for evidence of biological reactions to wear debris. In addition to the animals that received a Bryan disc, one goat did not receive any implant (control); four more goats received an anterior cervical plate and were followed for 12 months. Particulate material was characterized as polarizable (likely polyurethane debris from the disc) or nonpolarizable (e.g., Ti debris from the disc or from cervical plates). Polymeric debris was observed in the three periprosthetic tissue samples of one goat. However, the wear debris was located extracellularly and was not associated with an inflammatory reaction. Particulate wear debris was also observed in the epidural space of two animals but was not associated with an inflammatory reaction. Although some evidence of metallic wear debris, or its products (referred to as "nonpolarizable granular material" in the paper), was detected in two of the artificial disc-implanted goats, all of the goats implanted with a cervical plate exhibited far greater evidence of this type of particulate wear debris. Overall, the biological response to wear debris generated by the Bryan disc was judged to be "satisfactory without significant inflammatory reaction" [Anderson et al. 2003].

Retrieval analysis of six explanted Bryan discs has been performed after implantation periods ranging from 4 to 16 months [Anderson et al. 2004]. Dimensional measurements of the nucleus were found to be within the initial, as-manufactured tolerances of the components. Periprosthetic tissue was obtained in two cases, and showed evidence of extra-cellular and phagocytosed polymeric wear debris. No metallic wear debris was detected. When polymeric wear debris was identified histologically, it was associated with the presence of macrophages and foreign body giant cells. No evidence of acute inflammation, infection, or osteolysis was found. Qualitatively, the magnitude of the biological response was judged by the authors to be satisfactory.

The extent of bone ingrowth into the porous coating has also been evaluated from explanted Bryan discs [Jensen et al. 2005]. In two cases, the artificial discs were retrieved from chimpanzees after 12 weeks. Prior to revision, the primates were administered tetracycline hydrochloride for two days, after 7 and 11 weeks following initial implantation. Fluorochrome labeling was then able to successfully confirm new bone growth in the porous coating. Two artificial discs were also obtained by revision surgery from human patients after 8 to 10 months of implantation. Retrieved metal shells were embedded in polymer, sectioned, polished, and viewed under optical microscopy. The extent of bone ingrowth ranged between less than 10% and between 40% and 50% for the end plates revised from primates at 12 weeks. From the human patient retrievals, the average extent of ingrowth was 30% ±12%. Overall, the results of this study supported the hypothesis that new bone grows into the pores of the Bryan shells *in vivo*.

11.4.3 ProDisc-C

The ProDisc-C, produced by Synthes, is a cervical version of the lumbar ProDisc II and employs metal-on-UHMWPE articulation (CoCr alloy) (Figure 11.26). Like the ProDisc II, the ProDisc-C is a ball-and-socket CoCr/UHMWPE bearing. In contrast to the lumbar design, in the ProDisc-C the UHMWPE component is provided already inserted into the inferior end plate by the manufacturer. Bone-implant fixation is achieved by a combination of a keel and titanium plasma sprayed surface, similar to the ProDisc II. Naturally, the size and proportion of the keel and articulations are much smaller in the ProDisc-C as compared with the ProDisc II, but the technology underlying both designs is identical. Synthes has started a prospective randomized clinical trial with the ProDisc-C for the FDA, but no additional details are currently available.

Bertagnoli and associates have reported promising one-year clinical follow-up for the ProDisc-C [Bertagnoli et al. 2005]. Starting in December of 2002, the ProDisc-C study included 27 single-level patients who were implanted between C4-C5 and C6-C7. The average patient age was 49 years (range: 31 to 66 years). No device-related or procedure-related complications were reported. After one year, the patients' average range of motion had improved from 4.2 degrees (preoperative ROM) to 10.2 degrees. The patients' Neck Disability Index (NDI) also improved, on average, from 28.9 points (preoperatively) to 18.8 points at one year.

In vitro biomechanical testing of the ProDisc-C was performed by DiAngelo et al. [2004]. Six cervical spines (C2-C7) were tested sequentially in the intact state, following disc arthroplasty, and then after a simulated single-level fusion. The testing frame was a custom-built load frame attached to a servo-motor load actuator (International Device Corp., Novato, CA) with a robotic controller (Adept, Inc., San Jose, CA) in line with a load cell. Custom fixtures were then

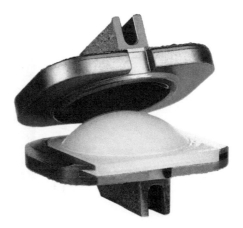

Fig. 11.26.
The ProDisc-C cervical disc replacement implant photograph. *(Reproduced with permission from Synthes Spine, Paoli, PA.)*

used to drive the cervical spine in displacement control to produce flexion/extension, lateral bending, or axial rotation. The authors justify their displacement control method by suggesting that their procedure is more physiologic than applied pure bending moments, and further opine that the use of a follower load "restricts the spine from following its natural path." They measured a significant difference in the extension range of motion of the intact spine (28 degrees ± 6 degrees) as compared with the ProDisc-C (39 degrees ± 2 degrees), but in all other degrees of freedom the flexibility of the intact spines and the disc replacement were not significantly different. The authors concluded that the ProDisc-C maintains the overall flexibility of the cervical spine, comparable to its intact state.

11.4.4 PCM (Cervitech)

The porous coated motion (PCM) artificial disc was invented by Paul McAfee, M.D., and design modifications were subsequently made by Link and Keller, who also commercialized the Charité artificial disc for the lumbar spine [Pimenta et al. 2004]. The PCM is manufactured by Cervitech, Inc. (Rockaway, NJ) (Figure 11.27). Like the Charité, the PCM is a "minimally constrained" bearing design [Link, McAfee, and Pimenta 2004]. The "gliding surfaces" of the PCM are intended to accommodate smooth translations and rotations. Consequently, the PCM strongly depends on the competency of the surrounding soft

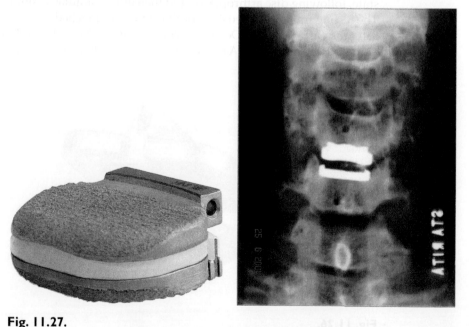

Fig. 11.27.
The PCM cervical disc replacement. (A) Implant photograph; (B) AP radiograph of the PCM implanted in the cervical spine. *(Reproduced with permission from Cervitech, Inc.)*

tissues for proper kinematics. In that respect, it is more analogous to a cruciate retaining total knee replacement than to a total hip replacement. The inventors compare the PCM with a "surface replacement."

The PCM uses the same well-established bearing and coating technologies as the Charité. The reader is referred to the earlier section for a more detailed description of the bearing materials and coating methods. The cephalad and caudal end plates of the PCM are CoCr alloy. The UHMWPE core is fixed to the caudal end plate, so that motion occurs between the concave cephalad end plate and the convex UHMWPE surface. The outer surfaces of the end plates have a serrated profile, for primary fixation, and have the same Ti/CaP coating as the Charité for long-term bone ongrowth [Link, McAfee, and Pimenta 2004]. The porosity of the Ti plasma spray with the PCM is smaller than the Charité, to account for the finer trabecular architecture in the cervical spine as opposed to the lumbar spine [Pimenta et al. 2004].

The anterior profile of the PCM varies with the low-profile and fixed designs. The low-profile design does not protrude beyond the anterior margins of the vertebral column. With the fixed design, on the other hand, the anterior face of the end plates is flanged for supplemental fixation using cancellous bone screws. The anterior flange protrudes over the surface of the vertebral body, much like the Prestige ST (discussed previously). The low profile is the standard implant that has been used in the majority of cases, whereas the fixed design is now only used in "extreme" cases, such as in revisions and adjacent to multilevel fusions [Wefers 2005].

One-year follow-up data are available for the PCM from a prospective pilot study conducted by Pimenta and associates in Brazil. The clinical study began in December of 2002 and included 52 patients who were implanted with 81 cervical discs, between C3-C4 and C7-T1. The average patient age was 45 years (range: 28 to 68 years). Two complications were reported, including one case of anterior migration and one case of heterotopic bone formation. By one year, the clinical success was good or excellent in 97% of the cases. The patients' Neck Disability Index (NDI) had improved, on average, to 15 points (range: 40 to 0) following one year. Preoperatively, the average NDI for the patients was 45 (range: 98 to 18). Interestingly, 10 of the procedures were revisions of previous anterior surgeries [Pimenta et al. 2004].

The range of motion of the PCM and role of the posterior longitudinal ligament (PLL) have been evaluated by McAfee and co-workers [McAfee et al. 2003] using the flexibility testing protocol developed by Cunningham et al. [Cunningham 2004]. Using this protocol, cervical spine sections between C3-C7 were tested from seven donors under applied pure moments in flexion, extension, left and right lateral bending, and left and right axial torsion. As described previously in the Charité section of this chapter, Cunningham's protocol does not include axial preload, and therefore assesses the maximum theoretical flexibility of the cervical spine column. At C5-C6, no significant difference was observed between the flexion-extension range of motion for the PCM versus the intact spine. In contrast, resecting the PLL had a significant effect on ROM in both flexion-extension, axial rotation, and lateral bending as compared with the intact spine. McAfee et al. also implanted the PCM into the

C3-C4 levels of 12 goats, which were followed for 6 months [McAfee et al. 2003]. No significant postoperative complications occurred, and no evidence of wear debris, osteolysis, or particle-related biological reactions was observed.

In a recent study, Dmitriev and co-workers tested the hypothesis that the cervical disc replacement preserves the segmental kinematics and disc pressures of adjacent levels [Dmitriev et al. 2005]. Ten cervical spines were obtained and treated at the C5-C6 level using the PCM disc replacement, allograft dowel, and allograft dowel with anterior cervical plate. The researchers focused their attention on the motion of adjacent segments, C4-C5 and C6-C7, in addition to the treated level. Disc pressures were monitored using miniature pressure transducers (width = 1.5 mm, height = 0.3 mm; Precision Measurement Co., Ann Arbor, MI) inserted into the C4-C5 and C6-C7 discs. The intact spine specimens were first loaded with pure moments (±5 Nm in flexion, extension, left/right lateral bending, and left/right axial rotation) to record the maximum ROM in each degree of the six degrees of freedom. The apparatus for applying the pure moments was similar to that used by Cunningham et al. [2004]. After each of the three interventions, the tests were rerun under displacement control at a rate of 3 degrees for all six degrees of freedom, using the maximum ROM in that particular degree of freedom as the limit for the test. The investigators observed no significant difference in adjacent level disc pressures or segmental motions between the intact and PCM-treated spines. In general, the greatest difference between treatments was observed in flexion and extension testing. Both fusion treatments resulted in higher disc pressures than the intact or TDR-treated spines during flexion/extension testing. Although limited by the lack of axial preload during the testing, the available data from this study support the hypothesis that cervical disc replacement preserves adjacent level disc pressures and segmental kinematics. According to Cervitech's web site (*http://www.cervitech.com*), the company has now started their prospective randomized clinical trial for the FDA, but no further details are available at the present time.

11.4.5 CerviCore

The CerviCore, produced by Stryker Spine, is a cervical version of the Flexi-Core and employs metal-on-metal articulation (CoCr alloy) [Phillips and Garfin 2005]. Bone-implant fixation is similar to the FlexiCore. No data describing either the biomechanical response or clinical performance of this device are available in the literature.

11.5 Many Unanswered Questions Remain

Total disc replacement is a new, promising field of spine implant technology that has the potential to revolutionize the treatment of degenerative disc disease. It is clear from both *in vitro* and clinical data that disc replacements can successfully preserve the motion of treated spinal level. Aside from patient satisfaction and the speed of recovery, there are few objective clinical benefits with disc replacement that manifest in the short-term as compared with fusion. Furthermore, unlike fusion procedures, disc replacements may also need to be revised due to poor implantation technique or failure of the device. On the other hand, over the long term the primary benefit of disc replacement is expected to be the reduced incidence of adjacent segment degeneration, which will hopefully offset the new, and as yet poorly quantified, risks associated with the technology. It will be many years, probably over a decade, before sufficient data have been generated to evaluate whether the promises inherent in total disc replacement have been fulfilled, and in turn whether the long-term benefits of the technology justify the additional risks inherent with their implantation and potential revision. The current technologies for disc replacement should be viewed, therefore, as still being in their infancy.

As we have seen, many different designs and biomaterials are currently being used in disc replacements. In this chapter we have focused primarily on designs that have reached advanced stages of clinical deployment. However, many more disc replacement designs, as yet unproven and unvalidated, are currently under development or in the early stages of animal or human clinical experimentation. All of these disc replacements have the potential to exhibit wear and particulate debris release, at some length scale, however microscopic. For materials with long-standing use in total joint replacements, such as UHMWPE, there may be a risk of osteolysis, albeit in a small patient population. For metal-on-metal disc designs—including the Maverick, FlexiCore, CerviCore, and Prestige—the risk of osteolysis from particulate wear debris is thought to be somewhat diminished because of their lower wear rates. However, the long-term biological consequences of the metallic wear debris and their soluble corrosion products in the spine are also unknown at the present time. Basic clinical data, such as the levels of metal ions in patients implanted with metal-on-metal disc replacements, have not yet been published, so that aspect of disc replacement performance cannot yet be compared with the metal-on-metal hip replacement literature. Furthermore, certain cervical disc designs—such as the Bryan and the Prestige—employ polymeric and metalloceramic biomaterials without any clinical precedence as long-term orthopedic bearings. Although these novel biomaterials appear to exhibit satisfactory short-term biocompatibility, their biological response over the long term is also simply unknown. At least 10 years of clinical follow-up will be needed to confirm that these novel bearing combinations are comparable to historical bearing materials that have a clinical history spanning five decades of continuous use.

This chapter clearly illustrates the crucial role played by the bioengineer in the refinement of artificial discs design, and even more importantly in the verification of the designs to show safety and effectiveness during pre-clinical testing. We have seen that prior to clinical investigations in humans, artificial disc designs are subjected to demanding *in vitro* static and fatigue testing, wear simulations, animal and biocompatibility testing, as well as biomechanical testing in cadavers. This chapter has focused in particular on the methodology employed in previous assessments of disc replacements, because these test methods are novel and currently undergoing continuous improvement. Assessments of artificial disc designs using numerical methods, such as finite element analysis, is a growing and equally promising field of inquiry for bioengineers that is covered in Chapter 14. In the following chapter, we turn to technologies for augmentation of vertebral bodies following compression fractures.

11.6 Acknowledgments

Supported in part by NIH R01 AR47192. This chapter was not written with the financial support of any manufacturer of total disc replacements. However, all of the producers of disc replacements, whose products are mentioned in this review, were contacted by the author, and given the opportunity to verify the factual accuracy of the information related to their products.

The author is indebted to Frank Chan, Ph.D., Medtronic Sofamor Danek, Inc., for his encouragement, assistance with locating figures, and many helpful discussions related to total disc arthroplasty, without which this chapter would not have been possible. Special thanks are also due to Jeffrey Rouleau, Ph.D.; Frank Bono; and Christopher Hughes (Medtronic Sofamor Danek, Inc.) for their assistance. Thanks to Hassan Serhan, Ph.D. (DePuy Spine, Inc.) for feedback about the *in vitro* testing, packaging, and end plate technology for the AcroFlex and Charité designs. I also thank Michael Bushelow, Synthes Spine, for helping to track down the historical details of the ProDisc-L and ProDisc-C. Thanks to Mike Wefers (Cervitech, Inc.) for providing images and clarifying details related to the PCM. The author is especially grateful to Ms. Ashlyn Sakona (Drexel University) and Lauren Ciccarelli and Marta Villarraga, Ph.D. (Exponent, Inc.) for their editorial assistance with this chapter. Special thanks are also extended to Christopher Espinosa and Michael Drzal, Exponent, for assistance with several of the figures.

11.7 References

Anderson, P. A., J. P. Rouleau, V. E. Bryan, and C. S. Carlson (2003). "Wear Analysis of the Bryan Cervical Disc Prosthesis," *Spine* 28:S186–S194.

Anderson, P. A., J. P. Rouleau, J. M. Toth, and K. D. Riew (2004). "A Comparison of Simulator-tested and -retrieved Cervical Disc Prostheses," Invited submission from the Joint Section Meeting on Disorders of the Spine and Peripheral Nerves, March 2004. *J. Neurosurg. Spine* 1:202–210.

Anderson, P. A., R. C. Sasso, et al. (2004). "The Bryan Cervical Disc: Wear Properties and Early Clinical Results," *Spine J.* 4:303S–309S.

Bertagnoli, R. (2005). *Complications and Rescue Strategies in TDR Procedures.* Proceedings of the NASS 20th Annual Meeting. Philadelphia, PA.

Bertagnoli, R., J. Zigler, A. Karg, and S. Voigt (2005). "Complications and Strategies for Revision Surgery in Total Disc Replacement," *Orthop. Clin. North Am.* 36: 389–395.

Bertagnoli, R., N. Duggal, et al. (2005). "Cervical Total Disc Replacement, Part Two: Clinical Results," *Orthop. Clin. North Am.* 36:355–362.

Bertagnoli, R., J. J. Yue, et al. (2005a). "Early Results After ProDisc-C Cervical Disc Replacement," *J. Neurosurg. Spine* 2:403–410.

Bertagnoli, R., J. J. Yue, et al. (2005b). "The Treatment of Disabling Multilevel Lumbar Discogenic Low Back Pain with Total Disc Arthroplasty Utilizing the ProDisc Prosthesis: A Prospective Study with 2-year Minimum Follow-up," *Spine* 30:2192–2199.

Bertagnoli, R., J. J. Yue, et al. (2005c). "The Treatment of Disabling Single-level Lumbar Discogenic Low Back Pain with Total Disc Arthroplasty Utilizing the Prodisc Prosthesis: A Prospective Study with 2-year Minimum Follow-up," *Spine* 30:2230–2236.

Blumenthal, S., P. C. McAfee, et al. (2005). "A Prospective, Randomized, Multicenter Food and Drug Administration Investigational Device Exemptions Study of Lumbar Total Disc Replacement with the Charité Artificial Disc Versus Lumbar Fusion. Part I: Evaluation of Clinical Outcomes," *Spine* 30:1565–1575; discussion E388–390.

Bono, C. M., and S. R. Garfin (2004). "History and Evolution of Disc Replacement," *Spine J.* 4:145S–150S.

Bryan, V. E. Jr. (2002). "Cervical Motion Segment Replacement," *Eur. Spine J.* 11(Suppl. 2):S92–S97.

Bushelow, M., H. Aberman, and C. Kaddick (2005). *Wear Testing of Artificial Total Disc Replacement Prostheses: A Comparison Between Two Wear Simulation Methods.* Global Symposium on Motion Preservation Technology (SAS). New York, NY.

Büttner-Janz, K. (2003). "History," in K. Buttner-Janz, S. H. Hochschuler, and P. C. McAfee (eds.). *The Artificial Disc.* Berlin: Springer.

Büttner-Janz, K., S. H. Hochschuler, and P. C. McAfee (2003). *The Artificial Disc.* Berlin: Springer.

Büttner-Janz, K., K. Schellnack, and H. Zippel (1989). "Biomechanics of the SB Charité Lumbar Intervertebral Disc Endoprosthesis," *International Orthopedics (SICOT)* 13:173–176.

Büttner-Janz, K., K. Schellnack, H. Zippel, and P. Conrad (1988). "Experience and Results with the SB Charite Lumbar Intervertebral Endoprosthesis," *Z. Klin. Med.* 43:1785–1789.

Chan, F. W., P. Pare, et al. (2005). *Is Unidirectional Wear Testing Appropriate for Total Disc Replacement Implants?* Global Symposium on Motion Preservation Technology (SAS). New York, NY.

Charnley, J. (1979). "Low Friction Principle," in *Low Friction Arthroplasty of the Hip: Theory and Practice.* J. Charnley (ed). Berlin: Springer-Verlag.

Cinotti, G., T. David, and F. Postacchini (1996). "Results of Disc Prosthesis After a Minimum Follow-up Period of 2 Years," *Spine* 21:995–1000.

Clarke, I. C., V. Good, et al. (2000). "Ultra-low Wear Rates for Rigid-on-rigid Bearings in Total Hip Replacements," *Proc. Inst. Mech. Eng. [H].* 214:331–347.

cms.hhs.gov (2005). "Medicare Program; Changes to the Hospital Inpatient Prospective Payment Systems and Fiscal Year 2006 Rates: Final Rule," Department of Health and Human Services, Centers for Medicare & Medicaid Services. Accessed at *https://www.cms.hhs.gov/providers/hipps/cms-1500f.pdf* on November 28, 2005:309–322.

Cummins, B. H., J. T. Robertson, and S. S. Gill (1998). "Surgical Experience with an Implanted Artificial Cervical Joint," *J. Neurosurg.* 88:943–948.

Cunningham, B. W. (2004). "Basic Scientific Considerations in Total Disc Arthroplasty," *Spine J.* 4:219S–230S.

Cunningham, B. W., A. E. Dmitriev, N. Hu, and P. C. McAfee (2003). "General Principles of Total Disc Replacement Arthroplasty: Seventeen Cases in a Nonhuman Primate Model," *Spine* 28:S118–S124.

Cunningham, B. W., J. D. Gordon, et al. (2003). "Biomechanical Evaluation of Total Disc Replacement Arthroplasty: An In Vitro Human Cadaveric Model," *Spine* 28:S110–S117.

Cunningham, B. W., G. L. Lowery, et al. (2002). "Total Disc Replacement Arthroplasty Using the AcroFlex Lumbar Disc: A Non-human Primate Model," *Eur. Spine J.* 11(Suppl. 2):S115–S123.

Currier, B. (2004). *Charite Core Oxidation (Shelf).* Charite Artificial Disc F.D.A. Panel Meeting. Gaithersburg, MD, June 2, 2004.

David, T. (1993). "Lumbar Disc Prosthesis," *Eur. Spine J.* 1:254–259.

David, T. (2005). "Revision of a Charite Artificial Disc 9.5 Years In Vivo to a New Charite Artificial Disc: Case Report and Explant Analysis." *Eur. Spine J.* 14:507–511.

de Kleuver, M., F. C. Oner, and W. C. Jacobs (2003). "Total Disc Replacement for Chronic Low Back Pain: Background and a Systematic Review of the Literature," *Eur. Spine J.* 12:108–116.

Delamarter, R. B., H. W. Bae, and B. B. Pradhan (2005). "Clinical Results of ProDisc-II Lumbar Total Disc Replacement: Report from the United States Clinical Trial," *Orthop. Clin. North Am.* 36:301–313.

Delamarter, R. B., D. M. Fribourg, L. E. Kanim, and H. Bae (2003). "ProDisc Artificial Total Lumbar Disc Replacement: Introduction and Early Results from the United States Clinical Trial," *Spine* 28:S167–S175.

DiAngelo, D. J., K. T. Foley, et al. (2004). "In Vitro Biomechanics of Cervical Disc Arthroplasty with the ProDisc-C Total Disc Implant," *Neurosurg. Focus* 17:E7.

DiAngelo, D. J., J. T. Roberston, et al. (2003). "Biomechanical Testing of an Artificial Cervical Joint and an Anterior Cervical Plate," *J. Spinal Disord. Tech.* 16:314–323.

Dmitriev, A. E., B. W. Cunningham, et al. (2005). "Adjacent Level Intradiscal Pressure and Segmental Kinematics Following a Cervical Total Disc Arthroplasty: An In Vitro Human Cadaveric Model," *Spine* 30:1165–1172.

Enker, P., A. Steffee, et al. (1993). "Artificial Disc Replacement: Preliminary Report with a 3-year Minimum Follow-up," *Spine* 18:1061–1070.

Errico, T. J. (2005). "Lumbar Disc Arthroplasty," *Clin. Orthop. Relat. Res.* 435:106–117.

Fernström, U. (1966). "Arthroplasty with Intercorporal Endoprothesis in Herniated Disc and in Painful Disc," *Acta Chir. Scand. Suppl.* 357:154–159.

Fraser, R. D., E. R. Ross, et al. (2004). "AcroFlex Design and Results," *Spine J.* 4:245S–251S.

Gamradt, S. C., and J. C. Wang (2005). "Lumbar Disc Arthroplasty," *Spine J.* 5:95–103.

Goffin, J., A. Casey, et al. (2002). "Preliminary Clinical Experience with the Bryan Cervical Disc Prosthesis," *Neurosurgery* 51:840–845; discussion 845–847.

Goffin, J., F. Van Calenbergh, et al. (2003). "Intermediate Follow-up After Treatment of Degenerative Disc Disease with the Bryan Cervical Disc Prosthesis: Single-level and Bi-level," *Spine* 28:2673–2678.

Griffith, S. L., A. P. Shelokov, et al. (1994). "A Multicenter Retrospective Study of the Clinical Results of the LINK SB Charite Intervertebral Prosthesis: The Initial European Experience," *Spine* 19:1842–1849.

Hilibrand, A. S., and M. Robbins (2004). "Adjacent Segment Degeneration and Adjacent Segment Disease: The Consequences of Spinal Fusion?," *Spine J.* 4: 190S–194S.

Hitchon, P. W., K. Eichholz, et al. (2005). "Biomechanical Studies of an Artificial Disc Implant in the Human Cadaveric Spine," *J. Neurosurg. Spine* 2:339–343.

Hoogland, T., A. D. Steffee, J. D. Black, and A. S. Greenwald (1978). *Total Lumbar Intervertebral Disc Replacement: Testing of New Articulating Spacer in Human Cadaver Spines.* Orthopaedic Research Society. Rosemont, IL.

Huang, R. C., and H. S. Sandhu (2004). "The Current Status of Lumbar Total Disc Replacement," *Orthop. Clin. North Am.* 35:33–42.

Huang, R. C., M. R. Lim, F. P. Girardi, and F. P. Cammisa Jr. (2004). "The Prevalence of Contraindications to Total Disc Replacement in a Cohort of Lumbar Surgical Patients," *Spine* 29:2538–2541.

Huang, R. C., F. P. Girardi, et al. (2005). "Correlation Between Range of Motion and Outcome After Lumbar Total Disc Replacement: 8.6-year Follow-up," *Spine* 30:1407–1411.

Jensen, W. K., P. A. Anderson, L. Nel, and J. P. Rouleau (2005). "Bone Ingrowth in Retrieved Bryan Cervical Disc Prostheses." *Spine* 30:2497–2502.

Kurtz, S. M. (2004). *The UHMWPE Handbook: Ultra-High Molecular Weight Polyethylene in Total Joint Replacement.* New York: Academic Press.

Kurtz, S. M., J. Peloza, R. Siskey, and M. L. Villarraga (2005). "Analysis of a Retrieved Polyethylene Total Disc Replacement Component," *Spine J.* 5:344–350.

Kurtz, S. M., A. van Ooij, et al. (2005). *Central Core and Rim Damage in Retrieved Polyethylene Total Disc Replacement Components.* Proceedings of the NASS 20th Annual Meeting. Philadelphia, PA.

Le Huec, J., Y. Basso, et al. (2005a). "The Effect of Single-level, Total Disc Arthroplasty on Sagittal Balance Parameters: A Prospective Study," *Eur. Spine J.* 14:480–486.

Le Huec, J. C., Y. Basso, et al. (2005b). "Influence of Facet and Posterior Muscle Degeneration on Clinical Results of Lumbar Total Disc Replacement: Two-year Follow-up," *J. Spinal Disord. Tech.* 18:219–223.

Le Huec, J. C., H. Mathews, et al. (2005). "Clinical Results of Maverick Lumbar Total Disc Replacement: Two-year Prospective Follow-up," *Orthop. Clin. North Am.* 36:315–322.

Le Huec, J. C., T. Kiaer, et al. (2003). "Shock Absorption in Lumbar Disc Prosthesis: A Preliminary Mechanical Study," *J. Spinal Disord. Tech.* 16:346–351.

Lemaire, J. P., H. Carrier, et al. (2005). "Clinical and Radiological Outcomes with the Charite Artificial Disc: A 10-year Minimum Follow-up," *J. Spinal Disord. Tech.* 18:353–359.

Leung, C., A. T. Casey, et al. (2005). "Clinical Significance of Heterotopic Ossification in Cervical Disc Replacement: A Prospective Multicenter Clinical Trial," *Neurosurgery* 57:759–763; discussion 759–763.

Link, H. D. (2002). "History, Design and Biomechanics of the LINK SB Charite Artificial Disc," *Eur. Spine J.* 11(Suppl. 2):S98–S105.

Link, H. D., and A. Keller (2003). "Biomechanics of Total Disc Replacement," in K. Büttner-Janz, S. H. Hochschuler, and P. C. McAfee (eds.). *The Artificial Disc.* Berlin: Springer.

Link, H. D., P. C. McAfee, and L. Pimenta (2004). "Choosing a Cervical Disc Replacement," *Spine J.* 4:294S–302S.

Lipman, J., D. Campbell, et al. (2003). *Mechanical Behavior of the Prodisc II Intervertebral Disc Prosthesis in Human Cadaveric Spines.* 49th Annual Meeting of the Orthopedic Research Society. New Orleans, LA.

McAfee, P. C. (2003). "An Explanation of Early, Suboptimal Results from Charité Hospital: Philosophical and Metallurgical Differences," in K. Büttner-Janz, S. H. Hochschuler and P. C. McAfee (eds.). *The Artificial Disc*. Berlin: Springer.

McAfee, P. C. (2004). "The Indications for Lumbar and Cervical Disc Replacement," *Spine J*. 4:177S–181S.

McAfee, P. C., B. Cunningham, et al. (2003). "Cervical Disc Replacement-porous Coated Motion Prosthesis: A Comparative Biomechanical Analysis Showing the Key Role of the Posterior Longitudinal Ligament," *Spine* 28:S176–S185.

McAfee, P. C., B. Cunningham, et al. (2005). "A Prospective, Randomized, Multicenter Food and Drug Administration Investigational Device Exemption Study of Lumbar Total Disc Replacement with the Charité Artificial Disc Versus Lumbar Fusion. Part II: Evaluation of Radiographic Outcomes and Correlation of Surgical Technique Accuracy with Clinical Outcomes," *Spine* 30:1576–1583; discussion E388–E390.

McAfee, P. C., F. Geisler, et al. (2005). *Revisability of the Charité Artificial Disc Replacement: Analysis of 347 Patients Enrolled in the US IDE Study of the Charité Artificial Disc*. Global Symposium on Motion Preservation Technology (SAS). New York, NY.

McKenzie, A. H. (1995). "Fernstrom Intervertebral Disc Arthoplasty: A Long Term Evaluation," *Orthopaedics International Edition* 3:313–324; supplement 154–159.

McMillin, C. R. (1987). "Characterization of Hexsyn, a Polyolefin Rubber," *J. Biomater. Appl*. 2:3–100.

Mathews, H. H., J. C. Lehuec, et al. (2004). "Design Rationale and Biomechanics of Maverick Total Disc Arthroplasty with Early Clinical Results," *Spine J*. 4:268S–275S.

Mayer, H. M., K. Wiechert, A. Korge, and I. Qose (2002). "Minimally Invasive Total Disc Replacement: Surgical Technique and Preliminary Clinical Results," *Eur. Spine J*. 11(Suppl. 2):S124–S130.

Mirza, S. K. (2005). "Point of View: Commentary on the Research Reports That Led to Food and Drug Administration Approval of an Artificial Disc," *Spine* 30: 1561–1564.

O'Leary, P., M. Nicolakis, et al. (2005). "Response of Charite Total Disc Replacement Under Physiologic Loads: Prosthesis Component Motion Patterns," *Spine J*. 5:590–599.

Papadopoulos, S. (2005). "The Bryan Cervical Disc System," *Neurosurg. Clin. N. Am*. 16:629–636.

Phillips, F. M., and S. R. Garfin (2005). "Cervical Disc Replacement." *Spine* 30:S27–S33.

Pickett, G. E., J. P. Rouleau, and N. Duggal (2005). "Kinematic Analysis of the Cervical Spine Following Implantation of an Artificial Cervical Disc," *Spine* 30:1949–1954.

Pimenta, L., P. C. McAfee, et al. (2004). "Clinical Experience with the New Artificial Cervical PCM (Cervitech) Disc," *Spine J*. 4:315S–321S.

Porchet, F., and N. H. Metcalf (2004). "Clinical Outcomes with the Prestige II Cervical Disc: Preliminary Results from a Prospective Randomized Clinical Trial," *Neurosurg. Focus* 17:E6.

Putzier, M., J. F. Funk, et al. (2005). "Charite Total Disc Replacement Clinical and Radiographical Results After an Average Follow-up of 17 Years," *Eur. Spine J*. In Press.

Reitz, H., and M. J. Joubert (1964). "Intractable Headache and Cervico-Brachialgia Treated by Complete Replacement of Cervical Intervertebral Discs with a Metal Prosthesis," *S. Afr. Med. J*. 38:881–884.

Robertson, J. T., and N. H. Metcalf (2004). "Long-term Outcome After Implantation of the Prestige I Disc in an End-stage Indication: 4-year Results from a Pilot Study," *Neurosurg. Focus* 17:E10.

Rouleau, J. P. (2005). Personal communication, Medtronic Sofamor Danek, Memphis, TN.

Sekhon, L. H. (2003). "Cervical Arthroplasty in the Management of Spondylotic Myelopathy." *J. Spinal Disord. Tech.* 16:307–313.

Sekhon, L. H. (2004). "Cervical Arthroplasty in the Management of Spondylotic Myelopathy: 18-month Results," *Neurosurg. Focus* 17:E8.

Serhan, H. (2005). Personal communication, DePuy Spine, Raynham, MA.

Serhan, H., A. Dooris, P. Ares, and S. M. Gabriel (2005). *Wear Characterization of the Charité Artificial Disc Using ASTM Guidelines.* Global Symposium on Motion Preservation Technology (SAS). New York, NY.

Shim, C. S., S. Lee, D. H. Maeng, and S. H. Lee (2005). "Vertical Split Fracture of the Vertebral Body Following Total Disc Replacement Using ProDisc: Report of Two Cases," *J. Spinal Disord. Tech.* 18:465–469.

Sott, A. H., and D. J. Harrison (2000). "Increasing Age Does Not Affect Good Outcome After Lumbar Disc Replacement," *Int. Orthop.* 24:50–53.

Steffee, A. D. (1992). "The Steffee Artificial Disc," in J. N. Weinstein (ed.). *Clinical Efficacy and Outcome in the Diagnosis and Treatment of Low Back Pain.* New York: Raven Press.

Stokes, K., R. McVenes, and J. M. Anderson (1995). "Polyurethane Elastomer Biostability," *J. Biomater. Appl.* 9:321–354.

Szpalski, M., R. Gunzburg, and M. Mayer (2002). "Spine Arthroplasty: A Historical Review," *Eur. Spine J.* 11(Suppl. 2):S65–S84.

Traynelis, V. C. (2004). "The Prestige Cervical Disc Replacement," *Spine J.* 4:310S–314S.

Traynelis, V. C. (2005). "The Prestige Cervical Disc," *Neurosurg. Clin. N. Am.* 16:621–628.

Tropiano, P., R. C. Huang, F. P. Girardi, and T. Marnay (2003). "Lumbar Disc Replacement: Preliminary Results with ProDisc II After a Minimum Follow-up Period of 1 Year," *J. Spinal Disord. Tech* 16:362–368.

Tropiano, P., R. C. Huang, et al. (2005). "Lumbar Total Disc Replacement: Seven to Eleven-year Follow-up." *J. Bone Joint Surg. Am.* 87:490–496.

Valdevit, A., and T. J. Errico (2004). "Design and Evaluation of the FlexiCore Metal-on-metal Intervertebral Disc Prosthesis," *Spine J.* 4:276S–288S.

van Ooij, A., and L. van Rhijn (2005). *Complications of the Charité Disc Prosthesis in 55 Patients and Retrieval in 6 Patients.* Back into Motion: NASS Spring Break. Bal Halbour, FL.

van Ooij, A., F. C. Oner, and A. J. Verbout (2003). "Complications of Artificial Disc Replacement: A Report of 27 Patients with the SB Charite Disc," *J. Spinal Disord. Tech.* 16:369–383.

Wang, A., A. Essner, et al. (1998). "Lubrication and Wear of Ultra-high Molecular Weight Polyethylene in Total Joint Replacements," *Tribology International* 31:17–33.

Wang, M. Y., C. H. Leung, and A. T. Casey (2005). "Cervical Arthroplasty with the Bryan Disc," *Neurosurgery* 56:58–65; discussion 58–65.

Wefers, M. (2005). Personal communication, Cervitech, Inc, Rockaway, NJ.

Wigfield, C. C., S. S. Gill, et al. (2002). "The New Frenchay Artificial Cervical Joint: Results from a Two-year Pilot Study," *Spine* 27:2446–2452.

Wittig, C., R. T. Muller, and H. W. Staudte (1989). "Bandscheibenprosthese SB Charite, Erfolge und Misserfolge an Hand von Fruhergebnisse," *Med. Orthop. Technik.* 109.

Zdrahala, R. J., and I. J. Zdrahala (1999). "Biomedical Applications of Polyurethanes: A Review of Past Promises, Present Realities, and a Vibrant Future," *J. Biomater. Appl.* 14:67–90.

Zeegers, W. S., L. M. Bohnen, M. Laaper, and M. J. Verhaegen (1999). "Artificial Disc Replacement with the Modular Type SB Charite III: 2-year Results in 50 Prospectively Studied Patients," *Eur. Spine J.* 8:210–217.

Zigler, J. E. (2003). "Clinical Results with ProDisc: European Experience and U.S. Investigation Device Exemption Study," *Spine* 28:S163–S166.

Zigler, J. E. (2004). "Lumbar Spine Arthroplasty Using the ProDisc II," *Spine J.* 4:260S–267S.

Zindrick, M. R., M. A. Lorenz, and W. H. Bunch (2005). "Editorial Response to Parts 1 and 2 of the FDA IDE Study of Lumbar Total Disc Replacement with the Charite Artificial Disc vs. Lumbar Fusion," *Spine* 30:E388–E390.

Chapter 12

Vertebral Compression Fracture Treatments

Karen Talmadge, Ph.D.

Executive Vice President, Co-Founder, and
Chief Science Officer, Kyphon Inc. Sunnyvale, CA

12.1 Vertebral Body Compression Fractures: The Clinical Problem

Each year, an estimated more than 700,000 osteoporotic vertebral compression fractures (VCFs) occur in the United States [Riggs and Melton 1995]. Osteoporosis is a disease wherein bone mineral loss couples with changes in bony microarchitecture. The disease can lead to fracture of vertebral bodies subjected even to normal loads. Other causes of VCFs include various conditions that lead to osteopenia (such as steroid treatment, cancer, or infection), as well as trauma.

Only 25 to 35% of fractures due to osteopenia come to medical attention [Cooper et al. 1992]. While some of the undiagnosed fractures may not be acutely symptomatic, there are other reasons for under-diagnosis. VCFs apparent on X-ray have been overlooked in up to 75% of cases [Delmas, van de Langerijt, and Watts 2005]. In addition, vertebral bodies that appear to have no or only mild deformity on initial X-ray can collapse with time. For example, in one study 42% (89/210) of patients with osteoporosis presenting with acute back pain had no or only mild vertebral body deformity initially, but follow-up imaging showed progressive collapse over 6 to 18 months, with the patients experiencing multiple episodes of intense pain [Lyritis et al. 1989]. More rapid changes have also been documented. Heggeness [1993] reported eight cases of

VCF in which the initial X-ray showed no or mild deformity, but the patients returned with neurologic symptoms within 1 to 12 weeks. X-rays revealed that the fractures had rapidly progressed to become osteoporotic burst fractures, with retropulsed bone and cord compression.

In patients with bone weakened by osteopenia, conventional surgery is generally not performed because the metal implants often fail to anchor in poor quality bone. In addition, many of these patients are elderly and/or debilitated. The large surgery required is invasive, with substantial recovery time, and generally contraindicated. Instead, care of patients with osteoporotic VCFs commonly consists of three options: nonoperative care, vertebroplasty, and balloon kyphoplasty.

12.2 Nonoperative Care of VCFs

12.2.1 Nonoperative Care Technique

Nonoperative care of painful VCFs is historically considered first line treatment for patients with painful VCFs, and usually includes bed rest, narcotic analgesia, and back braces. The goal of therapy is pain palliation until the bone heals. This is often followed by physical therapy to strengthen back muscles, as well as counseling for fall prevention and coping strategies for chronic pain [Gold et al. 1989; Papaioannou, Watts, and Kendler 2002].

12.2.2 Nonoperative Care Clinical Outcomes

It has been stated that bone healing occurs within 6 to 8 weeks after immobilization, though studies document that it can take much longer [Lyritis et al. 1989]. Indeed, patients with painful VCFs managed nonoperatively and followed prospectively show modest or no improvements in pain and/or measures of quality of life at six months [Grafe et al. 2005; Kasperk et al. 2005; Komp, Ruetten, and Godolias 2004; Zethraeus et al. 2002], one year [Grafe et al. 2005; Zethraeus et al. 2002], or two years [Hallberg et al. 2004]. They remain substantially below age-matched norms at five years after their last clinically evident fracture [Hall et al., 1999].

Importantly, nonoperative care does not prevent the kyphotic spinal deformity even in the presence of optimal drug therapy for osteoporosis treatment [Reginster et al. 2000]. Multiple studies show that the spinal deformity of an osteoporotic patient substantially impairs functioning and health independent of acute fracture pain.

Kyphotic deformity arising from osteoporotic spinal osteoporosis, *independent of acute fracture pain*, is associated with postural imbalance [Gold et al. 1989; Sinaki et al. 2005], impaired gait [Gold et al. 1989; Sinaki et al. 2005], reduced mobility and/or activities [Gold et al. 1989; Grafe et al. 2005; Nevitt et al. 1998; Pluijm et al. 2000; Sinaki et al. 2005], impaired physical performance [Greendale et al. 2000; Hallberg et al. 2004; Lyles et al. 1993; Nevitt et al. 1998;

Pluijm et al. 2000], decreased pulmonary function [Culham, Jimenez, and King 1994; Pluijm et al. 2000; Schlaich et al. 1998], bloating, eructation, and early satiety [Gold et al. 1996], chronic fatigue [Gold et al. 1996], chronic back pain [Grafe et al. 2005; Ismail et al. 1999; Nevitt et al. 1998], reduced quality of life [Greendale et al. 2000; Hail et al. 1999; Kasperk et al. 2005; Leidig-Bruckner et al. 1997; Oleksik et al. 2005; Pluijm et al. 2000; Silverman et al. 2001; van Schoor et al. 2005; Zethraeus et al. 2002], loss of independence [Gold et al. 1996; Greendale et al. 2000; Lyles et al. 1993], and clinical depression [Gold et al. 1989, 1996]. These decrements increase with increasing deformity [Gold et al. 1996; Ismail et al. 1999; Leidig-Bruckner et al. 1997; Lyles et al. 1993; Oleksik et al. 2005; Pluijm et al. 2000; Silverman et al. 2001; van Schoor et al. 2005]. As measured using SF-36, which allows comparisons among disease states [Ware 1993], patients with one or two VCFs have a quality of life similar to patients with COPD and heart disease, while patients with three or more VCFs have a quality of life similar to patients with stroke or cancer [van Schoor et al. 2005]. Patients with clinically evident and/or radiographic vertebral fractures also have an increased risk of death [Cauley et al. 2000; Ensrud et al. 2000; Johnell et al. 2004; Kado et al. 2004] that exceeds the excess mortality from hip fracture [Cauley et al. 2000; Johnell et al. 2004] and increases with increasing kyphotic deformity [Kado et al. 2004].

The direct relationship of these health and quality of life decrements to the spinal deformity is reviewed in Gold et al. [1996], Liebarman and Talmadge [2005] and Yuan et al. [2004]. In brief, with each additional vertebral body compression fracture the spine shortens, the head and thoracic spine move forward, the ribs angle downward, and the distance between the ribs and the pelvis can be reduced to the point that the twelfth rib rests on the iliac crest. Patients attempt to counterbalance the increasing forward bending moment of their kyphotic posture by flexing their hips and knees, and contracting the posterior musculature to tilt their pelvis. This brings their shoulders and head back up, but stresses the hips and knees, and tightens the hamstrings, which reduces gait velocity and mobility. It also fatigues the paraspinal muscles, contributing to chronic back pain. At the same time, the thoracic and abdominal spaces become restricted. The lungs cannot inflate fully, contributing to pulmonary problems. The abdomen protrudes and distends, contributing to early satiety, nutritional, and metabolic problems. The center of gravity shifts so far forward that the force pushes the patient forward and off balance, increasing the risk of falls and requiring the use of walking aids. Ultimately, the position of the head and neck over the pelvis becomes fixed so that an upright posture becomes impossible.

Biomechanical effects of kyphosis are prominent. As each thoracic fracture brings the spine above it forward, stresses on the anterior spine are increased. Each lumbar fracture has the same effect, by reducing lordosis (effectively, increasing lumbar kyphosis). The normal loads of daily living (such as bending or stepping off a curb) combined with the additional loads creating by the forward bending moment of the kyphosis lead to fracture of the weakened bone. The greater the curvature, the greater the effect, documented clinically in multiple studies [Klotzbuecher 2000; Lindsay, Pack, and Zhengqing 2005; Lindsay et al. 2001; Lunt et al. 2003]. For example, compared to patients with the same bone mineral density but no prior fracture, one prior fracture increases future fracture risk three fold, two prior fractures increase future fracture risk nine fold, and three prior fractures increase future fracture risk 23 fold [Lunt et al. 2003].

Spinal biomechanics would also suggest that subsequent fractures are more likely to be adjacent to preexisting fractures than at remote locations, because stresses are greatest at the apex of a curve, which will often be at the index fracture. Documentation of adjacent fracture risk in the natural history of osteoporosis is limited. However, in one large population of postmenopausal women enrolled in drug studies, among patients with at least two VCFs as detected by X-ray who had a subsequent fracture 58% of these fractures were adjacent [Silverman et al. 2001]. Thus, nonoperative care does not prevent spinal deformity, and spinal deformity has profound effects on patient health and quality of life.

12.3 Vertebroplasty

12.3.1 Vertebroplasty Technique

Vertebroplasty was developed in the 1980s in France by radiologists originally seeking to address vertebral pain without the burden of spine surgery by stabilizing the spine percutaneously [Cotten et al. 1998; Deramond et al. 1998]. The first patients had bony defects resulting from vertebral hemangioma [Galibert et al. 1987], and the technique was later applied to osteoporotic compression fractures [Debussche-Depriester et al. 1991]. The initial U.S. experience was published in 1997 [Jensen et al. 1997].

Conventionally, polymethylmethacrylate bone cement with added radiopacifier is injected into the vertebral body through 10- or 11-gauge spinal needles under X-ray imaging guidance [Cotten et al. 1998; Deramond et al. 1998; Jensen et al. 1997]. This requires relatively liquid bone cement and the use of small syringes [Jensen et al. 1997] to achieve the pressure needed to overcome resistance of the bone to insertion of the cement [Krebs et al. 2005]. Like any liquid, bone cement tends to follow the path of least resistance. One common extravasation pathway includes the venous plexus into the epidural, lateral, and anterior veins, with the potential for neurologic injury if the venous flow is epidural or foraminal [Cotten et al. 1998; Deramond et al. 1998; Jensen et al. 1997; Ryu et al. 2002]. All venous return from the vertebral bodies occurs via the vena cava, creating the risk of cement embolism. Another leak pathway involves the fracture lines themselves, with the potential for soft tissue, nerve root, or cord injury [Cotten et al. 1998; Deramond et al. 1998; Ryu et al. 2002; Yeom et al. 2003]. Cement extravasation is minimized by several maneuvers, including careful imaging, slow delivery of cement, stopping filling as soon as a leak is detected, using the smallest volume of cement required, and stopping the procedure if changing needle position or waiting for the cement to become more viscous does not prevent leaks [Deramond et al. 1998; Jensen et al. 1997; Krebs et al. 2005; Moreland, Landi, and Grand 2001; Ryu et al. 2002; Uppin et al. 2003; Yeom et al. 2003]. The procedure stops when there is a leak that cannot be addressed by using more viscous cement or repositioning the needle, or the vertebral body is judged to be adequately augmented. Vertebral angiograms have been used to assess the presence of potential leak pathways, although whether this predicts leaks is controversial [Gaughen et al. 2002a; Vasconcelos et al. 2002]. The use of CT [Gangi et al. 1999] and open procedures [Wenger and Markwalder 1999] have also been advocated.

Many practitioners now perform vertebroplasty through one pedicle unless medial cement flow appears inadequate [Kim, Jensen, and Dion 2002]. Biomechanical studies on fractured cadaver vertebral bodies treated by unipedicular vertebroplasty describe tests using a platen that could rotate from the center, providing central compression with a pivot point. As the bone cement-filled vertebral bodies resisted normal loads without failing more on one side, the authors concluded that unipedicular filling was sufficient to strengthen the vertebral body even where flow to the contralateral side was limited [Higgins et al. 2003; Tomeh et al. 1999]. However, the strength of vertebral bodies under loads during lateral (side-to-side) bending was not assessed in these two studies. Unlike the loads applied in the studies, lateral bending stresses lateral regions of the vertebral body. As lateral bending is a normal movement of the spine, these studies did not assess the most likely fracture mode arising from an asymmetric fill from a unilateral vertebroplasty failure through an unsupported lateral region during lateral bending.

Filling the vertebral body manually can require high manual pressures exerted on the syringe to overcome resistance to bone cement flow. A number of bone cement delivery systems are being marketed in the United States to facilitate cement delivery. These include the Plexis (Advanced Biomaterials Chatham, NJ), Parallax (Arthrocare Sunnyvale, CA), OsteoJect (Integra Life Sciences Plainsboro, NJ), Equestra (Medtronic Memphis, TN), and PCD (Stryker Kalamazoo, MI) bone cement delivery systems. These systems are fundamentally syringes threaded to provide a mechanical advantage, with the goal of making thick cement delivery easier, thereby presumably reducing the risk of cement leaks. However, turning the threaded handle typically pushes the cement against the narrow opening of the syringe, creating a pressure front. Because of this, cessation of handle rotation does not necessarily stop cement flow until the excess pressure dissipates. Rotating the handle in the opposite direction may reduce, but not stop, the leak once it begins.

The CDO bone cement delivery system (Biomet Interpore Cross) uses a larger bore cannula filled with cement that is then pushed into the vertebral body with a stylet. It is generally used in a unilateral, posterolateral approach to the vertebral body. This system allows for the use of thicker cement without creating a pressure front during delivery. It does not address fracture lines and venous flow pathways (which can lead to leaks), define where the cement will flow, or define how much cement to use.

12.3.2 Vertebroplasty Clinical Outcomes

The literature contains more than 30 retrospective case series with clinical follow-up [Amar et al. 2001; Barr et al. 2000; Cotten et al. 1998; Cyteval et al.

1999; Deramond et al. 1998; Evans et al. 2002; Fourney et al. 2003; Gangi et al. 1999; Gaughen et al. 2002b; Grados et al. 2000; Heini, Walchli, and Berlemann 2000; Hodler, Peck, and Gilula 2003; Jensen et al. 1997; Kallmes et al. 2002; Kaufmann et al. 2001; Martin et al. 1999; McGraw et al. 2002; Peh, Gilula, and Peck 2002; Weill et al. 1996; Wenger and Markwalder 1999] and seven prospective case series [Cortet et al. 1999; McGraw et al. 2002; McKiernan, Faciszewski, and Jensen 2004, 2005; Tsou et al. 2002; Zoarski et al. 2002] reporting single- or two-center experience with patients before and after vertebroplasty. These studies report rapid and sustained pain relief in a majority of patients, with more recent studies quantifying the pain relief as well as measuring function and/or quality of life. Differences in pain outcomes were not detected in patients with acute compared to chronic fractures [Kaufmann et al. 2001]. There is also one concurrently controlled prospective study comparing vertebroplasty to non-operative care showing superior pain relief at 24 hours postoperatively, but not at six weeks or six month follow-up [Diamond, Champion, and Clark 2003]. A randomized clinical trial (RCT) comparing vertebroplasty to nonoperative care is underway at the Mayo Clinic, but enrollment appears to be slow (D. Kallmes, personal communication).

Most studies document procedure-related safety and cement leak rates, although the measurement of leaks is not standardized, so that leak testing modality, leak definition, and method of quantification (per vertebral body or per patient) varies. Leak rates were as low as 8% per patient and 12.5% per vertebral body [McKiernan, Jensen, and Faciszewski 2003] and as high as 81% per patient and 65% per vertebral body [Cortet et al. 1999], including reports of more than one leak pathway per vertebral body [Hodler, Peck, and Gilula 2003; Ryu et al. 2002]. Fortunately, most of these leakages are clinically silent, as the complications of cement leakage during vertebroplasty (increased local pain, symptomatic pulmonary embolus, radiculopathy, cord compression) are estimated to be 1 to 3% in osteoporosis and 5 to 10% in cancer [Deramond 1998]. The higher risk of cement complications in cancer has been attributed to loss of cortex due to tumour [Fourney et al. 2003]. Because cement placement cannot always be controlled, and premature cement fill termination may be required due to a leak, the cement fill may not always be adequate to support the vertebral body, leading to further fracture of a treated level, increased kyphosis, decreased stability, and resumption of pain. This has been reported in 2.5% [Dansie et al. 2005] to 18% [Yoon, Qureshi, and Heller 2005] of fractures treated.

Correction of spinal deformity is usually not a goal of vertebroplasty. However, some authors have reported that postural reduction prior to cement placement can increase vertebral body height and/or reduce angular deformity in patients with "mobile" fractures; that is, those with clefts, usually due to pseudarthrosis [Jang, Kim, and Lee 2003; McKiernan, Jensen, and Faciszewski 2003; McKiernan, Faciszewski, and Jensen 2005; Peh et al. 2003; Teng et al. 2003]. These studies report no or limited change in spinal alignment in fractures that are not mobile. One study did not find improved quality of life using the Osteoporosis Quality of Life Questionnaire in patients undergoing vertebroplasty with mobile fractures that could be reduced compared to those who did not have mobile fractures [McKiernan, Faciszewski, and Jensen 2005]. However, the study noted that the number of patients was small, and the correction of spinal deformity using postural reduction was limited. Another issue in comparing studies is the lack of standardization in defining fracture (see Black et al. [1995] for this issue in osteoporosis drug studies) and measuring height change [McKiernan, Faciszewski, and Jensen 2003].

12.4 Balloon Kyphoplasty

12.4.1 Balloon Kyphoplasty Technique

In orthopedics, the principles of fracture management are [Schatzker 2001]:

- Anatomy restoration
- Rigid fixation
- Minimal tissue disruption
- Safe and early mobilization

The balloon kyphoplasty procedure was created by Mark Reiley (an orthopedic surgeon) and Arie Scholten (a device designer) to treat VCFs secondary to osteopenia following these four principles. The first procedures were performed in 1998.

Figures 12.1a through 12.1d illustrate the balloon kyphoplasty technique. In general, a posterior bilateral transpedicular (shown in Figure 12.1b) or

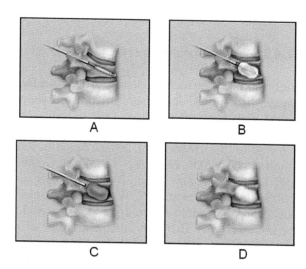

A

B

C

D

Fig. 12.1.

Balloon kyphoplasty procedure. (A) Minimally invasive bone access. (B) Balloon reduction. (C) Cavity creation. (D) Internal fixation.

extrapedicular approach is used to reach the vertebral body through a small cannula. Inflatable bone tamps are positioned under the fractured end plate, and slowly inflated with contrast medium under imaging guidance (Figure 12.1c). When fracture reduction is complete, the balloon tamps are removed, leaving a cavity that is filled with an appropriate material for internal fixation (Figure 12.1d).

Inflation of the Inflatable Bone Tamps increases its volume, which compacts the cancellous bone [Phillips et al. 2003; Togawa et al. 2003] to create a defined cavity while moving the outer cortices apart to restore vertebral anatomy. The process of fracture reduction using balloon tamps is finely controlled. The balloon tamp inflation medium is radiopaque for X-ray visualization. A digital pressure gauge allows the physician to precisely monitor pressure, which reflects the ability of the bone to respond to the IBT.

The degree of fracture reduction achievable for any fracture is not predictable because many osteoporotic fractures collapse slowly with time, with periods of healing [Lyritis et al. 1989], and the IBT is not designed to compress healed bone. Curettes with varying hinged tips can be brought through the introducer cannula and angled within the vertebral body to scrape and score healed bone before balloon placement and/or after initial balloon inflation.

After reduction, the cavity is filled with bone cement, which acts as an internal cast, fixing the fracture (Figure 12.1d). The most common filler today is polymethylmethacrylate bone cement. The creation of the void allows slow and controlled low-pressure manual placement of highly viscous bone cement using a cannula and stylet, avoiding the creation of a pressure wave. The volume to be delivered is known, defined by the final volume of the two balloons. The location for delivery is also known, because compaction of the cancellous bone fills in fracture lines and disrupts internal venous flow pathways [Phillips et al. 2002]. Thus, the path of least resistance for cement flow is generally the void itself.

12.4.2 Balloon Kyphoplasty Clinical Outcomes

There are more than 25 published articles on the outcomes of balloon kyphoplasty with clinical follow-up, including two prospective concurrently controlled trials comparing balloon kyphoplasty to nonoperative care [Grafe et al. 2005; Kasperk et al. 2005; Komp, Ruetten, and Godolias 2004] and 12 prospective studies [Berlemann et al. 2002; Coumans, Reinhardt, and Lieberman 2003; Crandall et al. 2004; Dudeney et al. 2002; Gaitanis et al. 2004; Gerszten et al. 2005; Lane, Hong, and Koob 2004; Lieberman and Reinhardt 2003; Lieberman et al. 2001; Phillips et al. 2002; Voggenreiter et al. 2004; Wilhelm 2003]. (Kasperk et al. report six-month follow-up and Grafe et al. report one-year follow-up in the same cohort.) There are also a number of retrospective series [Fourney et al. 2003; Garfin, Yuan, and Reiley 2001; Ledlie and Renfro 2003; Ledlie and Renfro 2005; Majd, Farley, and Holt 2005; Rhyne et al. 2004]. These studies all demonstrate marked improvements in pain, function, and/or quality of life after balloon kyphoplasty that are rapid (as soon as seven days) and sustained, with follow-up to 18–24 months [Coumans, Reinhardt, and Lieberman 2003;

Ledlie and Renfro 2005]. A multi-center randomized controlled clinical trial comparing balloon kyphoplasty and nonoperative care at 39 centers in the United States was initiated in 1999 but stopped in 2001 due to low enrollment. A 19-center prospective U.S. cohort study was conducted documenting the outcomes of balloon kyphoplasty, and has been submitted for publication. An international multi-center randomized controlled clinical trial comparing balloon kyphoplasty and nonoperative care is currently underway in 21 centers in Sweden, Germany, Austria, France, Belgium, Italy, and the United States, and enrollment was completed at the end of 2005. The patients will be followed for two years.

Cement leaks are reported in kyphoplasty studies with measurements that, as in the vertebroplasty literature, are not standardized. The range of reported leaks is 0% per patient per fracture treated [Fourney et al. 2003] up to 39% of levels treated during open decompressive surgery for patients with osteoporotic burst fractures [Boszcyk et al. 2004]. The VCFs treated with balloon kyphoplasty as reported by Fourney et al. [2003] had posterior cortical disruption with no leaks, yet VCFs without posterior cortical disruption were treated by vertebroplasty, with a leak rate of 8% per vertebral body. In patients undergoing balloon kyphoplasty, Phillips et al. [2002] compared the leak patterns of contrast medium delivered into a fractured vertebral body using a spinal needle (the vertebroplasty model) to the leak patterns of contrast medium delivered into the same vertebral body after fracture reduction and void creation with an inflatable bone tamp (the balloon kyphoplasty model). The number and severity of contrast medium leaks were greatly reduced after use of the inflatable bone tamp.

Two independent groups performed similar concurrently controlled studies in small cohorts, reporting follow-up at six months [Kasperk et al. 2005; Komp et al. 2004] and one year [Grafe et al. 2005, continuing the study of Kasperk et al.]. The patients in Komp et al. had acute fractures (mean age, 34 days), while the patients in Kasperk et al. and Grafe et al. had chronic fractures (minimum duration of symptoms, one year). Both studies showed that, consistent with the osteoporosis literature, patients undergoing nonoperative care did not improve significantly compared to baseline at six months [Kasperk et al. 2005; Komp, Ruetten, and Godolias 2004] or one year follow-up [Grafe et al. 2005]. In addition, the number of subsequent fractures was statistically significantly reduced compared to medical management alone at six months [Komp, Ruetten, and Godolias 2004] and one year [Grafe et al. 2005]. The subset of fractures adjacent to preexisting fractures was also lower, although not statistically significantly so [Grafe et al. 2005; Kasperk et al. 2005]. Komp et al. [2004] also demonstrated that balloon kyphoplasty was superior to nonoperative care in pain and function at six months, while Grafe et al. [2005] showed that balloon kyphoplasty was superior to nonoperative care in pain and mobility at six months, and pain at one year.

Vertebral body height restoration and/or improvements in angulation have been reported in multiple studies [Berlemann et al. 2002; Crandall et al. 2004; Fourney et al. 2003; Gaitanis et al. 2004; Garfin, Yuan, and Reiley 2001; Grafe et al. 2005; Kasperk et al. 2005; Komp et al. 2004; Lane, Hong, and Koob 2004; Ledlie and Renfro 2003, 2005a, 2005b; Lieberman et al. 2001; Majd, Farley, and

Holt 2005; Phillips et al. 2003; Rhyne et al. 2004; Voggenreiter et al. 2004]. Only one study reported that balloon kyphoplasty did not alter vertebral height in 13 patients treated [Feltes et al. 2005]. In an initial report, Lieberman et al. [2001] found that 70% of vertebral bodies had at least 10% of lost midline height restored. Recently, Lane et al. [2004] documented vertebral body height restoration using the same definition in 91% of anterior levels treated and 100% of midline levels treated in patients with fractures due to osteoporosis, and 76% of anterior levels treated and 84% of midline levels treated in patients with fractures due to multiple myeloma. There are no reports of further fracture after treatment, and maintenance of height has been demonstrated at one [Ledlie and Renfro 2003] and two [Ledlie and Renfro 2005b] years.

12.5 Bone Fillers

Both vertebroplasty and kyphoplasty involve the use of bone fillers to stabilize the spine. The ideal bone filler for kyphoplasty and vertebroplasty should:

- Be easy to deliver without leaks
- Be adequately radiopaque so that small volumes are visible on fluoroscopy
- Make excellent contact with the host bone
- Contain no toxic components and remain biocompatible long-term
- Become rapidly load bearing
- Provide sufficient strength to support the vertebral body against physiologic loads
- Become bone in a manner and time frame that maintains spinal stability, or perform in a manner indistinguishable from normal bone
- Serve its function for the lifespan of the patient
- Be on label

There are two classes of biomaterials currently in human use: the acrylic cements and the calcium-based cements. None of the cements on the market today or in development appear likely to meet all of the desired characteristics.

12.5.1 Acrylic Cements

12.5.1.1 PMMAs

Polymethyl methacrylate (PMMA) bone cements have been used since the early 1900s for cranial reconstruction, and since the 1940s in the spine (reviewed in [Cruikshank 1988]). PMMAs contain methyl methacrylate which polymerizes and hardens, achieving high compressive strength compared to cancellous bone. The compressive strength of PMMAs is typically 70 MPa or more, while the compressive strength of vertebral cancellous bone is generally 5 to 10 MPa (see Table 12.1). PMMAs are less able to resist torsion or shear loads compared to compressive loads, but are successfully used inside the vertebral body, where

Table 12.1.

Compressive strength and compressive modulus (stiffness) of bone, disc, and various bone fillers.

Material	Compressive Strength (MPa)	Compressive Modulus (MPa)	Reference No.
Cortical shell	200	5,000	Silva et al., 1997
Vertebral body end plate	—	1,000	Silva et al., 1997
Cancellous bone, normal	5–30	100	Goel et al., 1998
Cancellous bone, osteoporotic	1–10	25	Liebscher et al., 2001; Goel et al., 1998
Disc, normal	—	0.5–2.0	White et al., 1990
Disc, degenerated (grade II)	—	8.4	Kumanesem et al., 2001
PMMA	70–110	2,000–4,000	Lewis et al., 1997
Cortoss	210	8,000	www.orthovita.com
CP cements	30–80*	2,600	Data on file at Kyphon
CS cements	5–80**	2,700	Data on file at Kyphon

CP = calcium phosphate, CS = calcium sulfate, PMMA = polymethyl methacrylate, CP = calcium phosphate, CS = calcium sulfate, PMMA = polymethyl methacrylate.
*In an aqueous environment at 24 hours.
**In a dry environment at 2 to 24 hours.

the torsion and shear loads are also low. The chemical composition of the final polymer, and the means by which polymerization is initiated, varies from product to product. These types of differences alter the handling characteristics and the rate at which the polymer cures, but not the general mechanical properties after hardening. Radiopacity is achieved though the addition of various agents, generally barium sulfate. KyphX HV-R (Kyphon), Parallax with Tracers radiopacifier (Arthrocare), and Spineplex (Stryker) bone cements are currently cleared in the United States for kyphoplasty. Concert Spine VR (Advanced Biomaterial Systems Chatham, NJ), Parallax with Tracers radiopacifier (Arthrocare), and Spineplex (Stryker) bone cements are currently cleared in the United States for vertebroplasty. Ava-Tex bone cement (Cardinal Health Chatham, NJ) is currently cleared in the United States for fixation of pathological fractures. Despite their long-term human use, there are many questions raised about PMMA cements, including:

- *Control during placement:* Greater control is achieved through added radiopacifiers, creating a void to provide a defined location for placement as well as to reduce the force required for delivery, and delivering the cement late in its polymerization phase (while highly viscous).

- *Monomer toxicity:* An infrequent but well-known risk, monomer toxicity typically manifests as transient arterial hypotension. Its incidence can be reduced treating a limited number of levels per operation. Using less cement is an additional approach taken by vertebroplasty practitioners, while balloon kyphoplasty users are able to place the cement very late in its polymerization phase (when free monomer is at a lower level).

- *Exotherm:* Depending on volume and geometry, the core of a PMMA bolus during curing can transiently reach 70 to 100°C. Bench and animal studies, as well as autopsy retrievals, show that these elevated temperatures cause a local thermal necrosis (within a few millimeters). However, bone is a poor conductor of heat, and the vascularity of the vertebral body, along with fluid flow in the spinal cord, rapidly dissipate heat. Thus, no statistically (or clinically) significant change in temperature could be detected in a pig model with 3 mm of bone between a vertebral PMMA bolus and the spinal cord dura [Park et al. 1999]. Similar results were found *in vitro* [Deramond et al. 1998]. No published study provides definitive evidence that the exotherm leads to a clinically significant tissue injury.

- *Bone-cement interface:* A fibrous layer between PMMA and bone is formed in cemented prostheses and in autopsy retrievals after vertebral augmentation [Togawa et al. 2003]. Importantly, however, no published study has shown any clinical sequelae related to this, such as further inflammation, implant cracking, or implant failure.

- *Long-term stability:* Because PMMA does not remodel back into bone, questions remain about long-term stability. Long-term follow-up of vertebroplasty [Grados et al. 2000] and kyphoplasty [Coumans, Reinhardt, and Lieberman 2003; Ledlie and Renfro 2005] has begun to appear in the clinical literature, but there is more substantial long-term follow-up in patients with giant cell tumors (GCTs). GCTs create large metaphyseal cancellous bone defects, often in the tibial plateau and distal femur, areas that routinely experience compressive loads that are greater than those in the spine [Buckwalter, Einhorn, and Simon 2000]. The standard of care today for many GCTs is curettage, adjuvant treatment, and PMMA fixation [Blackley et al. 1999]. There are excellent outcomes in multiple studies reporting long-term follow-up to 18 years [Bini, Gill, and Johnston 1995; Dreinhofer et al. 1995; O'Donnell et al. 1994; Pals and Wilkins 1992; Segura et al. 1997; Wada et al. 2002]. There are also reports of long-term follow-up with PMMA in the anterior spine placed during open surgery [Boker, Schultheiss, and Probst 1989; Duff 1986]. In contrast, failures of PMMA in the spine have generally been associated with posterior fixation or anterior reconstruction involving multiple levels, where shear and torsion loads are high [McAfee et al. 1986]. The GCT and open spine surgery studies support the long-term stability of PMMA for vertebral body internal fixation.

- *Adjacent fracture:* PMMA is slightly than osteoporotic cancellous bone (see Table 12.1). A hypothesis has been proposed that placement of stiffer bone cement leads to adjacent fracture after vertebroplasty or balloon kyphoplasty. This issue is discussed after reviewing other bone fillers.

12.5.1.2 Composite Acrylic Bone Cements

Composite acrylic bone cements consisting of the dimethacrylates, combined with silica (glass) and/or hydroxyapatite, are in clinical use in Europe, and in development in the United States and Asia. The dimethacrylates have a long history in the dental field and allow mix-on-demand, enhancing ease of use compared to PMMAs. The composite acrylic bone cement on the market in Europe and in development in the United States, Cortoss bone cement (Orthovita Malvern, PA) is composed of three dimethacrylate polymers combined with three forms of silica. The mechanical strength after curing approximates cortical bone, around 200 MPa (see Table 12.1). Compared to PMMAs, dimethacrylate composite cements have greater radiopacity and a lower exotherm (~60° C, Orthovita web site). Animal data also suggest that they bond more tightly to bone than PMMAs, possibly because they are less likely to form a fibrous layer between the cement and bone [Erbe, Clineff, and Gualtieri 2001]. However, it has not been established that the exotherm, or a fibrous interface, affects the clinical performance of PMMA. Like PMMAs, these materials are stiffer than cancellous bone, but, unlike PMMA, they are also stiffer than cortical bone (Table 12.1). In contrast to PMMAs, the composites remain relatively liquid, then rapidly harden, and therefore cannot be delivered in the "doughy" (viscous) state. They also do not remodel back into bone. The risk of monomer toxicity, leak rates, complications from leaks, and stability/biocompatibility long-term will be established in clinical studies.

12.6 Calcium Cements

Calcium cements labeled for load-bearing applications in the spine are available in Europe and Japan but not in the United States, where they are under development. Calcium cements are generally prepared by mixing powdered calcium salts with appropriate salt solutions. This allows crystals of calcium salts to nucleate, precipitate, and ultimately entangle, creating a stable 3D lattice held together through strong ionic interactions. Calcium cements have attracted interest in this application because bench, animal, and/or human studies show they are biocompatible, form a tight interface with bone, have no exotherm, include no monomer, and have the potential to undergo remodeling into bone via the body's own metabolic processes. Like PMMA, calcium cements are stiffer than cancellous bone (see Table 12.1).

Calcium sulfate cements (plaster of Paris) have been used to augment bone for over 100 years. There are no calcium sulfate cement formulations labeled for balloon kyphoplasty or vertebroplasty in the United States. Presently available calcium sulfate cements (such as Osteoset, Wright Medical) have been used in long bone defects as an adjunct to hardware [Kelly 2001]. The compressive strength of these cements is generally 5 to 15 MPa, which is within the range of cancellous bone but not greater, although Wright Medical Technology (Memphis, TN) reported their newest calcium sulfate cements have compressive strengths within the range of PMMA cements (80 MPa) at 2 hours in a dry environment (Table 12.1 and Wright Medical Technology web site). However, calcium sulfate cements in general rapidly lose their strength in an aqueous environment due to dissolution, and animal models have shown that the dissolution rate *in vivo* can be faster than the rate at which the bone heals, with the potential for gaps and/or instability [Blaha 1998]. Mixtures of calcium sulfates with other calcium salts are currently being investigated.

Calcium phosphates have been formulated into injectable pastes whose crystalline forms dissolve slowly, including Biopex R (Mitsubishi Medical, Japan), Bone Source (Stryker), Calcibon (E. Merck, Germany), KyphOs (Kyphon), and Norian Skeletal Repair System (Synthes West Chester, PA). Animal studies show that these cements are replaced with bone through endochondral substitution, reducing the risk of gaps. The compressive strength of these cements varies by the specific salts being used, and within a given formulation by the ratio of liquid-to-powder components. Calcium phosphate cements on the market or in development have published compressive strengths in the range of 35 to 70 MPa, exceeding the compressive strength of cancellous bone. The first human studies using calcium phosphates in vertebroplasty (using Biopex R) [Nakano et al. 2002, 2005] and balloon kyphoplasty (using Calcibon) [Grafe et al. 2005; Kasperk et al. 2005] for osteoporotic VCFs have been published. Figure 12.2 is a case from Dr. Hillmeier, a co-author of Kaspek and Grafe, showing fracture reduction and Calcibon calcium cement fixation at six-month follow-up (Figure 12.2b) in a 55-year-old female with a traumatic vertebral compression fracture with a small anterior split component (Figure 12.2a). Oner et al. [2005] and Verlaan et al. [2005] have reported on the outcomes of using balloon kyphoplasty and Bone Source (Stryker) to strengthen the anterior

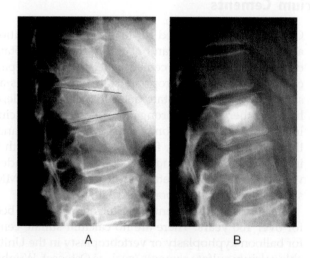

A   B

Fig. 12.2.

Balloon kyphoplasty in a 52-year-old woman with a traumatic L1 fracture. Pre-operative X-ray. Post six-month postoperative follow-up X-ray. Red lines show the angulation created by the fracture (pre) and the near correction of the end plates to parallel (post). (*Courtesy of Dr. Joachim Hillmeier, Heidelberg, Germany*).

column minimally invasively during open stabilization of the posterior column in traumatic burst fractures, avoiding second, open anterior, procedure. A similar study in traumatic burst fractures using Norian Skeletal Repair System has been conducted in the United States (Dr. Vivek Kushwaha, personal communication).

There are many differences between calcium and acrylic cements with respect to handling characteristics. Most calcium phosphate cements were formulated for use in open surgery, not for minimally-invasive delivery. Their flow properties were not optimized for delivery through a cannula. Some newer calcium cements have been formulated to address this issue. Unlike PMMA, which sets through polymerization rather than crystallization, if calcium cements are disturbed during crystallization inadequate final mechanical strength may result. Intra-operative manipulations that are benign with acrylic cements (such as using a device to test whether the cement has hardened inside the vertebral body, or using a mallet to push semi-hardened cement into the vertebral body) can disturb the crystallization process, and the entire cement mass, or a part of it, may not achieve the desired mechanical strength. Compared to PMMA polymerization, crystallization of calcium cements can occur relatively rapidly at body temperature. This reduces the potential for interdigitation, and can create delivery problems if the calcium phosphate cement has a short working time. As with bone grafting contact with the host bone throughout the void is important for maintaining the continuous interface between the bone and cement to promote remodeling. The creation of a void can enhance calcium cement delivery to bone [Nakano et al. 2002].

Since incorporation of calcium phosphate into bone requires active cellular processes, the rate at which this occurs is likely to be influenced by both the nature of calcium cement formulation as well as the healing and/or remodeling potential of the host bone. The suitability of calcium phosphate cements for balloon kyphoplasty and/or vertebroplasty is under active evaluation in Europe and Japan. With balloon kyphoplasty, the focus is using the operative technique for the reduction and internal fixation of traumatic vertebral compression fractures in patients without neurologic injury, replacing nonoperative care or open surgery in appropriate candidates. There are no published data in the spine on long-term outcomes or the rate of remodeling in various patient populations.

12.7 PMMA and the Potential for Adjacent Fracture

Case reports and case series document adjacent vertebral body fracture after placement of PMMA bone cement into osteoporotic vertebral bodies during kyphoplasty [Fribourg et al. 2004; Harrop et al. 2004] and vertebroplasty [Grados et al. 2000; Uppin et al. 2003]. It is commonly assumed that the stiffness of PMMA, being greater than bone, increases adjacent stresses and causes these fractures. As shown in Table 12.1, PMMA is more stiff than cancellous bone (although less stiff than cortical bone). It is also commonly assumed that there is a need for less stiff fillers, and that calcium cements or other compounds might solve this problem. These assumptions are not supported by mechanical testing, the principles of biomechanics, or the osteoporosis literature.

Reports of adjacent fracture, or any fracture, after balloon kyphoplasty or vertebroplasty cannot be interpreted without a matched control group to compare the fracture rate in the absence of cement. This is because there are multiple factors that influence the observed fracture rate, including varying definitions of fracture, even within the osteoporosis literature [Black 1995], as well as multiple independent variables for fracture risk, notably age, bone mineral density, the number of previous fractures, steroid use, and osteoporosis drug treatment. For example, studying the risk of an additional fracture within one year in patients matched for bone mineral density, Lunt et al. [2003] found that patients with a first fracture are three times more likely to have another fracture, patients with a second fracture are nine times more likely to have another fracture, and patients with a third fracture are 23 times more likely to have another fracture compared to patients who have never had a fracture. Moreover, the adjacent fracture rate is high in the natural history of osteoporosis: 58% of patients with more than one vertebral fracture had adjacent fractures in large osteoporosis drug studies [Silverman et al. 2001].

This acceleration of future fracture risk with increasing deformity and the increased likelihood of adjacent over remote fracture are predicted by the biomechanics of the spine (reviewed in Yuan et al. [2004] and discussed previously). Each successive fracture leads to a kyphotic deformity that pushes the spine anteriorly, shifting the center of gravity forward and down and increasing anterior stress. The added stress of the kyphotic deformity leads to fracture at lower and lower loads. The apex of the curve, often the site of the new fracture, experiences the highest stresses, particularly increasing the risk of further fracture in that region. Studies show that balloon kyphoplasty significantly decreases the rate of subsequent fractures compared to nonoperative management [Grafe et al. 2005; Komp, Ruetten, and Godolias 2004], and show a trend toward reducing the subset of subsequent fractures that are adjacent, supporting the role of kyphosis in creating these risks, and the role of deformity correction in reducing them.

The idea that PMMA has to lead to adjacent fracture is also not supported by the giant cell tumor literature, discussed previously. There is not one reported case of adjacent fracture in patients receiving large volumes of bone cement in areas of metaphyseal (and sometimes subchrondral) cancellous bone.

An analogy to fusion is often drawn when suggesting that PMMA in a vertebral body could lead to adjacent fractures. Fusion, however, is not the mechanical equivalent of filling a vertebral body with PMMA. The functional spine unit consists of a disc and the vertebra above and below. The response of any system, including the functional spine unit, is driven by its *least stiff* component. Table 12.1 summarizes the compressive modulus (stiffness in compression) of bone, disc, PMMA, and other cements. In the setting of a vertebral fracture filled with PMMA, the disc is the least stiff component, and therefore load transfer cannot be markedly altered by the presence of PMMA in the bone.

This mechanical principle is illustrated in Figure 12.3 with three springs in a series, the mechanical equivalent of the functional spine unit. In Figure 12.3a,

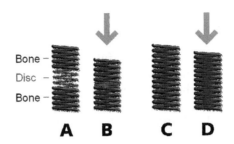

Fig. 12.3.

Three springs in a series. The functional spine unit (two vertebral bodies with a disc in between) represented as its mechanical equivalent, three springs in a series. (A) Two stiffer purple springs (vertebral bodies) with the less stiff orange spring (disc) in between. (B) The functional spine unit model loaded in compression (arrow), showing that the least stiff spring (the disc in orange) will respond while the more stiff components (the vertebral bodies in purple) remain largely unaffected. (C) Three stiff (bony) purple springs in a series represent the functional spine unit after fusion, where disc is replaced by bone (purple). (D) The fused functional spine unit under a compressive load (arrow). The vertebral bodies now respond, due to the loss of the least stiff component, the disc.

the top and bottom springs, which represent vertebral bodies, are stiffer than the middle spring, which represents the disc. Loaded in compression (Figure 12.3b), the response occurs through the least stiff component, which is the middle spring in this model and the disc in the functional spine unit. This mechanical setting can be contrasted with fusion, where the least stiff component (the disc) is replaced with something much more stiff (bone). This is illustrated in Figure 12.3c, showing three stiff springs in a row. This *does* alter load transfer through the bone, as illustrated in Figure 12.3d (three stiff springs loaded in compression).

At least 14 studies have assessed the stiffness of the vertebral body before fracture, after fracture, and after treatment—either vertebroplasty or kyphoplasty—using PMMA, composite acrylic, calcium phosphate, or calcium sulfate bone cements. The vast majority show that placement of bone cement stiffens the vertebral body compared to the fractured state, not that the vertebral body becomes stiffer than normal cancellous bone [Belkoff, Jasper, and Stevens 2002; Belkoff et al. 2001; Berlemann et al. 2002; Perry et al. 2005; Polikeit, Nolte, and Ferguson 2003; Tomita et al. 2003].

Thus, based on mechanical principles and mechanical testing the stiffness of bone cement does not explain the observation that patients suffer additional fractures after balloon kyphoplasty and vertebroplasty, and it does not support the search for a new filler. Instead, mechanical principles show that the kyphosis leads to increased loading, and the osteoporosis literature reflects this reality—the increasing risk of fractures in patients with increasing kyphotic deformity. Concurrently controlled studies show a significantly reduced rate of subsequent fracture in kyphoplasty-treated patients compared to non-operatively managed controls [Komp et al., 2004; Grafe et al., 2005]. These observations support the goal of correcting sagittal balance whenever possible.

12.8 Conclusions

Patients with acutely painful vertebral body compression fractures managed nonoperatively have impaired health and reduced quality of life caused by the resulting kyphotic deformity independent of acute fracture pain. The changes in spinal alignment increase future fracture risk, including adjacent fractures. Vertebroplasty and balloon kyphoplasty are minimally invasive procedures that stabilize the fractured vertebral body, while balloon kyphoplasty is also designed to correct the spinal deformity. Both procedures provide immediate and sustained relief of pain. Two concurrently controlled studies show that balloon kyphoplasty improves pain and quality of life outcomes compared to nonoperative management, while reducing the number of future (and adjacent) fractures. Similar studies for vertebroplasty have not been published. There are acrylic and calcium cements in use or in development for these procedures. None of the cements today have all the desired characteristics. While there are theoretical advantages of newer cements, PMMA has a long history of successful use in areas of compressive loading, including the vertebral body. Concerns that bone cement stiffness leads to adjacent fracture are not justified on mechanical principles. The biomechanics of the spine predict that kyphosis itself increases the risk of future fracture, especially adjacent fractures, and the osteoporosis literature demonstrates this. These studies support the goal of correcting sagittal alignment whenever possible.

12.9 References

Amar, A. P., D. W. Larsen, N. Esnaashari, et al. (2001). "Percutaneous Transpedicular Polymethylmethacrylate Vertebroplasty for the Treatment of Spinal Compression Fractures," *Neurosurgery* 49:1105–1114.

Barr, J., M. Barr, T. Lemley, et al. (2000). "Percutaneous Vertebroplasty for Pain Relief and Spinal Stabilization," *Spine* 25:923–928.

Belkoff, S., J. Mathis, E. Erbe, et al. (2000). "Biomechanical Evaluation of a New Bone Cement for Use in Vertebroplasty," *Spine* 25:1061–1064.

Belkoff, S. M., L. E. Jasper, and S. S. Stevens (2002). "An Ex Vivo Evaluation of an Inflatable Bone Tamp Used to Reduce Fractures Within Vertebral Bodies Under Load," *Spine* 27:1640–1643.

Belkoff, S. M., J. M. Mathis, D. C. Fenton, et al. (2001). "An Ex Vivo Biomechanical Evaluation of an Inflatable Bone Tamp Used in the Treatment of Compression Fracture," *Spine* 26:151–156.

Belkoff, S., J. Mathis, L. Jasper, et al. (2001). "An Ex Vivo Biomechanical Evaluation of a Hydroxyapatite Cement for Use with Vertebroplasty," *Spine* 26:1542–1546.

Berlemann, U., T. Franz, R. Orler, et al. (2004). "Kyphoplasty for Treatment of Osteoporotic Vertebral Fractures: A Prospective Non-randomized Study," *Eur. Spine J.* 13:496–501.

Berlemann, U., S. Ferguson, L. Nolte, et al. (2002). "Adjacent Vertebral Failure After Vertebroplasty: A Biomechanical Evaluation," *J. Bone Joint Surg.* 84B:745–752.

Bini, S., K. Gill, and J. Johnston (1995). "Giant Cell Tumor of Bone: Curettage and Cement Reconstruction," *Clin. Orthop.* 321:245–250.

Black, D. M., L. Palermo, M. C. Nevitt, et al. (1995). "Comparison of Methods for Defining Prevalent Vertebral Deformities: The Study of Osteoporotic Fractures," *J. Bone Miner. Res.* 10:890–902.

Blackley, H., J. Wunder, A. Davis, et al. (1999). "Treatment of Giant-cell Tumors of Long Bones with Curettage and Bone-grafting," *J. Bone Joint Surg.* 81A:811–820.

Blaha, J. D. (1998). Evolving Technologies: New Answers or New Problems? Calcium Sulfate Bone Void Filler," *Orthopedics* 21:1017–1019.

Boker, D., R. Schultheiss, and E. Probst (1989). "Radiologic Long-term Results After Cervical Vertebral Interbody Fusion with Polymethly Methacrylate (PMMA)," *Neurosurg. Rev.* 12:217–221.

Boszcyk, B., M. Bierschneider, K. Schmid, et al. (2004). "Microsurgical Interlaminary Vertebro- and Kyphoplasty for Severe Osteoporotic Fractures," *J. Neurosurg. (Spine 1)* 100:32–37.

Buckwalter, J., T. Einhorn, and S. Simon (2000). *Orthopaedic Basic Science Biology and Biomechanics of the Musculoskeletal System* (2nd ed.). Rosemont, IL: American Academy of Orthopedic Surgeons.

Cauley, J., D. Thompson, K. Ensrud, et al. (2000). "Risk of Mortality Following Clinical Fractures," *Osteoporos Int.* 11:556–561.

Cooper, C., E. J. Atkinson, W. M. O'Fallon, et al. (1992). "Incidence of Clinically Diagnosed Vertebral Fractures: A Population-based Study in Rochester, Minnesota, 1985–1989," *J. Bone Miner. Res.* 7:221–227.

Cortet, B., A. Cotten, N. Boutry, et al. (1999). "Percutaneous Vertebroplasty in the Treatment of Osteoporotic Vertebral Compression Fractures: An Open Prospective Study," *J. Rheumatol.* 26:2222–2228.

Cotten, A., N. Boutry, B. Cortet, et al. (1998). "Percutaneous Vertebroplasty: State of the Art," *Radiographics* 18:311–320; discussion 320–323.

Coumans, J. V., M. K. Reinhardt, and I. H. Lieberman (2003). "Kyphoplasty for Vertebral Compression Fractures: 1-year Clinical Outcomes from a Prospective Study," *J. Neurosurg. Spine* 99:44–50.

Crandall, D., D. Slaughter, P. J. Hankins, et al. (2004). "Acute Versus Chronic Vertebral Compression Fractures Treated with Kyphoplasty: Early Results," *Spine J.* 4: 418–424.

Cruickshank, J. W. (1988). "Interbody Spine Fusion Utilizing Methyl Methacrylate Bone Glue (MMG)," *J. Neurol. Orthop. Med. Surg.* 9:361–362.

Culham, E., H. Jimenez, and C. King (1994). "Thoracic Kyphosis, Rib Mobility, and Lung Volumes in Normal Women and Women with Osteoporosis," *Spine* 19:1250–1255.

Cyteval, C., M. P. B. Sarrabere, J. O. Roux, et al. (1999). "Acute Osteoporotic Vertebral Collapse: Open Study on Percutaneuos Injection of Acrylic Surgical Cement in 20 Patients," *Am. J. Roentgenology* 173:1685–1690.

Dansie, D. M., P. H. Luetmer, J. I. Lane, et al. (2005). "MRI Findings After Successful Vertebroplasty," *Am. J. Neuroradiol.* 26:1595–1600.

Debussche-Depriester, C., H. Deramond, P. Fardellone, et al. (1991). "Percutaneous Vertebroplasty with Acrylic Cement in the Treatment of Osteoporotic Vertebral Crush Fracture Syndrome," *Neuroradiology* 33:149–152.

Delmas, P., L. van de Langerijt, and N. B. Watts (2005). "Underdiagnosis of Vertebral Compression Fractures Is a Worldwide Problem: The IMPACT Study," *J. Bone Min. Res.* 20:557–563.

Deramond, H., N. Wright, and S. Belkoff (1999). "Temperature Elevation Caused by Bone Cement Polymerization During Vertebroplasty," *Bone* 25:17S–21S.

Deramond, H., C. Depriester, P. Galibert, et al. (1998). "Percutaneous Vertebroplasty with Polymethylmethacrylate: Technique, Indications, and Results," *Radiol. Clin. North Am.* 36:533–546.

Diamond, T. H., B. Champion, and W. A. Clark (2003). "Management of Acute Osteoporotic Vertebral Fractures: A Nonrandomized Trial Comparing Percutaneous Vertebroplasty with Conservative Therapy," *Excerpta Medica* 114:257–265.

Dreinhofer, K., A. Rydholm, H. Bauer, et al. (1995). "Giant-cell Tumours with Fracture at Diagnosis," *J. Bone Joint Surg.* 77B:189–193.

Dudeney, S., I. H. Lieberman, M-K. Reinhardt, et al. (2002). "Kyphoplasty in the Treatment of Osteolytic Vertebral Compression Fractures As a Result of Multiple Myeloma," *J. Clin. Oncol.* 20:2382–2387.

Duff, T. A. (1986). "Surgical Stabilization of Traumatic Cervical Spine Dislocation Using Methyl Methacrylate: Long-term Results in 26 Patients," *J. Neurosurg.* 64:39–44.

Ensrud, K., D. Thompson, J. Cauley, et al. (2000). "Prevalent Vertebral Deformities Predict Mortality and Hospitalization in Older Women with Low Bone Mass: Fracture Intervention Trial Research Group," *J. Am. Geriatr. Soc.* 48:241–249.

Erbe, E. M., T. D. Clineff, and G. Gualtieri (2001). "Comparison of a New Bisphenol-a-glycidyl Dimethacrylate-based Cortical Bone Void Filler with Polymethyl Methacrylate," *Eur. Spine J.* 10(Suppl. 2):S147–S152.

Evans, A. J., M. E. Jensen, K. E. Kip, et al. (2002). "Vertebral Compression Fractures: Pain Reduction and Improvement in Functional Mobility After Percutaneous Polymethyl Methacrylate Vertebroplasty: Retrospective Report of 245 Cases," *Radiology* 226:366–372.

Feltes, C., K. N. Fountas, T. Machinis, et al. (2005). "Immediate and Early Postoperative Pain Relief After Kyphoplasty Without Significant Restoration of Vertebral Body Height in Acute Osteoporotic Vertebral Fractures," *Neurosurg. Focus* 18:e5.

Fourney, D. R., D. F. Schomer, R. Nader, et al. (2003). "Percutaneous Vertebroplasty and Kyphoplasty for Painful Vertebral Body Fractures in Cancer Patients," *J. Neurosurg. Spine* 98:21–30.

Fribourg, D., C. Tang, P. Sra, et al. (2004). "Incidence of Subsequent Vertebral Fracture After Kyphoplasty," *Spine* 29:2270–2276; discussion 2277.

Gaitanis, I., A. Hadjipavlou, P. Katonis, et al. (2004). "Balloon Kyphoplasty for the Treatment of Pathological Vertebral Compressive Fractures," *European Spine J.* (published online.)

Galibert, P., H. Deramond, P. Rosat, et al. (1987). "A Preliminary Note on the Treatment of Vertebral Angiomas by Percutaneous Vertebroplasty with Acrylic Cement," *Neurosurg.* 33:166–168.

Gangi, A., J. L. Dietemann, S. Guth, et al. (1999). Computed Tomography (CT) and Flouroscopy-guided Vertebroplasty: Results and Complications in 187 Patients," *Sem. Intervent. Radiol.* 16:137–142.

Garfin, S. R., H. A. Yuan, and M. A. Reiley (2001). "New Technologies in Spine: Kyphoplasty and Vertebroplasty for the Treatment of Painful Osteoporotic Compression Fractures," *Spine* 26:1511–1515.

Gaughen, J. R., M. E. Jensen, P. A. Schweickert, et al. (2002a). "Relevance of Antecedent Venography in Percutaneous Vertebroplasty for the Treatment of Osteoporotic Compression Fractures," *Am. J. Neuroradiol.* 23:594–600.

Gaughen, J. R., M. E. Jensen, P. A. Schweickert, et al. (2002b). "Lack of Preoperative Spinous Process Tenderness Does Not Affect Clinical Success of Percutaneous Vertebroplasty," *J. Vasc. Interv. Radiol.* 13:1135–1138.

Gerszten, P. C., A. Germanwala, S. A. Burton, et al. (2005). "Combination Kyphoplasty and Spinal Radiosurgery: A New Treatment Paradigm for Pathological Fractures," *Neurosurg. Focus* 18:e8.

Goel, V. K., Y. H. Kim, T. H. Lim, et al. (1988). "An Analytical Investigation of the Mechanics of Spinal Instrumentation," *Spine* 13:1003–1011.

Gold, D., C. W. Bales, K. W. Lyles, et al. (1989). "Treatment of Osteoporosis: The Psychological Impact of a Medical Education Program on Older Patients," *J. Am. Ger. Soc.* 37:417–422.

Gold, D., K. Lyles, K. Shipp, et al. (1996). "Unexpected Consequences of Osteoporosis," in R. Marcus, D. Feldman, and J. Kelsey (eds.). *Osteoporosis.* San Diego: Academic Press.

Grados, F., C. Depriester, G. Cayrolle, et al. (2000). "Long-term Observation of Vertebral Osteoporotic Fractures Treated by Percutaneous Vertebroplasty," *Rheumatology* 39:1410–1414.

Grafe, I. A., K. Da Fonseca, J. Hillmeier, et al. (2005). "Reduction of Pain and Fracture Incidence After Kyphoplasty: One-year Outcomes of a Prospective Controlled Trial of Patients with Primary Osteoporosis," *Osteoporos Int.* (published online.)

Greendale, G., T. DeAmicis, A. Bucur, et al. (2000). "A Prospective Study of the Effect of Fracture on Measured Physical Performance: Results from the MacArthur Study (MAC)," *J. Am. Geriatr. Soc.* 48:546–549.

Hall, S., R. Criddle, T. Comito, et al. (1999). "A Case-Control Study of Quality of Life and Functional Impairment in Women with Long-Standing Vertebral Osteoporotic Fracture," *Osteoporos Int.* 9:508–515.

Hallberg, I., A. Rosenqvist, L. Kartous, et al. (2004). "Health-related Quality of Life After Osteoporotic Fractures," *Osteoporos Int.* 15:834–841.

Harrop, J., B. Prba, M-K. Reinhardt, et al. (2004). "Primary and Secondary Osteoporosis Incidence of Subsequent Vertebral Compression Fractures After Kyphoplasty," *Spine* 29:2120–2125.

Heggeness, M. (1993). "Spine Fracture with Neurologic Deficit in Osteoporosis," *Osteoporos Int.* 3:215–221.

Heggeness, M., and K. Mathis (1996). "An Orthopedic Perspective of Osteoporosis," in R. Marcus, D. Feldman, and J. Kelsey (eds.). *Osteoporosis.* San Diego: Academic Press.

Heini, P. F., B. Walchli, and U. Berlemann (2000). "Percutaneous Transpedicular Vertebroplasty with PMMA: Operative Technique and Early Results—A Prospective Study for the Treatment of Osteoporotic Compression Fractures," *Eur. Spine J.* 9:445–450.

Higgins, K., R. Harten, N. Langrana, et al. (2003). "Biomechanical Effects of Unipedicular Vertebroplasty on Intact Vertebrae," *Spine* 28:1540–1548.

Hodler, J., D. Peck, and L. A. Gilula (2003). "Midterm Outcome After Vertebroplasty: Predictive Value of Technical and Patient-related Factors," *Radiology* 227:662–668.

Ismail, A. A., C. Cooper, D. Felsenberg, et al. (1999). "Number and Type of Vertebral Deformities: Epidemiological Characteristics and Relation to Back Pain and Height Loss," European Vertebral Osteoporosis Study Group. *Osteoporos Int.* 9:206–213.

Jang, J-S., D-Y. Kim, and S-H. Lee (2003). "Efficacy of Percutaneous Vertebroplasty in the Treatment of Intravertebral Pseudarthrosis Associated with Noninfected Avascular Necrosis of the Vertebral Body," *Spine* 28:1588–1592.

Jensen, M. E., A. J. Evans, J. M. Mathis, et al. (1997). "Percutaneous Polymethylmethacrylate Vertebroplasty in the Treatment of Osteoporotic Vertebral Body Compression Fractures: Technical Aspects," *Am. J. Neuroradiol.* 18:1897–1904.

Johnell, O., J. Kanis, A. Oden, et al. (2004). "Mortality After Osteoporotic Fractures," *Osteoporos Int.* 15:35–42.

Kado, D. M., M. Huang, A. Karlamangla, et al. (2004). "Hyperkyphotic Posture Predicts Mortality in Older Community-dwelling Men and Women: A Prospective Study," *J. Am. Geriatr. Soc.* 52:1662–1667.

Kallmes, M. F., P. A. Schweikert, W. F. Marx, et al. (2002). "Vertebroplasty in the Mid- and Upper Thoracic Spine," *Am. J. Neuroradiol.* 23:1117–1120.

Kaufmann, T. J., M. E. Jensen, P. A. Schweikert, et al. (2001). "Age of Fracture and Clinical Outcomes of Percutaneous Vertebroplasty," *Am. J. Neuroradiol.* 22:1860–1863.

Kasperk, C., J. Hillmeier, G. Noldge, et al. (2005). "Treatment of Painful Vertebral Fractures by Kyphoplasty in Patients with Primary Osteoporosis: A Prospective Non-randomized Controlled Study," *J. Bone Miner. Res.* 20:604–612.

Kelly, C. M. (2001). "The Use of a Surgical Grade Calcium Sulfate As a Bone Graft Substitute: Results of a Multi-center Trial," *Clin. Orthop.* 382:42–50.

Kim, A. K., M. E. Jensen, J. E. Dion (2002). "Unilateral Transpedicular Percutaneous Vertebroplasty: Initial Experience," *Radiology* 222:737–741.

Klotzbuecher, C., P. Ross, P. Landsman, et al. (2000). "Patients with Prior Fractures Have an Increased Risk of Future Fractures: A Summary of the Literature and Statistical Synthesis," *J. Bone Miner. Res.* 15:721–726.

Komp, M., S. Ruetten, and G. Godolias (2004). "Minimally Invasive Therapy for Functionally Unstable Osteoporotic Vertebral Fracture by Means of Kyphoplasty: Prospective Comparative Study of 19 Surgically and 17 Conservatively Treated Patients," *J. Miner. Stoffwechs.* 11(Suppl. 1):13–15.

Krebs, J., S. J. Ferguson, M. Bohner, et al. (2005). "Clinical Measurements of Cement Injection Pressure During Vertebroplasty," *Spine* 30:E118–E122.

Kumaresan, S., N. Yoganandan, F. A. Pintar, et al. (2001). "Contribution of Disc Degeneration to Osteophyte Formation in the Cervical Spine: A Biomechanical Investigation," *J. Orthop. Res.* 19:977–984.

Lane, J. M., R. Hong, and J. Koob (2004). "Kyphoplasty Enhances Function and Structural Alignment in Multiple Myeloma," *Clin. Orthop. Relat. Res.* 426:49–53.

Ledlie, J. T., and M. Renfro (2003). "Balloon Kyphoplasty: One-year Outcomes in Vertebral Body Height Restoration, Chronic Pain, and Activity Levels," *J. Neurosurg.* 98:36–42.

Ledlie, J. T., and M. Renfro (2005). "Decreases in the Number and Severity of Morphometrically Defined Vertebral Deformities After Kyphoplasty," *Neurosurg. Focus* 18:e4.

Ledlie, J. T., and M. Renfro (2006). "Balloon Kyphoplasty: Two-year Outcomes in Vertebral Body Height Restoration, Chronic Pain, and Activity Levels," *Spine* 31(1):57–64.

Leidig-Bruckner, G., H. Minne, C. Schlaich, et al. (1997). "Clinical Grading of Spinal Osteoporosis: Quality of Life Components and Spinal Deformity in Women with Chronic Low Back Pain and Women with Vertebral Osteoporosis," *J. Bone Miner. Res.* 12:663–675.

Lewis, G. (1997). "Properties of Acrylic Bone Cement: State of the Art Review," *Appl. Biomater* 38:155–182.

Lieberman, I. H., and M-K. Reinhardt (2003). "Vertebroplasty and Kyphoplasty for Osteolytic Vertebral Collapse," *Clin. Orthop. Relat. Res.* 415:S176–S186.

Lieberman, I. H., and Talmadge, K. (2005). "Surgical Innovations: Kyphoplasty for Women with Compression Fractures," *Clin Rev Bone Min Metab* 3:149–156.

Lieberman, I. H., S. Dudeney, M-K. Reinhardt, et al. (2001). "Initial Outcome and Efficacy of Kyphoplasty in the Treatment of Painful Osteoporotic Vertebral Compression Fractures," *Spine* 26:1631–1638.

Liebschner, M., D. Kopperdahl, W. Rosenberg, et al. (2003). "Finite Element Modeling of the Human Thoracolumbar Spine," *Spine* 28:559–565.

Lindsay, R., S. Pack, and L. Zhengqing (2005). "Longitudinal Progression of Fracture Prevalence Through a Population of Postmenopausal Women with Osteoporosis," *Osteoporos Int.* 16:306–312.

Lindsay, R., S. Silverman, C. Cooper, et al. (2001). "Risk of New Vertebral Fracture in the Year Following a Fracture," *J. Am. Med. Assoc.* 285:320–323.

Lunt, M., T. O'Neill, D. Felsenberg, et al. (2003). "Characteristics of a Prevalent Vertebral Deformity Predict Subsequent Vertebral Fracture: Results from the European Prospective Osteoporosis Study (EPOS)," *Bone* 33:505–513.

Lyles, K., D. Gold, K. Shipp, et al. (1993). "Association of Osteoporotic Vertebral Compression Fractures with Impaired Functional Status," *Am. J. Med.* 94:595–601.

Lyritis, G., B. Mayasis, N. Tsakalakos, et al. (1989). "The Natural History of the Osteoporotic Vertebral Fracture," *Clin. Rheum.* 8(Suppl. 2):66–69.

Majd, M., S. Farley, and R. Holt (2005). "Preliminary Outcomes and Efficacy of the First 360 Consecutive Kyphoplasties for the Treatment of Painful Osteoporotic Vertebral Compression Fractures," *Spine J.* 5:244–255.

Martin, J. B., B. Jean, K. Sugiu, et al. (1999). "Vertebroplasty: Clinical Experience and Follow-up Results," *Bone* 25:11S–15S.

McAfee, P. C., H. H. Bohlman, T. Ducker, et al. (1986). "Failure of Stabilization of the Spine with Methylmethacrylate," *J. Bone Joint Surg. Am.* 68A:1145–1157.

McGraw, J. K., J. A. Lippert, K. D. Minkus, et al. (2002). "Prospective Evaluation of Pain Relief in 100 Patients Undergoing Percutaneous Vertebroplasty: Results and Follow-up," *J. Vasc. Interv. Radiol.* 13:883–886.

McKiernan, F., T. Faciszewski, and R. T. Jensen (2003). "Reporting Height Restoration in Vertebral Compression Fractures," *Spine* 28:2517–2521.

McKiernan, F., T. Faciszewski, and R. T. Jensen (2004). "Quality of Life After Vertebroplasty," *J. Bone Joint Surg. Am.* 86:2600–2606.

McKiernan, F., T. Faciszewski, and R. T. Jensen (2005). "Does Height Restoration Achieved at Vertebroplasty Matter?," *J. Vasc. Interv. Radiol.* 16:973–979.

McKiernan, F., R. Jensen, and T. Faciszewski (2003). "The Dynamic Mobility of Vertebral Compression Fractures," *J. Bone Miner. Res.* 18:24–29.

Moreland, D., M. Landi, and W. Grand (2001). "Vertebroplasty: Techniques to Avoid Complications," *Spine J.* 1:66–71.

Nakano, M., N. Hirano, H. Ishihara, et al. (2005). "Calium Phosphate Cement Leakage After Vertebroplasty for Osteoporotic Vertebral Fractures: Risk Factor Analysis for Cement Leakage," *J. Neurosurg. Spine* 2:27–33.

Nakano, M., N. Hirano, K. Matsuura, et al. (2002). "Percutaneous Transpedicular Vertebroplasty with Calcium Phosphate Cement in the Treatment of Osteoporotic Vertebral Compression and Burst Fractures," *J. Neurosurg. Spine* 97:293–297.

Nevitt, M., B. Ettinger, D. Black, et al. (1998). "The Association of Radiographically Detected Vertebral Fractures with Back Pain and Function: A Prospective Study," *Ann. Intern. Med.* 128:793–800.

O'Donnell, R., D. Springfield, H. Motwani, et al. (1994). "Recurrence of Giant-cell Tumors of the Long Bones After Curettage and Packing with Cement. *J. Bone Joint Surg.* 76-A:1827–1833.

Oleksik, A., S. Ewing, W. Shen, et al. (2005). "Impact of Incident Vertebral Fractures on Health Related Quality of Life (HRQOL) in Postmenopausal Women with Prevalent Vertebral Fractures," *Osteoporos Int.* 16:861–870.

Oner, F. C., W. J. Dhert, and J. J. Verlaan (2005). "Less Invasive Anterior Column Reconstruction in Thoracolumbar Fractures," *Injury* 36(Suppl. 2):B82–B89.

Orthovita web site. *http://www.orthovita.com/products/cortoss/ous/comparison.html*. Accessed 5 October 2005.

Pals, S., and R. Wilkins (1992). "Giant Cell Tumor of Bone Treated by Curettage, Cementation, and Bone Grafting," *Orthopedics* 15:703–708.

Papaioannou, A., N. B. Watts, and D. L. Kendler (2002). "Diagnosis and Management of Vertebral Fractures in Elderly Adults," *Excerpta Med.* 113:220–228.

Park, C. K., M. J. Allen, J. Schoonmaker, et al. (1999). "Gelfoam As a Barrier to Prevent Polymethylmethacrylate-induced Thermal Injury of the Spinal Cord: In Vitro and In Vivo Studies in Pigs," *J. Spin. Disord.* 12:496–500.

Peh, W. C. G., L. A. Gilula, and D. D. Peck (2002). "Percutaneous Vertebroplasty for Severe Osteoporotic Vertebral Body Compression Fractures," *Radiology* 223:121–126.

Peh, W. C. G., M. S. Gelbart, L. A. Gilula, et al. (2003). "Percutaneous Vertebroplasty: Treatment of Painful Vertebral Compression Fractures with Intraosseous Vacuum Phenomena," *Am. J. Roentgenology* 180:1411–1417.

Perez-Higueras, A., L. Alvarez, R. E. Rossi, et al. (2002). "Percutaneous Vertebroplasty: Long-term Clinical and Radiological Outcome," *Neuroradiology* 44:950–954.

Perry, A., A. Mahar, J. Massie, et al. (2005). "Biomechanical Evaluation of Kyphoplasty with Calcium Sulfate Cement in a Cadaveric Osteoporotic Vertebral Compression Fracture Model," *Spine J.* 5:489–493.

Phillips, F., M. Campbell-Hupp, T. McNally, et al. (2003). "Early Radiographic and Clinical Results of Balloon Kyphoplasty for the Treatment of Osteoporotic Vertebral Compression Fractures," *Spine* 28:2260–2265.

Phillips, F., F. Wetzel, I. H. Lieberman, et al. (2002). "An In Vivo Comparison of the Potential for Extravertebral Cement Leakage After Vertebroplasty and Kyphoplasty," *Spine* 27:2173–2179.

Pluijm, S., A. Tromp, J. Smit, et al. (2000). "Consequences of Vertebral Deformities in Older Men and Women," *J. Bone Miner. Res.* 15:1564–1572.

Polikeit, A., L. Nolte, and S. Ferguson (2003). "The Effect of Cement Augmentation on the Load Transfer in an Osteoporotic Functional Spinal Unit," *Spine* 28:991–996.

Reginster, J-Y., H. Minne, O. Sorensen, et al. (2000). "Randomized Trial of the Effects of Risedronate on Vertebral Fractures in Women with Established Postmenopausal Osteoporosis," *Osteoporos Int.* 11:83–91.

Rhyne, A., III, D. Banit, E. Laxer, et al. (2004). "Kyphoplasty: Report of Eighty-two Thoracolumbar Osteoporotic Vertebral Fractures," *J. Orthop. Trauma* 18:294–299.

Riggs, L. D., and J. Melton (1995). "The Worldwide Problem of Osteoporosis: Insights Provided by Epidemiology," *Bone* 17:505S–511S.

Ryu, K. S., C. K. Park, M. C. Kim, et al. (2002). "Dose-dependent Epidural Leakage of Polymethylmethacrylate After Percutaneous Vertebroplasty in Patients with Osteoporotic Vertebral Compression Fractures," *J. Neurosurg. (Spine 1)* 96:56–61.

Schatzker, G. (2001). "AO Philosophy and Principles", in T. P. Rüedi and W. M. Murphy (eds.). *AO Principles of Fracture Management*. Stuttgart, Germany: Thieme Medical Publishing.

Schlaich, C., H. Minne, T. Bruckner, et al. (1998). "Reduced Pulmonary Function in Patients with Spinal Osteoporotic Fractures," *Osteoporos Int.* 8:261–267.

Segura, J., J. Albareda, A. Bueno, et al. (1997). "The Treatment of Giant Cell Tumors by Curettage and Filling with Acrylic Cement: Long-term Functional Results," *Chir. Organi. Mov.* 52:373–380.

Silva, M., T. Keaveny, and W. Hayes (1997). Load Sharing Between the Shell and Centrum in the Lumbar Vertebral Body," *Spine* 22:140–150.

Silverman, S., M. Minshall, W. Shen, et al. (2001). "The Relationship of Health-related Quality of Life to Prevalent and Incident Vertebral Fractures in Postmenopausal Women with Osteoporosis," *Arthrit. & Rheum.* 44:2611–2619.

Sinaki, M., R. Brey, C. Hughes, et al. (2005). "Balance Disorder and Increased Risk of Falls in Osteoporosis and Kyphosis: Significance of Kyphotic Posture and Muscle Strength," *Osteoporos Int.* 16:1004–1010.

Teng, M. M. H., C-J. Wei, C-B. Luo, et al. (2003). "Kyphosis Correction and Height Restoration Effects of Percutaneous Vertebroplasty," *Am. J. Neurorad.* 24:1893–1900.

Togawa, D., H. Bauer, I. H. Lieberman, et al. (2003). "Histologic Evaluation of Human Vertebral Bodies After Vertebral Augmentation with Polymethyl Methacrylate," *Spine* 28:1521–1527.

Tomeh, A. G., A. M. Mathis, J. C. Fenton, et al. (1999). "Biomechanical Evaluation of the Efficacy of Unipedicular Versus Bipedicular Vertebroplasty for Management of Osteoporotic Compression Fractures," *Spine* 24:1772–1776.

Tomita, S., A. Kin, M. Yazu, et al. (2003). "Biomechanical Evaluation of Kyphoplasty and Vertebroplasty with Calcium Phosphate Cement in a Simulated Osteoporotic Compression Fracture," *J. Orthop. Sci.* 8:192–197.

Tsou, I. Y. Y., P. Y. T. Goh, W. C. G. Peh, et al. (2002). "Percutaneous Vertebroplasty in the Management of Osteoporotic Vertebral Compression Fractures: Initial Experience," *Ann. Acad. Med. Singapore* 31:15–20.

Uppin, A., J. Hirsch, L. Centenera, et al. (2003). "Occurrence of New Vertebral Body Fracture After Percutaneous Vertebroplasty in Patients with Osteoporosis," *Radiology* 226:119–124.

van Schoor, N., J. Smit, J. Twisk, et al. (2005). "Impact of Vertebral Deformities, Osteoarthritis, and Other Chronic Diseases on Quality of Life: A Population-based Study," *Osteoporos Intl.* 16:749–756.

Vasconcelos, C., P. Gailloud, N. J. Beauchamp, et al. (2002). "Is Percutaneous Vertebroplasty Without Pretreatment Venography Safe? Evaluation of 205 Consecutive Procedures," *Am. J. Neuroradiol.* 23:913–917.

Verlaan, J-J., W. J. Dhert, A. J. Verbout, et al. (2005). "Balloon Vertebroplasty in Combination with Pedicle Screw Instrumentation: A Novel Technique to Treat Thoracic and Lumbar Burst Fractures," *Spine* 30:E73–E79.

Voggenreiter, G. "Balloon hyphoplasty is effective in deformity correction of osteopartic vertebral compression fractures," *Spine* 30(24):2806–2812.

Wada, T., M. Kaya, S. Nagoya, et al. (2002). "Complications Associated with Bone Cementing for the Treatment of Giant Cell Tumors of Bone," *J. Orthop. Sci.* 7:194–198.

Ware, J. (1993). "Validity: Norm-Based Interpretation SF-36 Health Survey Manual and Interpretation Guide," The Health Institute, New England Medical Center. Boston, Massachusetts.

Weill, A., J. Chiras, J. M. Simon, et al. (1996). "Spinal Metastases: Indications for and Results of Percutaneous Injection of Acrylic Surgical Cement," *Radiology* 199:241–247.

Wenger, M., and T. M. Markwalder (1999). "Surgically Controlled Transpedicular Methyl Methacrylate Vertebroplasty with Fluoroscopic Guidance," *Acta Neurochirurgica* 141:625–631.

White, A., and M. Panjabi (1990). *Clinical Biomechanics of the Spine.* Phildelphia: J. B. Lippincott & Co.

Wilhelm, K., M. Stoffel, F. Ringel, et al. (2003). "Preliminary Experience with Balloon Kyphoplasty for the Treatment of Painful Osteoporotic Compression Fractures," *Fortschr. Rontgenstr.* 175:1690–1696.

Wright Medical Technology web site. *http://www.wmt.com/Physicians/Products/Biologics/MIIGX3HighStrengthInjectableGraft.asp.* Accessed 4 Oct 2005.

Yeom, J. S., W. J. Kim, W. S. Choy, et al. (2003). "Leakage of Cement in Percutaneous Transpedicular Vertebroplasty for Painful Osteoporotic Compression Fractures," *J. Bone Joint Surg*. 85B:83–89.

Yoon, S. T., A. A. Qureshi, J. G. Heller (2005). "Kyphoplasty for Salvage of a Failed Vertebroplasty in Osteoporotic Vertebral Compression Fractures: Case Report and Surgical Technique," *J. Spinal Disord. Tech*. 18:S129–S134.

Yuan, H. A., C. W. Brown, and F. M. Phillips (2004). "Osteoporotic Spinal Deformity: A Biomechanical Rationale for the Clinical Consequences and Treatment of Vertebral Body Compression Fractures," *J. Spinal Disord. Tech*. 17:236–242.

Zethraeus, N., F. Borgstrom, O. Johnell, et al. (2002). "Costs and Quality of Life Associated with Osteoporosis Related Fractures: Results from a Swedish Survey," Working Paper Series in Economics and Finance, No. 512, Stockholm School of Economics (published online).

Zoarski, G. H., P. Sno, W. J. Olan, et al. (2002). "Percutaneous Vertebroplasty for Osteoporotic Compression Fractures: Quantitive Prospective Evaluation of Long-term Outcomes," *J. Vasc. Interv. Radiol*. 13:139–148.

Chapter 13

Standard Test Methods for Spine Implants

Jove Graham, Ph.D.

Mechanical Engineer, Office of Science and
Engineering Laboratories, Center for Devices and
Radiological Health, Food and Drug Administration

Author's Note: Any opinions expressed are those of the author and do not necessarily reflect those of the U.S. Public Health Service or the Food and Drug Administration.

13.1 Introduction

As you read in Chapter 5, spinal implants must withstand a wide range of variable loads during daily activities in the human body. These loads can be static or dynamic, and their magnitudes can differ drastically depending on their position in the spine (cervical, thoracic, or lumbar) and the patient's activity level. Static compressive loads in the upper cervical spine are limited mainly to the weight of the human head. Static compressive loads in the lower lumbar spine may be significantly higher, supporting not only the weight of the head and the rest of the spine but the trunk and arms as well.

Whereas the static compressive loads on the spine are body weight dependent, dynamic loads on the spine are primarily posture or activity dependent. The position of the spine and the angle of flexion of the body during the activity can have significant effects on spinal loading. The primary orientation of most of the loads on the spine can be considered axial, or vertical along the length of the spine, for a person who is standing upright. Spinal curvature causes the axis of the spine at each level to be oriented at a different angle with respect to the vector of gravity. This mismatch in alignment means that there can be significant shear components of load, particularly in the lumbar spine, even when a person is at a state of rest and standing still in a neutral position. When a person begins to engage in activities, further non-axial loads can be introduced.

The three primary directions of motion for the spine are flexion-extension (bending forward or backward), lateral bending (bending from side to side), and axial rotation (twisting from side to side). Motions in each of these directions will introduce multidirectional shear loads, increased bending moments, and torsion in addition to the purely axial compressive loads that are ordinarily present.

How, then, can we hope to evaluate the mechanical performance of a spinal implant device in a laboratory knowing it will be subjected to such complex, multi-axial, weight-dependent and activity-dependent loads in the body? How can we capture this complex loading environment in an *in vitro* mechanical bench test? The simple answer is that we cannot. Fortunately, we have several decades of clinical and historical experience with spinal implants. We also have a considerable body of literature describing musculoskeletal biomechanics that has provided us with estimates of expected *in vivo* spinal loads. With this background information, we can design and develop a series of more limited tests focused on various aspects of a device's mechanical performance. We can use these tests to compare different devices to each other and to expected loads. Some of these tests are described in published consensus standards.

13.2 Using Testing Standards

This chapter explores and describes several of the important standards used for mechanical testing of spinal implants. Biocompatibility standards that were discussed in Chapter 2 should also be used to address issues of biocompatibility, carcinogenicity, and immunogenicity of novel materials. The descriptions in this chapter are general overviews of the key concepts and parameters of each standard and are not intended as a substitute for the published standards themselves. Investigators should obtain and familiarize themselves with the original standards before conducting actual tests.

13.2.1 The Voluntary/Consensus Standards Concept

The standards development process can be described as both voluntary and consensus oriented. Three major standards organizations with an interest in medical devices are the American Society for Testing of Materials International (ASTM), the International Standards Organization (ISO), and the Association for the Advancement of Medical Instrumentation (AAMI). Members of these groups include representatives from health care organizations, academic laboratories, government agencies, manufacturers, testing companies, and trade associations. The development and publishing of a standard, therefore, is a consensus process with these persons of varied backgrounds working together to agree on a standard method or practice. A standard is typically initiated by a technical committee or subcommittee of members with a shared interest in a particular area who then write and vote on a series of drafts until a final document can be agreed upon and published.

Standards are described as voluntary because the organizations that issue them have voluntary membership and they have no legal authority to impose or enforce their implementation. Although some standards published by ISO, for example, have been adopted by some governments as part of their legislative or regulatory framework, such decisions are made by individual governments and not by ISO. In the United States, the Food and Drug Administration's Center for Devices and Radiological Health (FDA/CDRH) has a standards recognition program by which consensus standards may be evaluated by the FDA and recognized for use in satisfying a regulatory requirement. The goal of standards recognition is to allow manufacturers the option to declare partial or total conformity to a recognized standard. This conformity is voluntary but is intended to reduce the time and burden necessary for clearance or approval of a device, in that both parties (the manufacturer and FDA) are already familiar with the techniques or protocols described in the standard. The manufacturer should therefore not need to provide as detailed an explanation of those methods in their reporting as they would have to do for an original test protocol.

The FDA updates the list of recognized standards in the Federal Register approximately once per year and more frequently, if necessary. National or international standards that do not conflict with any statute, regulation, or policy under which the FDA operates and that are developed by an organization using a transparent development process (i.e., open to public scrutiny) are eligible for recognition. Standards may be proposed for recognition from within the agency based on regulatory needs or by outside persons. More information is available through the FDA/CDRH web site by consulting the guidance documents titled "Frequently Asked Questions on the Recognition of Consensus Standards: Guidance for Industry and for FDA Staff" and "CDRH Standard Operating Procedures for the Identification and Evaluation of Candidate Consensus Standards for Recognition: Final Guidance for Industry."

13.2.2   Goals and Scope of Standards

It is important to read the sections of any standard that lay out the assumptions and expectations for use of the methods or practices described. Standards used for materials and devices often need to be very specific in their scope, focusing on the measurement of a specific property or set of properties. Rarely can they be all things to all people. For mechanical testing standards, the primary goal is often to apply a set of very well-defined loading conditions to a device or component. These loading conditions may or may not be an accurate representation of the loading conditions that are expected in the body. If different devices or designs are subjected to identical loading conditions as described in the standard, however, this provides a powerful means of comparing designs with respect to a particular characteristic. It is not uncommon, therefore, for a standard (e.g., ASTM F1717) to include statements such as these:

> These test methods are used to quantify the static and dynamic mechanical characteristics of different designs and spinal implant assemblies. The mechanical tests are conducted *in vitro* using simplified load schemes and do not attempt to mimic the complex loads of the spine. . . .
> The results obtained here cannot be used directly to predict *in vivo* performance. The results can be used to compare different component designs in terms of the relative mechanical parameters.

It is important, therefore, to keep in mind the specific goals and intended application of a particular standard before implementing it.

13.2.3 Benefits of Using Standards

The primary benefit of the standards development process is the establishment of a consensus in the technical community as to the best currently available test procedure for a specific application. A fully developed standard should ideally be supported by experience and data obtained from testing so users have some confidence that the techniques described can produce repeatable, reliable results. The need for every investigator to constantly "reinvent the wheel" should be reduced.

Another important benefit specific to the regulatory process is a streamlining of the information that must be communicated between a manufacturer (which must always report on their test methodologies and results) and the regulatory agency, which must interpret those results. Other nonstandard methods can be developed and employed to test a particular device. When a manufacturer chooses to use a standard, however, this decision should reduce the amount of time and discussion needed for a regulatory official to understand which tests were done and how they were performed. Even if the user must make modifications or adaptations to a standard to fit their specific device design, beginning with a published standard method or practice gives the manufacturer and the reviewer a common point of reference. Outside of the regulatory domain, standards play a similar role in giving experimentalists and testing professionals a common ground for discussion.

Finally, it is the goal of many standards to allow comparisons of data not only among different device designs tested at the same facility but devices tested at different facilities. The certainty with which these data can be compared is defined in terms of the precision and bias of that particular test. *Precision* describes the variability that can be expected between test results for a given method, even when repeated by the same user under the same conditions. *Bias* describes a systematic error in a particular investigator's experiment that may contribute to the difference between his or her results and an accepted reference value. Unfortunately, numerical values of precision and bias are not included in many standards because of the complexity involved in establishing such values.

Despite their importance in demonstrating repeatability, estimates of precision and bias require multi-laboratory or "round-robin" testing, which can be time and labor intensive. As a result, this type of robust testing is sometimes delayed until after the publication of a standard, if it takes place at all. It is important to remember, therefore, that the development of a standard test method is not finished upon its initial publication. Standards require ongoing multi-laboratory testing as well as periodic review in light of technological advances in order to maintain their usefulness as living, functional, and relevant documents.

13.2.4 Limitations of Standards

Several limitations of standards have already been discussed. Standards are typically focused on methods of measuring specific characteristics of a device or material *in vitro*. They provide useful tools for comparison of devices, but results cannot necessarily be extrapolated to predict clinical performance because of the complexity of the *in vivo* loading environment compared to rigidly controlled laboratory conditions. While a well-designed method should provide repeatability (high precision) and minimize variation between investigators using the method (low bias), numerical estimates of these variability measures are often unavailable. The consensus process does not deliver instantaneous results, and it can therefore be a challenge to insure that standards are updated frequently enough to reflect the current technology innovations and breadth of designs for a particular category of device. Occasionally, a duplication of effort exists when multiple standards organizations publish methods for the same purpose but with different techniques or parameters. Despite these limitations and challenges, however, standards provide not only useful practical information about how to set up an experiment but also effective communication tools for researchers with similar areas of interest.

13.2.5 Basic Organizational Structure of a Testing Standard

ASTM International suggests 25 subject headings to be used in the organization of an ASTM document, seven of which are mandatory. These mandatory headings are title, designation, scope, significance and use, procedure, precision and bias, and keywords. In appropriate cases, a hazards section may also be mandatory. This uniformity of subject headings among ASTM documents is intended to help orient the reader and make information easy to locate within the text. ISO likewise acknowledges a need for uniformity of structure and style among documents, although their drafting guidelines point out the difficulty in requiring specific subject headings given the diversity of subject matter. Even so, ISO encourages subdivisions with names similar to those suggested by ASTM (e.g., title, scope, requirements, sampling, test methods, apparatus, and so forth). AAMI documents typically follow the ISO formatting guidelines.

Before implementing a standards method or practice, an investigator's first task should be to examine the sections that discuss the purpose, scope, and significance of use for the method. These sections should help to determine whether the method is appropriate for the desired application and whether it can be expected to yield the desired results. From there, the investigator should continue to familiarize himself or herself with any definitions or terminology and read the more technical sections of the document (e.g., apparatus, methods, procedure) to determine what materials and equipment will be necessary to perform the tests described. The investigator should make sure that all pertinent information will be collected during testing for inclusion in the final report. Descriptions of the components tested and their intended spinal locations and all test parameters should be recorded, especially if any deviations were made from the recommendations in the standard. Results should typically include descriptions of all failures, plots such as load-displacement curves, and tables of the mean values and standard deviations for all mechanical properties of interest, and thus all of this information should be collected during the test. Finally, before beginning an experiment an investigator should always pay attention to any annexes or appendices, as these often provide helpful background information and underlying assumptions of the test method that may be helpful in choosing specific test parameters.

13.2.6 Adapting or Modifying Standards to Fit Your Device

In order for a standard test method to be useful, it must be specific enough to reproducibly measure a property of a type of device yet broad enough to allow testing of a wide variety of designs. Innovation and competition demand that no two devices be exactly the same in terms of geometry, materials, and other design characteristics. Standards must be flexible enough to evaluate and compare all of these different designs, yet not so open-ended that they prohibit meaningful comparisons among them. As technology evolves, it becomes more common for a device manufacturer to discover that a standard test method must be modified or adapted to fit their particular new design. Some modifications will obviously have greater consequences than others. It becomes of paramount importance that the investigator understand the goal of the testing and how each modification of the method will affect his or her ability to compare the results with data from devices tested using the original, unmodified method.

Consider the following common example: ASTM F1717 describes a method for testing spinal fusion systems in a corpectomy model, discussed in Section 13.4.3. The device system is anchored at the top and bottom to two polymeric blocks representing vertebral bodies with a gap between them. This gap represents the space that would be left after removal of a vertebra, or corpectomy, and therefore the test represents a worst-case scenario where the device must transfer all of the axial and bending loads across this empty space. The standard specifies that the longitudinal gage length, or the vertical distance between the top and bottom anchors that span this gap, should be either 35.0 mm (for cervical devices) or 76.0 mm (for thoraco lumbar devices). These dimensions were chosen based on anatomical measurements of the gap actually created by a corpectomy.

Of course, there is vast anatomic variability among real patients and a market demand for plates and rods of lengths other than just 35.0 mm and 76.0 mm! Does this mean that these products of alternative lengths cannot be tested using the ASTM F1717 method? No, but an investigator should understand and be prepared to justify the consequences of any changes they make to fit their design. If the test setup is properly aligned, the only loads on the plate or rod should be a purely axial compressive load and a pure bending moment. Small-deformation beam theory tells us that neither of these loads should be affected by the longitudinal gage length. However, in non-ideal laboratory conditions a large deformation of the test blocks or a small deviation in alignment between the longitudinal axis and the vertical axis could introduce shear components of load that would indeed cause gage length to affect the stress state. It should also be noted that there are other dimensions in the F1717 standard, such as the horizontal block moment arm distance, that are much more critical to the resultant stress state regardless of whether the test alignment is ideal or not. A distinction should be drawn between modifications that will significantly affect the load or stress state, which should be avoided, and those that will not.

In some cases, a device that seems like it would not fit the standard can still be gripped or fixtured in a way that conforms to the standard's recommendations. In the previous example, even if a particular lumbar plate is longer than the desired gage length of 76.0 mm perhaps it may be anchored so that only a reduced section of 76.0 mm is tested. In other cases, conformity to the standard is not possible but it may still be possible to perform side-by-side testing of two designs under the same conditions to ensure a valid comparison is being made. If a particular cervical plate is shorter than the desired 35.0-mm gage length, the investigator should consider testing as long a section as possible (e.g., 25.0 mm) and then testing another plate design anchored such that it is constrained to the same gage length of 25.0 mm. Consistency and the ability to compare data should always be a priority, and deviations from any test parameters in the standard should always be described and justified in test reports.

13.2.7 Defining Acceptance Criteria and Interpreting Results

In general, a standard test method describes the materials and methods an investigator will need in order to carry out a test and describes the measurements that will be taken as a result. Standard methods do not prescribe how to interpret those results, however, or whether a particular result should be considered a "pass" or "failure." It is the responsibility of the user to define the *acceptance criteria* for the test, and to compare the final results to these acceptance criteria to determine whether or not the test yielded an acceptable result.

Acceptance criteria for mechanical testing of spinal implants are generally developed from two types of sources: results from similar, previously tested devices or biomechanical literature data.

The majority of medical devices reviewed by the FDA are cleared through the 510(k) notification process, the goal of which is to establish that the device in question is "substantially equivalent" to a previously cleared device. The previously cleared device is known as the *predicate*, and in these cases it makes the most sense for the developer of the new device to base their acceptance criteria on data from side-by-side testing of the predicate device. An alternative approach is to use acceptance criteria based on the expected physiologic loads or motions that will be applied to the device *in vivo*. Various estimates of spinal loads and kinematics can be found in the biomechanics literature, and a test should demonstrate that the device can withstand expected loads with an appropriate factor of safety. When constructing an acceptance criterion based on literature values, the investigator should pay special attention to the underlying assumptions and limitations of each specific study to make sure that the data are applicable to the particular location, application, and loading mode of the current device. If the assumptions and testing conditions in the literature study are not sufficiently conservative for the new device being studied, additional factors of safety may be incorporated into the acceptance criteria.

13.3 Terminology (ASTM F1582)

ASTM F1582, titled "Standard Terminology Relating to Spinal Implants," while not absolutely necessary for the conduct of actual experimental tests is a good starting place for those investigators who may be new to the spine or spinal implants. In addition to providing functional definitions for the different categories of spinal implants (bolts, posts, screws, hooks, plates, rods, and so on), it provides helpful terminology in describing a test or test setup itself. For example, the terms *assembly* or *subassembly* should be used to describe implant configurations that are tested by themselves without being attached to any skeletal structures (real or simulated), whereas *construct* or *subconstruct* should be used to describe a testing configuration that includes both the implant and a representative skeletal structure such as a spinal motion segment. This chapter will use standard terminology as it is defined in ASTM F1582 wherever possible.

13.4 Standards for Fusion Systems

Fusion systems, discussed in Chapters 7 and 8, are multiple-component systems that typically consist of longitudinal elements, attachment elements, and interconnection mechanisms. Ultimately, we are most interested in the mechanical strength and stability of this entire system because it is the whole system that will be implanted into a patient. But naturally it makes sense to have methods of evaluating smaller subsets of the system as well. If a system includes transverse bars that connect to the longitudinal plating or rod components, we may be interested in the strength of those connections, their resistance to slipping, or their resistance to twisting. We may be interested in the flexural bending strength of the pedicle screws alone, irrespective of what system they are used in.

Testing on multiple scale levels helps to characterize the system both as a construct and as a collection of individual parts. Because surgeons often have an "Erector set" of various screws and components to work with, this approach to testing also helps to compare those individual components and contrast different designs. ASTM has published three standards that describe testing of fusion systems on three scales: ASTM 2193 (component level), ASTM 1798 (subassembly level), and ASTM F1717 (whole system level).

13.4.1 Component-level Testing (ASTM F2193)

ASTM F2193, titled "Standard Specifications and Test Methods for Components Used in the Surgical Fixation of the Spinal Skeletal System," describes methods for testing screws, plates, rods, and other individual components of a fusion system. This document also refers heavily to two other published standards that were developed for osteosynthesis devices not specific to the spinal column: ASTM F382 ("Standard Specification and Test Method for Metallic Bone Plates") and ASTM F543 ("Standard Specification and Test Methods for Metallic Medical Bone Screws"). Familiarity with all three of these standards is suggested for anyone wishing to evaluate spinal plates or screws. This chapter, however, focuses on ASTM F2193 because it is limited in scope to spinal devices.

Various sections of this standard provide a bibliography of other ASTM standards for test methods and materials that may be useful, a glossary of terminology specific to testing of spinal components, a listing of the information that should be included in component packaging and directly on the components, and some examples of materials that have been used for spinal components in the past. Several of these materials are described separately in published ASTM specifications and they include primarily titanium and titanium alloys (F67, F136, F1295, F1341, and F1472) or stainless steels (F138, F1314).

Annex A1 is a specification for metallic spinal screws, listing the information used to describe a screw and its performance characteristics. Overall screw shape should be classified into one of four categories depending on the head shape and thread symmetry. Specific dimensions such as screw length, thread length, pitch, core diameter, and thread diameter should be provided along with their tolerances and should follow the nomenclature as defined in F543. The shape and dimensions of the screw's drive connection (i.e., the recess in the head into which the driving tool is inserted) should be classified according to the descriptions in Annex A6 of F543. Testing should be performed to determine the insertion and removal torque and the axial pull-out load, using test methods described in Annexes A2 and A3 of F543, respectively. These tests are used to identify the potential stress that could be placed on the screw during insertion or removal and the ability of the screw to transfer load from the longitudinal element to the bone without loosening.

Static and fatigue test methods are also described in Annex A4 of both F543 and F2193 to test the bending properties of metallic screws. Screws should be loaded in cantilever bending with a monotonic or sinusoidal load to measure the mechanical response. The screw head should be rigidly fixed or constrained while the threaded region of the screw is embedded into a test block made of synthetic material such as stainless steel, polyethylene, or polyurethane foam. A load is applied through the center of this test block, transverse to the longitudinal axis of the screw and at a fixed moment arm distance L from the center of the screw head to produce a known bending moment.

All screws having the same nominal length should be tested with the same moment arm of either 10 mm or one-third of the screw's nominal length, whichever is smaller. Static testing should use a minimum sample size of five (unless otherwise justified using the methods in ASTM Practice E122) and a loading rate of 25 mm/min. or less. Fatigue tests should use at least two specimens at each of three different maximum moment levels (the standard suggests initial moments of 75, 50, and 25% of the ultimate bending moment as measured in the static testing). Fatigue testing should use a sinusoidal load and a test frequency to be determined by the user but no more than 30 Hz. For lumbar and thoracic plates, which are expected to experience fluctuating loads in one direction only, a minimum-to-maximum load ratio R of 0.10 should be used. For cervical plates that are expected to experience fully reversed loading, a load ratio R of −1.0 should be used. Fatigue testing should determine the maximum moment level at which specimens do not fail before 2.5 million cycles, referred to as the "run-out moment." The standard suggests that this runout moment be determined to within 10% of the device's ultimate bending moment.

Similarly, Annex A2 is a specification for metallic spinal plates, listing the information used to describe a plate and its performance characteristics. Plates should be classified depending on the indicated spinal region, position, and type of surgical procedure. Specific dimensions such as length, width, and thickness should be provided along with tolerances, following the nomenclature as defined in ASTM F382. Testing methods are described to measure the static and fatigue bending properties of the plate. Plates should be tested in four-point bending, and the distance between the inner rollers (test gage section) as well as the distance between the inner and outer roller on each side should be either 35.0 mm for cervical plates or 76.0 mm for thoracic and lumbar plates. Static tests should be performed on a minimum sample size of five specimens using a loading rate of 10 mm/min. or less. Fatigue tests should use the same sample sizes, load ratios, frequencies, and moment levels as previously suggested for screws.

Annex A3 is a specification for metallic spinal rods, listing the information used to describe a rod and its performance characteristics. Rods should be classified depending on their indicated spinal region, position, and type of surgical procedure. Testing methods, similar to those in ASTM F382, are described to test the static and fatigue bending properties of the rod. Rods should be tested in four-point bending using notched rollers in order to allow testing of a range of rod sizes and to prevent a load concentration point where the outer circumferences of the rod and a cylindrical roller would meet. The distance between the inner rollers, as well as the distance between the inner and outer rollers on each side, should be either 35.0 mm for cervical rods and 76.0 mm for thoracic or lumbar rods. Static tests should use a minimum sample size of five and a loading rate of 10 mm/min. or less. Fatigue tests should use the same sample sizes, load ratios, frequencies, and moment levels as previously suggested for screws and plates.

The appendices of standard ASTM F2193 provide more details on the various rationales behind the overall specification and the particular details of each specification for screws, plates, and rods. In general, this section emphasizes the importance of giving a surgeon standardized, reliable information about a particular component on which he or she can base a selection. It is acknowledged that these test methods have limited ability to define performance levels for spinal implants or to address long-term mechanical issues, particularly if the device does not lead to fusion of the spine.

13.4.2 Subassembly-level Testing (ASTM F1798)

ASTM F1798, titled "Standard Guide for Evaluating the Static and Fatigue Properties of Interconnection Mechanisms and Subassemblies Used in Spinal Arthrodesis Implants," describes a series of methods for testing subgroups of fusion system components. These tests can be considered "mid-scale," in contrast with the small-scale (individual component) testing of ASTM F2193 or the large-scale (whole system) testing of ASTM F1717. The standard assumes that hooks and screws are the most common connectors that will be tested, although the methods could be adapted for use with other novel connector designs. In general, an interconnection component such as a hook, screw, or transverse element is attached to a longitudinal element to form a subassembly for testing. The standard uses a right-handed global coordinate system in which the x axis is aligned with the anterior-posterior direction of the vertebra, the y axis is aligned with the medial-lateral direction, and the z axis is aligned with the superior-inferior direction. For an individual hook or screw, this global coordinate system is translated into a local coordinate system by centering the z axis through the longitudinal element and centering the x axis through either the axis of a screw or the inferior surface of a hook. The standard describes a total of six test methods in which either a load or bending moment is applied to the subassembly in each of these three directions (x, y, and z).

For all test methods, a subassembly is formed by attaching a connector (e.g., hook or screw) to a longitudinal element using the tightening, crimping, or locking method specified by the manufacturer for use during surgery. If set screws or nuts must be tightened, the torques required to tighten them should be measured and recorded. If a transverse element such as a cross bar is to be tested, it should also be attached using the manufacturer's recommended method. For most tests, these connectors will be attached at the center of a 50-mm exposed length of the longitudinal element which is then rigidly clamped on both ends. The two exceptions are the first and last test methods, which evaluate the interconnection strength along and about the z axis. In these cases, the connector is placed near one end of the longitudinal element but with at least 5 mm of longitudinal element exposed above and below.

In all cases, static testing should be performed on a minimum of five samples. Static loads should be applied using a loading rate of no more than 20 N/s or 25 mm/min. for loads and no more than 25 Nm/min. or 25°/min. for moments until failure occurs. It is the responsibility of the user to define what constitutes a failure although the standard suggests, for example, that a 1.5-mm permanent displacement or 5 degrees permanent rotation between connected components during axial gripping tests should be considered a functional failure. Fatigue testing should determine the maximum run-out load or moment at which at least three consecutive specimens show run out to 2.5 million cycles. The choice of test frequency and environment is left to the user, although the recommended maximum frequency is 16 Hz. The user should also determine for each loading mode whether the components are designed to withstand fluctuating loads in one direction or fully reversed loading in both directions. For components that will experience fluctuating loads in one direction only, a minimum-to-maximum load ratio R of 10 or greater should be used (e.g., a minimum load of −200 N and a maximum load of −20 N, which would yield a load ratio of R = 10). For components that will experience fully reversed loading, a load ratio R of −1 should be used (e.g., a minimum load of −100 N and a maximum load of +100 N). After testing is completed, the torques required to loosen any set screws or other tightening mechanisms during disassembly should also be measured and recorded.

Figure 13.1 illustrates the six testing setups described in ASTM F1798. The first test setup is used to evaluate the strength of the interconnection mechanism in axial gripping along the z axis. The user has the option of rigidly holding the longitudinal element and applying an axial load to the connector as illustrated in Figure 13.1a, or vice versa (i.e., rigidly holding the connector and applying a load to the longitudinal element instead). The end result of either strategy is to measure the failure load at which the gripping capacity of the connector is overcome, causing it to slide up or down along the longitudinal element. The connector should be attached at least 5 mm from either end of the longitudinal element. If the longitudinal element is rigidly held (using the first option, mentioned previously), loads should be applied to the connector via a sleeve or collar that freely surrounds the longitudinal element and distributes the load evenly around it.

The second test setup, shown in Figure 13.1b, is used to evaluate the strength of the interconnection mechanism in the anterior-posterior direction along the x axis. A 50-mm section of the longitudinal element is rigidly clamped on both ends with the connector attached at the midpoint between the two clamps. (25 mm from each end). An anterior load in the positive-x direction and cen-

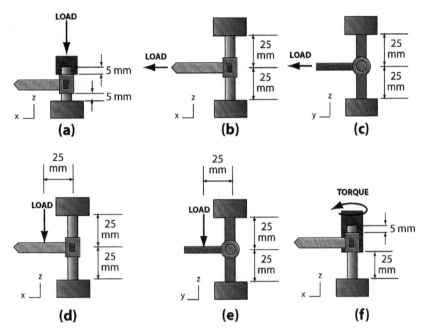

Fig. 13.1.

Schematic of the six testing setups described in ASTM F1798 for static and dynamic testing of inter-connection mechanisms and subassemblies. A screw (yellow) with a transverse element (brown) is attached to the longitudinal element (pink) and rigidly clamped on one or both ends (green). For the first and last tests, load is applied via a sleeve or collet (blue). The six tests are (a) axial gripping, (b) anterior-posterior strength, (c) lateral strength, (d) flexion-extension bending, (e) lateral bending, and (f) axial torque.

tered on the local *x*-coordinate axis of the connector should be applied to the connector via a clamp. Static and fatigue testing should be performed using this setup to test the static failure strength and the maximum run-out load at which devices can survive 2.5 million loading cycles.

The third test setup, shown in Figure 13.1c, is used to evaluate the strength of the interconnection mechanism in the medial-lateral direction along the *y* axis in cases where a transverse element is to be used. As before, a 50-mm exposed length of the longitudinal element is rigidly clamped on both ends and a connector with a transverse element is attached at the section's midpoint. A mediolateral load in the positive-*y* direction and centered on the local *y*-coordinate axis of the connector should be applied to the interconnection. Static and fatigue testing should be performed using this setup to test the static failure strength and the maximum run-out load at which devices can survive 2.5 million loading cycles.

The fourth test setup is used to evaluate the interconnection mechanism's resistance to bending moment in flexion-extension about the *y* axis. Again, the connector is attached at the center of a 50-mm section of the longitudinal element that has been rigidly clamped on both ends. An inferiorly directed load (parallel to the negative-z axis and to the axis of the longitudinal element) is applied to the interconnection. For a hook, this load may be applied via a cylinder set into the hook notch. For a screw, the load should be applied to the screw such that the moment arm distance along the x axis between the central axis of the longitudinal element and the point of load application is 25 mm, as shown in Figure 13.1d.

The fifth test setup, shown in Figure 13.1e, is used to evaluate the interconnection mechanism's resistance to a lateral bending moment about the x axis. This test is nearly identical to the previous one (flexion-extension about the y axis), except that the inferiorly directed load is applied to the transverse element (or to the connector via a clamp if there is no transverse element) at a moment arm distance of 25 mm along the y axis, not the x axis, to simulate lateral bending.

The sixth and final test setup is similar to the first one and is used to evaluate the axial torque gripping capacity of the interconnection mechanism about the z axis. The connector is attached to the longitudinal element so that a 25-mm length of longitudinal element is always exposed between the rigidly fixtured end and the end to which a torque is applied. The user is given several options of how to apply this axial torque to the interface between the connector and longitudinal element. In the first option, the longitudinal element is rigidly held at one end and a pure torque is applied to the connector via a sleeve or collar, as illustrated in Figure 13.1f. Alternatively, the connector may be rigidly fixed and a torque applied to the longitudinal element via a clamp or collet. A third option would be to clamp both ends of the longitudinal element and create a torque by applying a horizontal load to the connector (at a fixed moment arm distance D from the origin, along the x axis) via a block or clamp.

13.4.3 Whole System-level Testing (ASTM F1717)

ASTM F1717, titled "Standard Test Methods for Spinal Implant Constructs in a Vertebrectomy Model," describes a method for testing fusion systems using a vertebrectomy (or corpectomy) model. The model assumes a worst-case loading situation in which a patient's vertebra has been completely removed and the fusion system must transfer all of the loads across this empty gap. In the testing setup, the fusion system is anchored at the top and bottom (at the *anchor points*) to two polymeric blocks representing the vertebral bodies above and below this gap. The first section of the standard explains that the scope of the document is to measure the displacements, yield load, stiffness, and strength of a spinal implant assembly using three static tests (tension, compression, and torsion) and one fatigue test (compression).

A considerable portion of ASTM F1717 is devoted to illustrations and descriptions of the various test blocks that must be fabricated in order to test differently-configured systems. These test blocks, which simulate the vertebral bodies to which the system will be anchored, are to be machined from ultra-high molecular weight polyethylene (UHMWPE). The standard specifies that only UHMWPE with an ultimate tensile strength of $40 \pm 3\,MPa$ (per ASTM D638) should be used, although for the purposes of strength testing it is probably sufficient to choose any UHMWPE material that is strong enough not to fail during the test and provide uniformity among specimens. If the user is primarily concerned with comparing the stiffnesses of different systems, the specific choice of UHMWPE formulation may become more important.

Figures 13.2a and b show a sample set of test blocks with a plating system attached. The particular construct shown here is for a cervical, bilateral plating system with screws. Like all test blocks described in the standard, these blocks are intended to be loaded into a uniaxial load frame via metal pins that are inserted through the large pinholes in each block. Figure 13.3 is a schematic of the system pictured in the previous figure, showing some of the key dimensions of the system. The dimensions of the UHMWPE blocks will vary greatly depending on whether the system is intended for the cervical or lumbar spine,

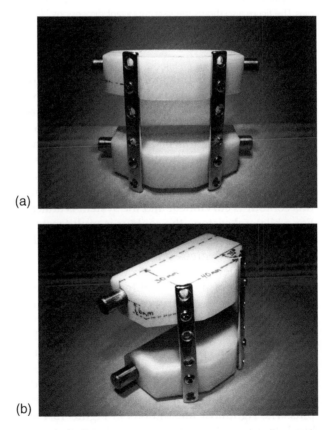

(a)

(b)

Fig. 13.2.
Sample set of cervical, bilateral test blocks as described in ASTM F1717 with a plate and screw system attached. Loads are applied via the upper and lower stainless steel hinge pins, inserted into the test blocks as seen here. (a) Posterior view of the system. (b) Oblique lateral-posterior view, with selected dimensions labeled.

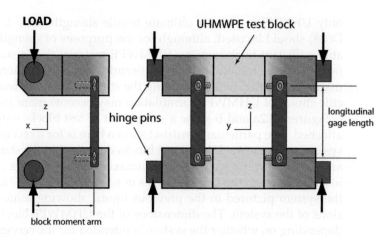

Fig. 13.3.
Schematic of the test setup showing how a compressive load is applied to the system via the hinge pins. The figure also shows the two important dimensions: block moment arm and longitudinal gage length.

if it is unilateral or bilateral, and if it is anchored with screws or bolts as opposed to hooks, cables, or wires. The anterior-posterior depth of the blocks is designed so that the anchor points are located at a specific displacement along the x axis from the hinge pins (referred to as the *block moment arm*). For a cervical construct, this block moment arm distance should be 30 mm, and for a lumbar construct it should be 40 mm to represent typical anatomic dimensions. Additionally, the contour of the anterior surface of the blocks is dependent on whether the system is unilateral or bilateral. For a unilateral system, this contour is curvilinear and the system is attached to the block at its midline. For a bilateral system, the contour is multifaceted and the attachment anchors are placed to the left and right of the midline, angled inward at either 35 degrees (cervical) or 15 degrees (lumbar) from the normal. Figure 13.4 shows a horizontal plane view (*xy*) of the six different test blocks described in the standard and how some of their critical features (including the block moment arm and posterior surface geometry) compare with one another.

A variation on the test block design may be required for systems using hooks, cables, or wires that do not rigidly attach to the pedicles and cannot resist bending moments or rotation around the anchor points. For these attachment mechanisms, it is necessary to add a second set of pinholes and metal pins (referred to as "roll pins") to each test block, and recesses in the faceted anterior surfaces to allow the hooks, wires, or cables to be attached to these roll pins. The rightmost illustrations in Figure 13.4 show a cervical and a lumbar block that have been modified in this way to include roll pins for attaching hooks. Section 6.9 of the standard discusses other adjustments to the method that must be made for such a system. Because the hooks, wires, or cables are able to rotate around the roll pins, and the UHMWPE test blocks are able to

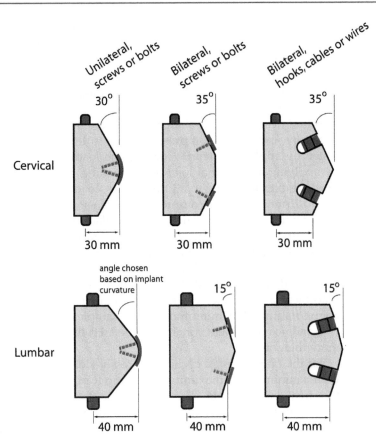

Fig. 13.4.
Horizontal (*xy*) plane view of six UHMWPE test block designs described in ASTM F1717. The top row shows cervical blocks for three system configurations: unilateral screws or bolts, bilateral screws or bolts, and bilateral hooks, cables, or wires. The bottom row shows lumbar blocks for the same three system configurations.

rotate around the main loading pins, the test construct is less stable than it is with a rigidly anchored system. The standard recommends placing one aluminum block between the modified test block and the base plate of the testing machine to help eliminate this rotational degree of freedom. The standard points out in several places that if modified test blocks and aluminum spacer blocks are used on both the top and bottom, all bending moment is eliminated and the test becomes pure axial tension or compression. This should be avoided where possible by using hooks, wires, or cables on only one end of the system (preferably the superior end) and using rigid anchors at the other end. The use of these aluminum spacer blocks is only appropriate with hook, cable, or wire anchors and is inappropriate for any system that will be expected to carry both bending moments and axial loads. The final critical aspect of the testing construct is the vertical displacement between the upper and lower anchor points (referred to as the *active length of the longitudinal element*, or longitudinal gage length). As mentioned earlier in this chapter, the standard specifies that this gage length should be either 35 mm (for a cervical system) or 76 mm (for a lumbar system) to represent typical anatomical distances.

Compared to all these details of designing the test blocks and the test construct, the actual testing procedure itself is relatively straightforward. The standard describes three static tests and one fatigue test. Static compression is tested by applying a compressive force to the loading pins. Static tension is tested by applying a tensile force to the loading pins. Static torsion is tested by applying a rotational load to the loading pins about the longitudinal axis of the testing machine. In all three cases, loading is applied at a constant rate (up to 25 mm/min. for compression or tension, or up to 60°/min. for torsion) until failure of the construct. Load-displacement or torque-angular displacement curves are constructed from which mechanical properties can be calculated. For compression and tension, these properties include displacement at 2% offset yield, elastic displacement, yield load, stiffness, ultimate displacement, and ultimate load. For torsion, these properties include angular displacement at 2% offset yield, elastic angular displacement, yield torque, and angular stiffness. A minimum of five samples should be used for each static test, and no components (including the UHMWPE test blocks) should be tested more than once.

For the fatigue test, a cyclic compressive load is applied to the loading pins with a minimum-to-maximum load ratio R of greater than 10 and a maximum test frequency of 5 Hz. The purpose of the fatigue test is to establish the maximum load at which no specimens fail before reaching five million cycles. The standard recommends that this run-out load be determined to within an accuracy of 10% of the compression bending ultimate load of the system, although in practice it is more important to justify that the maximum run-out load is sufficient to withstand the worst-case expected physiologic loads than it is to achieve this goal of 10% accuracy. The run-out load is typically determined by testing pairs of specimens at different load levels until an appropriately high load is established at which both specimens survive five million cycles. Section 7.5 suggests that the user begin by testing at 75, 50, and 25% of the ultimate strength as determined in the static testing, but alternative testing schemes are possible.

13.5 Standards for Intervertebral Body Fusion Devices (Cages)

Intervertebral body fusion devices, broadly referred to as "cages" because many of them are designed to be porous or hollow in order to allow bone grafting material to be packed inside, were discussed in Chapters 7 and 8. In this chapter, interbody fusion devices are simply referred to as cages. ASTM has published two testing standards that specifically address the testing of cages. ASTM F2077 covers the static and dynamic testing of these implants, whereas ASTM F2267 describes a method for evaluating their resistance to subsidence.

13.5.1 Static and Dynamic Testing of Cages (ASTM F2077)

ASTM F2077, titled "Test Methods for Intervertebral Body Fusion Devices," describes testing setups and methods that should be used for the static and dynamic testing of interbody fusion devices or cages. The standard emphasizes that the methods are intended to allow mechanical comparisons of cage designs but are not intended to directly predict *in vivo* performance or establish performance standards for these devices. Resistance to expulsion is not addressed by the standard, and the user is warned that not all cage designs may be testable in all of the test configurations described. Testing should be conducted in a dry ambient environment, although it is suggested that the user may wish to conduct additional testing in saline or other fluid media to subsequently investigate the effect of these environments on the device's performance. If the materials are already known at the outset to be temperature or environment dependent, a physiologic solution such as saline should be used. Fluid media may also be desirable in cases where the device is expected to generate wear debris, either through abrasion or articulating motion, and the user wishes to collect this debris by filtering the fluid.

For all tests, the device should be placed between two test blocks simulating the vertebral bodies. Figure 13.5 illustrates how a device fits into these test blocks. Test blocks are manufactured from either stainless steel or polyacetal (commonly referred to by the trade name Delrin Dupont). Metallic blocks are used for static testing so that the test blocks will not fail under very high loads and so that stiffness measurements of the whole construct accurately reflect the stiffness of the device itself. Softer, low-friction polyacetal blocks are used for dynamic testing to avoid wear of the device during the test. The standard recommends that the stainless steel used for the test blocks (and for other fixtures described elsewhere) have a minimum ultimate tensile strength of 1,310 MPa

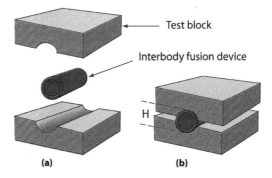

Fig. 13.5.
Schematic of test blocks to be used for testing of interbody fusion devices or cages. (a) Expanded view of test blocks and device. Note that surfaces of the test blocks are contoured to interface with the device. (b) Test blocks with device in place. Intradiscal height, *H*, between test block surfaces at the device's center should be constant for all devices of the same nominal size. Similar test blocks are also used for testing of total disc replacements.

and that the polyacetal have a minimum ultimate tensile strength of 61 MPa. For the purposes of strength testing, it is probably more important to choose a material that is strong enough to withstand the tests without failure and provide uniformity among specimens than to choose a material with a specific tensile strength, unless determining the stiffness of the system is of high importance. The test blocks should have inner surfaces that are contoured to mate with the device, simulating the way in which the device will interface with the vertebral end plates *in vivo*. When the device is placed between these test blocks and the construct is in its unloaded state, it is specified that the intradiscal height H, or the vertical distance between the test blocks at the device's midline be consistent for all devices of the same nominal size (see Figure 13.5). Recommended values of H are 4, 6, or 10 mm for cervical, thoracic, and lumbar cages, respectively, although this variable will depend mostly on the height of the specific design being tested. These recommended values are based on morphometric data and if a height of less than 4 mm or greater than 18 mm is used, it should be justified as being anatomically relevant.

A significant portion of F2077 is devoted to descriptions and illustrations of the testing fixtures that should be designed to apply the desired loads to the device (pure compression, compression-shear or torsion) without introducing any additional off-axis bending moments that could be highly sensitive to small misalignments or geometric features of the testing setup and could confound the test results. Figure 13.6 illustrates the setup recommended for axial compression testing. For all three testing setups, the load should be transferred to the device via a long, hollow pushrod. This pushrod is to be at least 38 cm in length, 25 mm in diameter, and manufactured from stainless steel (with a rec-

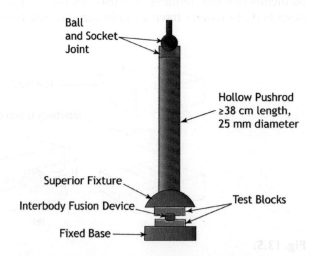

Fig. 13.6.
Testing setup described in ASTM F2077 for axial compression testing of interbody fusion devices or cages. The hollow pushrod and superior fixture are manufactured from stainless steel, and the test blocks are either stainless steel (for static testing) or polyacetal (for dynamic testing). The ball-and-socket joint at the top of the pushrod may be replaced with a universal joint.

ommended minimum ultimate tensile strength of 1,310 MPa). It is intended to provide a long, narrow "two-force member" that can apply a pure compression or torsional load along its central axis without transferring any shear or bending moments. The top of the pushrod should be connected to the testing machine via a minimal friction universal joint (for any of the tests) or a ball-and-socket joint (for axial compression or compression-shear tests only). Universal joints are multi-hinged fixtures that allow transfer of compressive and torsional loads but are unconstrained in bending about other axes and are therefore unable to transmit loads in those directions. Ball-and-socket joints are able to transfer compressive loads to a surface but not torsion or bending moments.

The bottom of the pushrod must interface with the superior test fixture, which transfers the applied load to the device/test block construct. The superior fixture is also manufactured from stainless steel and should be in the shape of a 50-mm-diameter (or larger) sphere that has been truncated so that the sphere's center will coincide with the geometric center of the device. For axial compression and compression-shear testing, the bottom of the pushrod should have a concave spherical end with a 25-mm radius so that it may interface with the superior fixture via a minimal friction sphere joint. This type of interface will further ensure that bending and torsion loads will not be applied to the device. For torsional testing, the bottom of the pushrod must have a slightly different design so that torsion about the pushrod axis can be transferred to the device via a gimbal mechanism. Two example designs (a pin-slot gimbal or a spherical gimbal) are illustrated in the standard. The underside of the superior fixture should mate with the upper test block, and the lower test block should rest on a base that is rigidly fixed to the load cell or testing machine frame.

Like ASTM F1798, this standard uses a right-handed coordinate system with the origin of the three axes located at the geometric center of the device, the positive-z axis directed superiorly, the positive-x axis directed anteriorly, and the y axis directed laterally to the left. Static and fatigue testing should be conducted in each of the three loading modes described: axial compression, compression-shear, and torsion. For axial compression testing, the device and test blocks should be placed into the test fixtures so that the local coordinate z axis (superior-inferior axis) of the device is parallel to, and collinear with, the axis of the pushrod and the loading axis of the testing machine. The intradiscal height, H, between the inner surfaces of the test blocks should be measured and should be constant for all devices of a given size. For the static axial compression testing, a minimum of five samples should be tested by applying an axial load via the pushrod at a rate of 25 mm/min. or less until failure occurs. The load displacement curve should be recorded and used to calculate mechanical properties such as stiffness, yield load, and ultimate load. For dynamic axial compression testing, a minimum of six samples should be tested to construct a plot of load versus cycles to failure and to establish the maximum run-out load at which devices can withstand five million loading cycles without failure. The standard suggests that this maximum run-out load be determined to within 10% of the static strength of the device. Dynamic axial compression testing should use a minimum-to-maximum load ratio R of 10. The test frequency is not specified, although the user is cautioned that frequencies above 10 Hz may cause melting of the polyacetal test blocks.

The setup and test methods used for compression-shear testing are very similar to those for axial compression testing with one major exception. The inferior fixture should be designed so that the z axis of the device is rotated 45 degrees in flexion relative to the axis of the pushrod. This 45-degree rotation ensures that the load being applied by the testing machine results in both a compressive load component and an anterior shear load component on the device, each of equal magnitude. The device should still be positioned so that its geometric center is in line with the loading axis of the pushrod and the testing machine. All other details of static and dynamic testing such as sample size, loading rate, and load ratios should be the same as those used during axial compression testing.

For torsion testing, the specimen should be placed in the same upright position that it was for axial compression testing (with the local z axis parallel to the loading axis of the testing machine). The interface between the pushrod and superior fixture, as previously mentioned, should be designed so that torsion and compression can be applied to the device without introducing additional shear forces or bending moments. A compressive preload of 100, 300, or 500 N (for cervical, thoracic, or lumbar devices, respectively) is suggested in order to ensure that the device is well seated in the test blocks and to avoid separation of the blocks during the test. For static torsional testing, a torsional moment should be applied via the pushrod at a rate of 60°/min. or less until failure occurs. A plot of moment-versus-angular rotation should be generated and used to calculate static properties such as rotational stiffness, yield moment, and ultimate moment. For dynamic torsional testing, a minimum of six samples should be tested to construct a plot of applied moment versus cycles-to-failure and to establish the maximum run-out moment at which devices can withstand five million loading cycles without failure. It is suggested that this moment be determined to within 10% of the static torsional strength of the device. Dynamic torsional testing should use a fully reversed applied moment with a minimum-to-maximum load ratio R of −1. Again, it is left to the user to choose a test frequency, but it is mentioned in the appendix that frequencies above 10 Hz may melt the polyacetal test blocks.

13.5.2 Subsidence Testing of Cages (ASTM F2267)

ASTM F2267, titled "Standard Test Method for Measuring Load Induced Subsidence of Intervertebral Body Fusion Device Under Static Axial Compression," describes a test method that is used in conjunction with ASTM F2077 to evaluate the implant's resistance to subsidence. Subsidence is defined as the process of a vertebral body deforming around an implanted device (or the device "sinking into" the vertebral body), resulting in a loss of disc space height.

Unlike the other standards for fusion systems or cages that describe a series of static and dynamic tests, this standard is limited to a single static axial compression test. As in F2077, the interbody fusion device or cage is placed between two test blocks that simulate the vertebral bodies. For subsidence testing purposes, the blocks should closely resemble the stiffness and subsidence resistance of vertebral bone and it is thus recommended that they be manufactured from grade 15 rigid polyurethane foam conforming to ASTM specification F1839 (nominal density of $240 \pm 16 \, \text{kg/m}^3$, compressive modulus of 111 to 136 MPa). As before, the intradiscal height H, or the distance between the inner surfaces of the test blocks, is recommended to be 4, 6, or 10 mm for cervical, thoracic, and lumbar cages, respectively. The standard also recommends that the total height of the test construct (test blocks and device combined) be 40, 60, or 70 mm for cervical, thoracic, or lumbar devices, respectively. These are recommendations based on anatomical data and should be used as guidelines, although deviations may be necessary depending on the device design. The most important consideration is that the intradiscal heights and total construct heights should be constant for all tested devices of the same nominal size.

The rest of the testing setup and fixtures closely resemble those described in ASTM F2077 for static axial compression testing. The axial load should be applied to the device via a long, hollow stainless steel pushrod (at least 38 cm in length), the top of which is connected to the testing machine via a universal joint and the bottom of which interfaces with the superior test fixture via a low friction sphere joint. This pushrod ensures that the axial compressive force is transferred from the testing machine to the device with negligible shear loads or bending moments in other directions.

It is specified that the user should first follow the ASTM 2077 standard to conduct destructive static axial compression testing of their device using metallic blocks in order to establish the yield load and stiffness of the device, Kd. Then, a minimum sample size of five new specimens should be tested in static axial compression using the polyurethane foam test blocks described previously. Static load is to be applied at a rate of 0.1 mm/s, and the load-displacement curve should be recorded to determine the yield load and stiffness of this system, Ks. By modeling the system as two springs in series (the device and the test blocks), a value for the stiffness of the polyurethane foam blocks, Kp, can be calculated. This stiffness Kp is an indicator of the device's potential to cause subsidence of the vertebral end plate bodies. For two given devices, the design that yields a higher Kp will be less likely to cause subsidence (or will subside a smaller distance into the vertebral bodies). While this method uses both a simplified loading configuration and a calculated theoretical value of subsidence resistance, it provides a useful benchmark statistic by which various designs can be compared.

13.5.3 Testing of Vertebral Body Replacements

Vertebral body replacements (VBRs) are a separate category of interbody devices that are intended to replace a diseased vertebral body that has been resected or removed due to a tumor, trauma, or fracture. They are typically made from titanium and are similar in geometry (though taller in height) than interbody fusion cages. As a result, it is reasonable to use testing methods that are similar to those developed for interbody fusion devices and described in ASTM F2077. No separate published standard exists for the testing of vertebral body replacements, and F2077 does not specifically mention that it may be used for them. Nonetheless, those methods can easily be adapted for the testing and evaluation of VBRs.

Briefly, the device is placed between two test blocks and loaded in axial compression or torsion. These test blocks can be manufactured from either stainless steel (for static testing) or polyacetal (for dynamic testing) and be similar to those described in ASTM F2077. The FDA guidance document for spinal system 510(k)s recommends that static and dynamic axial compression testing, static and dynamic torsion testing, and expulsion testing be performed on VBR devices to demonstrate substantial equivalence between a new device and a predicate device. It is also noted that depending on the novelty of the design or materials additional shear or off-axis compression loading may also be necessary. In general, the testing parameters and guidelines discussed in ASTM F2077 should be used or taken into consideration when evaluating a vertebral body replacement.

13.6 Standards for Total Disc Replacements

Artificial intervertebral discs or total disc replacements, discussed in Chapter 11, are intended to mimic the mechanical properties and range of motion of a natural disc. Although total disc replacements have been in use in Europe for decades, the first total disc replacement (Depuy Spine's Charité Artificial Disc) was approved by the FDA for the U.S. market in 2004. Numerous new designs are currently under development. As a result, disc replacements are a diverse, fledgling category of device and standardized test methods are still being developed and tried. As of this writing (March of 2006), the ASTM and ISO standards organizations have published or are developing three standard test methods for static and fatigue testing (ASTM F2346) and wear testing (ASTM F2423, ISO/DIS 18912-1). This section discusses current thinking on the important elements of disc replacement testing.

13.6.1 Static and Fatigue Testing of Total Disc Replacements (ASTM F2346)

Although a disc replacement is a motion-preserving device, it is subjected to the same static and dynamic loads as other spinal implants, and therefore uniaxial static and fatigue testing should be important aspects of its mechanical evaluation. The ASTM standard for this static and fatigue testing (F2346), titled "Standard Test Methods for Static and Dynamic Characterization of Spinal Artificial Discs," is similar in many respects to ASTM F2077 for fusion cages in its format and approach. In general, an investigator should always keep the goals of their testing in mind. Static testing should establish the maximum loads the device can withstand before failure in axial compression, compression-shear, and torsion. Fatigue testing should establish the maximum run-out loads at which all specimens can withstand ten million cycles of loading in these same three modes.

The test setup and testing parameters described in ASTM F2346 for static and dynamic testing of artificial discs are similar to those used in ASTM F2077. Devices are placed between a pair of test blocks simulating the vertebral bodies, made from either stainless steel (for static testing) or polyacetal (for fatigue testing). Fixtures should be designed to eliminate any transverse bending moments on the device. All static loads should be applied at a rate of no more than 25 mm/min. or 60°s/min. until failure. Compression-shear may be applied by rotating the specimen so that its vertical axis is at a 45-degree angle in the sagittal plane from the loading axis of the testing machine. During static torsion tests, a compressive preload of 100, 300, or 500 N should be applied (for cervical, thoracic, or lumbar discs, respectively) to seat the device in its test blocks. During fatigue testing, loads should be applied with a minimum-to-maximum load ratio R of either 10 (for compression and compression-shear) or −1 (for fully reversed torsion). Fatigue testing should be conducted in a 0.9% saline test fluid at body temperature (37° C) and with a frequency of no more than 2 Hz.

13.6.2 Wear Testing of Total Disc Replacements (ASTM F2423 and ISO/DIS 18192-1)

Currently, both ASTM and ISO have published or are developing their own standard test methods for wear testing of intervertebral disc replacements. The fact that there is this dual effort highlights the great interest and need for standards in this area, although unfortunately it is not usually desirable to have two competing standards for the same type of test. Further complicating matters is the difficulty in validating any wear test method given the fact that disc replacements are still in their early stages of clinical use, and there has not been substantial reporting in the literature of retrieved devices and clinically observed wear mechanisms. The goal of a "wear simulator" is not to mimic physiologic conditions perfectly but to produce the same type and amount of wear on a specimen that is seen on an explanted device. Hip and knee simulators have been able to draw these comparisons to some extent, but spinal disc simulators thus far have not because of the relative lack of long-term clinical experience with these devices. Therefore, it is still too early to define the best or optimal test conditions for a disc replacement wear test. Because this ultimate goal of correlation between test samples and clinically retrieved devices cannot be achieved at the present time, the current goal should be to simulate spinal loading conditions well enough so that a design that will have poor resistance *in vivo* can be identified.

In general, wear testing is performed by applying an axial compressive load to the device and then applying rotational motions in displacement control about the three axes. These three axes are based on a global coordinate system with its origin at either the geometric center of the device or the center of rotation of the total disc replacement. The z axis is directed superiorly relative to the specimen's initial position and parallel to the loading axis, with the x axis directed anteriorly and the y axis directed laterally to the left. The three applied motions are flexion-extension (rotation in the sagittal plane about the y axis), lateral bending (rotation in the frontal plane about the x axis), and axial rotation (rotation in the horizontal plane about the z axis). Wear is assessed by weighing the specimens at various intervals during the test to determine the weight loss of the device due to wear. This approach is similar in many respects to gravimetric assessment of wear in hip prostheses (ASTM F1714) and knee prostheses (ASTM F1715), but these ASTM and ISO drafts specify load and motion profiles and other parameters tailored for spinal disc replacements.

ASTM's standard F2423 is titled "Standard Test Method for the Functional and Kinematic Wear Assessment of Total Disc Prostheses" and describes a testing method for wear testing of total disc replacements, including parameters such as loads, motions, frequency, and test environment. In the opening section, it explains that this method is not intended for partial disc, nucleus, or facet joint replacements and not intended to assess the fixation of the device to the vertebral body end plates. Because the ASTM test method is not intended to evaluate the bone-implant interface, it is specified that device components should be rigidly mounted to the testing machine fixtures in a way that does not interfere with periodic weight measurements, even if this requires a modification of the bone-contacting surfaces. Adhesives or glues, unless they can be removed completely from the implant surfaces before weighing, may leave residual material on surfaces and may ruin the precise weight measurements that are needed for wear assessment. Although the potential for *in vivo* wear or damage to bone-contacting surfaces should be considered and evaluated separately (e.g., if the surface includes a sintered bead or plasma-sprayed coating), it is not necessary to incorporate that evaluation into this wear test, the purpose of which is to focus on the articulating surfaces or other interfaces that may produce wear debris.

The ASTM draft standard specifies that specimens should be mounted in a noncorrosive test chamber and submerged in a bovine serum solution diluted to a protein concentration of $20\,\text{g}/\text{L}$ in phosphate buffered saline and maintained at $37°\text{C}$. (Newborn calf serum is suggested to achieve greater consistency between lots.) It is suggested that additives such as 0.2% sodium azide (or other antibiotic) and 20-mM ethylene-diaminetetraacetic acid (EDTA) be added to the test fluid to minimize bacterial growth and calcium phosphate precipitation onto the surfaces. Unless the investigator is certain that the device will not absorb any of this fluid (e.g., an all metal device), additional "soak control" specimens subjected to the same static load for the same time intervals should also be used. These soak control specimens are not subjected to motion but are removed and weighed at the same intervals as the test specimens in order to correct for weight gain of those specimens due to fluid sorption. All specimens should be weighed and relevant dimensions (such as disc height, circumference, or bearing area) should be measured prior to the start of testing.

All tests are conducted for a minimum of ten million cycles, with a cycle defined as one complete excursion through the range of motion, beginning and ending at the starting position. Testing should be interrupted at a minimum of once every million cycles to remove, clean, dry, and weigh the components to measure weight loss. Specimens should be weighed three times in rotation at each interval using a balance with a sensitivity of $\pm 10\,\mu g$. Other relevant dimensions or geometric features may also be measured at these intervals, surfaces should be inspected for signs of wear, and any failures should be noted. After weighing and inspection, the test specimens and soak controls are replaced into the testing machine for continued testing. Weight measurements taken at each testing interval can be used to calculate the net wear (in mg) at the end of each cycle and the average net wear rate (in mg per million cycles). These weight measurements can be converted to volumetric wear and volumetric wear rate by dividing the weights by the nominal density of the material, assuming the material has a constant density.

Another important task that must be performed at each of these inspection intervals is to change and filter the test fluid to isolate particulate debris that has been generated from the bearing surfaces. The draft standard references standard practice ASTM F1877, which provides information on characterizing particulate debris in terms of size and morphology. ASTM F561 provides more information on particle isolation techniques. Particle collection and analysis should be considered an integral part of the wear evaluation process.

ASTM suggests that all motions should use a test frequency of no more than 2 Hz unless it can be justified that the machine accuracy, device properties, and testing environment are not being affected by a higher frequency. The static preload should be maintained with an accuracy of $\pm 3\%$, and motions should be controlled with an accuracy of ± 0.5 degrees. The draft standard provides illustrations of apparatus designs that can maintain the constant preload throughout a full range of motion.

For cervical disc replacements, ASTM suggests that each device be tested for ten million cycles in flexion/extension, followed by another ten million cycles of combined lateral bending and axial rotation. Alternatively, all three motions may be tested simultaneously if the investigator's equipment is capable of this. Regardless of testing sequence or motion coupling, each device should complete ten million cycles of motion in every direction, and a minimum of five devices should be tested. Table 13.1 lists the loads and ranges of motion that are suggested by the ASTM standard and ISO draft standard, with the ASTM parameters for cervical discs in the first column. If lateral bending and axial rotation are the only motions being combined, they should be in phase with each other (0-degree phase angle). If all three motions are to be combined, it is left to the user to select and justify the phase angles. A minimum sample size of five specimens should be tested, and if all three motions are not combined into a single test the same devices should be used for each sequential test.

For lumbar disc replacements, ASTM suggests three options for testing sequences. Devices may be tested in each of the three motions sequentially (flexion-extension, lateral bending, and axial rotation) for ten million cycles each. Alternatively, devices may be tested for ten million cycles of lateral bending, followed by another ten million cycles of combined flexion-extension and axial rotation. As a third option, all three motions may be tested simultaneously if the

Table 13.1.

Loads and ranges of motion specified by ASTM standard and ISO draft standard for wear testing of cervical and lumbar disc replacements. Note that ASTM specifies a constant axial load, whereas ISO specifies a sinusoidally varying load.

	Cervical		Lumbar	
	ASTM	**ISO**	**ASTM**	**ISO**
Axial Load (N)	100	50–150	1,200	600–2,000
Flexion-extension range of motion (°)	±7.5	±7.5	±8.5	–3/+6
Lateral bending range of motion (°)	±6	±6	±6	±2
Axial rotation range of motion (°)	±6	±4	±3	±2

investigator's equipment is capable of doing this. Regardless of testing sequence or motion coupling, each device should complete ten million cycles of motion in every direction, and a minimum of five devices should be tested. The ASTM parameters for lumbar discs are listed in the third column of Table 13.1. If flexion-extension and axial rotation are the only motions being combined, they should be 90 degrees out of phase with each other. If all three motions are to be combined, it is left to the user to select and justify the phase angles.

ISO's draft standard (ISO/DIS 18192-1) is titled "Implants for Surgery: Wear of Total Intervertebral Spinal Disc Prostheses. Part 1: Loading and Displacement Parameters for Wear Testing and Corresponding Environmental Conditions for Tests," and it differs from the ASTM method in several fundamental ways. First, it specifies that all three axes of motion are to be tested simultaneously and does not allow for separate sequential motion testing as mentioned in the ASTM standard. Graphs are provided showing how these motion cycles should be phased in relation to each other. More significantly, it specifies that a sinusoidally varying axial compressive load should be applied to the device instead of the static axial load used in the ASTM method. All loads and motions should use the same test frequency of 1 Hz, unless a higher frequency can be justified by the user in which case frequencies up to 2 Hz may be used. For lumbar devices constrained in the horizontal (xy) plane, it is also recommended that they be placed into the testing machine at an inclined angle in the sagittal plane to generate a shear load component on the device. Collection and analysis of the particulate debris are outside the scope of the document and are not discussed.

Otherwise, the ISO and ASTM methods are similar in testing approach but contain different test parameters in several significant places. These different parameters are shown in Table 13.1 for comparison. For cervical discs, the ranges of motion are the same as the ASTM method for flexion-extension and lateral bending but smaller for axial rotation. For lumbar discs, all three ranges of motion suggested are smaller than those in the ASTM method, particularly for lateral bending. The ISO draft also suggests that weight measurements be taken at least once every 500,000 cycles, instead of once per million cycles. A slightly different formulation of bovine calf serum fluid is specified as well (diluted with deionized water to a 30 g/L protein concentration instead of diluted with saline to 20 g/L).

Unlike most other standards that are codified descriptions of a method that has already been developed and used (and the validity of which has already been demonstrated), standards for disc wear testing satisfy an immediate need to provide researchers and device manufacturers with common test methods for safety evaluation and comparison purposes. Regardless of whether an agreed-upon method is an ideal simulation of spinal wear, in the short term it will at least allow comparisons between designs—something that will never be possible if common test methods are never adopted.

13.7 Other Nonfusion Devices

In addition to total disc replacements, other devices are being developed in an effort to eliminate the source of pain in a degenerated disc and provide structural support to the spinal column while allowing "normal" flexibility. New designs of nonfusion devices—including partial disc replacements, nucleus replacements, and other dynamic systems or spacers—are expected to emerge because of the rapidly growing interest in the nonfusion approach. With all of these novel nonfusion devices, the investigator has great freedom in the design of testing but also great responsibility to perform a risk analysis, consider all possible loading modes and scenarios to which the device will be subjected, consider all possible failure modes, and ensure that testing demonstrates that there will be low risk of these failure modes occurring. In addition to insuring static and fatigue strength of the implant, other characteristics such as its resistance to expulsion, migration, and wear may be very important to consider, depending on the geometry and the materials being used.

If a device is expected to generate wear debris during typical use, it is just as important to characterize the nature of that debris in terms of size, shape, composition, and potential for biological activity as it is to measure the overall wear rate of the device. Particle size distribution, including the numbers or proportions of particles that are above and below the phagocytosable range, should be considered important elements of characterizing a device's wear behavior. If the device is expected to generate wear debris particles of a material that is novel for the spine, the FDA often recommends that a small animal study may be needed to evaluate the local and systemic responses to particulate debris of the same size, shape, and composition as that which the device will generate. These evaluations, while separate from mechanical testing, are important components of device evaluation that should not be overlooked because an untoward reaction to wear debris could have a significant impact on the device's performance and function. As described in Chapter 2, materials that are novel for spinal implants should also be evaluated for biocompatibility, carcinogenicity, and immunogenicity using other applicable ASTM and ISO standards.

For mechanical testing of partial disc replacements or nucleus replacements, there are no ASTM or ISO standards currently in published form, although ASTM has formed a working group with the goal of writing such a standard. Designing a mechanical testing apparatus for a partial disc or nucleus replacement is more difficult than designing one for a total disc replacement because there is an implicit assumption that there will be other structures in the disc space. The most important of these structures is the annulus fibrosus, a multi-layer composite ring of collagen fibers that surrounds and constrains the gel-like nucleus pulposus. There may also be some nucleus pulposus material remaining in the disc space alongside the implant. These structures will have an impact on the device function by sharing some of the load across the segment but also by constraining the motion of the implant.

If a nucleus device is made from a very compliant, gel-like material, it may be desirable to incorporate a simulated annulus into the *in vitro* testing model in order to prevent it from "flattening out" or deforming in a way that would not realistically occur *in vivo*. In this case, care should be taken to use a material that consistently simulates the compressive properties of the annulus in the intended patients. It is important to keep in mind that a patient undergoing spinal surgery of any type is most likely suffering from severe degenerative disc disease and it is unlikely that remaining structures will retain the strength and stability of normal, healthy tissues. When in doubt, appropriate factors of safety or conservatively modified values for those material properties should be used to avoid underestimating the loads on the device. For a partial disc or nucleus replacement design that does not use a very compliant, gel-like or viscous material that requires an annulus to maintain its shape, a simulated annulus may not be necessary.

Besides total and partial disc replacements, other types of nonfusion spinal implants are being developed. Some of these are similar in geometry to fusion systems (rod or plating systems), but they include components that are designed to remain mobile and allow for flexibility. Other devices are intended to be inserted between the spinous processes and prevent collapse of the disc space while still allowing motion at the affected segment. In many cases, the investigator may begin with a published standard for a similar device and adapt it as necessary for their novel implant. For a dynamic system that resembles the geometry of a fusion system, the investigator should begin with a setup similar to that described in ASTM F1717, determine what modifications must be made to allow testing of their dynamic system while still yielding meaningful results, and make those modifications. For a device that is truly novel in its geometry and intended location, more work may be necessary in order to develop a battery of original test methods that addresses all potential failure mechanisms.

13.8 Controversies and Challenges

In the beginning of this chapter, we discussed some of the benefits and limitations of using standard test methods to evaluate devices. In addition to these general limitations, there are a number of controversial or challenging issues related to specific tests or specific device types. Some of these issues have already been mentioned, but the remainder of this chapter discusses some of the other important issues and points to consider when designing or implementing a spinal implant test method.

13.8.1 Relevance of the Corpectomy Model to All Fusion Systems

ASTM F1717 is designed to test the static and dynamic failure loads of a fusion system in a corpectomy model, in which it is assumed that one entire vertebral body will be removed. This model represents a worst-case loading scenario because the implant system is solely responsible for transferring the loads across the segment. Some would argue, however, that this is not clinically realistic for all devices. While fusion devices are sometimes used in conjunction with a corpectomy, at other times they are used in situations where some or all of the anatomical structures are preserved. While these structures can be considered non-healthy, thus requiring surgery, it may be overly pessimistic to assume that they will be unable to share any of the loads across the segment. If a system is intended for use in patients who will retain some of their load-bearing bony structures, it might be more realistic to test a construct that better represents this situation instead of assuming a corpectomy will be performed.

On the other hand, the difficulty in designing an alternative model is in ensuring that the stress being applied to the device is unique and determinable. If a device is tested in parallel with other elements representing the remaining intact anatomic structures, the investigator must be able to determine exactly how the load is being shared and be satisfied that the end result is not more dependent on the testing configuration than on the properties of the device itself! In order to calculate how the loads are being shared between the device and these parallel elements, the parallel elements would have to be added in such a way that their location, moment arm, cross-sectional area, and material properties were precisely known. Otherwise, the loads on the device may be indeterminable or unpredictable and the test results would be difficult to interpret or compare with other devices. Using a corpectomy model not only represents a worst-case scenario but also avoids these complications. Although a corpectomy model may not be clinically realistic for all devices, it has the distinct advantage of having a one-to-one relationship between the load being applied to the entire construct and the load being applied across the device itself. This relationship, while it requires a simplified clinical scenario, makes it much easier to determine the exact stress state on the implant components and compare the results from various designs.

13.8.2 Difficulties in Comparing Different Geometries

In Section 13.2.6, it was mentioned that there is often a need to modify specific numbers or parameters within standards in order to fit a specific device design that may not conform to the "standard" size or geometry, but that the investi-gator should always be aware of what consequences these modifications may have on the final results. ASTM F1717 specifies that the longitudinal gage length of the testing construct should be either 35 or 76 mm, based on reported anatomic measurements of the gap created by a corpectomy [Cunningham et al. 1993]. If a device is designed to be another size, it may still be possible to conform to the standard by fixturing it so that only a 35- or 76-mm section is tested. If this is not possible, alternative gage lengths may be chosen, but in that case it may be necessary to perform side-by-side testing with another design that has been tested at the same alternate gage length to ensure that a valid comparison is being made. Similarly, if significant differences in other dimen-sions or the overall geometry of a design make it impossible to conform to the testing conditions described in a standard test method, modifications to the standard may be warranted. In those instances, the investigator should always consider testing a known device under the same, modified testing conditions for comparison purposes. Additionally, test reports should describe the modi-fications that were made to the standards and discuss any effects or conse-quences the modifications may have had on the test results. The ability to properly interpret test results and compare the device performance to well-defined acceptance criteria should always be of the highest priority.

13.8.3 Relevance of Bench Testing to *In Vivo* Expulsion

There is a substantial mismatch, unfortunately, between the high importance of ensuring that a spinal implant will not be expulsed from the spinal column *in vivo*, and the relative inability of *in vitro* bench testing to evaluate this impor-tant design consideration. When a device or system is implanted into the spinal column, it is tremendously important that it and all of its components stay in place. For devices that are attached to the vertebral bodies or inserted into the disc space, the surgeon and patient will undoubtedly be interested in where the devices might end up if they are expulsed from their intended location. Pos-terior to the vertebral bodies lay the spinal cord and the branching nerve roots. Anterior to the vertebral bodies along most of the spinal column's length are the aorta and vena cava, the major vessels of the circulatory system. Obviously, it is critical that a spinal implant component should not be expulsed in either of these directions where it could potentially impinge on these important anatomic structures. Evaluating the resistance to expulsion is particularly important for nucleus replacements or other devices that are not designed to be rigidly fixed within the disc space and therefore have the potential to be squeezed out. The process by which a device or component could migrate, however, is a very design-specific, dynamic, and complex process and one that is not easily understood or simulated on a testing bench.

Lateral "push-out" testing is a common technique to try and address the issue of device expulsion. There is no ASTM or ISO standard for this type of push-out testing but it is typically performed by placing a device between two test blocks simulating the vertebral bodies. These blocks can be of a variety of materials, although the polyacetal or polyurethane foam recommended in ASTM F2077 or F2267 are logical choices. A static axial compressive preload may be applied to this construct to simulate the physiologic load and increase friction between the device and test blocks that would help to hold the device in place. Then, a transverse load (in the lateral, anterior, or posterior direction) is increased until the device is completely expulsed or until some predetermined amount of displacement is observed. Such a displacement is defined as a failure criterion prior to testing based on a clinical evaluation of the displacement *in vivo* that would be detrimental to the patient or to the device's function (typically on the order of a few millimeters). For an interbody device with multiple stacked components, push-out testing may be performed on individual components. For example, a three-piece total disc replacement with metal end plates and a polymeric core may be tested by rigidly holding its end plates to the test machine and applying a horizontal load to the core to measure the force needed to cause its expulsion or displacement.

It may be difficult to predict the potential for *in vivo* expulsion using only lateral push-out tests, however, for a number of reasons. A pure horizontal load will seldom if ever be applied to a spinal implant in the body, and thus this loading mode could be considered either "very worst case" or "completely unrealistic," depending on the user's point of view. The magnitude of an applied compressive preload, zero or otherwise, will undoubtedly have a significant impact on the test results and therefore its selection could affect whether or not the test accurately represents the expected loading environment. The frictional characteristics and homogeneity of the test blocks differ from those of vertebral end plates and therefore may offer a different amount of resistance to expulsion than the *in vivo* spinal structures. Many authors have suggested that expulsion of cages often occurs not because of a static load but after long-term migration of the device in conjunction with non-ideal surgical conditions such as insufficient annular tension, inadequate sizing, or cages placed too far laterally [Eshkenazi et al. 2001; McAfee et al. 1999]. These non-ideal conditions are prohibitively difficult to simulate on the testing bench. A lateral push-out test is also a short-term test of the implant's resistance to expulsion immediately after implantation and does not evaluate the effectiveness of the implant surfaces and/or coatings to promote bony fixation. Springer et al. have previously provided an excellent and more thorough discussion of these issues [Springer et al. 2003]. While push-out testing is recommended for comparison of designs and as a part of the design and development process, a functional animal study or other approach to testing is probably more likely to effectively answer questions about a new device's risk for expulsion.

13.8.4 Relevance of Bench Testing to *In Vivo* Subsidence

Similarly, it should be recognized that subsidence of an interbody device into the vertebral body end plates is another complex, dynamic process that is challenging to simulate on the testing bench. Certain design aspects of interbody devices may have a significant effect on subsidence and these should be evaluated using methods such as ASTM F2267 to ensure that a new design does not pose an unreasonable risk of causing subsidence of the vertebral end plates. Attachment features on the device surfaces (e.g., keels, pegs, or teeth), the overall surface contour, and especially the surface contact area will all play a role in determining the stress distribution at the interface between the device and end plate, and these will consequently affect the device's potential to cause subsidence.

It is important to recognize the limitations of this testing, however, as it applies to devices with substantially new geometric features, materials, or surfaces that cannot easily be compared to existing designs. The stiffness parameter, Kp, obtained from the ASTM F2267 testing method is a benchmark that is useful for comparing designs. This Kp value is a relative benchmark, however, and is difficult to correlate directly with some absolute measure in the *in vivo* loading environment. The potential for subsidence depends on the health and quality of the patient's trabecular bone as well as the device itself. Bone tissue in general can demonstrate a tremendous variation in composition, structure, and mechanical properties depending on age, gender, body weight, disease, and a host of other patient-related factors. This variability, along with its susceptibility to chemical breakdown with increased exposure to the ambient laboratory environment, makes bone a very difficult material to use in models for *in vitro* laboratory testing. The standard therefore specifies a synthetic material (grade 15 polyurethane foam) to be used in place of bone tissue in order to provide greater consistency from sample to sample during subsidence testing. The variability of vertebral bone *in vivo*, however, also makes it more challenging to directly predict a device's performance based on the results of an *in vitro* test using foam blocks. For a design with a substantially new geometry, material, surface, or fixation mechanism, the potential for subsidence is probably better evaluated using a functional animal study or other type of model.

13.8.5 Number of Cycles

A recurring issue with all devices, particularly nonfusion devices, is the number of cycles that should be used for dynamic fatigue or wear testing. In general, the number of cycles should be based on the intended use of the device as well as the expected service lifetime and estimates of physiologic loading frequency. Fusion devices are intended to support all or most of the load across a spinal segment immediately following implantation, but eventually a new bony fusion mass should form and share a significant portion of that load, reducing the load on the device. Nonfusion devices are intended to support the same loads over their entire lifetimes and therefore should be evaluated to a higher number of testing cycles. Ideally, the lifetime of an implanted device should be maximized and should equal or exceed the expected lifetime of the patient in order to minimize or eliminate the need for re-operation and revision surgery. This ideal goal is not always possible, even with current technology, particularly if the patient is young and physically active. Total hip and knee replacements typically demonstrate survival rates of 90% or more after 10 years of implantation, particularly for older patients [Joshi, Markovic, and Gill 2003], and various designs have been reported to have survival rates of over 70% after 20 years or more [Brown et al. 2002; Emery et al. 1997]. For an octogenarian, a 20-year service lifetime for an orthopedic implant is probably more than adequate. In contrast, a 60-year-old patient who receives an implant with a 20-year expected service life may require a revision surgery within his or her lifetime. An even younger, 20- or 30-year-old patient who receives an implant with only a 20-year service lifetime will probably require multiple re-operations and replacements. If a spinal device intended to aid in fusion is successful, its expected implantation time should be very long, although it may be fully loaded for only a portion of that lifetime. The average or expected survival rates of newer nonfusion spinal implants (e.g., total and partial disc replacements) will not be known until more long-term clinical experience is obtained.

Estimating the number of cycles that a human spine is loaded per year is a difficult task, and currently no definitive data have been published. Several pedometer-based studies on walking activity have estimated that an average person takes between one and two million strides per year [Wallbridge and Dowson 1982]. A 1991 paper by Hedman et al. is frequently quoted as suggesting that an average person takes two million strides and makes 125,000 significant bends per year [Hedman et al. 1991]. The authors calculated these numbers by compiling a list of several types of daily bending activities and estimating their frequency in a person of moderate activity. These estimates would suggest that a spinal implant would experience over 40 million loading cycles during a 20-year service lifetime and that a device intended to last 20 years should be tested to 40 million cycles or more. For the purposes of wear testing, it can be argued that walking cycles should not have as much of an impact as "significant bends" because the angular displacement and load amplitude associated with an individual spinal segment during a gait cycle may be small. On the other hand, the small range of motion associated with walking results in the load being concentrated on a relatively small region of the bearing surface, and these cycles could have a deleterious effect on wear, particularly for materials that may exhibit cold flow or fretting wear [Hedman 2005].

Even though there is an obvious need and desire for measurement-based estimates of spinal loading cycles per year, this information is not readily available in the literature. Even without such data, it is important to keep in mind that the goal of fatigue and wear testing should be to evaluate and predict a device's performance over its intended lifetime. At the very least, fatigue and wear testing should simulate periods of time that are longer than the 24-month clinical trials typically conducted prior to FDA device approval. Fatigue and wear testing are often the most time-intensive aspects of pre-clinical testing, however, and there is a strong motivation to restrict the length of testing to a limited but scientifically valid timeframe. Traditionally, published fatigue and wear testing of other joint replacements has been carried out to a maximum of 10 million cycles, and so it has been the position of the FDA that 10 million cycles is a reasonable timeframe for dynamic testing of spinal nonfusion devices. The ASTM and ISO standard methods being developed for artificial disc replacements similarly suggest that fatigue and wear testing be carried out to 10 million cycles for those devices.

For testing of fusion systems and interbody fusion devices, the ASTM standards suggest that fatigue run-out loads be established to five million cycles. The appendix to ASTM F2077 for interbody fusion devices explains that a successful fusion should occur well within one year of implantation and the device ought to withstand normal spinal loads until this fusion occurs. The standard suggests a factor of safety of 2.5 and an estimate of two million loading cycles per year, yielding a recommended test duration of five million cycles. Similarly, ASTM F1717 for fusion systems arrives at the same end result by assuming that a patient with a moderate activity level will experience approximately 7,000 cycles per day and that testing should simulate two years of activity, or five million cycles. For individual components or subassemblies, the ASTM standards suggest that cycle numbers lower than five million can be used to evaluate and compare different designs, presumably because it is assumed that the complete systems or assemblies will also be evaluated (using higher cycle numbers) as a part of the overall battery of tests. The appendix of ASTM F1798 for interconnection mechanisms mentions that the estimated number of loading cycles per year ranges from 1 to 2.5 million, and therefore 2.5 million cycles is chosen as the recommended test duration.

13.8.6 Test Frequency

From a device developer's perspective, there is an understandable incentive to complete any test as quickly as possible. Static tests may require long setup times but the tests themselves are relatively short in duration. For a dynamic fatigue or wear test, the testing itself (which may run for 2.5 million, five million, or 10 million cycles) requires a much longer time to complete. The most important variable for determining this duration is the test frequency. If a test is run at one cycle per second (1 Hz), it takes approximately 11.5 days of continuous, round-the-clock testing to complete a million cycles of testing on a specimen. For a 10 million cycle test, this means approximately 115 days of testing or longer because it is impractical to run tests for that amount of time without interruption. Increasing the frequency from 1 to 2 Hz cuts the time in half, to approximately 58 days. Obviously, further increases in test frequency can greatly reduce the test duration.

On the other hand, there are reasons test frequency cannot be increased indefinitely. The chief considerations that should be taken into account when choosing a test frequency are the accuracy of the test machine at high frequencies, time-dependent behavior of any viscoelastic components, hysteretic heating and temperature effects on the components and test environment, and effects of sliding velocity on wear. The first technical limitation depends on the controller of the test machine, the accuracy of which could be more difficult to maintain at very fast frequencies. The ASTM standards for hip and knee wear testing specify that the test machine should be able to control the load on the device to within ±3% of the peak load throughout the testing. Currently, both the ASTM standard and ISO draft standard for disc wear testing have adopted similar recommendations regarding controller accuracy. If a testing machine cannot maintain this level of control over the loads or angles being applied to the device at a high frequency, the test should be slowed down until greater control is achieved.

A second consideration is the materials used in the device and whether any of them have viscoelastic, time-dependent properties. Metallic or ceramic components may be exempted from this consideration because they do not exhibit time-dependent behavior, but polymeric components in particular should not be subjected to very high test frequencies because their mechanical properties can be both time dependent and temperature dependent. The relationship between storage and loss modulus, or the proportion of strain energy stored in the polymer as opposed to being dissipated by viscous flow, depends on the time or the frequency with which loading is applied. A high frequency can therefore affect the structure and mechanical behavior of a polymer because of its time-dependent nature and can affect the validity of test results, even in the absence of heating or temperature effects.

It is also important to consider that an increased test frequency can cause increased energy dissipation and hysteretic heating of a polymer that will in turn raise the internal temperature and further change the polymer's structure and behavior. Thermocouples or other transducers are sometimes applied to the surface of the polymer or to the testing fluid chamber to monitor any changes in temperature during the course of testing and ensure that the temperature does not get too high. While this technique is relatively simple to implement and useful for detecting large temperature changes, it may be difficult to interpret whether or not a smaller temperature change detected in this fashion is having an appreciable effect on the test results. The relationship between frequency and viscoelastic properties for any raw material can be determined in the laboratory using dynamic mechanical analysis (DMA) testing equipment, and knowledge of this relationship for materials in the device may provide the user with a better assurance of the frequency and temperature ranges that can be used without affecting mechanical behavior.

In addition to adverse effects of temperature on the devices and components themselves, the user should also be aware of the consequences of elevated temperatures on the rest of the testing setup and test environment. ASTM F2077 and F2346 for cage and disc replacement testing, which use polymeric test blocks, warn that frequencies over 10 Hz could heat and soften the test blocks in addition to affecting the device itself. If a test is being conducted in a physiological fluid with proteins such as bovine serum, higher temperatures could cause the proteins to denature and degrade, negating any added benefit of using the serum [Lu and McKellop 1997].

Even if a high frequency is determined to be appropriate for fatigue testing, it may not be appropriate for wear testing. During fatigue testing, the device is not in motion and the only thing that changes with time is the stress state. If the constitutive properties of the materials are not affected by the test frequency, the test results will probably not be affected. Wear testing, on the other hand, involves a more complex process in which asperities of each material's surface are sliding past each other and interacting through abrasive, adhesive, fatigue, and fluid-film or boundary lubrication mechanisms that could depend highly on the relative sliding velocities of those surfaces. For this reason, even if the individual component materials are not expected to exhibit frequency-dependent behavior wear testing should not be accelerated beyond a physiologic range unless data can be generated to show that increasing the frequency does not affect the wear mechanisms for that device.

If frequency may have an effect on the device's mechanical behavior, investigators may be interested in knowing how their test frequency compares to the expected physiologic frequency at which their device will be used *in vivo*. What is a physiologic frequency range? The appendix of ASTM F2346 for disc replacement testing mentions that a physiologic range of frequencies is typically between 0.1 and 8 Hz, but no specific sources are cited. Normal walking speeds, during which there is limited spinal motion but a time-varying load, have been reported in the range of 1 to 3 Hz for various age groups [Al-Obaidi et al. 2003]. Data on the frequency of spinal motion cycles (flexion-extension, lateral bending, or axial rotation) are more difficult to find in the medical literature. World records for sit-up exercises, during which athletes attempt to perform a maximum number of flexion-extension cycles in a fixed period of time, may help to suggest a maximum achievable frequency for that particular spinal motion. The *Guinness Book of World Records* [2004] states that the current record for most sit-ups in an hour using an assistive abdominal frame device is 8,367, yielding an equivalent frequency of approximately 2.4 Hz. While sit-up exercises may be an atypical activity, this information suggests that even in a competitive athletic situation human beings can only achieve maximal flexion-extension frequencies of 2.4 Hz or below.

Currently, standards for spinal implants suggest a wide range of maximum test frequencies, from 1 to 2 Hz (for wear testing of discs) to 16 Hz (for interconnection mechanisms) to 30 Hz (for metallic screws and plates). It is the responsibility of the user to consider each of the factors discussed previously (machine accuracy, time-dependent material behavior, temperature effects on the device, temperature effects on the environment and wear mechanisms, comparison of test frequency to physiologic frequency) and choose a frequency for dynamic testing that will be economical without interfering with the validity of the test results.

13.8.7 Testing Fluid Environment

An important aspect of any wear test of any device or material couple is choice of whether to test in a fluid environment—and if so, which fluid to use. The human body, made up of approximately 60 to 70% water, is a very moist environment, and thus wear simulator testing in air should probably not be used except in preliminary screening studies. Selection of a fluid will affect the wear rate and wear mechanisms because the viscosity and composition of a fluid will affect the overall lubrication regime (boundary, fluid-film, or mixed-mode lubrication).

Fluids that have traditionally been used for wear testing of other orthopedic devices include water, saline, or serum, each of which come in many varieties. These different test fluids have been shown to significantly affect wear testing results for total hip and knee replacements [Good, Clarke, and Anissian 1996;

Wang et al. 1995). Bovine serum is currently the optimal choice for testing of these devices because it has resulted in wear mechanisms and debris morphology that compare well with retrieved implants [Cooper, Dowson, and Fisher 1993; McKellop et al. 1978; Wang, Stark, and Dumbleton 1996]. One of the reasons serum is thought to provide a good simulation of *in vivo* conditions for total joint prostheses is its protein content. Hip and knee joints are assumed to contain synovial fluid, which has been reported to have a protein concentration of 15 to 25 g/L in healthy joints and protein concentrations of 29 to 39 g/L or 36 to 54 g/L in osteoarthritic and rheumatoid arthritic patients, respectively [Mazzucco, Scott, and Spector 2004]. These concentrations are much lower than that of bovine serum, but the serum can easily be diluted using deionized water or saline to a protein concentration that more closely resembles synovial fluid. Wang et al. have studied a wide range of serum lubricants with different protein types and concentrations and described a complex dependence of wear rate on total protein content, albumin/globulin ratio, and protein precipitation [Wang, Essner, and Schmidig 2004]. Liao et al. [1999] have discussed the fact that very low concentrations of serum have led to nonphysiologic wear mechanisms such as pitting and flaking, which they attribute to the inability of soluble proteins to provide complete boundary lubrication at the surface. These authors also point out that precipitation of proteins out of the fluid, which can be accelerated by increasing temperatures, should also be minimized so that these proteins do not form a protective coating on the bearing surface but also so that the boundary lubrication properties of the serum are not degraded.

The intervertebral disc joint does not contain a synovial capsule or synovial fluid, and thus it is questionable whether it is necessary to use serum, which was originally employed to simulate synovial fluid, for wear testing of artificial disc replacements. Again, the limited clinical experience with these devices has not yet allowed comparisons to be drawn between wear patterns on retrieved implants and *in vitro* specimens that have been tested in different lubricants. The disc joint space most likely contains interstitial fluid, a category of extracellular fluid that surrounds the body tissues and allows transfer of oxygen, nutrients, wastes, and cytokines. This fluid is similar in composition to lymph and it does contain proteins, although its protein concentration is very low compared to blood plasma. This author is not aware of published data on protein concentration of interstitial fluid taken from the spinal column, but other authors have reported the protein concentration of interstitial fluid from other regions as high as 35 to 42 g/L [Bates, Levick, and Mortimer 1993]. Clinical retrieval results are needed to provide more information as to the optimal choice of lubricant and whether or not proteins are necessary. The ASTM and ISO draft standards currently suggest that bovine calf serum with a protein concentration of 20 to 30 g/L be used.

13.8.8 Loads and Angles for Wear Testing

As you read in Chapter 5 and at the beginning of this chapter, loads in the spine can vary greatly depending on factors such as spinal region, body weight, posture, and activity. Many measurements and modeling estimates of loads in the cervical [Moroney, Schultz, and Miller 1988; Snijders, Hoek van Dijke, and Roosch 1991] and lumbar spine [Nachemson 1963, 1965, 1975, 1981] during different activities can be found in the literature. Ranges of motion in three dimensions at various spinal levels have also been reported and compiled by other authors. The graphs in Figure 13.7 show some of these reported ranges of motion and how they compare with the wear testing ranges of motion suggested by ASTM (red lines) and ISO (blue lines). In general, the range of motion in flexion-extension is larger than that of lateral bending or axial rotation, particularly in the lumbar spine. Axial rotation is very small in the lumbar spine but much larger in the cervical spine. Lateral bending does not vary much with spinal level but is slightly larger in the cervical spine than the lumbar spine.

Defining the loading and range of motion conditions for a wear test is a subject of much debate. Choosing appropriate conditions for a wear test is more difficult than for a static or fatigue test, because a balance must be struck between "physiologic" and "worst-case" parameters in order to simulate the expected wear patterns. In a static test, for example, a very severe or worst-case load can be applied to cause a catastrophic failure of the device, and from there it is relatively straightforward to justify that the device will be able to withstand physiologically realistic loads without failing. Similarly, a fatigue test is usually repeated at a number of different load levels until a maximum run-out load is established, and then it can be justified that the run-out load exceeds the expected loads on the device. For a wear simulation test, if the testing conditions are too severe or worst-case, unrealistic wear patterns could result—and, more importantly, all designs might perform poorly and the ability to identify a bad design would be lost. At the same time, conditions should be conservatively chosen to represent the spectrum of patients who may be receiving and using the device. The temptation to pick only "average" or "typical" loads or motions from the literature could produce a wear test that does a very good job of predicting a device's wear performance for an "average" patient (average weight, medium build, average level of activity) but does not identify a design that might have very poor performance for a person who is "above average" in any of those categories. Unless the surgical inclusion criteria or indications for a particular device are narrowly defined so as to include only "average" patients (which is unlikely), a wear test should be designed with appropriate loads and motions to insure good wear performance of a device in any of its potential recipients.

13.8.9 Multidirectional Versus Unidirectional Motion

The spine is subjected to complex loading patterns during everyday living. Our motions can be broken down into orthogonal components and described in terms of flexion-extensions, lateral bends, and axial rotations. Unless we are performing a very repetitive task or attending an aerobics class, however, we are probably experiencing these different motions in various simultaneous combinations and sequences throughout the day. In fact, the facet joints of the

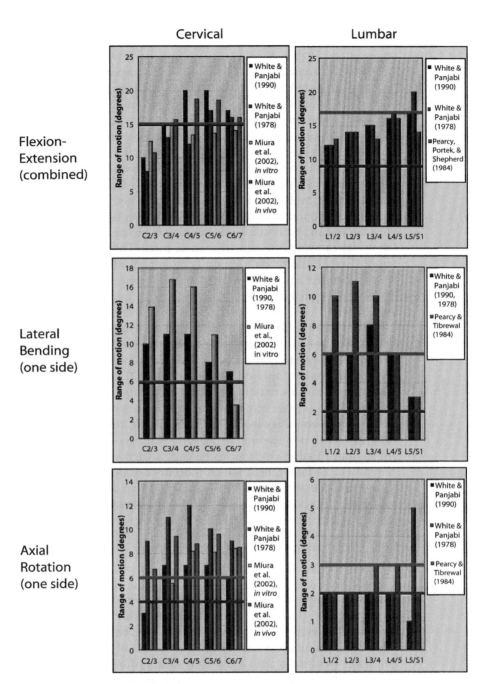

Fig. 13.7.

Ranges of motion in the cervical and lumbar spine as reported by White and Panjabi [1978, 1990]; Miura et al. [2002]; Pearcy, Portek, and Shepherd [1984]; and Pearcy and Tibrewal [1984] shown in comparison to ASTM and ISO recommendations for wear testing of total disc replacements. The left-hand column shows ranges of motion for the cervical spine in three motions: combined flexion/extension, one-sided lateral bending, and one-sided axial rotation. The right-hand column shows ranges of motion for the lumbar spine in the same three motions. The red lines represent the ranges of motion suggested by ASTM F2423 and the blue lines represent the ranges of motion suggested by ISO/DIS 18192-1.

vertebrae in some regions of the spine are shaped in such a way that it is very difficult to completely uncouple these spinal motions from each other. In the cervical and upper thoracic spine, lateral bending to one side causes an axial rotation of the spinous processes toward the opposite side.

In the lumbar spine, lateral bending to one side causes axial rotation of the spinous processes toward the same side, and vice versa [Miles and Sullivan 1961]. For example, if you twist around to your left using only your lumbar spine your right shoulder will naturally dip slightly forward in a right lateral bend. Spinal implants will therefore be expected to withstand a high degree of multiaxial motion in addition to more simple, uniaxial motions. For purposes of wear testing, however, it is much simpler to design and use a testing machine that rotates about one axis instead of three. Therefore, we must ask the question, "Even if multiaxial motion is more clinically relevant, what impact does it have on the results of wear testing?" Although we do not yet know this answer for spinal disc replacements, we can make educated guesses based on the history of wear testing of other total joint replacements.

The effect of multidirectional motion on wear depends greatly on the materials being tested. For ultrahigh molecular weight polyethylene (UHMWPE), multidirectional motion has been shown in simulator studies to produce higher wear than uniaxial motion [Barnett et al. 2001; Bragdon et al. 1996]. While all the reasons for this may not be fully understood, the predominant hypothesis is that when polymer chains at the surface are subjected to a unidirectional force they align themselves in the direction of that force over time. This molecular alignment can be measured using soft X-ray absorption [Sambasivan et al. 2004] or by transmission electron microscopy [Kurtz et al. 1999], and the amount of alignment and the rate at which it occurs can depend on many factors including the degree of cross linking. This orientation of the surface molecules causes the material to become hardened and quasi-glassy, and although it may be more susceptible to tensile cracking it is more wear resistant in general [Wright and Goodman 2001]. Therefore, simulator testing that applies motion in only one direction may underestimate the amount of wear that could be generated under more physiologic (i.e., multidirectional) motion.

It is interesting to note that this correlation of lower wear rates with unidirectional motion may not be the case for all device designs or material combinations, particularly metal-on-metal devices. Tipper et al. conducted pin-on-plate reciprocating wear testing of cobalt chrome alloys and showed that bi-axial motion (rotation and translation of the pin on the plate) resulted in lower wear rates than a uniaxial sliding motion [Tipper et al. 1999]. These results, although the study used a simplified testing geometry rather than a finished device, suggest that uniaxial motion will not always have a favorable effect on wear resistance when compared to combined motions. If uniaxial motions are applied sequentially instead of simultaneously (flexion-extension, then lateral bending, then axial rotation), wear performance could theoretically be even worse if a "wear track" or unidirectional scratches are formed on a surface and then during the next phase of testing asperities of the opposing surface are dragged across these scratches in the transverse direction. Because multidirectional motion has been shown to have effects on wear under many different conditions, the ASTM and ISO draft standards suggest that wear testing should incorporate coupled motions and that the same devices should be subjected to all motions rather than testing separate devices in separate directions.

13.9 Conclusions

In this chapter, we have discussed various methods for mechanical testing of spinal implant devices, focusing on methods that have been developed by standards organizations such as ASTM and ISO. We have also discussed how these voluntary standards are developed and the benefits and limitations of using a standard method for a new device design as opposed to developing an original test method. The goal of this chapter was not to teach the reader the particular details of individual methods, which are better learned by reading and implementing the standards themselves, but to give a better understanding of the larger issues and considerations to be kept in mind when choosing a test method and interpreting its results.

For any device, whether or not published standards are available as guidelines the investigator should always begin planning a testing regimen with a basic risk analysis of the device in mind. This risk analysis should take into account all the types of loading the device will be subjected to and all the potential failure mechanisms. Static tests should then be designed to measure the maximum loads or moments, in all relevant loading modes, the device can withstand without failure for comparison with other similarly indicated devices or estimates of physiologic loads. Dynamic tests should be designed to measure the maximum loads or moments in these same directions that the device can withstand without failing before an acceptable number of loading cycles have been reached. Failures should be defined prior to testing to include not only catastrophic fractures of components but also deformations, wear loss, or other changes to the device that could compromise its intended function.

In any case, the investigator should always keep in mind that the all-important goal of testing is to evaluate the device's ability to withstand physiologic conditions without failure. If a test method, standardized or not, can achieve this goal it will have been a successful and useful test regardless of whether the results are favorable.

13.10 References

The published ASTM standards discussed in this chapter are available in the 2006 *Annual Book of Standards, Volume 13.01, Medical and Surgical Materials and Devices; Anesthetic and Respiratory Equipment*, ASTM International, West Conshohocken, PA.

Al-Obaidi, S., J. Wall, A. Al-Yaqoub, and M. Al-Ghanim (2003). "Basic Gait Parameters: A Comparison of Reference Data for Normal Subjects 20 to 29 Years of Age from Kuwait and Scandinavia," *J. Rehab. Res. Develop.* 40:361–366.

Barnett, P., J. Fisher, et al. (2001). "Comparison of Wear in a Total Knee Replacement Under Different Kinematic Conditions," *J. Mater. Sci. Mater. Med.* 12:1039–1042.

Bates, D., J. Levick, and P. Mortimer (1993). "Change in Macromolecular Composition of Interstitial Fluid from Swollen Arms After Breast Cancer Treatment, and Its Implications," *Clin. Science (London)* 85:737–746.

Bragdon, C., D. O'Connor, et al. (1996). "The Importance of Multidirectional Motion on the Wear of Polyethylene," *Proc. Inst. Mech. Engrs. H.* 210:157–165.

Brown, S., W. Davies, D. DeHeer, and A. Swanson (2002). "Long-term Survival of McKee-Farrar Total Hip Prostheses," *Clin. Orthop. Rel. Res.* 402:157–163.

Cooper, J., D. Dowson, and J. Fisher (1993). "The Effect of Transfer Film and Surface Roughness on the Wear of Lubricated Ultra-high Molecular Weight Polyethylene," *Clin. Materials* 14:295–302.

Cunningham, B., J. Sefter, Y. Shono, and P. McAfee (1993). "Static and Cyclic Biomechanical Analysis of Pedicle Screw Spinal Constructs," *Spine* 18:1677–1688.

Emery, D., A. Britton, H. Clarke, and M. Grover (1997). "The Stanmore Total Hip Arthroplasty: A 15- to 20-year Follow-up Study," *J. Arthroplasty* 12:727–735.

Eshkenazi, A., D. Dabby, E. Tolessa, and J. Finkelstein (2001). "Early Retropulsion of Titanium-threaded Cages After Posterior Lumbar Interbody Fusion: A Report of Two Cases," *Spine* 26:1073–1075.

Good, V., I. Clarke, and L. Anissian (1996). "Water and Bovine Serum Lubrication Compared in Simulator PTFE/CoCr Wear Model," *J. Biomed. Mater. Res.* 33:275–283.

Guinness World Records. (2004). Guinness Book of World Records: Special 50th Anniversary Edition. Claire Folkard (ed.). New York: Bantam Books.

Hedman, T., J. Kostuik, G. Fernie, and W. Hellier (1991). "Design of an Intervertebral Disc Prosthesis," *Spine* 16:S256–S260.

Hedman, T. P. (2005). Personal Communication, UCLA, Los Angeles.

Joshi, A., L. Markovic, and G. Gill (2003). "Knee Arthroplasty in Octogenarians: Results at 10 Years," *J. Arthroplasty* 18:295–298.

Kurtz, S., L. Pruitt, et al. (1999). "Radiation and Chemical Crosslinking Promote Strain Hardening Behavior and Molecular Alignment in Ultra High Molecular Weight Polyethylene During Multi-axial Loading Conditions," *Biomaterials* 20:1449–1462.

Lu, Z., and H. McKellop (1997). "Frictional Heating of Bearing Materials Tested in a Hip Joint Wear Simulator," *Proc. Inst. Mech. Engrs. H.* 211:101–108.

McAfee, P., B. Cunningham, et al. (1999). "Revision Strategies for Salvaging or Improving Failed Cylindrical Cages," *Spine* 24:2147–2153.

McKellop, H., I. Clarke, K. Markolf, and H. Amstutz (1978). "Wear Characteristics of UHMW Polyethylene: A Method for Accurately Measuring Extremely Low Wear Rates," *J. Biomed. Mater. Res.* 12:895–927.

Mazzucco, D., R. Scott, and M. Spector (2004). "Composition of Joint Fluid in Patients Undergoing Total Knee Replacement and Revision Arthroplasty: Correlation with Flow Properties," *Biomaterials* 25:4433–4445.

Miles, M., and W. Sullivan (1961). "Lateral Bending at the Lumbar and Lumbosacral Joints," *Anat. Rec.* 139:387.

Moroney, S., A. Schultz, and J. Miller (1988). "Analysis and Measurement of Neck Loads," *J. Orthop. Res.* 6:713–720.

Nachemson, A. (1963). "The Influence of Spinal Movement on the Lumbar Intra Discal Pressure and on the Tensile Stresses in the Annulus Fibrosus," *Acta Orthop. Scand.* 33:183.

Nachemson, A. (1965). "In Vivo Discometry in Lumbar Discs with Irregular Radiograms," *Acta Orthop. Scand.* 36:418.

Nachemson, A. (1975). "A Critical Look at the Treatment for Low Back Pain: The Research Status of Spinal Manipulative Therapy," Bethesda: DHEW Publication No. (NIH) 76-998:21B.

Nachemson, A. (1981). "Disc Pressure Measurements," *Spine* 6:94–99.

Sambasivan, S., D. Fischer, M. Shen, and S. Hsu (2004). "Molecular Orientation of Ultra-high Molecular Weight Polyethylene Induced by Various Sliding Motions," *J. Biomed. Mater. Res.* 70B:278–285.

Snijders, C., G. Hoek van Dijke, and E. Roosch (1991). "A Biomechanical Model for the Analysis of the Cervical Spine in Static Postures," *J. Biomechanics* 24:783–792.

Springer, S., S. Campbell, et al. (2003). "Is Push-out Testing of Cage Devices Worthwhile in Evaluating Clinical Performance?," in M. Melkerson, J. Kirkpatrick, and S. Griffith (eds.). *Spinal Implants: Are We Evaluating Them Appropriately?* West Conshohocken, PA: ASTM International.

Tipper, J., P. Firkins, E. Ingham, and J. Fisher (1999). "Quantitative Analysis of the Wear and Wear Debris from Low and High Carbon Content Cobalt Chrome Alloys Used in Metal on Metal Total Hip Replacements," *J. Mater. Sci. Mater. Med.* 10:353–362.

Wallbridge, N., and D. Dowson (1982). "The Walking Activity of Patients with Artificial Hip Joints," *Eng. Med.* 11:95–96.

Wang, A., C. Stark, and J. Dumbleton (1996). "Mechanistic and Morphological Origins of Ultra-high Molecular Weight Polyethylene Wear Debris in Total Joint Replacement," *Proc. Inst. Mech. Engrs. H.* 210:141–155.

Wang, A., A. Essner, and G. Schmidig (2004). "The Effects of Lubricant Composition on In Vitro Wear Testing of Polymeric Acetabular Components," *J. Biomed. Mater. Res. (Appl. Biomat.)* 68B:45–52.

Wang, A., A. Essner, C. Stark, and J. Dumbleton (1995). "Comparsion of the Size and Morphology of UHMWPE Wear Debris Produced by a Hip Joint Simulator Under Serum and Water Lubricated Conditions," *Biomaterials* 17:865–871.

Wright, T., and S. Goodman (2001). "What Design and Material Factors Influence Wear in Total Joint Replacement?," in T. M. Wright and S. B. Goodman (eds.). *Implant Wear in Total Joint Replacement*. Rosemont, IL: American Academy of Orthopaedic Surgeons.

Chapter *14*

Finite Element Modeling of the Spine

Anton Bowden, Ph.D.
Exponent, Inc., Philadelphia, PA

14.1 Introduction to the Finite Element Method

Finite element analysis (FEA) was first proposed by Richard Courant in 1922 [Hurwitz and Courant 1922], ironically during an era in which the method was impractical due to the laborious process of solving linear systems of equations by hand. It was not until the advent of the digital computer in 1942 [Burks and Burks 1989] that the method became practical. Indeed, John Argyris is usually credited with making the method suitable for nontrivial problems in the early 1950s when he published a series of papers outlining the technique and realized the critical role that computers would play in the viability of the method [Argyris 1954, 1955]. Although the finite element method gained popularity in many engineering disciplines throughout the 1950s and 1960s, it was not until 1973 that the technique was applied to the human spine [Liu and Ray 1973]. Since that time, the finite element method has played an increasingly important role in improving our understanding of the fundamental biomechanics of the spine. Several key review articles of finite element analysis of the spine are Yoganandan et al. [1987], Goel and Gilbertsom [1995], Yoganandan et al. [1996], and Natarajan et al. [2004].

Like many numerical techniques, the finite element method converts a single very complex problem into hundreds, thousands, or millions of very simple problems (Figure 14.1). Dramatic improvements in computational speed and greater availability of robust and accurate modeling software have permitted ever more complex models to be developed. In 1965, Intel co-founder Gordon Moore made a much-cited prediction, commonly referred to as Moore's law [Moore 1965], which predicted that computational capacity would roughly

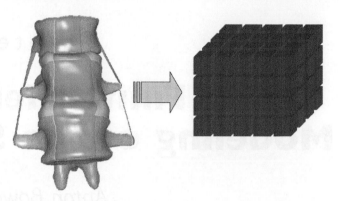

Fig. 14.1.

Overall goal of numerical modeling. The goal of numerical modeling is to convert a single very complex problem into many very simple problems.

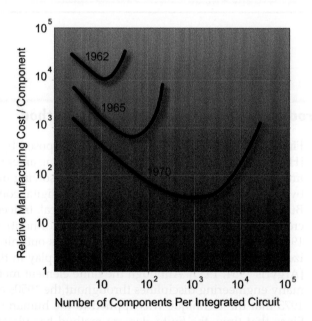

Fig. 14.2.

Moore's Law. In 1965, Gordon Moore accurately predicted that computational capacity would approximately double every one to two years, with an associated decrease in production costs.

double every one to two years, with an associated decrease in production costs (Figure 14.2). The prediction has held true for the past 40 years. Fueled by dramatic increases in computational capacity and by the proliferation of commercial software with user-friendly interfaces, finite element analysis has become part of the standard toolkit of engineering.

This chapter provides an overview of the use of the finite element method to study the normal and pathological biomechanics of the spine. First, general considerations with regard to the appropriate application of the method to spinal biomechanics are presented. Second, a basic hierarchy of numerical modeling is presented and described in the context of the spine. Third, a survey of significant numerical models from the literature. Last, the chapter concludes with a brief discussion of future trends in numerical modeling of the spine.

14.2 Application of the Finite Element Method to the Spine

Along with the increase in use of the finite element method has come a corresponding increase in its potential misapplication. There are several important keys to the proper application of any numerical method. In this section we address key components essential to proper numerical modeling of the spine.

14.2.1 Appropriate Solution Technique

The choice of solution technique is directly related to the formulation of the problem, particularly whether the problem addresses small or large deformations. For small-strain simulations of a single vertebral body a linear solution technique may (or may not) be appropriate [Langrana et al. 2002; Teo and Ng 2001; Whyne et al. 1998]. For multisegmental simulations, only nonlinear large deformation methods are adequate to address the large strains that develop in the intervertebral discs, as well as the highly nonlinear contact conditions that exist at the facets [Brolin and Halldin 2004; Chen et al. 2001; Chosa, Totoribe, and Tajima 2004; Ezquerro et al. 2004; Goel and Clausen 1998; Goto et al. 2002; Hong-Wan, Ee-Chon, and Qing-Hang 2004; Kumaresan, Yoganandan, and Pintar 1998; Lim et al. 2001; Natarajan et al. 2003; Polikeit et al. 2003; Ng and Teo 2005; Puttlitz et al. 2000; Shirazi-Adl and Parnianpour 2000; Rohlmann, Zander, and Bergmann 2005]. Many important research questions can be answered using quasi-static solution techniques, whereas others require dynamic simulations to properly address the inertial loading of the spine. Only dynamic simulations can evaluate problems that include super-physiologic velocities [Tropiano et al. 2004; Tschirhart, Nagpurkar, and Whyne 2004; Wang et al. 1998, 2000; Wilcox et al. 2003, 2004].

14.2.2 Model Geometry

Individuals vary in regards to geometry, size, density, and composition of their respective tissue structures. Additionally, like most structures in the body the components of the spine do not function in isolation—they draw additional mechanical stability from the surrounding tissue. Unfortunately, modeling every component is often not feasible, and determining which components are essential is difficult. Inter-subject variation in ligaments and musculature can be especially challenging.

In addition to inter-subject variation, intra-subject variation must be considered in any biological simulation. Over short time scales, boundary conditions change due to respiration, circulation, gait, posture, and even hydration level. Over long time scales, material and geometric changes due to growth, age, disease, and natural renewal must be considered. For example, bone architecture is continually in flux in response to specific activity levels.

14.2.3 Adequate Material Models

Biologic tissues are decidedly nonlinear [Dolan and Adams 2001; Hou et al. 1998; Hukins et al. 1990; Morgan and Keaveny 2001; Panjabi et al. 2001; Morgan, Bayraktar, and Keaveny 2003; Natarajan, Williams, and Andersson 2004; Panjabi, Goel, and Takata 1982; Przybylski et al. 1998]. However, in some instances linear assumptions may be appropriate to answer simple questions. The challenge is that often times this determination cannot be resolved *a priori*. For instance, it has been shown that linear models can effectively determine the sites of crack initiation during vertebral collapse [Crawford, Cann, and Keaveny 2003; Crawford, Rosenberg, and Keaveny 2003; Silva, Keaveny, and Hayes 1997; Hayes 1998]. However, a much richer nonlinear material model with specific failure criteria is required to simulate the actual process of vertebral collapse [Bowden et al. 2005]. Material models can be valid macroscopically or microscopically. However, very few models can adequately address behavior in both regimes [Baer et al. 2003; Ulrich et al. 1998; Yeni et al. 2003]. Multiphasic models have been used to study the behavior of the intervertebral disc [Ayotte et al. 2000; Chen, Lin, and Chang 2003; Chen et al. 2005; Ferguson, Ito, and Nolte 2004; Lee and Teo 2004; Lee et al. 2000; Lotz et al. 1998; Natarajan, Williams, and Andersson 2004; Whyne, Hu, and Lotz 2001, 2003; Wu and Chen 1996] and occasionally even the vertebral body [Lee and Teo 2004]. Very few models of the spine to date have incorporated pre-stress in the ligaments, even though ligament pre-stress plays an important role in the biomechanics of the knee [Weiss and Gardiner 2001]. Although bone is both nonhomogeneous and anisotropic [Hou et al. 1998; Morgan and Keaveny 2001; Morgan, Bayraktar, and Keaveny 2003], many models poetry bone as homogeneous and isotropic.

14.2.4 Boundary Conditions

Unlike engineering problems in many other fields, such as bridge or automotive design, determination of *in vivo* boundary conditions in biological systems can be extremely challenging. The spine is a flexible structure that bears the weight of the upper body and carries loads derived from human activity [Wilke et al. 2001], while also permitting a considerable range of motion. When modeling the spine, one needs to consider the physiologic boundary conditions (attachments to the head, sacrum, ribs, and so on), the effects of muscle forces, and kinematic constraints. Additionally, for models that simulate nonconservative material behavior, load history and loading rate are relevant. Disagreement remains as to what constitutes "physiologic" loading of the spine, especially as to what loads and moments should be applied to simulate typical quasi-static loads in both experimental and numerical models. On the other hand, the range of the motion of the spine has been relatively well established [White and Panjabi 1990].

14.3 In Search of a Better Model

The basic hierarchy of numerical modeling includes four key elements (Figure 14.3). These are discussed in the sections that follow.

14.3.1 Generation

Although phenomenological (lumped parameter) models can be used to study spinal biomechanics, it is generally accepted that models based on the underlying physics are superior [Griffin 2001] and are more likely to be developed into predictive models (stage IV on the hierarchy). Naturally, there are different levels of fidelity to the underlying physics. A brief summary of common approaches for each component of the spine follows.

14.3.1.1 Vertebrae

The key features of a vertebrae model are geometry, material properties, and facet contact properties for multisegment models. Geometry is usually derived from surface representation of the relevant anatomical structures. Generic vertebrae bone surface models can be purchased in several formats from vendors such as Digimation, Inc. (St. Rose, LA). Using these types of models reduces the effort required to extract surfaces from medical image data [Goto et al. 2003;

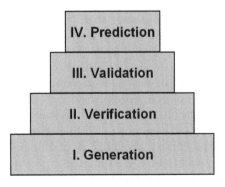

Fig. 14.3.
The basic hierarchy of numerical modeling.

Villarraga et al. 2005]. However, the selection of specimens of varied sizes is limited, and no information is available regarding the cancellous bone structure and topology. Alternatively, direct digitization of dried or embalmed cadaveric bones can provide excellent geometric fidelity at the cost of being time consuming [Guo et al. 2005; Ng and Teo 2001, 2004, 2005; Ng, Teo, and Lee 2004; Ng, Teo, and Zhang 2005; Ng et al. 2003; Teo and Ng 2001; Teo et al. 2004]. The most flexible and rigorous source of geometric data is subject-specific medical imaging, typically computed tomography (CT). Even though surface extraction is required, the technique allows for selection of a subject based on the specific requirements of the problem (age, gender, pathology, and so on) [Camacho, Nightingale, and Myers 1999; Chen, Cheng, and Liu 2002; Chen, Lin, and Chang 2003; Chen et al. 2001, 2005; Chosa et al. 2004; Hong-Wan, Ee-Chon, and Qing-Hang 2004; Crawford, Cann, and Keaveny 2003; Crawford, Rosenberg, and Keaveny 2003; Kawahara et al. 2003; Kong and Goel 2003; Kumaresan, Yoganandan, and Pintar 1999; Kumaresan et al. 1999, 2001; Liebschner, Rosenberg, and Keaveny 2001; Liebschner et al. 2003; Lim et al. 2001; Lin et al. 2004; Natarajan et al. 2000, 2002, 2003; Perie et al. 2001; Pitzen et al. 2001; Polikeit, Nolte, and Ferguson 2003, 2004; Polikeit et al. 2003; Puttlitz et al. 2000; Shirazi-Adl and Parnianpour 2000; Shirazi-Adl et al. 2002, 2004; Templeton, Cody, and Liebschner 2004; Wu and Chen 1996; Yoganandan et al. 1996]. Use of quantitative computed tomography (QCT) also provides additional information regarding bone density and structure.

Choice of material property formulation is often dependent on the complexity of the problem under consideration. For instance, in determination of gross spinal kinematics a rigid body assumption may be appropriate [Shirazi-Adl and Parnianpour 2000], and can greatly reduce the degrees of freedom (and associated computational complexity) of the model and allow for decreased solution time. The most commonly used material representation for bone is a homogeneous isotropic elastic formulation. Often the interior cancellous bone and surrounding cortical shell are given distinct material properties, sometimes with an assumption of preferred direction along the caudal-cranial axis [Polikeit, Nolte, and Ferguson 2004; Silva, Keaveny, and Hayes 1997; Tschirhart, Nagpurkar, and Whyne 2004].

The relationship between bone mineral density and cancellous bone modulus has been well established in the literature [Currey 1984, 1988; Ford and Keaveny 1996; Gibson 1985; Hodgskinson and Currey 1990; Jorgensen and Kundu 2002; Morgan and Keaveny 2001; Morgan, Bayraktar, and Keaveny 2003; Rho, Hobatho, and Ashman 1995; Rice, Cowin, and Bowman 1988; Schaffler and Burr 1988]. Some of the most advanced models of the spine incorporate inhomogeneous material properties based on bone mineral density [Crawford, Cann, and Keaveny 2003; Crawford, Rosenberg, and Keaveny 2003; Liebschner, Rosenberg, and Keaveny 2001; Liebschner et al. 2003; Pankoke, Hofmann, and Wolfel 2001; Perie et al. 2001]. Bone mineral density is approximated based on the same calibrated QCT data used to generate the model geometry. An even stronger correlation has been established between cancellous bone material properties and trabecular orientation [Ford and Keaveny 1996; Fyhrie and Carter 1986; Jensen, Madsen, and Linde 1991; Lasser and Pugh 1977; Martin and

Boardman 1993; Sevostianov and Kachanov 2000]. Trabecular orientation can be established based on very high resolution CT scans, such as those obtained using micro-CT scanners. Such trabecular orientation information can then be incorporated into continuum level finite element models by assigning orthotropic material properties. Alternatively, the individual voxels of these very high resolution images can be directly converted to cubic finite elements, and used to establish extremely detailed correlations of cancellous bone modulus and anisotropy to location [Ito et al. 2002; Jaasma et al. 2002; Pothuaud et al. 2002].

There are several computational methods for modeling facet contact conditions for multisegmental models, of which the most commonly employed technique is a penalty approach algorithm [Bathe 1996]. This approach is appropriate for both implicit and explicit nonlinear solution techniques and is available in most commercial nonlinear finite element packages.

14.3.1.2 Discs

The geometric features of the intervertebral discs have been shown to play only a minor role in overall biomechanics of a multisegment model [Lu, Hutton, and Gharpuray 1996; Natarajan and Andersson 1999]. Instead, the primary consideration when modeling the intervertebral discs is material property formulation [Ayotte et al. 2000; Baer et al. 2003; Ferguson, Ito, and Nolte 2004; Gu and Yao 2003; Kumaresan et al. 1999, 2001; Lee et al. 2000; Natarajan, Williams, and Andersson 2004; Ng, Teo, and Zhang 2005; Polikeit, Nolte, and Ferguson 2004; Yoganandan, Kumaresan, and Pintar 2001]. Although isotropic elastic formulations have been used in some finite element models, a more sophisticated formulation is required when accurate prediction of disc kinematics and pressures are required, or when studying the biomechanics of vertebral end plates.

The annulus fibrosus comprises the peripheral portion of the intervertebral disc and is composed of fibrocartilage and type I collagen. The fibers of the annulus run in concentric layers around the central nucleus pulposus with alternating oblique angles of 30 and 60 degrees. Various techniques have been used to model this highly anisotropic structure. Many researchers have used an isotropic continuum representation, with overlaying cable elements layered along the fiber directions [Goel and Gilbertson 1995; Lu, Hutton, and Gharpuray 1996; Maurel, Lavaste, and Skalli 1997; Natarajan and Andersson 1999; Pitzen et al. 2001; Shirazi-Adl et al. 2004], while others have used a continuum approach with an anisotropic material formulation [Elliott and Setton 2000, 2001].

The nucleus pulposus has also been represented using various techniques, including simple isotropic elastic properties [Chen et al. 2001; Guo et al. 2005; Qiu et al. 2003], a rubber-like hyperelastic formulation [Tschirhart, Nagpurkar, and Whyne 2004], or an incompressible fluid formulation [Calisse, Rohlmann, and Bergmann 1999; Goel and Clausen 1998; Kumaresan et al. 2001; Shirazi-Adl and Parnianpour 2000; Tropiano et al. 2004; Wilcox et al. 2004]. It is important to accurately consider the defining boundaries of the nucleus and its corresponding volume fraction (typically 30 to 40%) of the intervertebral disc.

In addition, researchers have observed that material properties for both the annulus and the nucleus change dramatically as the disc degenerates [Kumaresan et al. 2001; Natarajan, Williams, and Andersson 2004; Ng, Teo, and Zhang 2005].

14.3.1.3 Ligaments

In contrast to the intervertebral discs, both the geometry and material property formulation of the ligamentous structures of the spine contribute significantly to the fidelity of the model [Brolin and Halldin 2004; Hukins et al. 1990; Ng and Teo 2004; Ng, Teo, and Lee 2004; Panjabi, Goel, and Takata 1982; Przybylski et al. 1998; Zander, Rohlmann, and Bergmann 2004]. To date, the author is unaware of any subject-specific ligament geometries that have been used in models of the spine. However, recent advances in ligament modeling techniques for the knee may be applicable to the spine as well [Weiss and Gardiner 2001]. These techniques utilize magnetic resonance imaging (MRI) or dissected marked cadaveric CT imaging to identify ligament geometry. Material property formulation is also important for these structures, although they are often treated as simple elastic beam elements. A standard beam formulation for these elements imposes nonphysiologic loading during compression, and tension-only cable elements are preferred when using discrete elements to represent the ligaments [Chen et al. 2001; Chosa et al. 2004; Dooris et al. 2001; Ezquerro et al. 2004; Goel and Clausen 1998; Goto et al. 2002; Hong-Wan, Ee-Chon, and Qing-Hang 2004; Kong and Goel 2003; Kumaresan et al. 2001; Lee and Teo 2004; Natarajan and Andersson 1999; Ng and Teo 2001; Polikeit, Nolte, and Ferguson 2003; Rohlmann, Zander, and Bergmann 2005; Shirazi-Adl et al. 2004; Yoganandan et al. 1996]. Alternatively, both shell elements and volumetric elements have also been used, with cross-sectional properties based on values from representative cadaveric specimens or from the literature [Weiss and Gardiner 2001; Weiss et al. 2005]. Linear, bi-linear, and nonlinear elastic properties have been used with each of these element formulations.

Most ligaments contain an inherent tensile *in situ* strain, which is evidenced by the immediate retraction observed when the ligament is cut [Weiss et al. 2005]. However, there is some disagreement regarding whether this is indeed the case in the spinal ligaments [Brolin and Halldin 2004; Hukins et al. 1990; Przybylski et al. 1998]. It appears that the magnitude of this prestrain is relatively small and can possibly be ignored in most finite element simulations of the spine.

14.3.1.4 Cartilage

Physiologically, cartilage serves an important role at the facet joints by cushioning the contact between the articular processes. In addition, in combination with the capsular synovial fluid, it can serve to reduce the coefficient of friction of the joint. In previous finite element models of the spine, cartilage has been represented as both shell elements and volumetric elements [Kumaresan, Yoganandan, and Pintar 1998, 1999; Natarajan et al. 2000].

14.3.1.5 Muscles

The spinal musculature plays an important role in posture stabilization, as well as controlling motion. Shirazi-Adl [Shirazi-Adl and Parnianpour 2000; Shirazi-Adl et al. 2002, 2004] has studied the redundant active-passive segmental muscle forces developed during different postures using discrete beam representations for each muscle. The problem of determining the relative muscle forces is a challenging one as there are significant inter-subject differences, not only in the magnitude of muscle forces but in the relative distribution of forces among redundant musculature. Muscles have different mechanical properties during passive stretching, during activation, and post activation. There are several muscle representations that have been used in finite element models of other joints, such as the Hill muscle model [Hill 1938; Winters 1990]. However, the application of muscle forces to finite element models is a relatively recent development. Some of the recent work in applying muscles to finite element models has been reviewed elsewhere [Calisse, Rohlmann, and Bergmann 1999; Ezquerro et al. 2004; Kiefer, Shirazi-Adl, and Parnianpour 1998; Kong et al. 1996; Pankoke, Hofmann, and Wolfel 2001; Seidel, Bluthner, and Hinz 2001; Shirazi-Adl and Parnianpour 2000; Shirazi-Adl et al. 2002, 2004; Tropiano et al. 2004; Zander et al. 2001].

14.3.2 Verification

There are many sources of potential error in a numerical model. Verification is the process of eliminating as many of these sources of error as possible. Some sources of error in finite element models are universally applicable. Others are more specific to models of the spine.

Despite the wide use and acceptance of the finite element method (or perhaps because of it), it is the author's experience that there are far too many instances of the method being poorly applied. The comments of Cook, Malkus, and Plesha [1989] are equally applicable today:

> Powerful computer programs cannot be used without training. Their results cannot be trusted if users have no knowledge of their internal workings and little understanding of the physical theories on which they are based. An error caused by misunderstanding or oversight is not correctible by mesh refinement or by use of a more powerful computer. . . . Although the finite element method can make a good engineer better, it can make a poor engineer more dangerous.

Even though linear finite element methods have fewer pitfalls than nonlinear methods, the limitations of using a linear finite element method must be clearly understood or the results will have very little meaning. The major criteria for verification of a linear model are:

- Is the model truly linear? A linear finite element model is only valid for small strains and small deformations of linear elastic materials. As discussed in the previous section, these assumptions are often not appropriate for models of the spine.

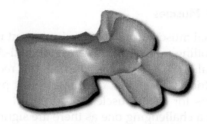

Fig. 14.4.

A single vertebral body. Even when modeling a relatively simple compression load on a single vertebral body, careful consideration must be given to developing accurate boundary conditions.

- Is the mesh discretization adequate? Does the addition of more elements to high stress/high strain areas of the model significantly influence the results? A general rule of thumb is that doubling the mesh density should not change the maximum stresses by more than 5%.
- Are the boundary conditions appropriately applied to the model? In general, point loads should be avoided, as they induce local stress concentrations that are not representative of physiologic loading. Similarly, rigidly fixed boundary conditions can induce local stress concentrations. As an example, consider simple compression loading of a single vertebral body (Figure 14.4). A casual approach to modeling the boundary conditions might be to apply a uniform pressure load to the cranial (superior) end plate, while rigidly fixing the caudal (inferior) end plate. However, under physiologic conditions pressure loading is transferred nonuniformly to the cranial end plate through the intervertebral disc (as well as through the facets), while the caudal end plate is supported on the elastic foundation of another intervertebral disc and the posterior elements are supported by a thinner viscoelastic cartilage layer that is attached to the posterior elements of the next inferior vertebral body. Each of these loadings will yield decidedly different results.

The use of nonlinear finite element methods opens the user to a much broader class of problem. With that freedom comes a larger number of solution options, many of which can significantly impact analysis results. Even though solution options can vary dramatically between software packages, many equivalent techniques are implemented in most commercially available packages. The major criteria for verification of a nonlinear model include the following, in addition to that already described for linear models.

- Is the solution numerically stable and converged? Although many standard nonlinear finite element problems are well-posed in the sense of Hadamard [1902], this is not always the case [Bowden 2003]. When a problem is ill posed, local minima solutions can be obtained that do not represent the global solution to the underlying physics of the problem. Aside from these unusual cases, the most common source of numerical convergence problems is due to "shortcuts" implemented to reduce solution time of nonlinear problems. These include features such as "mass scaling" in explicit simulations and quasi-Newton stiffness matrix updates in implicit simulations. Note that use of these techniques does not invalidate the solution process, but does impose a greater responsibility on the analyst to ensure that the problem correctly converges to an accurate solution.

- Is the choice of element formulation appropriate for the problem? Hexahedral (brick) elements are generally recognized to be superior for 3D nonlinear strain calculations [Benzley et al. 1995]. However, an automatic purely hexahedral mesh generator does not currently exist. Semiautomatic hexahedral mesh generation usually accounts for a large portion (50 to 90%) of the budget for a large nonlinear model. Because of the time and costs associated with mesh creation, many researchers are content to use automatically generated tetrahedral meshes, or mixed hexahedral/tetrahedral meshes. These element formulations often yield satisfactory results, but must be carefully examined for mesh discretization convergence. Instead of just increasing the number of mesh elements, the use of higher order elements can sometimes be more computationally effective [Bathe 1996].

- Is the material model appropriate for large deformation and large strain simulations? As discussed previously, biological materials exhibit nonlinear material behavior even under typical physiologic loading conditions. Additionally, physiologic loading conditions (e.g., flexion, extension, lateral bending, axial rotation) violate the small strain, small deformation requirements of some of the most commonly used material formulations. Despite this, isotropic linear elastic material formulations are still commonly used for representing many of the components of the spine.

14.3.3 Validation

In its simplest sense, a validated model is one that matches previously observed experimental behavior. There are many ways to validate a spine model, and not all carry the same weight. The most important model parameters to validate are those that will be studied later during the "prediction" phase of modeling. For example, if the model will only be used to predict spinal kinematics, then validation of cortical strains is neither sufficient not necessary. A model that will be used to study ligament strains must be validated against both kinematics and ligament strains [Griffin 2001].

An important consideration during the validation phase is directly related to the subject-specific nature of biological modeling. Subject-specific experimental validation studies are entitled to a higher measure of confidence than statistically significant experimental studies of different subjects. Obviously, this entitlement is only true when the methodology and results are rigorously examined. The large variation in material and geometric considerations between individuals warrant such considerations. Despite this advantage, it is difficult to perform subject-specific validation experiments and most models are validated against published experimental data from different subjects. The standard error measurements associated with these studies are usually high, due to the intersubject differences, making validation of gross kinematics difficult. As such, more rigorous (and more difficult) validation is obtained by comparing results that depend on both kinematic and material considerations, such as end plate strains and intervertebral disc pressures.

Another important consideration in validation studies is that finite element methods give more highly discretized field results than current experimental methods. For example, intervertebral disc pressure results are generally measured experimentally using a single needle-type pressure gage, inserted into the nucleus pulposus. When comparing pressure results from a finite element simulation, it is important to validate these results by using a local average within the corresponding area of the model, rather than by looking at global max/min values which potentially lie outside the region measured by the sensor.

14.3.4 Prediction

The highest tier in the hierarchy of numerical modeling is reserved for models that can not only accurately describe the behavior against which they were validated but accurately predict nonmeasurable behavior. Even though this is the goal of many finite element models, it is unrealistic to expect accurate predictive capability unless a numerical model can accurately simulate numerous high-level validation studies. Predictive models allow us a glimpse into the behavior of the spine under situations that are difficult or impossible to measure experimentally.

For example, numerous models of the spine have been developed with the primary purpose of studying the biomechanics of high velocity impacts, such as those experienced during automotive accidents [Langrana et al. 2002; Lee et al. 2000; Tencer, Mirza, and Bensel 2002; Wilcox et al. 2003, 2004; Yoganandan et al. 1987]. Other models allow us to study the response of the spine to novel surgical techniques [Baroud et al. 2003; Goto et al. 2003; Kosmopoulos and Keller 2004; Lee and Teo 2004; Lim et al. 2001; Polikeit, Nolte, and Ferguson 2003; Sun and Liebschner 2004]. Much of this handbook has been developed to better understand the behavior of medical implants *in vivo*. Predictive finite element models can allow us to accurately simulate the biomechanical response of the spine to currently available implants, as well as guide future development efforts. Recently, the U.S. Food and Drug Administration (FDA) has recognized the benefits of having such predictive models of device (non-spine) behavior prior to entering investigational clinical trials or to 510(k) submission [FDA 2004; U.S. DHHA 2001, 2003]. The American Society for Testing and Materials (ASTM) is also considering the adoption of standard guides for finite element analysis of orthopedic implants.

14.4 Current Numerical Models of the Spine

Finite element modeling of the spine has blossomed over the past two decades, and due to length considerations in this chapter it is impossible to review each

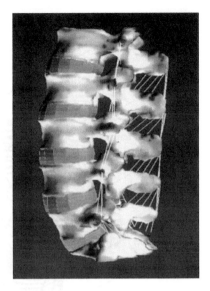

Fig. 14.5.
Detailed CT-based finite element model of the ligamentous lumbar spine. (Reprinted from Shirazi-Adl et al. [2000] with permission from Elsevier, Ltd.)

of them. It is appropriate, however, to review a few of the recent detailed numerical models of the spine and to give some of the details of each.

Shirazi-Adl et al. have an established track record for generating detailed, validated numerical models of the spine (e.g., Shirazi-Adl and Parnianpour [2000], Shirazi-Adl et al. [2002, 2004]). More recent publications have used the model shown in Figure 14.5. The geometry for the model was generated based on CT imaging of a cadaveric specimen of a 65-year-old man, and includes six vertebrae (L1 to S1), with five intervertebral discs, bilateral articulating facet surfaces at each level, and numerical representations of eight separate ligamentous structures at each segmental level. Each vertebra was modeled as two independent rigid bodies: one for the anterior body and the other for the posterior elements, interconnected by deformable beam elements oriented along the pedicles. At each segmental level, the disc annulus is modeled of an isotropic material, reinforced by membrane fibers oriented at 27 degrees. The nucleus is represented as a fluid filled cavity. Contact interaction at the facets is modeled using cap elements with no resistance in tension, and a stiffening resistance in compression. Nonlinear cable elements are used to define the ligamentous structures.

Goel et al. have developed several models of various spinal regions (e.g., Goel and Clausen [1998]; Goel and Gilbertson [1995]). These models have similar features. As an example, a recent model of the cervical spine [Goel and Clausen 1998] was developed based on the geometry of a 68-year-old man as obtained through CT scans at slice intervals of 1.5 mm (Figure 14.6). The full model consisted of 4,219 nodes and 5,577 elements representing various

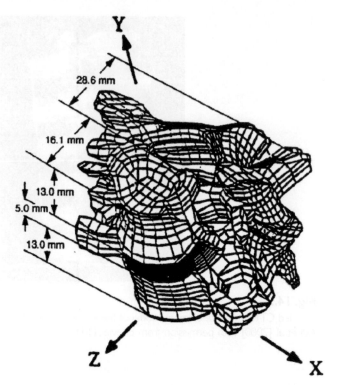

Fig. 14.6.

CT-based finite element model of the ligamentous spine. (Reprinted from Goel et al. [1998] with permission from Lippincott, Williams & Wilkins.)

structures of the C5-C6 motion segment. The model employed bi-linear elastic, tension-only cable elements for ligamentous structures. Facet surfaces were oriented manually at 45 degrees from the transverse plane, and articulation was modeled using gap elements. The annulus fibrosus was modeled using a linear elastic hexahedral matrix representation, with tension-only cable elements that defined six distinct layers of fiber reinforcement. The nucleus pulposus was modeled as an incompressible fluid. Hexahedral elements, with isotropic, linear elastic material properties were used for cortical, cancellous, and end plate structures.

Ng, Teo, and colleagues have published several recent articles outlining the development and application of a nonlinear model of the lower cervical spine [Ng and Teo 2001, 2004, 2005; Ng, Teo, and Lee 2004; Ng, Teo, and Zhang 2005; Ng et al. 2003; Teo and Ng 2001; Teo et al. 2004]. The geometry of their C2-C7 model was developed using a high-definition digitizer of a dried cadaveric specimen (Figure 14.7). The model assumes symmetry about the sagittal plane. Each vertebra modeled using solid brick elements included the cortical bone, cancellous bone, and posterior structures. Posterior articular facets were simulated using 3D nonlinear contact elements. Each intervertebral disc consisted

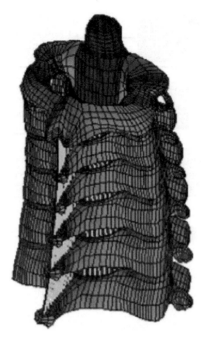

Fig. 14.7.
Finite element model of the cervical spine based on high-resolution direct digitization. (Reprinted from Ng et al. [2005] with permission from ASME.)

of disc annulus, disc nucleus, unconvertebral joint, annulus fibers, and end plates. All ligaments approximating the ligamentous structures in the cervical spine were incorporated into the finite element model using nonlinear two-node tension-only cable elements. Isotropic linear-elastic material properties were assigned to the hard tissue structures, as well as for the matrix of the annulus fibrosus. Tension-only cable ligaments were used to model the fiber reinforcement of the annulus fibrosus. A fluid material representation was used for the nucleus pulposus.

Bowden et al. [2005] have recently presented a subject-specific model of the thoraco lumbar (T12-L2) spine of a 60-year-old female. Vertebral geometry was obtained from bone mineral density-calibrated CT imaging. Spatially variant (nonhomogeneous) anisotropic material parameters for the cancellous bone were assigned to each element of the model based on bone mineral density values as obtained from the calibrated CT intensities (Figure 14.8). Linear elastic shell elements were used to model the surrounding cortex. The model uses a penalty approach for modeling contact at the facet joints. The seven major ligaments were modeled using shell elements that were assigned a tension-only "fabric" material representation. The annulus fibrosus was modeled as a continuum, with transversely anisotropic material properties that were discretely defined for the inner and outer regions of the annulus [Elliott and Setton 2001]. The nucleus pulposi were modeled using an incompressible

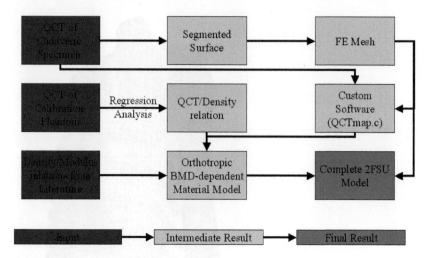

Fig. 14.8.
Methodology employed by Bowden et al. for assigning nonhomogeneous bone mineral density dependent moduli to a finite element model.

fluid material model. The highly discretized model consisted of 402,404 nodes, with 379,677 solid hexahedral elements and 19,080 shell elements (Figure 14.9). This model was validated with experimental data reported in the literature [Frei 2001].

14.5 Simulating Pathological and Post-surgical Biomechanics of the Spine

Development of a validated model of the normal spine with biological fidelity is a necessary precursor to accurate simulation of pathological or post-surgical spinal biomechanics. This baseline model is used for comparison purposes, and can be exercised with precisely the same loading modes and boundary conditions as the pathological model. This paradigm has been used to study situations such as vertebroplasty [Baroud et al. 2003; Kosmopoulos and Keller 2004; Liebschner, Rosenberg, and Keaveny 2001], kyphoplasty [Villarraga et al. 2005], prophylactic vertebral body reinforcement [Sun and Liebschner 2004], interbody fusion [Adam, Pearcy, and McCombe 2003; Epari, Kandziora, and Duda 2005; Kim 2001; Lee et al. 2004; Lin et al. 2004; Palm, Rosenberg, and Keaveny 2002], posterolateral fusion [Chen et al. 2005; Totoribe, Chosa, and Tajima 2004; Totoribe, Tajima, and Chosa 1999], laminectomy and facetectomy [Lee and Teo 2004; Zander et al. 2003], discectomy [Lim et al. 2001], pedicle screw fixation [Chen, Lin, and Chang 2003; Lim et al. 2001; Lin, Chen, and Sun 2003; Zhang, Tan, and Chou 2004], and even total disc replacement [Moumene and Geisler 2004; Rohlmann, Zander, and Bergmann 2005]. Additionally, when simulating

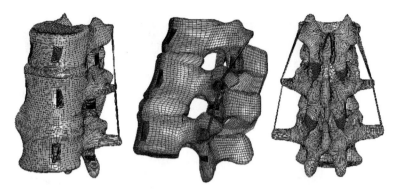

Fig. 14.9.
Highly discretized CT-based finite element model of the thoraco-lumbar spine employing tension-only shell elements for ligamentous structures.

the biomechanics of implanted medical devices it is often useful to separately validate the discretization and material behavior of the device model.

14.5.1 Modeling Device Failure Mechanisms

Analyzing medical device designs to improve performance in medical implants presents a unique challenge to engineers and clinicians. Unlike products created for use outside the body, medical implants are difficult to test in a realistic environment. Products are validated in increasingly lifelike scenarios, including computer models such as those described throughout this chapter, as well as experimental testing and clinical investigational trials. Nonetheless, despite best efforts by both regulatory agencies and industry, device failures can and do occur. Medical device failures in the spine are especially risky to the patients, due to the close proximity of these devices to the central nervous system and its associated structures. Thus, when an implanted device fails there is a strong motivation to determine the cause of failure, so that present and future design efforts can be improved.

The use of FEA as a tool for examining medical device failure is relatively novel, and despite the valuable information it can provide the results are very often kept proprietary and guarded by confidentiality agreements. An example is provided demonstrating the use of this technique to understand failure modes in retrieved Charité total disc replacements, which have demonstrated rim deformation and fracture, in manners analogous to failure modes already documented in other total joint replacements [Kurtz 2004; Mow and Huiskes 2005]. See Chapter 11 for more details about disc replacement and the Charité design in particular.

For this analysis, the finite element method was used to gain insight into the deformation and fracture mechanisms. In order to accurately develop the geometry for the model, a retrieved polyethylene core was scanned using

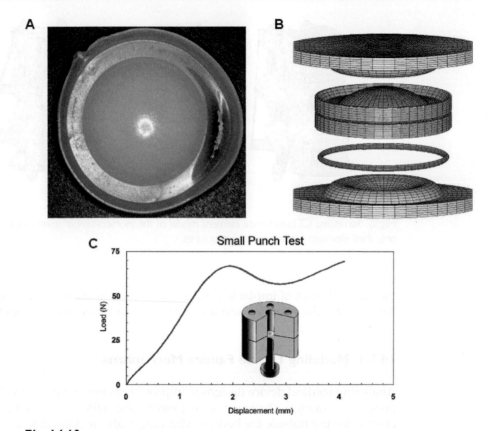

A

B

C

Small Punch Test

Fig. 14.10.
Finite-element-based failure mode analysis of a retrieved Charité total disc replacement. (A) The polyethylene core of a retrieved implant. (B) A detailed hexahedral finite element mesh was constructed based on microCT data of the polyethylene core, and direct digitization of the CoCr end plates. (C) Specimen-specific material properties were measured using small punch testing, and assigned to the model using a validated plasticity model for polyethylene.

micro-CT with a uniform voxel resolution of 74 microns. The undamaged portion of the retrieval was used to establish the axisymmetric cross section, then rotated to provide accurate surfaces for use in modeling the undeformed implant (Figure 14.10b). The geometry of the cobalt-chrome end plates was obtained using 3D point digitization. Specimen-specific material property data for the polyethylene core was obtained from mechanical test data using the small punch test method (Figure 14.10c) [Kurtz, Foulds, and Jewett 1997; Kurtz et al. 1999], and modeled numerically using a validated nonlinear plasticity model [Bergström, Rimnac, and Kurtz 2003]. The model was evaluated under direct compression loading and compression/flexion loading. Results from the FE analysis showed that the maximum effective stress in the implant was coincident with observed plastic deformation and fracture patterns in retrieved components (Figure 14.11), and that stress magnitudes were similar to those

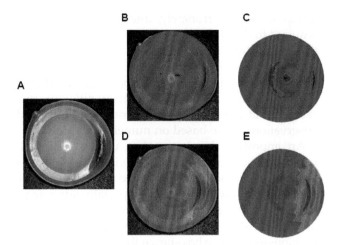

Fig. 14.11.
Finite element results matched well with observed failure modes. (A) The polyethylene core of a retrieved implant. (B-C) Minimum principal stress contours as predicted by the model (transparent overlay onto the retrieved implant). (C-D) Maximum principal stress contours as predicted by the model (transparent overlay onto the retrieved implant).

observed in total knee replacement [Mow and Huiskes 2005]. The information gained from these analyses helped determine the modes of rim failure for this particular implant design, as well as postulate likely modes of failure for similar implants.

14.6 Looking Forward

One of the largest challenges with regard to subject-specific modeling is that there is a tremendous variation in geometry, material properties, and even boundary conditions between individuals. Constructing detailed models of biological systems is a time-consuming (and usually expensive) process but can give valuable insights into the biomechanics of the system. Nevertheless, one model cannot adequately predict behavior for all individuals.

One direction of broadening the application of a particular model is by using stochastic methods [Dar, Meakin, and Aspden 2002]. Stochastic methods use statistical representations of the range of material properties for each component of the model. A random choice of material property is selected from the acceptable range for each component. The process is repeated multiple times using identical boundary conditions until a statistically significant range of model response can be identified.

To quantify the effects of anatomical variation, we present the concept of the "virtual clinic." In a laboratory setting, inter-subject variations in geometry and specimen composition are addressed by using statistically significant study group sizes. Unfortunately, due to the large amount of time and resources required to develop even a single complex subject-specific numerical model of the ligamentous spine numerical modeling studies generally are not used to address inter-subject variations in any meaningful sense. The expense and time required to build complex FE models dictate that in practice the same model geometry is used repetitively for many different studies. Obviously, such application could potentially have a dramatic effect on the general applicability of observations made based on numerical models.

An important development in understanding the variation in individual response would be to develop a "virtual clinic" composed of a pool of subject-specific spine models that could be subjected to identical boundary conditions. A clinic of this type would be especially advantageous to the medical device industry, in that it would allow evaluation of the effectiveness of spinal treatment options prior to subjecting human subjects to treatments in clinical trials. Previous experience has shown that it is very seldom the "average" patient who reacts poorly to a medical device. The exception, in addition to the rule, is of major concern. By having an established bank of models representing patients with certain pathologies, more certainty in the broad applicability of a particular candidate device could be obtained. At present no such virtual clinic exists, but developments in the generation of FE models allow the possibility of their existence in the immediate future.

14.7 Acknowledgments

Special thanks to Daniel Balint, Ph.D., and Marta Villarraga, Ph.D., of Exponent, Inc., for their editorial review, and to the editors for their helpful advice regarding the outline of this chapter.

14.8 References

Adam, C., M. Pearcy, and P. McCombe (2003). "Stress Analysis of Interbody Fusion: Finite Element Modeling of Intervertebral Implant and Vertebral Body," *Clin. Biomech. (Bristol, Avon)* 18:265–272.

Argyris, J. H. (1954). "Energy Theorems and Structural Analysis," *Aircraft Engineering* 26:347–356, 383–387.

Argyris, J. H. (1955). "Energy Theorems and Structural Analysis," *Aircraft Engineering* 27:42–58, 80–94, 125–134, 145–158.

Ayotte, D. C., K. Ito, S. M. Perren, and S. Tepic (2000). "Direction-dependent Constriction Flow in a Poroelastic Solid: The Intervertebral Disc Valve," *J. Biomech. Eng.* 122:587–593.

Baer, A. E., T. A. Laursen, F. Guilak, and L. A. Setton (2003). "The Micromechanical Environment of Intervertebral Disc Cells Determined by a Finite Deformation, Anisotropic, and Biphasic Finite Element Model," *J. Biomech. Eng.* 125:1–11.

Baroud, G., J. Nemes, P. Heini, and T. Steffen (2003). "Load Shift of the Intervertebral Disc After a Vertebroplasty: A Finite-element Study," *Eur. Spine J.* 12:421–426.

Bathe, K.-J. (1996). *Finite Element Procedures.* Upper Saddle River, NJ: Prentice-Hall, Inc.

Benzley, S. E., E. Perry, et al. (1995). *A Comparison of All Hexahedral and All Tetrahedral Finite Element Meshes for Elastic and Elasto-plastic Analysis.* 4th International Meshing Roundtable. Sandia National Laboratories Albuguerque, NM.

Bergström, J. S., C. M. Rimnac, and S. M. Kurtz (2003). "Prediction of Multiaxial Behavior for Conventional and Highly Crosslinked UHMWPE Using a Hybrid Constitutive Model," *Biomaterials* 24:1365–1380.

Bowden, A. E. (2003). "Tools for Deformable Image Registration," *Bioengineering.* Salt Lake City, University of Utah.

Bowden, A. E., M. L. Villarraga, A. A. Edidin, and S. M. Kurtz (2005a). *Advanced Numerical Modeling of Spinal Biomechanics.* Spine Research Symposium. Philadelphia, PA.

Bowden, A. E., M. V. Villarraga, A. A. Edidin, and S. M. Kurtz (2005b). *Numerical Simulation of Vertebral Collapse.* Philadelphia Spine Research Symposium. Philadelphia, PA.

Brolin, K., and P. Halldin (2004). "Development of a Finite Element Model of the Upper Cervical Spine and a Parameter Study of Ligament Characteristics," *Spine* 29:376–385.

Burks, A. R., and A. W. Burks (1989). *The First Electronic Computer: The Atanasoff Story.* Ann Arbor, MI: University of Michigan Press.

Calisse, J., A. Rohlmann, and G. Bergmann (1999). "Estimation of Trunk Muscle Forces Using the Finite Element Method and In Vivo Loads Measured by Telemeterized Internal Spinal Fixation Devices," *J. Biomech.* 32:727–731.

Camacho, D. L., R. W. Nightingale, and B. S. Myers (1999). "Surface Friction in Near-vertex Head and Neck Impact Increases Risk of Injury," *J. Biomech.* 32:293–301.

Chen, B. H., R. N. Natarajan, H. S. An, and G. B. Andersson (2001). "Comparison of Biomechanical Response to Surgical Procedures Used for Cervical Radiculopathy: Posterior Keyhole Foraminotomy Versus Anterior Foraminotomy and Discectomy Versus Anterior Discectomy with Fusion," *J. Spinal Disord.* 14:17–20.

Chen, C. S., C. K. Cheng, and C. L. Liu (2002). "A Biomechanical Comparison of Posterolateral Fusion and Posterior Fusion in the Lumbar Spine," *J. Spinal Disord. Tech.* 15:53–63.

Chen, C. S., C. K. Cheng, C. L. Liu, and W. H. Lo (2001). "Stress Analysis of the Disc Adjacent to Interbody Fusion in Lumbar Spine," *Med. Eng. Phys.* 23:483–491.

Chen, C. S., C. K. Feng, et al. (2005). "Biomechanical Analysis of the Disc Adjacent to Posterolateral Fusion with Laminectomy in Lumbar Spine," *J. Spinal Disord. Tech.* 18:58–65.

Chen, S. I., R. M. Lin, and C. H. Chang (2003). "Biomechanical Investigation of Pedicle Screw-vertebrae Complex: A Finite Element Approach Using Bonded and Contact Interface Conditions," *Med. Eng. Phys.* 25:275–282.

Chosa, E., K. Goto, K. Totoribe, and N. Tajima (2004). "Analysis of the Effect of Lumbar Spine Fusion on the Superior Adjacent Intervertebral Disk in the Presence of Disk Degeneration, Using the Three-dimensional Finite Element Method," *J. Spinal Disord. Tech.* 17:134–139.

Chosa, E., K. Totoribe, and N. Tajima (2004). "A Biomechanical Study of Lumbar Spondylolysis Based on a Three-dimensional Finite Element Method," *J. Orthop. Res.* 22:158–163.

Cook, R. D., D. S. Malkus, and M. E. Plesha (1989). *Concepts and Applications of Finite Element Analysis.* New York, NY: John Wiley & Sons.

Crawford, R. P., C. E. Cann, and T. M. Keaveny (2003). "Finite Element Models Predict In Vitro Vertebral Body Compressive Strength Better Than Quantitative Computed Tomography," *Bone* 33:744–750.

Crawford, R. P., W. S. Rosenberg, and T. M. Keaveny (2003). "Quantitative Computed Tomography-based Finite Element Models of the Human Lumbar Vertebral Body: Effect of Element Size on Stiffness, Damage, and Fracture Strength Predictions," *J. Biomech. Eng.* 125:434–438.

Currey, J. D (1984). "Effects of Differences in Mineralization on the Mechanical Properties of Bone," *Philos. Trans. R. Soc. Lond. B. Biol. Sci.* 304:509–518.

Currey, J. D (1988). "The Effect of Porosity and Mineral Content on the Young's Modulus of Elasticity of Compact Bone," *J. Biomech.* 21:131–139.

Dar, F. H., J. R. Meakin, and R. M. Aspden (2002). "Statistical Methods in Finite Element Analysis," *J. Biomech.* 35:1155–1161.

Dolan, P., and M. A. Adams (2001). "Recent Advances in Lumbar Spinal Mechanics and Their Significance for Modelling," *Clin. Biomech. (Bristol, Avon)* 16(Suppl. 1):S8–S16.

Dooris, A. P., V. K. Goel, et al. (2001). "Load-sharing Between Anterior and Posterior Elements in a Lumbar Motion Segment Implanted with an Artificial Disc," *Spine* 26:E122–E129.

Elliott, D. M., and L. A. Setton (2000). "A Linear Material Model for Fiber-induced Anisotropy of the Anulus Fibrosus," *J. Biomech. Eng.* 122:173–179.

Elliott, D. M., and L. A. Setton (2001). "Anisotropic and Inhomogeneous Tensile Behavior of the Human Anulus Fibrosus: Experimental Measurement and Material Model Predictions," *J. Biomech. Eng.* 123:256–263.

Epari, D. R., F. Kandziora, and G. N. Duda (2005). "Stress Shielding in Box and Cylinder Cervical Interbody Fusion Cage Designs," *Spine* 30:908–914.

Ezquerro, F., A. Simon, M. Prado, and A. Perez (2004). "Combination of Finite Element Modeling and Optimization for the Study of Lumbar Spine Biomechanics Considering the 3D Thorax-pelvis Orientation," *Med. Eng. Phys.* 26:11–22.

FDA (Food and Drug Administration) (2004). "FEA Software Enables Study of Tissue Ablation Dynamics," *NASA Tech Briefs.*

Ferguson, S. J., K. Ito, and L. P. Nolte (2004). "Fluid Flow and Convective Transport of Solutes Within the Intervertebral Disc," *J. Biomech.* 37:213–221.

Ford, C. M., and T. M. Keaveny (1996). "The Dependence of Shear Failure Properties of Trabecular Bone on Apparent Density and Trabecular Orientation," *J. Biomech.* 29:1309–1317.

Frei, H., T. R. Oxland, G. C. Rathonyi, L. P. Nolte (2001). "The Effect of Nucleotomy on Lumbar Spine Mechanics in Compression and Shear Loading," *Spine* 26:2080–2089.

Fyhrie, D. P., and D. R. Carter (1986). "A Unifying Principle Relating Stress to Trabecular Bone Morphology," *J. Orthop. Res.* 4:304–317.

Gibson, L. J (1985). "The Mechanical Behaviour of Cancellous Bone," *J. Biomech.* 18:317–328.

Goel, V. K., and J. D. Clausen (1998). "Prediction of Load Sharing Among Spinal Components of a C5-C6 Motion Segment Using the Finite Element Approach," *Spine* 23:684–691.

Goel, V. K., and L. G. Gilbertson (1995). "Applications of the Finite Element Method to Thoracolumbar Spinal Research: Past, Present, and Future," *Spine* 20:1719–1727.

Goto, M., N. Kawakami, et al. (2003). "Buckling and Bone Modeling As Factors in the Development of Idiopathic Scoliosis," *Spine* 28:364–370; discussion 371.

Goto, K., N. Tajima, et al. (2002). "Mechanical Analysis of the Lumbar Vertebrae in a Three-Dimensional Finite Element Method Model in Which Intradiscal Pressure in the Nucleus Pulposus Was Used to Establish the Model," *J. Orthop. Sci.* 7:243–246.

Goto, K., N. Tajima, et al. (2003). "Effects of Lumbar Spinal Fusion on the Other Lumbar Intervertebral Levels (Three-dimensional Finite Element Analysis)," *J. Orthop. Sci.* 8:577–584.

Griffin, M. J. (2001). "The Validation of Biodynamic Models," *Clin. Biomech. (Bristol, Avon)* 16(Suppl. 1):S81–S192.

Gu, W. Y., and H. Yao (2003). "Effects of Hydration and Fixed Charge Density on Fluid Transport in Charged Hydrated Soft Tissues," *Ann. Biomed. Eng.* 31:1162–1170.

Guo, L. X., E. C. Teo, K. K. Lee, and Q. H. Zhang (2005). "Vibration Characteristics of the Human Spine Under Axial Cyclic Loads: Effect of Frequency and Damping," *Spine* 30:631–637.

Hadamard, J. (1902). "Sur les Problemes aux Derives Partielles et Leur Signification Physique," *Bull. Univ. Princeton* 13 pp 49–52.

Hill, A. V (1938). "The Heat of Shortening and the Dynamic Constraints of Muscle," *Proc. Roy. Soc.* B126:136–195.

Hodgskinson, R., and J. D. Currey (1990). "Effects of Structural Variation on Young's Modulus of Non-human Cancellous Bone," *Proc. Inst. Mech. Eng. [H]* 204:43–52.

Hong-Wan, N., T. Ee-Chon, and Z. Qing-Hang (2004). "Biomechanical Effects of C2-C7 Intersegmental Stability Due to Laminectomy with Unilateral and Bilateral Facetectomy," *Spine* 29:1737–1745; discussion 1746.

Hou, F. J., S. M. Lang, et al. (1998). "Human Vertebral Body Apparent and Hard Tissue Stiffness," *J. Biomech.* 31:1009–1015.

Hukins, D. W., M. C. Kirby, et al. (1990). "Comparison of Structure, Mechanical Properties, and Functions of Lumbar Spinal Ligaments," *Spine* 15:787–795.

Hurwitz, A., and R. Courant (1922). *Vorlesunger über Allgemeine Funcktionen Theorie.* (4th Ed, vol 3, Grundlehren der mathematischer Wissenschaften, Springer, 1964).

Ito, M., A. Nishida, et al. (2002). "Contribution of Trabecular and Cortical Components to the Mechanical Properties of Bone and Their Regulating Parameters," *Bone* 31:351–358.

Jaasma, M. J., H. H. Bayraktar, G. L. Niebur, and T. M. Keaveny (2002). "Biomechanical Effects of Intraspecimen Variations in Tissue Modulus for Trabecular Bone," *J. Biomech.* 35:237–246.

Jensen, N. C., L. P. Madsen, and F. Linde (1991). "Topographical Distribution of Trabecular Bone Strength in the Human Os Calcanei," *J. Biomech.* 24:49–55.

Jorgensen, C. S., and T. Kundu (2002). "Measurement of Material Elastic Constants of Trabecular Bone: A Micromechanical Analytic Study Using a 1-GHz Acoustic Microscope," *J. Orthop. Res.* 20:151–158.

Kawahara, N., H. Murakami, et al. (2003). "Reconstruction After Total Sacrectomy Using a New Instrumentation Technique: A Biomechanical Comparison," *Spine* 28:1567–1572.

Kiefer, A., A. Shirazi-Adl, and M. Parnianpour (1998). "Synergy of the Human Spine in Neutral Postures," *Eur. Spine J.* 7:471–479.

Kim, Y. (2001). "Prediction of Mechanical Behaviors at Interfaces Between Bone and Two Interbody Cages of Lumbar Spine Segments," *Spine* 26:1437–1442.

Kong, W. Z., and V. K. Goel (2003). "Ability of the Finite Element Models to Predict Response of the Human Spine to Sinusoidal Vertical Vibration," *Spine* 28:1961–1967.

Kong, W. Z., V. K. Goel, L. G. Gilbertson, and J. N. Weinstein (1996). "Effects of Muscle Dysfunction on Lumbar Spine Mechanics: A Finite Element Study Based on a Two Motion Segments Model," *Spine* 21:2197–2206; discussion 2206–2207.

Kosmopoulos, V., and T. S. Keller (2004). "Damage-based Finite-element Vertebroplasty Simulations," *Eur. Spine J.* 13:617–625.

Kumaresan, S., N. Yoganandan, and F. A. Pintar (1998). "Finite Element Modeling Approaches of Human Cervical Spine Facet Joint Capsule," *J. Biomech.* 31:371–376.

Kumaresan, S., N. Yoganandan, and F. A. Pintar (1999). "Finite Element Analysis of the Cervical Spine: A Material Property Sensitivity Study," *Clin. Biomech. (Bristol, Avon)* 14:41–53.

Kumaresan, S., N. Yoganandan, F. A. Pintar, and D. J. Maiman (1999). "Finite Element Modeling of the Cervical Spine: Role of Intervertebral Disc Under Axial and Eccentric Loads," *Med. Eng. Phys.* 21:689–700.

Kumaresan, S., N. Yoganandan, et al. (2001). "Contribution of Disc Degeneration to Osteophyte Formation in the Cervical Spine: A Biomechanical Investigation," *J. Orthop. Res.* 19:977–984.

Kurtz, S. M (2004). *The UHMWPE Handbook.* San Diego, Elsevier Academic Press.

Kurtz, S. M., J. R. Foulds, and C. W. Jewett (1997). "Validation of a Small Punch Testing Technique to Characterize the Mechanical Behavior of Ultra-high Molecular Weight Polyethylene," *Biomaterials* 18:1659–1663.

Kurtz, S. M., C. W. Jewett, J. R. Foulds, and A. A. Edidin (1999). "A Miniature-specimen Mechanical Testing Technique Scaled to the Articulating Surface of Polyethylene Components for Total Joint Arthroplasty," *J. Biome. Mater. Res. (Appl. Biomater.)* 48:75–81.

Langrana, N. A., R. R. Harten, et al. (2002). "Acute Thoracolumbar Burst Fractures: A New View of Loading Mechanisms," *Spine* 27:498–508.

Lasser, S., and J. Pugh (1977). "Preferred Orientations in Cancellous Bone: Techniques for Determination and Possible Biomechanical Significance [Proceedings]," *Bull. Hosp. Joint. Dis.* 38:8–9.

Lee, C. K., Y. E. Kim, et al. (2000). "Impact Response of the Intervertebral Disc in a Finite-element Model," *Spine* 25:2431–2439.

Lee, K. K., and E. C. Teo (2004a). "Effects of Laminectomy and Facetectomy on the Stability of the Lumbar Motion Segment," *Med. Eng. Phys.* 26:183–192.

Lee, K. K., and E. C. Teo (2004b). "Poroelastic Analysis of Lumbar Spinal Stability in Combined Compression and Anterior Shear," *J. Spinal Disord. Tech.* 17:429–438.

Lee, K. K., E. C. Teo, et al. (2004). "Finite-element Analysis for Lumbar Interbody Fusion Under Axial Loading," *IEEE Trans. Biomed. Eng.* 51:393–400.

Liebschner, M. A., D. L. Kopperdahl, W. S. Rosenberg, and T. M. Keaveny (2003). "Finite Element Modeling of the Human Thoracolumbar Spine," *Spine* 28:559–565.

Liebschner, M. A., W. S. Rosenberg, and T. M. Keaveny (2001). "Effects of Bone Cement Volume and Distribution on Vertebral Stiffness After Vertebroplasty," *Spine* 26:1547–1554.

Lim, T. H., J. G. Kim, et al. (2001). "Biomechanical Evaluation of Diagonal Fixation in Pedicle Screw Instrumentation," *Spine* 26:2498–2503.

Lim, T. H., H. Kwon, et al. (2001). "Effect of Endplate Conditions and Bone Mineral Density on the Compressive Strength of the Graft-end plate Interface in Anterior Cervical Spine Fusion," *Spine* 26:951–956.

Lin, C. Y., C. C. Hsiao, P. Q. Chen, and S. J. Hollister (2004). "Interbody Fusion Cage Design Using Integrated Global Layout and Local Microstructure Topology Optimization," *Spine* 29:1747–1754.

Lin, L. C., H. H. Chen, and S. P. Sun (2003). "A Biomechanical Study of the Cortex-anchorage Vertebral Screw," *Clin. Biomech. (Bristol, Avon)* 18:S25–S32.

Liu, Y., and G. Ray (1973). "A Finite Element Analysis of Wave Propagation in the Human Spine," *Technical Report F33615-72-C-1212.* Wright Patterson A.F.B. Fairborn, OH.

Lotz, J. C., O. K. Colliou, et al. (1998). "Compression-induced Degeneration of the Intervertebral Disc: An In Vivo Mouse Model and Finite-element Study," *Spine* 23:2493–2506.

Lu, Y. M., W. C. Hutton, and V. M. Gharpuray (1996). "Can Variations in Intervertebral Disc Height Affect the Mechanical Function of the Disc?," *Spine* 21:2208–2216; discussion 2217.

Martin, R. B., and D. L. Boardman (1993). "The Effects of Collagen Fiber Orientation, Porosity, Density, and Mineralization on Bovine Cortical Bone Bending Properties," *J. Biomech.* 26:1047–1054.

Maurel, N., F. Lavaste, and W. Skalli (1997). "A Three-dimensional Parameterized Finite Element Model of the Lower Cervical Spine: Study of the Influence of the Posterior Articular Facets," *J. Biomech.* 30:921–931.

Moore, G. E (1965). "Cramming More Components onto Integrated Circuits," *Electronics* 38:114–117.

Morgan, E. F., and T. M. Keaveny (2001). "Dependence of Yield Strain of Human Trabecular Bone on Anatomic Site," *J. Biomech.* 34:569–577.

Morgan, E. F., H. H. Bayraktar, and T. M. Keaveny (2003). "Trabecular Bone Modulus-density Relationships Depend on Anatomic Site," *J. Biomech.* 36:897–904.

Moumene, M., and F. H. Geisler (2004). *Effect of Artificial Disc Placement on Facet Loading.* Global Symposium on Intervertebral Disc Replacement & Non-fusion Technology. Vienna, Austria.

Mow, V. C., and R. Huiskes (2005). *Basic Orthopaedic Biomechanics and Mechano-biology.* Philadelphia, PA Lippincott Williams & Wilkins.

Natarajan, R. N., and G. B. Andersson (1999). "The Influence of Lumbar Disc Height and Cross-sectional Area on the Mechanical Response of the Disc to Physiologic Loading," *Spine* 24:1873–1881.

Natarajan, R. N., J. R. Williams, and G. B. Andersson (2004). "Recent Advances in Analytical Modeling of Lumbar Disc Degeneration," *Spine* 29:2733–2741.

Natarajan, R. N., G. B. Andersson, A. G. Patwardhan, and S. Verma (2002). "Effect of Annular Incision Type on the Change in Biomechanical Properties in a Herniated Lumbar Intervertebral Disc," *J. Biomech. Eng.* 124:229–236.

Natarajan, R. N., B. H. Chen, H. S. An, and G. B. Andersson (2000). "Anterior Cervical Fusion: A Finite Element Model Study on Motion Segment Stability Including the Effect of Osteoporosis," *Spine* 25:955–961.

Natarajan, R. N., R. B. Garretson, et al. (2003). "Effects of Slip Severity and Loading Directions on the Stability of Isthmic Spondylolisthesis: A Finite Element Model Study," *Spine* 28:1103–1112.

Ng, H. W., and E. C. Teo (2001). "Nonlinear Finite-element Analysis of the Lower Cervical Spine (C4-C6) Under Axial Loading," *J. Spinal Disord.* 14:201–210.

Ng, H. W., and E. C. Teo (2004). "Probabilistic Design Analysis of the Influence of Material Property on the Human Cervical Spine," *J. Spinal Disord. Tech.* 17:123–133.

Ng, H. W., and E. C. Teo (2005). "Influence of Preload Magnitudes and Orientation Angles on the Cervical Biomechanics: A Finite Element Study," *J. Spinal Disord. Tech.* 18:72–79.

Ng, H. W., E. C. Teo, and V. S. Lee (2004). "Statistical Factorial Analysis on the Material Property Sensitivity of the Mechanical Responses of the C4-C6 Under Compression, Anterior and Posterior Shear," *J. Biomech.* 37:771–777.

Ng, H. W., E. C. Teo, and Q. Zhang (2005). "Influence of Cervical Disc Degeneration After Posterior Surgical Techniques in Combined Flexion-extension: A Nonlinear Analytical Study," *J. Biomech. Eng.* 127:186–192.

Ng, H. W., E. C. Teo, K. K. Lee, and T. X. Qiu (2003). "Finite Element Analysis of Cervical Spinal Instability Under Physiologic Loading," *J. Spinal Disord. Tech.* 16:55–65.

Palm, W. J. T., W. S. Rosenberg, and T. M. Keaveny (2002). "Load Transfer Mechanisms in Cylindrical Interbody Cage Constructs," *Spine* 27:2101–2107.

Panjabi, M. M., V. K. Goel, and K. Takata (1982). "Physiologic Strains in the Lumbar Spinal Ligaments: An In Vitro Biomechanical Study," *Spine* 7:192–203.

Panjabi, M. M., N. C. Chen, E. K. Shin, and J. L. Wang (2001). "The Cortical Shell Architecture of Human Cervical Vertebral Bodies," *Spine* 26:2478–2484.

Pankoke, S., J. Hofmann, and H. P. Wolfel (2001). "Determination of Vibration-related Spinal Loads by Numerical Simulation," *Clin. Biomech. (Bristol, Avon)* 16(Suppl. 1):S45–S56.

Perie, D., J. Sales De Gauzy, C. Baunin, and M. C. Hobatho (2001). "Tomodensitometry Measurements for In Vivo Quantification of Mechanical Properties of Scoliotic Vertebrae," *Clin. Biomech. (Bristol, Avon)* 16:373–379.

Pitzen, T., F. H. Geisler, et al. (2001). "The Influence of Cancellous Bone Density on Load Sharing in Human Lumbar Spine: A Comparison Between an Intact and a Surgically Altered Motion Segment," *Eur. Spine J.* 10:23–29.

Polikeit, A., L. P. Nolte, and S. J. Ferguson (2003). "The Effect of Cement Augmentation on the Load Transfer in an Osteoporotic Functional Spinal Unit: Finite-element Analysis," *Spine* 28:991–996.

Polikeit, A., L. P. Nolte, and S. J. Ferguson (2004). "Simulated Influence of Osteoporosis and Disc Degeneration on the Load Transfer in a Lumbar Functional Spinal Unit," *J. Biomech.* 37:1061–1069.

Polikeit, A., S. J. Ferguson, L. P. Nolte, and T. E. Orr (2003a). "Factors Influencing Stresses in the Lumbar Spine After the Insertion of Intervertebral Cages: Finite Element Analysis," *Eur. Spine J.* 12:413–420.

Polikeit, A., S. J. Ferguson, L. P. Nolte, and T. E. Orr (2003b). "The Importance of the Endplate for Interbody Cages in the Lumbar Spine," *Eur. Spine J.* 12:556–561.

Pothuaud, L., B. Van Rietbergen, et al. (2002). "Combination of Topological Parameters and Bone Volume Fraction Better Predicts the Mechanical Properties of Trabecular Bone," *J. Biomech.* 35:1091–1099.

Przybylski, G. J., P. R. Patel, G. J. Carlin, and S. L. Woo (1998). "Quantitative Anthropometry of the Subatlantal Cervical Longitudinal Ligaments," *Spine* 23:893–898.

Puttlitz, C. M., V. K. Goel, C. R. Clark, and V. C. Traynelis (2000). "Pathomechanisms of Failures of the Odontoid," *Spine* 25:2868–2876.

Puttlitz, C. M., V. K. Goel, et al. (2000). "Biomechanical Rationale for the Pathology of Rheumatoid Arthritis in the Craniovertebral Junction," *Spine* 25:1607–1616.

Qiu, T. X., E. C. Teo, et al. (2003). "Validation of T10-T11 Finite Element Model and Determination of Instantaneous Axes of Rotations in Three Anatomical Planes," *Spine* 28:2694–2699.

Rho, J. Y., M. C. Hobatho, and R. B. Ashman (1995). "Relations of Mechanical Properties to Density and CT Numbers in Human Bone," *Med. Eng. Phys.* 17:347–355.

Rice, J. C., S. C. Cowin, and J. A. Bowman (1988). "On the Dependence of the Elasticity and Strength of Cancellous Bone on Apparent Density," *J. Biomech.* 21:155–168.

Rohlmann, A., T. Zander, and G. Bergmann (2005a). "Comparison of the Biomechanical Effects of Posterior and Anterior Spine-stabilizing Implants," *Eur. Spine J.*

Rohlmann, A., T. Zander, and G. Bergmann (2005b). "Effect of Total Disc Replacement with ProDisc on Intersegmental Rotation of the Lumbar Spine," *Spine* 30:738–743.

Schaffler, M. B., and D. B. Burr (1988). "Stiffness of Compact Bone: Effects of Porosity and Density," *J. Biomech.* 21:13–16.

Seidel, H., R. Bluthner, and B. Hinz (2001). "Application of Finite-element Models to Predict Forces Acting on the Lumbar Spine During Whole-body Vibration," *Clin. Biomech. (Bristol, Avon)* 16(Suppl. 1):S57–S63.

Sevostianov, I., and M. Kachanov (2000). "Impact of the Porous Microstructure on the Overall Elastic Properties of the Osteonal Cortical Bone," *J. Biomech.* 33:881–888.

Shirazi-Adl, A., and M. Parnianpour (2000). "Load-bearing and Stress Analysis of the Human Spine Under a Novel Wrapping Compression Loading," *Clin. Biomech. (Bristol, Avon)* 15:718–725.

Shirazi-Adl, A., M. El-Rich, D. G. Pop, and M. Parnianpour (2004). "Spinal Muscle Forces, Internal Loads and Stability in Standing Under Various Postures and Loads-application of Kinematics-based Algorithm," *Eur. Spine J.* 14(4):381–392.

Shirazi-Adl, A., S. Sadouk, et al. (2002). "Muscle Force Evaluation and the Role of Posture in Human Lumbar Spine Under Compression," *Eur. Spine J.* 11:519–526.

Silva, M. J., T. M. Keaveny, and W. C. Hayes (1997). "Load Sharing Between the Shell and Centrum in the Lumbar Vertebral Body," *Spine* 22:140–150.

Silva, M. J., T. M. Keaveny, and W. C. Hayes (1998). "Computed Tomography-based Finite Element Analysis Predicts Failure Loads and Fracture Patterns for Vertebral Sections," *J. Orthop. Res.* 16:300–308.

Sun, K., and M. A. Liebschner (2004). "Biomechanics of Prophylactic Vertebral Reinforcement," *Spine* 29:1428–1435; discusssion 1435.

Templeton, A., D. Cody, and M. Liebschner (2004). "Updating a 3-D Vertebral Body Finite Element Model Using 2-D Images," *Med. Eng. Phys.* 26:329–333.

Tencer, A. F., S. Mirza, and K. Bensel (2002). "Internal Loads in the Cervical Spine During Motor Vehicle Rear-end Impacts: The Effect of Acceleration and Head-to-head Restraint Proximity," *Spine* 27:34–42.

Teo, E. C., and H. W. Ng (2001a). "Evaluation of the Role of Ligaments, Facets and Disc Nucleus in Lower Cervical Spine Under Compression and Sagittal Moments Using Finite Element Method," *Med. Eng. Phys.* 23:155–164.

Teo, E. C., and H. W. Ng (2001b). "First Cervical Vertebra (Atlas) Fracture Mechanism Studies Using Finite Element Method," *J. Biomech.* 34:13–21.

Teo, E. C., K. K. Lee, et al. (2004). "The Biomechanics of Lumbar Graded Facetectomy Under Anterior-shear Load," *IEEE Trans. Biomed. Eng.* 51:443–449.

Teo, E. C., K. Yang, et al. (2004). "Effects of Cervical Cages on Load Distribution of Cancellous Core: A Finite Element Analysis," *J. Spinal Disord. Tech.* 17:226–231.

Totoribe, K., E. Chosa, and N. Tajima (2004). "A Biomechanical Study of Lumbar Fusion Based on a Three-dimensional Nonlinear Finite Element Method," *J. Spinal Disord. Tech.* 17:147–153.

Totoribe, K., N. Tajima, and E. Chosa (1999). "A Biomechanical Study of Posterolateral Lumbar Fusion Using a Three-dimensional Nonlinear Finite Element Method," *J. Orthop. Sci.* 4:115–126.

Tropiano, P., L. Thollon, et al. (2004). "Using a Finite Element Model to Evaluate Human Injuries Application to the HUMOS Model in Whiplash Situation," *Spine* 29:1709–1716.

Tschirhart, C. E., A. Nagpurkar, and C. M. Whyne (2004). "Effects of Tumor Location, Shape and Surface Serration on Burst Fracture Risk in the Metastatic Spine," *J. Biomech.* 37:653–660.

Ulrich, D., B. van Rietbergen, H. Weinans, and P. Ruegsegger (1998). "Finite Element Analysis of Trabecular Bone Structure: A Comparison of Image-based Meshing Techniques," *J. Biomech.* 31:1187–1192.

U.S. DHHS (U.S. Dept. of Health and Human Services) (2001). "Guidance for Annuloplasty Rings 510(k) Submissions: Final Guidance for Industry and FDA Staff," U.S. Dept. of Health and Human Services, Food and Drug Administration.

U.S. DHHS (U.S. Dept. of Health and Human Services) (2003). "Class II Special Controls Guidance Document: Knee Joint Patellofemorotibial and Femorotibial Metal/Polymer Porous-Coated Uncemented Prosthesis: Guidance for Industry and FDA," U.S. Dept. of Health and Human Services, Food and Drug Administration.

Villarraga, M. L., A. J. Bellezza, et al. (2005). "The Biomechanical Effects of Kyphoplasty on Treated and Adjacent Nontreated Vertebral Bodies," *J. Spinal Disord. Tech.* 18:84–91.

Wang, J. L., M. Parnianpour, A. Shirazi-Adl, and A. E. Engin (1998). "The Dynamic Response of L(2)/L(3) Motion Segment in Cyclic Axial Compressive Loading," *Clin. Biomech. (Bristol, Avon)* 13:S16–S25.

Wang, J. L., M. Parnianpour, A. Shirazi-Adl, and A. E. Engin (2000). "Viscoelastic Finite-element Analysis of a Lumbar Motion Segment in Combined Compression and Sagittal Flexion: Effect of Loading Rate," *Spine* 25:310–318.

Weiss, J. A., and J. C. Gardiner (2001). "Computational Modeling of Ligament Mechanics," *Crit Rev Biomed Eng* 29:1–70.

Weiss, J. A., J. C. Gardiner, et al. (2005). "Three-dimensional Finite Element Modeling of Ligaments: Technical Aspects," *Med. Eng. Phys* 27:895–861.

White, A. A., and M. M. Panjabi (1990). *Clinical Biomechanics of the Spine.* Philadelphia, PA Lippincott Williams & Wilkins.

Whyne, C. M., S. S. Hu, and J. C. Lotz (2001). "Parametric Finite Element Analysis of Vertebral Bodies Affected by Tumors," *J. Biomech.* 34:1317–1324.

Whyne, C. M., S. S. Hu, and J. C. Lotz (2003a). "Biomechanically Derived Guideline Equations for Burst Fracture Risk Prediction in the Metastatically Involved Spine," *J. Spinal Disord. Tech.* 16:180–185.

Whyne, C. M., S. S. Hu, and J. C. Lotz (2003b). "Burst Fracture in the Metastatically Involved Spine: Development, Validation, and Parametric Analysis of a Three-dimensional Poroelastic Finite-element Model," *Spine* 28:652–660.

Whyne, C. M., S. S. Hu, S. Klisch, and J. C. Lotz (1998). "Effect of the Pedicle and Posterior Arch on Vertebral Body Strength Predictions in Finite Element Modeling," *Spine* 23:899–907.

Wilcox, R. K., D. J. Allen, et al. (2004). "A Dynamic Investigation of the Burst Fracture Process Using a Combined Experimental and Finite Element Approach," *Eur. Spine J.* 13:481–488.

Wilcox, R. K., T. O. Boerger, et al. (2003). "A Dynamic Study of Thoracolumbar Burst Fractures," *J. Bone Joint Surg. Am.* 85-A:2184–2189.

Wilke, H., P. Neef, et al. (2001). "Intradiscal Pressure Together with Anthropometric Data: A Data Set for the Validation of Models," *Clin. Biomech. (Bristol, Avon)* 16(Suppl. 1):S111–S126.

Winters, J. M (1990). "Hill-based Muscle Models: A Systems Engineering Perspective," in Winters, J. M., Wu, S. L.-Y. (eds.). *Multiple Muscle Systems: Biomechanics and Movement Organization.* New York, Springer-Verlag.

Wu, J. S., and J. H. Chen (1996). "Clarification of the Mechanical Behaviour of Spinal Motion Segments Through a Three-dimensional Poroelastic Mixed Finite Element Model," *Med. Eng. Phys.* 18:215–224.

Yeni, Y. N., F. J. Hou, et al. (2003). "Trabecular Shear Stresses Predict In Vivo Linear Microcrack Density But Not Diffuse Damage in Human Vertebral Cancellous Bone," *Ann. Biomed. Eng.* 31:726–732.

Yoganandan, N., S. Kumaresan, and F. A. Pintar (2001). "Biomechanics of the Cervical Spine. Part 2. Cervical Spine Soft Tissue Responses and Biomechanical Modeling," *Clin. Biomech. (Bristol, Avon)* 16:1–27.

Yoganandan, N., S. Kumaresan, L. Voo, and F. A. Pintar (1996). "Finite Element Applications in Human Cervical Spine Modeling," *Spine* 21:1824–1834.

Yoganandan, N., J. B. Myklebust, G. Ray, and A. Sances (1987). "Mathematical and Finite Element Analysis of Spine Injuries," *CRC Crit Rev Biomed Eng* 15:29–93.

Yoganandan, N., S. C. Kumaresan, et al. (1996). "Finite Element Modeling of the C4-C6 Cervical Spine Unit," *Med. Eng. Phys.* 18:569–574.

Zander, T., A. Rohlmann, and G. Bergmann (2004). "Influence of Ligament Stiffness on the Mechanical Behavior of a Functional Spinal Unit," *J. Biomech.* 37:1107–1111.

Zander, T., A. Rohlmann, J. Calisse, and G. Bergmann (2001). "Estimation of Muscle Forces in the Lumbar Spine During Upper-body Inclination," *Clin. Biomech. (Bristol, Avon)* 16(Suppl. 1):S73–S80.

Zander, T., A. Rohlmann, C. Klockner, and G. Bergmann (2003). "Influence of Graded Facetectomy and Laminectomy on Spinal Biomechanics," *Eur. Spine J.* 12:427–434.

Zhang, Q. H., S. H. Tan, and S. M. Chou (2004). "Investigation of Fixation Screw Pull-out Strength on Human Spine," *J. Biomech.* 37:479–485.

Chapter *15*

FDA Regulation of Spinal Implants

Janice M. Hogan, Esq.
Hogan & Hartson, LLP
Philadelphia, PA

15.1 Introduction

This chapter provides an overview of the FDA's current framework for the regulation of spinal implants. The principal focus is on FDA regulation of medical devices, which encompass the majority of spinal implants. However, because medical devices may incorporate drug or biological components, the Agency's regulation of products that combine medical devices drugs with biological or drug components is also addressed.

Orthopedic devices represented nearly one-third of the over $50 billion U.S. market for medical devices in 2003, and spinal implants are a rapidly growing part of the orthopedics market segment. Orthopedic device manufacturers have generally outperformed the S&P 500 index by a wide margin, as shown below. The spinal implant segment is expected to grow at a rate of over 20% per year through the end of the decade [Vfinance 2004, Morgan Stanley 2003]. A major reason for this growth is the aging of the population, which directly impacts the incidence of spinal and other orthopedic disorders. Investment in the spinal implant market drives the proliferation of new technologies, which in turn directs FDA review resources to these products.

A comprehensive regulatory approach to spinal implants must address the total product life cycle, from product inception through pre-market clearance to commercial sale. This chapter focuses solely on the pre-market phase of the product life cycle, which is generally of the greatest interest and importance to engineers and scientists involved in product development. This section describes the overall process for obtaining marketing clearance of spinal implants from the FDA. Section I focuses on the general mechanisms for obtaining premarket clearance of spinal implants; Section II provides a review of the FDA's regulation of specific types of spinal implants. Finally, Section III provides a review of current trends and expected changes in the FDA's regulation of spinal implants.

15.2 Overview of FDA Regulatory Framework

The FDA's legal authority over spinal implants derives from the Federal Food, Drug, and Cosmetic Act (the "FDC Act"), which authorizes the Agency to regulate four discrete product categories: medical devices, human and animal drugs, foods and dietary supplements, and cosmetics [21 U.S.C. § 321]. In addition, the FDA has responsibility for the oversight of biological products, such as blood products and derivatives, cellular products, and gene therapies, as defined under section 351 of the Public Health Service Act ("PHS Act") [42 U.S.C. § 262].

As noted, the majority of spinal implants today are regulated solely as medical devices. The FDA applies a "tiered" approach to the regulation of devices, in which devices that present the highest degree of risk are subject to the highest level of regulation, while devices that present a lesser degree of risk are subject to a lesser degree of regulation. Devices are generally classified by the FDA in one of three classes, with Class I representing the lowest level of risk and Class III representing the highest level of risk.

The level of risk presented by a medical device, as reflected in its classification, impacts the degree of both premarket and postmarket regulation. With respect to pre-market regulatory requirements, there are two principal pathways for obtaining FDA clearance: the first is a 510(k) notice, named for the section of the FDC Act that created this mechanism, and the second is a premarket approval ("PMA") application. Each of these mechanisms is described below. Although there are alternative mechanisms that may be used in some instances, as discussed below, the vast majority of medical devices are cleared via one of these two pathways.

Devices that present relatively low risk are generally placed in Class I or Class II and require the manufacturer to seek 510(k) clearance from the FDA prior to marketing, unless exempted from this requirement by regulation. In recent years, the FDA has exempted a substantial number of Class I and Class II devices from the premarket clearance requirement, but because the vast majority of spinal implants are not exempt, this chapter focuses on devices that require some form of premarket clearance. The FDA will grant clearance of a 510(k) if the submitted information establishes that the new device is "substantially equivalent" to one or more "predicate devices." The term "substantial equivalence" requires that the new device be similar to the predicate(s) in both intended use and technological features. The "predicate device(s)" that can be used to establish substantial equivalence are limited to legally marketed devices that do not require premarket approval; a PMA approved product cannot be used as a predicate for purposes of establishing substantial equivalence.

Many 510(k) notices are cleared on the basis of mechanical testing and other types of non-clinical testing, without the need for clinical evaluation. The difficulty of simulating the loading conditions of the human spine in an animal model has led to reliance principally on sophisticated mechanical testing models for pre-clinical evaluation of spinal implants, as described in Chapter 13. However, animal tests are used to assess certain aspects of the performance of spinal implants, such as biocompatibility, biological response to implant wear debris, etc. Approximately 5–10% of all 510(k) submissions also must include clinical data, and clinical data also are required to support 510(k) clearance for certain types of spinal implants, as discussed in Section 15.2.1 below.

A medical device that does not qualify for 510(k) clearance is placed in Class III, which is reserved for devices classified by the FDA as posing the greatest risk (e.g., life-sustaining, life-supporting or implantable devices, or devices that are not substantially equivalent to a predicate device). A Class III device generally requires FDA approval of a PMA application, which requires the manufacturer to submit valid scientific evidence of safety and effectiveness. Unlike 510(k) notices, PMA applications almost always require supporting clinical data, in addition to pre-clinical data. PMA applications also must include detailed information about the device and its components, as well as comprehensive information about the manufacturing methods, labeling, and promotion. As part of the PMA review, the FDA will inspect the manufacturer's facilities for compliance with the Quality System Regulation ("QS Reg."), 21 C.F.R. Part 820, which includes elaborate testing, control, documentation, and other quality assurance procedures.

Generally, most device manufacturers prefer to pursue 510(k) clearance rather than PMA approval, if possible, because it is typically less costly and time-consuming. The number of PMA applications per year is only a small fraction of the number of 510(k)s, as illustrated in Figures 15.1.

The more burdensome nature of the PMA application process is also illustrated by the longer review time compared to 510(k) notices. In fiscal year 2004, total time from submission to approval averaged 436 days for PMA applications, compared to 100 days for 510(k) notices [Office of Device Evaluation 2004]. Thus, there is a significant incentive for manufacturers to seek 510(k) clearance or other alternatives to the PMA application pathway for regulatory clearance.

The FDA has issued a detailed framework to assist reviewers in determining whether a new device is "substantially equivalent" and, thus, may be cleared via the 510(k) notification process [21 U.S.C. § 360]. According to this framework, the first question that a reviewer should ask in making a substantial equivalence decision is whether the device has the same intended use as one or more "predicate" product(s), which generally must be previously 510(k)-cleared or 510(k)-exempt products. It should be noted that PMA approved products cannot be used as predicates in a 510(k) submission. If the intended use differs from any predicates, the analysis stops, and the device is deemed "not substantially equivalent" ("NSE"), requiring PMA approval.

While the new device must have the same general intended use as a predicate to be substantially equivalent, the new device need not be labeled with exactly the same specific claims as the predicate device. Generally, differences in the specific indication statements will not render a new device NSE, provided that the differences do not alter the intended diagnostic or therapeutic effect of the device, considering the impact of the differences on safety and effectiveness.

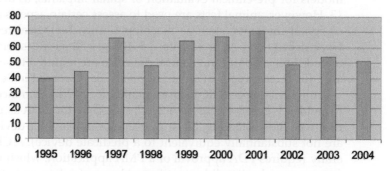

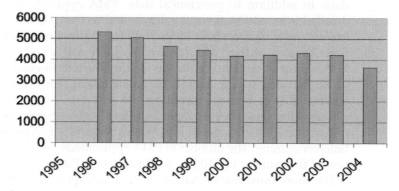

Fig. 15.1.

The next question that must be asked in the substantial equivalence evaluation is whether the new device has the same technological characteristics, such as design, materials, and energy sources, as the predicate device. Devices whose characteristics are the same or very similar to a predicate may be found substantially equivalent. However, if there are new characteristics, the reviewer must further ask whether they could affect safety or effectiveness and, if so, whether they raise new types of safety or effectiveness questions. If the new technological characteristics raise different types of safety or effectiveness issues from the predicates, the device is NSE. If the device does not raise any new types of questions of safety or effectiveness, it may be found SE if accepted scientific methods exist to assess the effects of the new characteristics, and if data are available to demonstrate that the new characteristics do not impact safety or effectiveness. If performance data generated by accepted *in vitro* test methods are not available, the FDA may request the submission of animal or human clinical data to demonstrate equivalence. A detailed chart illustrating the FDA's review process for 510(k) notices is provided in Figure 15.2 below [510(k) Memorandum #K86-3].

510(k) "SUBSTANTIAL EQUIVALENCE"
DECISION-MAKING PROCESS (DETAILED)

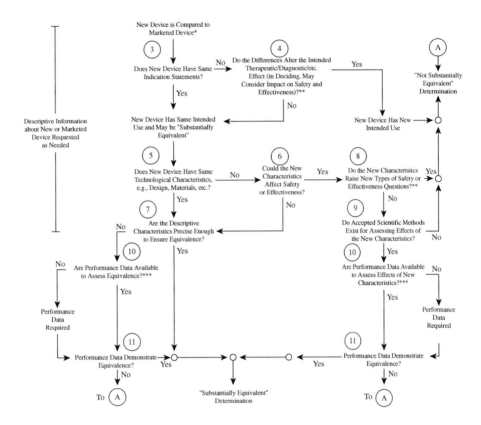

*   510(k) submissions compare new devices to marketed devices. FDA requests additional information if the relationship between marketed and "predicate" (pre-Amendments or reclassified post-Amendments) devices is unclear.

**   This decision is normally based on descriptive information alone, but limited testing information is sometimes required.

*** Data may be in the 510(k), other 510(k)s, the Center's classification files, or the literature.

Fig. 15.2.

After a product receives initial FDA clearance via either a 510(k) notice or a PMA application, the manufacturer may need to submit additional filings to the FDA for subsequent modifications. For a 510(k) cleared product, a new 510(k) submission must be filed for a modification that could *significantly* impact safety or effectiveness [21 C.F.R. § 807.81; 510(k) Memorandum #K97-1 1997], while for a PMA approved product, a supplemental application is required for any change that affects safety or effectiveness [21 C.F.R. § 814.39]. Thus, the difference in the standard for new submissions is more stringent for PMA approved products, requiring more supplemental filings, commensurate with the higher level of risks these products present. Various types of supplemental filing mechanisms are available for different types of changes, with different associated review times. For 510(k) cleared products, a "Special 510(k) Notice" may be filed for changes that are relatively minor in nature; this type of submission is typically reviewed in 30 days rather than the 90-day period for review of a "traditional" 510(k) notice [The New 510(k) Paradigm 2000]. Similarly, for PMA approved products, there are a variety of types of PMA supplements, including "Real Time" supplements, which are intended to provide expeditious review of relatively minor changes ["Real-Time" Review Program 1997].

15.2.1 Alternatives to 510(k) Clearance or PMA Approval

One alternative to PMA approval for a product that is intended for use in a limited patient population is to seek a humanitarian device exemption ("HDE"). FDA defines a Humanitarian Use Device ("HUD") as a device that is intended to treat or diagnose diseases that affect fewer than 4,000 individuals in the United States per year [21 C.F.R. § 814.3(n)]. It should be noted that this threshold for eligibility is much lower than the corresponding 200,000 patient threshold for orphan drug designation. Devices designated as HUDs by the FDA are eligible for approval under an HDE [*Id*. § 814.100]. An HDE is similar to a PMA in terms of the content of the application, with the exception that an HDE requires proof of safety but not effectiveness. As such, HDE device labeling is required to carry a disclaimer stating that the effectiveness of the device has not been established. Additionally, the FDA's review timeframe for an HDE review is shorter than for a PMA, 75 days (excluding the time required to obtain the initial HUD designation) compared to 180 days.

Prior to submitting an HDE for marketing approval of an HUD, an applicant must submit a written request for HUD designation from the FDA through the Agency's Office of Orphan Products Development. The written request must include:

- a statement that an HUD designation is being requested for a rare disease or condition;
- the name, address, and contact information for the applicant;
- a description of the disease or condition, the proposed indications for use of the device, and an explanation on why the device treatment is needed;
- a description of the device and a scientific rationale for use of the device in the treatment of the disease or condition; and
- documentation, including copies of authoritative references, that the device is designed to treat a disease or condition that occurs in fewer than 4,000 people in the United States per year.

The FDA will make a determination on the HUD designation request within 45 days of receipt.

If an HUD designation is obtained from the FDA, then an applicant can submit an HDE for marketing approval of the HUD. The HDE must include:

- an explanation of why the device would not be available unless an HDE were granted;
- a statement that no comparable device is available to treat the condition or disease;
- risk/benefit analysis (taking into account other alternative treatments that are available for the condition or disease);
- all of the information required in a PMA application with the exception of the clinical study details, which may be replaced by summaries, conclusions, and any results from clinical experience or investigations that are relevant to the use of the device in the HUD condition to permit assessment of risks and benefits;
- the amount that will be charged for the device, which if greater than $250 must be supported by a report from an independent certified public accountant, or an attestation from a responsible individual within the applicant's organization, that verifies that the charge does not exceed the costs of the device's research, development, fabrication, and distribution; and
- the labeling for the device, which must carry the following statement: "Humanitarian Device, Authorized by Federal law for use in the treatment of (state disease or condition). The effectiveness of this device for this use has not been demonstrated."

The agency will review the HDE application and make a determination of whether it is approvable within 75 days of receipt.

After an HDE is approved, there are substantial ongoing restrictions on its commercialization. In addition to the price limitation described above, prior to HUD use at any facility, the HDE holder is required to obtain approval from the facility's institutional review board ("IRB"), which is the body responsible for oversight of clinical research. Additionally, the HDE holder is required to maintain files that contain records of the names and addresses of the facilities to which the HUD is shipped and all IRB correspondence. No informed consent is required. However, if at any time the HDE holder decides to collect safety and effectiveness data to support a PMA, then both IRB approval and informed consent are required. The FDA has the discretion to rescind approval of the HDE if another device that is the same as the HUD receives 510(k) clearance or PMA approval, or if the FDA determines that more than 4,000 individuals in the United States per year are affected with the disease or condition [HDE Regulation 2001].

15.2.2 Product Development Protocols

For class III products that are ineligible for 510(k) clearance, there is an alternative mechanism to a PMA application known as a product development protocol or PDP. The principal difference between a PDP and a PMA application is that for a PDP application, the applicant and the FDA negotiate an up-front agreement as to the information that will be required to obtain approval, including both detailed test procedures and acceptance criteria for these tests. The PDP is divided into several phases: preparation of a PDP Summary Outline; review of the PDP by the FDA and, if applicable, the Advisory Panel; the manufacturer then executes the agreed protocol. Once the FDA declares that the PDP has been declared completed, the applicant is considered to have an approved PMA [21 C.F.R. § 814.19].

The PDP process is designed to be well suited to established products for which test methods and acceptance criteria are generally well known. The protocol as agreed with the FDA is intended to serve as a "contract" that provides the manufacturer with certainty early in the development process as to the type of data needed for approval. Data are reported to the FDA throughout the execution of the PDP. Despite these potential advantages, however, the PDP process has been used relatively rarely. Only one PDP was completed in fiscal year 2004, and prior to that, no PDPs were approved in the preceding three years. Thus, PDPs represent a small minority of all class III product approvals, with the vast majority still approved via PMA applications.

Some of the reasons that the PDP process has not been more widely used may relate to the increasing availability of other FDA mechanisms that provide similar advantages. For example, availability of early planning meetings prior to initiating clinical studies, as discussed below, offers some of the same benefits as the PDP, as does the opportunity to submit modular PMA applications. Moreover, although the PDP is intended to provide near-contractual certainty of FDA approval requirements, other mechanisms were introduced under the Food and Drug Administration Modernization Act of 1997, such as formal pre-IDE "Agreement Meetings" and "Determination Meetings," that were intended to serve a similar purpose. Furthermore, scientific understanding may evolve over the years that may be required to complete clinical studies can impact the approval process, particularly in the case of spinal implants, where multi-year clinical studies may be required. Significant changes in scientific understanding over time make it difficult to achieve absolute certainty as to the data requirements to achieve approval, regardless of the mechanism of approval.

15.2.3 Reclassification and Automatic Downclassification

Manufacturers of class III devices that require PMA approval may petition the FDA to downclassify a category of devices to class II to permit 510(k) clearance. In order to support downclassification, the petition must demonstrate that the risks presented by the device category can be adequately managed through the controls that are available for class I or class II devices. Such petitions must typically summarize all available information about the device type, including prior clinical studies. The FDA has in the past downclassified a number of types of orthopedic implants from class III to class II, and is presently considering whether to downclassify spinal fusion cages, which would permit them to be 510(k) cleared [Transcript 2003].

Another mechanism was created in Section 207 of the Food and Drug Administration Modernization Act of 1997 to permit "automatic downclassification" of class III devices. This provision permits *"de novo"* downclassification of novel class III devices for which there is no predicate device to support a finding of substantial equivalence, but which presents low risk and, therefore, does not warrant the onerous process required for PMA approval.

To pursue de novo downclassification under this provision, the applicant must first submit a 510(k) notice and receive a "not substantially equivalent" determination. Within 30 days, a petition must be filed under the de novo downclassification provision, and the FDA will decide whether the product is eligible for downclassification within 60 days. If the FDA agrees that the device meets the criteria for de novo downclassification, then it will grant the petition, which effectively renders the device 510(k) cleared. It should be noted that the device can then be used as a predicate in future 510(k) submissions.

Comparing the de novo downclassification process to a conventional reclassification petition, as discussed above, there are several key differences. First, the applicant does not need to first submit a 510(k) notice and have it found not substantially equivalent before a reclassification petition may be filed. Second, the review time for a reclassification petition is typically much longer than for a de novo petition (180 days versus 60 days). Thus, these mechanisms may have utility under somewhat different circumstances, although they have a common objective.

15.2.4 Clinical Studies of Medical Devices

Regardless of which of the regulatory pathways that a manufacturer pursues to obtain medical device clearance, if clinical data are required, it must be determined whether or not the study requires prior FDA approval of an investigational device exemption ("IDE") application. Clinical studies of "significant risk" ("SR") investigational devices require prior FDA approval of an IDE application, while nonsignificant risk ("NSR") studies do not. A "significant risk" device study is defined as a study of a device that presents a potential for serious risk to the health, safety, or welfare of a subject and (1) is intended as an implant; or (2) is used in supporting or sustaining human life; or (3) is of substantial importance in diagnosing, curing, mitigating, or treating disease, or otherwise prevents impairment of human health; or (4) otherwise presents a potential for serious risk to the health, safety, or welfare of a subject [21 C.F.R. 812.3(m)]. Examples of devices that the FDA views as presenting significant risk in investigational studies include sutures, cardiac pacemakers, hydrocephalus shunts, and nearly all orthopedic implants. Both SR and NSR studies require prior approval by the participating hospitals' institutional review boards ("IRBs"), and informed consent of participating patients.

Under § 812.7 of the IDE regulations, sponsors are permitted to charge for investigational devices, provided that the amount does not exceed the costs of research, development, manufacture, and distribution. Thus, unlike for drugs and biologics, it is not uncommon for devices to be sold during the investigational phase, within the limits of the IDE approval.

15.2.4.1 Expedited Review

For 510(k)s and PMAs, expedited review status is available for devices that provide for more effective treatment or diagnosis of life-threatening or irreversibly debilitating diseases or conditions than do currently available alternative clinical treatments. When expedited review status is assigned to a device, its marketing application moves to the front of the agency's application review queue and receives priority review by the FDA over other pending marketing applications. The FDA uses the following criteria to determine a device's eligibility for expedited review:

- The device is a breakthrough technology, defined to mean that the device is demonstrated to provide a clinical improvement in the treatment or diagnosis of a life-threatening or irreversibly debilitating condition.
- There is no approved alternative.
- The device provides significant, clinically meaningful advantages over existing approved alternatives.
- Device availability serves the best interest of the patients. The guidance specifies that this criterion requires the device to provide a specific public health benefit or meet the needs of a well-defined patient population. Examples of devices meeting this criterion include those that are designed or modified to overcome an unanticipated serious failure occurring in a critical component of an approved device for which there are no alternatives, or for which alternative treatment would involve a substantial risk of patient morbidity.

See *Guidance for Industry and FDA Staff: Expedited Review of Premarket Submissions for Device*.[1] The guidance notes that combination products containing a device are also eligible for expedited review if either CDRH or CBER is designated as the lead center.

A device may be granted expedited review status if it meets any of these four criteria. Expedited review status may be rescinded once another device that offers similar advantages or advances is approved by the agency. It should be noted, however, that the FDA's statistics on approval times show no significant reduction in the mean review time for "expedited" applications compared to all others. In fact, mean review times for "expedited review" applications are somewhat longer, likely due to the novelty of the clinical issues they may present. However, the Agency has committed to Medical Device User Fee and Modernization Act performance goals that would require at least 70% of

---

1. This guidance has replaced the FDA's previous guidance on expedited review of devices, *PMA/510(k) Expedited Review—Guidance for Industry and CDRH Staff* (March 20, 1998). Although the criteria for expedited review in the new guidance are very similar to those set forth in the 1998 guidance, the new guidance also establishes performance goals with respect to review time for expedited submissions, as noted above.

expedited review PMA decisions to be reached within 300 days by 2005, provided certain administrative requirements are satisfied. Nonetheless, even without a review time advantage, there may be some commercial advantages to the expedited review designation because it connotes to investors and the marketplace an important, highly innovative product.

15.2.4.2 Alternative Pathways

(1) Humanitarian Device Designation and Exemption

One alternative to PMA approval for a product that is intended for use in a limited patient population is to seek a humanitarian device exemption ("HDE"). The FDA defines a Humanitarian Use Device (HUD) as a device that is intended to treat or diagnose diseases that affect fewer than 4,000 individuals in the United States per year [21 C.F.R. § 814.3(n)]. It should be noted that this threshold for eligibility is much lower than the corresponding 200,000 patient threshold for orphan drug designation. Devices designated as HUDs by the FDA are eligible for approval under an HDE. [*Id.* § 814.100]. An HDE is similar to a PMA in terms of the informational content of the application, with the exception that an HDE requires proof of safety but not effectiveness. As such, HDE device labeling is required to carry a disclaimer stating that the effectiveness of the device has not been established. Additionally, the FDA's review timeframe for an HDE review is shorter than for a PMA, 75 days (excluding the time required to obtain the initial HUD designation) compared to 180 days.

Prior to submitting an HDE for marketing approval of an HUD, an applicant must submit a written request for HUD designation from the FDA through the Agency's Office of Orphan Products Development. The written request must include:

- a statement that an HUD designation is being requested for a rare disease or condition;
- the name, address, and contact information for the applicant;
- a description of the disease or condition, the proposed indications for use of the device, and an explanation on why the device treatment is needed;
- a description of the device and a scientific rationale for use of the device in the treatment of the disease or condition; and
- documentation, including copies of authoritative references, that the device is designed to treat a disease or condition that occurs in fewer than 4,000 people in the United States per year.

The FDA will make a determination on the HUD designation request within 45 days of receipt.

If an HUD designation is obtained from the FDA, then an applicant can submit an HDE for marketing approval of the HUD. The HDE must include:

- an explanation of why the device would not be available unless an HDE were granted;

- a statement that no comparable device is available to treat the condition or disease;
- risk/benefit analysis (taking into account other alternative treatments that are available for the condition or disease);
- all of the information required in a PMA application with the exception of the clinical study details, which may be replaced by summaries, conclusions, and any results from clinical experience or investigations that are relevant to the use of the device in the HUD condition to permit assessment of risks and benefits; and
- the amount that will be charged for the device, which if greater than $250 must be supported by a report from an independent certified public accountant, or an attestation from a responsible individual within the applicant's organization, that verifies that the charge does not exceed the costs of the device's research, development, fabrication, and distribution; and
- the labeling for the device, which must carry the following statement: "Humanitarian Device, Authorized by Federal law for use in the treatment of (state disease or condition). The effectiveness of this device for this use has not been demonstrated."

The Agency will review the HDE application and make a determination of whether it is approvable within 75 days of receipt.

After an HDE is approved, there are substantial ongoing restrictions on its commercialization. In addition to the price limitation described above, prior to HUD use at any facility, the HDE holder is required to obtain approval from the facility's IRB. Additionally, the HDE holder is required to maintain files that contain records of the names and addresses of the facilities to which the HUD is shipped and all IRB correspondence. No informed consent is required. However, if at any time the HDE holder decides to collect safety and effectiveness data to support a PMA, then both IRB approval and informed consent are required. The FDA has the discretion to rescind approval of the HDE if another device that is the same as the HUD receives 510(k) clearance or PMA approval, or if the FDA determines that more than 4,000 individuals in the United States per year are affected with the disease or condition. Additional information regarding the HDE process is provided in the FDA's *Humanitarian Device Exemption (HDE) Regulation; Questions and Answers; Final Guidance for Industry* (2001).

15.2.4.3 Pediatric Devices

The FDA reviews pediatric indications for medical devices through all of the regulatory clearance pathways described above. The Medical Device User Fee and Modernization Act of 2002 ("MDUFMA"), which was signed into law on October 26, 2002, added three provisions to the FDC Act concerning the regulation of pediatric medical devices. First, Section 210 of MDUFMA amends Section 515(c) of the FDC Act (premarket approvals) by requiring an advisory panel reviewing a PMA to include or consult with pediatric expert(s), where appropriate. Second, MDUFMA requires the FDA to request that the Institute of Medicine conduct a study to determine whether the FDA's postmarket surveillance program provides adequate safeguards for the use of devices in pediatric populations. The results of this study must be reported to Congress no later than October 26, 2006. Finally, the FDA is required to develop guidance on: (1) the type of information required to provide reasonable assurance of the safety and effectiveness of medical devices intended for use in pediatric populations; and (2) protections for pediatric subjects in clinical investigations of the safety or effectiveness of such devices. Additionally, MDUFMA has specifically exempted premarket applications for pediatric medical devices from user fee requirements provided that the proposed conditions of use for the device involved are solely for a pediatric population.

The FDA recently issued two guidance documents related to pediatric medical devices: (1) *Draft Guidance for Industry and FDA Staff—Pediatric Expertise for Advisory Panels,* June 3, 2003, ("Pediatric Advisory Panel Guidance"); and (2) *Draft Guidance for Industry and FDA Staff—Premarket Assessment of Pediatric Medical Devices*, July 24, 2003, ("Pediatric Premarket Review Guidance"). The Pediatric Advisory Panel Guidance describes the FDA's internal procedures for ensuring that, where appropriate, pediatric experts are consulted for development of pediatric regulatory documents and that these experts participate in the review of premarket submission review of pediatric devices. An overview of the Pediatric Premarket Review Guidance is set forth below.

The purpose of the FDA's Pediatric Premarket Review Guidance is to assist in defining: (1) pediatric populations, pediatric uses, and clinical trials; (2) the type of information necessary to assure the safety and effectiveness of pediatric medical devices; and (3) protections for pediatric patients enrolled in clinical studies. The FDA views medical devices for which the primary indication is in a pediatric population as pediatric use devices. The FDA also considers that for devices with a general indication, if it is expected that the device will have wide application to a pediatric population, then this type of device is a pediatric use device. Table 15.1 includes a list of the FDA's proposed pediatric population subgroups.

The FDA, however, also recognizes that factors other than chronological age, e.g., physiological and neurological development, weight, body size, etc., may need to be considered in defining the appropriate pediatric patient population for use with specific medical devices.

Table 15.1.
FDA's Proposed Age Ranges of Pediatric Subgroups for Medical Devices.

Pediatric Subgroup	Approximate Age Range
Newborn	Birth to 1 month of age
Infant	1 month to 2 years of age
Child	2 to 12 years of age
Adolescent	12 to 21 years of age

In general, the type of information required to demonstrate and assure safety and effectiveness is the same for medical devices used in pediatric populations as in other populations, e.g., biocompatibility, sterility, stability and, where applicable, pre-clinical animal and clinical studies. For clinical studies, when determined to be necessary for a specific pediatric medical device, the FDA has recommended that the design of these studies should take into consideration the following characteristics that may be unique to this population:

- effects of the device on the growth and development of the subject as well as the effects of growth and development on the device, e.g., will the subject outgrow the device, will additional intervention be needed to adjust for growth, will the device alter normal growth patterns
- impact of subject's activity and maturity level on the effectiveness of the device as well as the impact of the device on the subject's activity
- influence of hormonal status, maturity or immaturity of organ systems, etc.

Additionally, since the Agency views pediatric subjects as a vulnerable group of individuals, as noted above, clinical trial sponsors, investigators, and IRBs must conform to 21 C.F.R. Part 50, Subpart D, which provides additional safeguards for children involved in clinical investigations. As discussed above, these additional procedures include: (1) assessment of risk to the subject; (2) justification of the anticipated direct benefit for the subject of a study that presents a greater than minimal risk to the pediatric subject; (3) justification for those studies that have no direct benefit to the subject that any increased risk presents only a minor increase over minimal risk and is likely to yield general information about the subject's condition; (4) expert and public review of studies that present greater than minimal risk and do not provide direct benefit to or yield information on the subject's condition; and (5) assent by subjects, when capable of providing such assent, or permission from parents or guardians.

The first step in determining the FDA jurisdictional assignment of a product is to compare it to the statutory definitions of each of the above categories. The definition of a "biologic" in the PHS Act is as follows:

a virus, therapeutic serum, toxin, antitoxin, vaccine, blood, blood component or derivative, allergenic product, or analogous product, or arsphenamine or derivative of arsphenamine (or any other trivalent organic arsenic compound), applicable to the prevention, treatment, or cure of a disease or condition of human beings [42 U.S.C. §262(i)].

The definition of a medical device under the FDC Act is:

an instrument, apparatus, implement, machine, contrivance, implant, in vitro reagent, or other similar or related article, including any component, part, or accessory, which is—
(1) recognized in the official National Formulary, or the United States Pharmacopeia, or any supplement to them,
(2) intended for use in the diagnosis of disease or other conditions, or in the cure, mitigation, treatment, or prevention of disease, in man or other animals, or

(3) intended to affect the structure or any function of the body of man or other animals, and which does not achieve its primary intended purposes through chemical action within or on the body of man or other animals and which is not dependent upon being metabolized for the achievement of its primary intended purposes [21 U.S.C. §321(h)].

Comparing these two definitions, in some instances, it may be unclear whether a product falls within one or more of these categories. In addition, in some cases, a product may encompass more than one element, combining, for example, drug and device or drug and biologic elements.

The FDC Act provides relatively little guidance on how jurisdictional assignments should be made for products that do not fall squarely within the definition of a device, drug or biologic. The Act does specify that the Agency must make a jurisdictional assignment for combination products, i.e., those that are "comprised of two or more regulated components, i.e., drug/device, biologic/device, drug/biologic, or drug/device/biologic, that are physically, chemically, or otherwise combined or mixed and produced as a single entity." In addition, the Agency's framework for jurisdictional assignment of combinations also provides some insight on how jurisdiction is determined for single-entity products that do not fall clearly within one of the above-referenced definitions. Under Section 503(g) of the FDC Act [21 U.S.C. 353(g)], the FDA must assign administrative responsibility for a combination based on the product's "primary mode of action." For example, if the primary mode of action of a drug-device combination is based on the activity of the drug, then the entire combination will be assigned for premarket review to the Agency's Center for Drug Evaluation and Research ("CDER"). However, the statute does not define the term "primary mode of action," and its interpretation by the FDA is currently under active debate and reevaluation, as discussed below.

Section 503(g) also does not specify the regulatory requirements that will apply to combination products—i.e., whether the product will be regulated solely by one center and require only one form of approval, or whether dual approvals by two separate centers will be necessary. Instead, the Act authorizes the Agency to use "any agency resources . . . necessary to ensure adequate review of the safety, effectiveness, or substantial equivalence of an article" within the combination [21 U.S.C. 353(g)(2)]. It should be noted that the Act gives any Center within the FDA the authority to issue any form of approval; thus, CDRH can issue not only medical device approvals, but approval of biologics license applications, and CBER can issue not only biologics approvals, but also approvals of medical device applications. The Agency has considerable latitude and flexibility under the law to use the various regulatory mechanisms at its disposal to assign jurisdiction and issue approvals in the manner that it deems most appropriate and efficient.

To clarify the jurisdictional assignment of combination products and certain other types of products that do not clearly fall within one of the above statutory definitions of drug, device, or biologic, the FDA has relied on guidance documents, known as "Intercenter Agreements" or "ICAs" between each of the Centers (CDER, CDRH, and CBER), to outline the Agency's general approach to review of various categories of products.

As an illustration of the manner in which the Intercenter Agreements are applied, the *Intercenter Agreement Between the Center for Biologics Evaluation and Research and the Center for Devices and Radiological Health* (1991) ("CBER/CDRH Agreement" or "the Agreement") outlines a number of general principles that the centers apply in making jurisdictional determinations about medical devices, biologics, and device/biologic combinations. The Agreement states, for example, that "[c]ellular and tissue implants, including infused cells and encapsulated cells or tissues, will be regulated by CBER under the PHS Act and the FD&C Act (as amended), as appropriate." The Agreement also provides that "medical devices intended to serve as *in vivo* delivery systems or implants for licensed biologicals which are either impregnated with a licensed biological or combined with a licensed biological as part of the manufacturing process" are regulated by CBER under the PHS Act.

The Agreement does not, however, explicitly address products made of animal-derived collagen with no cellular components. Thus, the best available information regarding the likely regulatory jurisdiction over animal-derived collagen products is the Agency's past precedent. Our experience is that virtually all animal-derived collagen products that have no cellular components have been regulated by CDRH as devices, while CBER has taken responsibility for certain types of xenograft products.[2] Collagen products that have been regulated by CDRH as devices include implanted bovine or porcine collagen surgical meshes, injectable bovine collagen for use as a urethral bulking agent for treatment of incontinence or as a dermal contouring agent for correction of wrinkles, collagen-derived hemostatic/sealant products such as CoSeal, collagen corneal shields, collagen-hydroxyapatite bone void fillers for orthopedic use, collagen combined with bone morphogenetic proteins ("BMPs") for orthopedic uses, and many others. Notably, a number of implanted bovine collagen sponges and pastes, with or without additional therapeutic components, have been regulated as medical devices by CDRH. Although the past precedent with respect to jurisdiction over collagen products is clear, it should be noted that CBER has had a substantial consulting role in several of these submissions where components other than bovine collagen, such as BMPs, were involved. Additional information regarding the regulatory pathway for these products is provided below.

In the past, when a request was submitted to the FDA for a jurisdictional assignment, the Agency generally did not make public its decisions. However, among the recent changes that have been implemented, Office of Combination Products has begun more frequent publication of its jurisdictional decisions. A list of past jurisdictional determinations has also been published. Nonetheless, with the proliferation of many novel types of combination products, direct consultation with the FDA in some cases is the only reliable means to resolve a jurisdictional question. For a combination product, the FDA regulations set forth a procedure for submission of a "request for designation" ("RFD"), which requires the Agency to make a jurisdictional assignment [21 C.F.R. Part 3]. Within 60 days from the filing of the RFD, the agency will issue a "designation

---

2. CBER retains jurisdiction over "products composed of human or animal cells or from physical parts of those cells."

letter" identifying the "lead Center" for the product and specifying whether any of the other Centers will be consulting on the review of the product and, in most cases providing information about the premarket review requirements that will apply. For a product that is not a combination, the same type of request for a jurisdictional decision may be made via a letter to the Office of Combination Products ("OCP") or via a Request for Classification ("RFC") Pursuant to Section 563 of the FDC Act [21 U.S.C. § 360bbb-2]. Informal consultation with the FDA on jurisdictional issues also may be appropriate in certain cases, which can be accomplished by communications with the Product Jurisdiction Officer for the involved centers.

There have been two recent changes in the FDA's approach to jurisdictional issues. First, pursuant to the Medical Device User Fee and Modernization Act of 2002 ("MDUFMA") [P.L. 107–250], the FDA recently revised the organizational structure responsible for jurisdictional assignments, with official establishment of the OCP in December 2002. One of the stated objectives of this reorganization was to improve the efficiency and consistency of jurisdictional decisions. The OCP has already held public meetings discussing the process by which these determinations are made, and it is currently considering substantial revision of the Agency's policies as articulated in the Intercenter Agreements [Regulation of Combination Products 2002]. Among other issues that are presently under active consideration by OCP are the interpretation of the term "primary mode of action."

Second, the FDA has recently made substantial changes in the jurisdictional assignment of therapeutic biological products, with many of these products now transferred to CDER rather than CBER. The key product categories that were transferred to CDER are as follows:

- Monoclonal antibodies for *in vivo* use.
- Proteins intended for therapeutic use, including cytokines (e.g., interferons), enzymes (e.g., thrombolytics), and other novel proteins, except for those that are specifically assigned to CBER (e.g., vaccines and blood products). This category includes therapeutic proteins derived from plants, animals, or microorganisms, and recombinant versions of these products.
- Immunomodulators (non-vaccine and non-allergenic products intended to treat disease by inhibiting or modifying a pre-existing immune response).
- Growth factors, cytokines, and monoclonal antibodies intended to mobilize, stimulate, decrease, or otherwise alter the production of hematopoietic cells *in vivo*.

Key products that remain under CBER's jurisdiction include, for example, cellular and gene therapies and blood products [Transfer of Therapeutic Biological Products 2003].

15.3 Overview of Product Clearance Pathways for Biologics and Drugs

Because spinal implants may incorporate drug or biological ingredients, pathways to obtain FDA clearance of both biologics and drugs are summarized below.

15.3.1 Pathways for Clearance of Biologics

The FDC Act defines a "drug" in relevant part as an article "intended for the diagnosis, cure, mitigation, treatment, or prevention of disease in man and articles (other than food) intended to affect the structure or any function of the body of man" [21 U.S.C. § 321(g)]. The definition of a drug implicitly includes biologics, because both drugs and biologics are intended for the prevention, treatment, or cure of diseases. Although this part of the definition also is common to medical devices, the definition of a device expressly excludes products that are metabolized or that achieve their action chemically.

As previously stated, a biologic is defined as

> a virus, therapeutic serum, toxin, antitoxin, vaccine, blood, blood component or derivative, allergenic product, or analogous product, or arsphenamine or derivative of arsphenamine (or any other trivalent organic arsenic compound), applicable to the prevention, treatment, or cure of a disease or condition of human beings [42 U.S.C. § 262i].

Due to the typical difficulty of manufacture of biologics, there are also lot-by-lot release requirements, unlike other drugs, among other differences. However, both drugs and biologics are subject to the requirement for an investigational new drug ("IND") application prior to beginning U.S. human clinical trials, as discussed below.

15.3.1.1 INDs

Before a new drug can lawfully be marketed, it must be the subject of an approved marketing application [21 U.S.C. § 505(a)]. Such applications generally include results from clinical research studies of the drug. Biologics are usually marketed pursuant to an approved biologics license application (BLA) [42 U.S.C. § 262(a)]. Clinical research of unapproved new drugs/biologics may only be conducted in the United States in accordance with FDA regulations governing IND applications [21 U.S.C. § 505i, 21 C.F.R. Part 312]. When preclinical testing of a drug/biologic is considered adequate by the sponsor to demonstrate the safety and the scientific rationale for initial human studies, an IND is filed with the FDA to seek authorization to begin human testing of the drug candidate. The IND becomes effective if not put on clinical hold by the FDA within 30 days after filing. The IND must provide data on previous experiments; how, where and by whom the new human studies will be conducted; the chemical structure of the compound; the method by which it is believed to work in the human body; any toxic effects of the compound found in the animal studies; and how the compound is manufactured. The FDA may, at any time during the 30-day period after filing of an IND or at any future time, impose a clinical hold on proposed or ongoing clinical trials. If the FDA imposes a clinical hold, clinical trials cannot commence or recommence without FDA authorization and then only under terms authorized by the FDA.

15.3.1.2 New Drug Application/Biologics License Application

If the sponsor concludes that there is substantial evidence, primarily from clinical studies, that the drug candidate is effective and that the drug/biologic is safe for its intended use, a BLA may be submitted to FDA. BLAs contain all of the information on the biologic gathered to that date, including data from the clinical trials and animal studies, a description of how the product is manufactured and controlled to make it reproducibly from batch-to-batch, the composition of the final product, the analytical tests conducted on each batch of product to ensure they are pure and potent before releasing them, and other information [21 C.F.R. §§ 601.2]. Applicants also must pay a "user fee" when submitting a BLA. The fee for fiscal year 2004 for applications containing clinical data is $573,500 [68 Fed. Reg. 45249].

Generally, the FDA also conducts an inspection of the manufacturing facility to ensure it complies with current good manufacturing practices (cGMPs) and that the new drug/biologic will be made in a controlled manner according to the description in the BLA. Such inspections are known as "pre-approval inspections" or "PAIs." Before making a final decision, the FDA typically refers the application to an appropriate advisory committee, usually a panel of clinicians, for a public review, evaluation, and recommendation. The FDA is not bound by the recommendation of an advisory committee, although such advice carries great weight and often is followed by the Agency.

If the FDA's evaluation of the BLA and the manufacturing facility is favorable, the Agency may issue an approval letter authorizing commercial marketing of the biologic for specified indications. The FDA also could issue an approvable letter, which usually contains a number of conditions that must be met in order to secure final approval of the BLA. When and if those conditions have been met to the FDA's satisfaction, the agency issues an approval letter. On the other hand, if the FDA's evaluation of the BLA submission or manufacturing facility is not favorable, the FDA may issue a non-approvable letter.

15.3.1.3 Priority Review

FDA reviews of NDAs/BLAs are designated as either Standard or Priority. A Standard designation sets the target date for completing all aspects of a review and the FDA taking an action on the application (i.e., to approve or disapprove) at 10 months after the date it was filed. A Priority designation sets the target date for the FDA action at 6 months. The FDA assigns a Priority designation in cases where

The drug product, if approved, would be a significant improvement compared to marketed products [approved (if such is required), including non-"drug" products/ therapies] in the treatment, diagnosis, or prevention of a disease. Improvement can be demonstrated by, for example: (1) evidence of increased effectiveness in treatment, prevention, or diagnosis of disease; (2) elimination or substantial reduction of a treatment-limiting drug reaction; (3) documented enhancement of patient compliance; or (4) evidence of safety and effectiveness of a new subpopulation [CBER 2003].

15.3.1.4 Charging for Investigational Products

FDA regulations permit the sale of investigational biological products distributed in accordance with the FDA's IND regulations only if the sponsor receives prior FDA approval of such sales [21 C.F.R. § 601.21]. In requesting FDA approval to charge for an investigational drug, which is part of a traditional IND, the sponsor is required to justify why charging for the drug or biologic is necessary to undertake or continue the clinical study, e.g., why distribution of the investigational product for clinical trials is not part of the normal cost of doing business [21 C.F.R. 312.7]. It is the exception rather than the rule for the FDA to allow such charges under an IND. If approval is granted to charge for an investigational biological product, the sponsor is prohibited, under the IND regulations, from commercializing the product by charging a price "larger than that necessary to recover the costs of manufacture, research, development and handling of the investigational drug" [21 C.F.R. § 312.7]. Generally, the ability to charge for an investigational device or biologic is less common than for medical devices, as discussed in more detail below.

15.3.1.5 Orphan Drug Exclusivity for NDAs/BLAs

In 1983, Congress added the Orphan Drug Amendments to the FDC Act [21 U.S.C. 360aa–360dd] to provide incentives for the development of products for the treatment of rare diseases and disorders that affect only small patient populations (i.e., generally 200,000 patients or less).

To be eligible for orphan drug exclusivity, a sponsor must submit a request to the FDA for orphan "designation" [21 U.S.C. 360]. If the FDA determines that the disease or condition for which the drug is intended affects fewer than 200,000 people as of the time of the sponsor's request, or if the sponsor shows that there is no reasonable expectation that the cost of developing and making the drug available in the United States will be recovered, the drug qualifies for orphan designation for the orphan indication [21 U.S.C. 360b; 21 C.F.R. 316.10].

Because orphan designations are made prior to drug approval,[3] more than one applicant may receive orphan designation for the "same drug" intended to treat the same disease or condition (21 U.S.C. 360b). Once a drug that has obtained orphan designation is approved for the designated indication, however, the Agency is precluded from granting final marketing approval for any other application for the "same drug" intended for the same use for a period of seven years [21 U.S.C. 360cc(a); 21 C.F.R. 316.3(b)(13)].

The Agency has outlined in regulations what the sponsor of a second drug must demonstrate to the FDA to establish that its drug is different from a previously approved orphan drug [21 C.F.R. 316.3(b)(13)]. If a drug is different, it may be approved for marketing during the first drug's exclusivity period—i.e., it may "break" the first drug's orphan drug exclusivity.

---

3. In fact, by statute, the request for orphan drug designation must be made before the sponsor submits an NDA/BLA to the agency for marketing approval.

Essentially, a subsequent drug is different from the original orphan drug if the subsequent drug (1) has a different molecular structure than the original or a different "intended use," or (2) is shown to be clinically superior to the original orphan product [21 C.F.R. 316.3]. This approach is intended to preserve the market exclusivity incentive while giving patients the benefit of a sponsor's innovation, should someone develop a better product.

A subsequent sponsor can show its product's clinical superiority by demonstrating any of the following:

- That it is safer;
- That it is more effective; or
- That it makes a major contribution to patient care.

Generally, head-to-head comparative studies are required to show superiority.

Applications for orphan drugs designated as such under Section 526 of the FDC Act are not subject to these user fees unless the application includes indications other than the "orphan" use. A supplement proposing to include a new indication for a rare disease or condition also is exempt from the user fee if the drug has been designated a drug for a rare disease or condition with regard to the indication proposed in the supplement.

15.3.1.6 Pediatric Drugs/Biologic Products

There are two guidance documents relevant to pediatric drug and biologic applications. The first is a document developed by the International Conference on Harmonisation of the Technical Requirements for Registration of Pharmaceuticals for Human Use ("ICH"), which has been adopted by both CBER and CDER, *Clinical Investigation of Medicinal Products in the Pediatric Population* (2000) ("ICH Pediatric Investigation Guidance"). This document provides that "medicinal products" (i.e., drugs or biologics) that are labeled for pediatric use typically will require supporting data from that population, but that these data must be collected without compromising the well-being of pediatric patients, which it defines as a "vulnerable subgroup." Accordingly, the ICH Pediatric Investigation Guidance suggests that "special measures" be taken to protect the rights of pediatric subjects and shield them from undue risk. Specifically, Institutional Review Boards ("IRB") approving clinical trials involving pediatric subjects are urged to include experts knowledgeable in pediatric ethical, clinical, and psychosocial issues, or to consult with such experts. In addition, recruitment of study participants must be free of any inappropriate inducements to the parent or guardian or the participant. Reimbursement and subsistence costs may be covered, but should be reviewed by the IRB.

Finally, because pediatric subjects may be legally unable to provide informed consent, full informed permission must be obtained from the parent or guardian and affirmative assent should be obtained from the child or adolescent.

The ICH guidance includes an age classification for pediatric patients—described as "one possible categorization"—that would include 16-year-old,

Table 15.2.
ICH Proposed Age Classification of Pediatric Patients.

Pediatric Subgroup	Approximate Age Range
Preterm Newborn	
Term Newborn	0 to 27 days
Infants and Toddlers	28 days to 23 months
Adolescent	12 to 16–18 years of age (depending on region)

and potentially 17- and 18-year-old, subjects in its "adolescent" category (see Table 15.2). However, the guidance notes that there is considerable overlap in developmental (e.g., physical, cognitive, and psychosocial) issues across age groups, and as discussed below, CDRH has promulgated a slightly different categorization for pediatric devices. The guidance describes the adolescent period as one involving "rapid growth" and evolving cognitive and emotional changes that "could potentially influence the outcome of clinical studies." The upper age limit is described as varying by region. Investigators are warned to specifically consider the impact on clinical studies involving adolescents of recreational use of unprescribed drugs, alcohol, and tobacco and to consider studying adolescent patients in centers with special knowledge of this population.

To minimize risk in studies involving pediatric subjects, those conducting the study should be properly trained and experienced in studying this population, including the evaluation and management of potential pediatric adverse effects. Finally, protocols for studies involving children should be specifically designed to minimize distress and discomfort. Examples include (1) topical anesthesia to place IV catheters, (2) indwelling catheters rather than repeated venipunctures for blood sampling, and (3) collection of some protocol-specified blood samples when routine clinical samples are obtained.

The second relevant guidance document on pediatric use of drugs and bio-logics is the Agency's *Guidance for Industry—The Content and Format for Pediatric Use Supplements* (1996) ("Pediatric Use Supplement Guidance"). This document describes the circumstances in which a drug manufacturer may be able to rely on clinical data from adults to support labeling related to use in a pediatric population. It should be noted that the Pediatric Use Supplement Guidance defines the "adolescent" category slightly differently than the ICH Pediatric Clinical Investigation Guidance, specifying an upper limit of 16 years on the adolescent age range.

There is no general exemption from user fees for pediatric use biological or drug products. In fact, even pediatric *supplements* to general applications, which had been exempt from user fees prior to 2002, are now subject to fees [Prescription Drug User Fee 2005].

In addition, it is important to note that pediatric exclusivity only is available to drugs approved through an NDA under section 505(b) of the FDC Act and is not available to products approved through a BLA under the PHS Act.

15.4 FDA Regulation of Specific Types of Spinal Implants

Relatively few FDA regulations have been issued that govern spinal implants. The FDA has issued regulations governing only three specific categories of spinal implant hardware, as summarized in the table below. Thus, other types of spinal implants remain unclassified and are presumptively in class III, which generally requires premarket approval. Some of the principal categories of spinal implants that remain unclassified include spinal fusion cages, artificial discs, and a number of other types of motion-preserving spinal implants such as disc nucleus replacements and posterior stabilization systems. Although these product categories are not covered by specific regulations, the FDA has stated in a 2004 guidance document that "interbody fusion and non-fusion devices (i.e., cages or disc replacement devices) or other non-fusion spinal devices . . . are class III devices and require the submission of premarket approval applications (PMAs) before they may be marketed" [Guidance for Industry- Spinal System 2004]. Thus, these devices are regulated as class III products and presently require premarket approval although, as noted above, downclassification of spinal fusion cages is presently under consideration.

Type Implant	Regulation	Definition	Classification
Spinal inter-laminal fixation orthosis	21 CFR 888.3050	a device intended to be implanted made of an alloy, such as stainless steel, that consists of various hooks and a posteriorly placed compression or distraction rod. The device is implanted, usually across three adjacent vertebrae, to straighten and immobilize the spine to allow bone grafts to unite and fuse the vertebrae together. The device is used primarily in the treatment of scoliosis (a lateral curvature of the spine), but it also may be used in the treatment of fracture or dislocation of the spine, grades 3 and 4 of spondylolisthesis (a dislocation of the spinal column), and lower back syndrome.	Class II

Continued

Type Implant	Regulation	Definition	Classification
Spinal inter-vertebral body fixation orthosis	21 CFR 888.3060	a device intended to be implanted made of titanium. It consists of various vertebral plates that are punched into each of a series of vertebral bodies. An eye-type screw is inserted in a hole in the center of each of the plates. A braided cable is threaded through each eye-type screw. The cable is tightened with a tension device and it is fastened or crimped at each eye-type screw. The device is used to apply force to a series of vertebrae to correct "sway back," scoliosis (lateral curvature of the spine), or other conditions.	Class II
Pedicle screw systems	21 CFR 888.3070	multiple component devices, made from a variety of materials, including alloys such as 316L stainless steel, 316LVM stainless steel, 22Cr-13Ni-5Mn stainless steel, Ti-6Al-4V, and unalloyed titanium, that allow the surgeon to build an implant system to fit the patient's anatomical and physiological requirements. Such a spinal implant assembly consists of a combination of anchors (e.g., bolts, hooks, and/or screws); interconnection mechanisms incorporating nuts, screws, sleeves, or bolts; longitudinal members (e.g., plates, rods, and/or plate/rod combinations); and/or transverse connectors	Class II (special controls), when intended to provide immobilization and stabilization of spinal segments in skeletally mature patients as an adjunct to fusion in the treatment of the following acute and chronic instabilities or deformities of the thoracic, lumbar, and sacral spine: severe spondylolisthesis (grades 3 and 4) of the L5-S1 vertebra; degenerative spondylolisthesis with objective evidence of neurologic impairment; fracture; dislocation; scoliosis; kyphosis; spinal tumor; and failed previous fusion (pseudarthrosis).
Pedicle screw systems	21 CFR 888.3070	Same as above	Class III (premarket approval), when intended to provide immobilization and stabilization of spinal segments in the thoracic, lumbar, and sacral spine as an adjunct to fusion in the treatment of degenerative disc disease and spondylolisthesis other than either severe spondylolisthesis (grades 3 and 4) at L5-S1 or degenerative spondylolisthesis with objective evidence of neurologic impairment

As indicated in the proceeding table, some types of spinal implants may fall into different classifications and require different premarket clearance pathways depending on the use for which they are intended. For example, pedicle screws are classified in class II for some uses but class III for others (although no call for PMAs has yet been issued for the class III uses of pedicle screws). Posterior stabilization systems, such as the Centerpulse Spine Tech, Inc. DYNESYS® Spinal System (Warsaw, IN), have received 510(k) clearance for use in spinal fusion but, according to the language from the FDA guidance cited above, presumably would be classified in class III and require premarket approval for nonfusion applications.[4] The rationale for classifying the same device in different categories depending on its intended use is generally risk-based. For example, in the case of posterior stabilization systems, although the FDA has long experience with the use of pedicle-screw based systems in the spine for fusion, the issues presented by long-term use of these devices with continuing movement of the spine over an extended period are less well known.

In addition to the spinal "hardware" products discussed above, various materials that are used in the spine in conjunction with hardware are also regulated as medical devices. These include, for example, bone void fillers, bone cements, and other bone graft substitutes such as demineralized bone matrix. Each of these product categories is subject to differing levels of FDA regulation, as discussed below.

Although there are relatively few regulations governing specific types of spinal implants, the FDA has been active in issuing guidance documents that cover spinal implants over the past five years. The Agency has recently updated its guidance document governing spinal implants that are eligible for 510(k) clearance, entitled *Guidance for Industry and FDA Staff—Spinal System 510(k)s*, issued May 3, 2004. The Agency also issued in 2004 a guidance document that governs procedures for treatment of vertebral fractures, entitled *Clinical Trial Considerations: Vertebral Augmentation Devices to Treat Spinal Insufficiency Fractures—Guidance for Industry and FDA Staff*. The FDA also issued in 2000 a guidance document that described IDE study requirements for spinal implants, principally focusing on fusion devices, entitled *Guidance Document for the Preparation of IDEs for Spinal Systems* ("Spinal System IDE Guidance"). Although this guidance document briefly addresses nonfusion devices, the Agency is presently reported to be developing a new guidance that focuses solely on motion-preserving devices. The FDA's current regulatory approach to each of these types of devices is summarized below.

15.4.1 Spinal Fusion Cages

The Spinal System IDE Guidance describes in detail the data required to support approval of devices such as spinal fusion cages. As for many other

4. In the letter to Centerpulse Spine Tech regarding clearance of the DYNESYS® Spinal System for use in fusion, the FDA required the company to state expressly in its labeling that "the safety and effectiveness of this device for the indication of spinal stabilization without fusion have not been established." See http://www.fda.gov/cdrh/pdf3/k031511.pdf.

orthopedic implants, the FDA typically requires clinical studies with extended follow-up, typically up to 24 months. Evaluation of the success of spinal fusion devices in clinical studies is based not only on achievement of fusion, but also on multicomponent scales that assess the patient's degree of functional and symptomatic improvement. Safety is principally determined based on freedom from adverse events, as well as the incidence of re-operations.

Early studies of spinal fusion cages were based in substantial part on data from nonrandomized clinical studies. However, more recently approved products have required randomized, controlled clinical investigations. Although historically controlled studies can provide valid scientific evidence under the FDA regulations, the Agency's acceptance of these types of studies as a basis for device approval has decreased over the past five to 10 years, and it is now uncommon for products to be approved based solely on this type of investigation.

Another important aspect of the regulatory approval process for spinal implants is the choice of indication for which the manufacturer seeks clearance. As noted above, the indication can even in some cases determine whether the device is class II or class III. In the case of spinal fusion cages, the indication under investigation is typically degenerative disc disease. However, the region of the spine and the number of levels that can be treated may vary. Generally, the broader the indications for use the manufacturer wishes to pursue, the larger the clinical study that may be required. Thus, many spinal implants are only studied and, therefore, only approved by the FDA for use at a single spinal level.

15.4.2 Bone Cements and Bone Void Fillers

Bone cements and other filler materials have long been used in orthopedic surgery. Until 1999, the FDA regulated polymethylmethacrylate cements as class III devices; historically, PMMA products had even been regulated as drugs. The principal risks related to PMMA that resulted in a high degree of initial regulation included the exothermic nature of the setting reaction *in vivo*, as well as the potential risks of material leakage and migration. However, in 1999, the Agency determined that these risks could be adequately addressed through the special controls described in its guidance document, *Class II Special Controls Guidance Document: Polymethylmethacrylate (PMMA) Bone Cement; Guidance for Industry and FDA* (2002). As defined in the FDA regulations, PMMA bone cements are "intended for use in arthroplastic procedures or the hip, knee, and other joints for the fixation of polymer or metallic prosthetic implants to living bone" [21 C.F.R. § 888.3027]. Although the regulation does not specifically address the use of PMMA in the spine, PMMA materials have recently been cleared for use in vertebral augmentation procedures, as discussed below.[5]

5. As indicated by the FDA in a public health notification, some safety issues have been associated with use of PMMA bone cements in the spine [Jurisdictional Update 2001].

In addition to PMMA, a number of other bone void filler materials have been developed for use as an alternative or supplement to bone autograft or allograft. Many of these fall within the classification of "calcium salts." These products also are classified in class II and are the subject of a special controls guidance document, *Class II Special Controls Guidance Document: Resorbable Calcium Salt Bone Void Filler Device; Guidance for Industry and FDA* (2002). As defined in the regulation, these products are "intended to fill bony voids or gaps of the extremities, spine, and pelvis that are caused by trauma or surgery and are not intrinsic to the stability of the bony structure" (21 C.F.R. § 888.3045). Although the meaning of the term "not instrinsic to the stability of the bony structure" suggests that calcium salt bone void fillers are not for load-bearing use, this limitation is somewhat paradoxical in light of the fact that the products are intended for replacement by new bone ingrowth over time. Fundamental principles of biomechanics suggest that some load sharing is necessary to produce new bone growth. This issue was noted by the Advisory Panel in reviewing the proposed downclassification but remains unresolved in the regulations and guidance.

Other available bone void filler materials include demineralized bone. Demineralized bone matrix products have in the past typically been regulated as human tissues, which are subject to regulation only under 21 CFR Part 1270 and do not require FDA premarket clearance. The FDA issued a document in 1997 that was intended to clarify the regulatory status of human tissue products, including bone products [Jurisdictional Update 2001]. According to the criteria set forth in this guidance, human tissue products are regulated only under Part 1270 if they are both "minimally manipulated" and "homologous in use," i.e., intended for the same use as the tissues served in their original place in the body, among other factors.

Because demineralized bone matrix products may be mixed with other materials that are currently regulated as devices (e.g., sodium hyaluronate, calcium phosphate, etc.), the FDA's Office of Combination Products recently issued a jurisdictional update that defines the regulatory status of these products [Jurisdictional Update 2001]. Demineralized bone products that are mixed with these other materials are now regulated as medical devices and require premarket clearance. The jurisdictional update specifies that in order to be regulated only as a human tissue, not a medical device, the demineralized bone matrix must meet the following requirements:

- The product is minimally manipulated;
- The product is intended for homologous use only;
- The manufacture of the Human Cell, Tissues and Cellular and Tissue-Based Products does not involve the combination of the cell or tissue component with a drug or device, except for a sterilizing, preserving, or storage agent, if the addition of the agent does not raise new clinical safety concerns with respect to the HCT/P; and
- Either:
    - The HCT/P does not have a systemic effect and is not dependent upon the metabolic activity of living cells for its primary function; or

- ■ The HCT/P has a systemic effect or is dependent upon the metabolic activity of living cells for its primary function, and:
  - ● is for autologous use
  - ● is for allogeneic use in a first or second degree relative; or
  - ● is for reproductive use.

Several combination products of this type have received premarket clearance from the FDA [510(k) Summary of Safety and Effectiveness 2005].

Notably, for most other bone void filler materials that are cleared through the 510(k) notification process, the FDA has not cleared claims related to osteoinduction. However, for demineralized bone matrix products, osteoinduction potential claims based on animal testing have been permitted. Osteoinductive products containing bone morphogenetic proteins are discussed below.

15.4.3 Vertebroplasty and Kyphoplasty Products

The FDA regulates several types of products that are used in the treatment of osteoporotic compression fractures. Both the hardware that is used to compress the osteoporotic bone and create a void to be filled in kyphoplasty procedures and the filler materials that are used in vertebroplasty and kyphoplasty procedures are regulated as medical devices. Filler materials include polymethylmethacrylate based bone cements, as well as calcium phosphate bone void fillers and other materials. Generally, hardware products for use in osteoporotic compression fractures have received 510(k) clearance with little or no supporting clinical testing, based on comparison to simple bone tamping devices. In contrast, filler materials for use in osteoporotic compression fractures have required supporting clinical testing. To date, several PMMA bone cements have received 510(k) clearance for use in osteoporotic compression fractures, and other materials are under study but have not yet received 510(k) clearance.

In 2004, the FDA issued a guidance document that describes the type of clinical testing necessary to support clearance of bone void fillers for use in vertebroplasty or kyphoplasty. This guidance, *Clinical Trial Consideration: Vertebral Augmentation Devices to Treat Spinal Insufficiency Fractures* (October 24, 2004) ("Vertebral Augmentation Guidance"), recommends conducting randomized, concurrently controlled studies over a two-year time period to assess device performance. In addition to measuring pain and function, the guidance recommends evaluations of key complications such as infection, re-operation, neurological damage, and material leakage/migration.

Although previously class III devices, PMMA bone cements are now classified in class II (21 C.F.R. 888.3027) and are the subject of a special controls guidance document, *Class II Special Controls Guidance Document: Polymethylmethacrylate Bone Cement* ("PMMA Special Controls Guidance"). Thus, for PMMA products intended for use in vertebral augmentation, requirements of both the Special Controls Guidance and the PMMA Special Controls Guidance may be applicable. However, as is often the case where multiple products of the same type have received 510(k) clearance with supporting clinical data, in the future, it is possible that similar PMMA products will require less clinical data to support 510(k) clearance, or may be cleared with no supporting clinical data requirements. Data requirements will likely vary depending on similarity to previously 510(k)-cleared materials.

15.4.4 Motion-preserving spinal implants

A variety of motion-preserving spinal implants are currently under development, generally for use in degenerative disc disease, stenosis, and spondylolisthesis as alternatives to spinal fusion. Although many motion-preserving devices have been used in Europe for more than a decade, the first such product, the Depuy Spine CHARITÉ® Disc, received FDA approval in 2004.

The FDA has in the past applied the same general principles described in the spinal implant IDE guidance, as discussed above, in determining the clinical data requirements for nonfusion devices. However, with the emergence of nonfusion technologies, new guidance is being developed that will presumably address the clinical considerations that are unique to nonfusion. Among other things, the new guidance may address the need for more detailed radiographic evaluation of nonfusion devices to determine if they accomplish their design objective of preserving a "normal" or "near-normal" degree of motion. However, it is expected that similar measures of device safety and effectiveness will be utilized, including validated measures of both pain and function.

In addition, one of the principal theoretical justifications for motion-preserving spinal implants is that they may prevent the load-shifting that otherwise may cause degeneration of adjacent spinal levels over time. Hilibrand et al. have reported that the rate of surgery for degeneration at adjacent levels may be 2–3% per year. Thus, future FDA guidance may require evaluation of whether motion-preserving implants do reduce the adverse impact on adjacent levels, although it is likely that this impact will not be measurable over study durations of two years. Continuing postmarket evaluation or cooperative registry studies may afford the mechanism to generate this information over time.

Other concerns associated with motion-preserving spinal implants include the potential adverse impact to wear debris generated over time. For implants that include polymer materials, the potential for osteolysis is a key consideration. For metal-metal implants, long-term risks of tumorigenicity and carcinogenicity may be raised by the FDA, although there is relatively little indication of increased risk associated with larger hip and knee implants that generate greater volumes of wear. Nonetheless, these issues may require evaluation and testing to obtain FDA approval in the future.

15.4.5 Orthopedic Implants with Drug or Biologic Components

Increasing development of combination products is expected to continue in the future, and these products are logically extended to use in the spine. Among the first spinal implants containing a biological ingredient to be approved by the FDA is Medtronic's INFUSE®, which combines the company's fusion cage with a bone morphogenetic protein. This product was regulated by the FDA as a medical device because its primary mode of action was to promote fusion mechanically, while the BMP component served to enhance this function. Nonetheless, the review of INFUSE also required input from the FDA's Center for Biologics Evaluation and Research, as would be expected for future device/biologic combinations. For many biological products, concerns about processing and consistency of the biological ingredient as manufactured require substantial documentation in an application for approval, and postmarket requirements related to manufacturing and quality also may be required to satisfy device requirements for device components, but biological/drug requirements for those components. Thus, combination products present a higher degree of complexity in both the premarket and postmarket phases. Stand alone use of BMPs in the spine has also been approved by the FDA, but thus far only via a humanitarian device exemption for limited use in patients with risk factors that compromise the ability to achieve fusion by other means [Summary of Safety and Probable Benefit 2002].

Other combination orthopedic products include antibiotic bone cements, which have recently been cleared by the FDA after years of negotiation to determine what type of data would be required to demonstrate benefit of the antibiotic. Although these have not received clearance for specific use in the spine, it is anticipated that antibiotics and other drug ingredients may be used in spinal implants in the future.

15.4.6 Pediatric Orthopedic Implants

One of the categories of spinal implants that has not yet been significantly developed is for pediatric patients. Although various types of spinal hardware have been used in children for years, e.g., to correct scoliosis, many of the types of implants discussed above are not intended for pediatric use and are designed to address disorders that result from the aging process. Nonetheless, consistent with the FDA's directive to develop more efficient procedures for the clearance of pediatric medical devices, the future development of spinal implants may include more specific guidance on, for example, studies in pediatric populations. HDEs also will likely continue to be used for adaptation of implants to pediatric patients who may require them, where the population is sufficiently small. One example of this is the recently approved Vertical Expandable Prosthetic Titanium Rib pictured below, which is intended for use to treat thoracic insufficiency syndrome in pediatric patients.

15.5 Current Trends in the Regulation of Spinal Implants

With the proliferation of spinal implant technology, increasing FDA resources will be required to address the review of each implant expeditiously and effectively. The proportion of the FDA's workload devoted to review of orthopedic implants is increasing, and further increases may be expected in the near future.

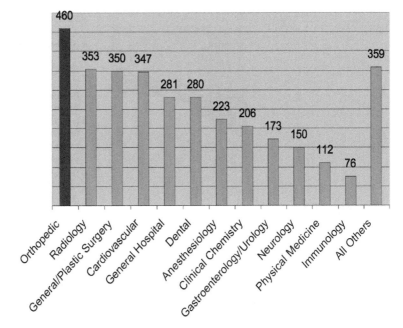

Fig. 15.3.
510(k) Clearances in 2004 by Therapeutic Area.[6]

Of the over three thousand 510(k) notices submitted in 2004, nearly 500 were classified as orthopedic products. As indicated in Figure 15.3, this represented the largest number of 510(k) notices in any single therapeutic area, and over 100 more orthopedics 510(k) notices were cleared by the FDA than in any other therapeutic category.

Between one-third and one-half of these orthopedic 510(k) notices were spinal devices. These were roughly equally divided across a number of different types of internal fixation products, as shown in the figure below.

The above 510(k) clearances are in addition to approval of 4 original PMA applications, 21 PMA supplements, and other submissions such as IDE applications. In recognition of the increasing need for spinal implant review resources, the FDA has recently created a specialized subgroup within CDRH responsible for the review of spinal devices.

With increasing new product development, spinal implants are also likely to draw a high level of scrutiny from both public and private sector entities. The FDA has indicated that it will devote significant enforcement resources to bioresearch monitoring generally, and orthopedic clinical studies specifically. Bioresearch monitoring is intended to ensure the quality, accuracy, and integrity of data from clinical studies that are submitted in support of product marketing applications. Failure to meet the requisite standards of clinical study

6. The figures represent the number of 510(k) clearances in calendar year 2004 categorized by advisory panel.

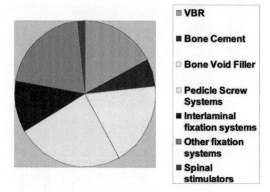

Fig. 15.4.
510(k) Submissions for Spinal Implant Devices in 2004.

oversight can delay or even prevent the approval of experimental devices. In recent years, FDA has used its authority under the Application Integrity Policy (AIP) to place several manufacturers "on hold" for data integrity issues related to FDA submissions. This policy allows not only the submission in question to be put on hold, but stops further review of *all* pending FDA submissions, and thus can have a severe impact. FDA also has taken action to disbar several investigators, three of whom were orthopedic surgeons, from conduct of future clinical studies due to noncompliance with the BIMO regulations. Thus, adherence to good clinical practices in the conduct of clinical investigations will continue to be of high importance to spinal and orthopedic companies in the future.

In recent years, CDRH has moved toward increasing reliance on randomized, concurrently controlled clinical studies with long-term follow-up for most types of orthopedic implants that require supporting clinical data. This paradigm, which has largely been carried over from the Agency's approach to regulation of drugs, has arguably presented some significant challenges as applied to medical devices. Although such studies may provide optimal data from a scientific perspective, the time and cost requirements are prohibitive for many medical device companies, which are often smaller than their pharmaceutical counterparts.

There are also inherent challenges in randomizing patients to studies of spinal implants. Given the fact that clinical studies of orthopedic implants by definition are intended to provide a patient with a lifelong implant, there is often greater resistance to randomization than in studies of shorter-acting pharmaceutical products. If a patient in a pharmaceutical study is randomized to a placebo or other "control" intervention, that patient generally will be able to use the experimental product once it becomes commercially available. However, the same is not true of a permanent implant such as most spinal devices; selection into the "control" group generally will render it impossible for the patient to receive the experimental device even after it is approved, at least for an extended period of time.

The challenges of randomization are heightened by the increasing awareness of new medical therapies by consumers, and the desire of many patients who are willing to participate in clinical trials to seek novel treatments. Thus, there is an implicit difficulty in seeking patients who are willing to participate in an experimental study, but also are willing to allow their treatment to be left to chance via randomization, with an equal chance of receiving the experimental treatment or standard medical care. Orthopedic studies also typically require patients to return for multiple follow-up visits and tests over a period of years, which creates further disincentives to study participation. Internationalization in health care also allows some patients the opportunity to seek treatment in countries where devices not yet available in the United States are already commercially marketed. All of these challenges will likely contribute to increasing difficulty in the coming years in performing randomized, controlled clinical studies of orthopedic implants.

Although Congress directed the FDA in the Food and Drug Administration Modernization Act of 1997 [P.L. 107–250][7] ("FUAMA") to consider the "least burdensome" means necessary in determining the data required to support product approval, this provision does not appear to have substantially reduced the need for randomized, controlled clinical trials. In fact, since enactment of FDAMA, the number of nonrandomized studies that have been found sufficient to support approval of orthopedic implants appears to have decreased.

One method that manufacturers have employed to attempt to address the long duration and associated costs of orthopedic clinical studies is the use of predictive statistical modeling methods, such as Bayesian analysis. Some of the potential advantages of these techniques are that they may permit earlier submission of a marketing application, before all patients complete the full duration of follow-up, by predicting overall outcomes based on data at earlier time points. These techniques have already been used successfully to support several spinal implant approvals, as well as other types of medical devices. The FDA has conducted a workshop on the application of these techniques and is reportedly preparing a guidance document on the use of Bayesian methods. Other innovative statistical techniques also may be developed to try to maximize the information derived from orthopedic clinical studies without unduly burdensome sample size and/or follow-up requirements.

As new spinal technologies gain FDA approval, enter the marketplace, and develop a database of broader clinical experience, it is likely that additional regulations may be issued governing specific implant types. This has been the typical evolution of FDA regulations governing other types of orthopedic implants, such as hip implants and knee implants, for which there are many more device-specific regulations than for spinal implants. For hip implants, for example, there are 14 separate FDA regulations governing different types of

---

7. See also *The Least Burdensome Provisions of the FDA Modernization Act of 1997: Concept and Principles; Final Guidance for FDA and Industry* 2002.

implants and components. There are also 14 regulations governing knee implants. These regulations generally differentiate implant types based on the degree of constraint, i.e., the degree to which the implant limits motion compared to the native joint, and the type of bearing (mobile versus fixed), along with other factors such as use with or without cement, types of implant materials, etc. Thus, in the foreseeable future, the four regulations governing spinal implants may be supplemented by additional regulations for motion-preserving implants such as artificial discs, posterior stabilization systems, nucleus replacements, etc. Also as in the case of hip and knee implants, further subdivision of spinal implant categories and issuance of new regulations may be followed by downclassification of additional spinal implant types, once sufficient clinical knowledge has been developed.

Finally, in addition to the above trends, increasing development of combination drug/device, biologic/device, or drug/biologic/device combinations can be expected over the coming years, because such products offer the opportunity to combine mechanical and biological solutions to physiologic problems. Market incentives may also favor the development of higher "value added" combination products, as opposed to more conventional orthopedic hardware. Growth factors, biomimetic coatings, and antibiotics likely represent only the first wave of drug and biologic components to be studied for use with spinal implants, with many more technologies likely to be studied in the future. Evolution in the FDA's regulation of combination products should facilitate these developments, although involvement of multiple centers at the FDA in the review may continue to present greater information requirements than single-center review, with associated increases in review time.

As spinal implants continue to develop over the coming years, a successful FDA regulatory approach will require consideration of the total product life-cycle, from clinical study and premarket review through commercialization. In the post-Vioxx era, it is likely that the clinical study of spinal implants may in many cases continue past the point of device approval. In 2004, the FDA transferred responsibility for oversight of medical device postmarket surveillance studies from the Office of Device Evaluation, which is responsible for premarket reviews, to the Office of Surveillance and Biometrics ("OSB") [The Gray Sheet 2004]. OSB has recently indicated that it plans to implement a publicly available tracking system to indicate whether or not companies are fulfilling their postmarket research commitments, and has also indicated that it may take tougher enforcement action against companies for failure to complete postmarket studies per the agreed protocols, including the potential use of civil money penalties and possible withdrawal of approval [The Gray Sheet 2005]. Together with other public pronouncements by Agency officials, it appears that increasing importance will be placed on completion of postmarket studies to avoid undetected safety issues that may arise only in large-scale commercialization. Further emphasis may also be placed on physician training in implantation methods for spinal implant devices to minimize the risk of patient injury. Spinal implant manufacturers will therefore increasingly need to plan for ongoing research, monitoring, and training activities over the lifetime of the device.

15.6 References

21 C.F.R. Part 3.

21 C.F.R. Part 312.

21 C.F.R. 312.7(d) and d(3).

21 C.F.R. 316.3.

21 C.F.R. 316.3(b)(13).

21 C.F.R. 316.10.

21 C.F.R. §§ 601.2.

21 C.F.R. § 807.81

21 C.F.R. 812.3(m).

21 C.F.R. § 814.19 (2004).

21 C.F.R. § 814.39.

21 C.F.R. § 814.3(n).

21 C.F.R. § 888.3027.

21 C.F.R. § 888.3045.

21 U.S.C. § § 321(f), (g), (h), (i), and (ff).

21 U.S.C. § 505(a) and (i).

21 U.S.C. 353(g) and (g)2.

21 U.S.C. § 360bbb-2.

21 U.S.C. § 360c(i)(1)(A).

21 U.S.C. 360cc(a).

42 U.S.C. § 262 (a) and (i).

510(k) Memorandum #K86-3: Guidance on the CDRH Premarket Notification Review Program. 1986.

510(k) Memorandum #K97-1: Deciding When to Submit a 510(k) for a Change to an Existing Device. 1997. Food and Drug Administration. http://www.fda.gov/cdrh/ode/510kmod.html.

510(k) Summary of Safety & Effectiveness: DBX Demineralized Bone Matrix. 2005. Food and Drug Administration. http://www.fda.gov/cdrh/pdf4/k040501.pdf.

510(k) Summary of Safety & Effectiveness: DBX Demineralized Bone Matrix. 2005. Food and Drug Administration. http://www.fda.gov/cdrh/pdf4/k040262.pdf.

68 Fed. Reg. 45249 (2003).

Can Bayesian Approaches to Studying New Treatments Improve Regulatory Decision-Making? 2004. Food and Drug Administration. *http://www.cfsan.fda.gov/~frf/bayesdl.html*.

Can Bayesian Approaches to Studying New Treatments Improve Regulatory Decision-Making? 2004. Prous Science. *www.prous.com/bayesian2004*

CBER, Manual on Policies and Procedures (MAPP) 6020.3.

Class II Special Controls Guidance Document: Polymethylmethacrylate (PMMA) Bone Cement; Guidance for Industry and FDA. 2002. Food and Drug Administration. http://www.fda.gov/cdrh/ode/guidance/668.html.

Class II Special Controls Guidance Document: Resorbable Calcium Salt Bone Void Filler Device; Guidance for Industry and FDA Staff. 2002. Food and Drug Administration. http://www.fda.gov/cdrh/ode/guidance/855.html.

Firms to Be Held More Accountable for Completing Postmarket Studies—FDA. In *The Gray Sheet*. 2004.

Guidance for Industry and FDA Staff Spinal System 510(k)s. 2004. Food and Drug Administration. http://www.fda.gov/cdrh/ode/guidance/636.html.

Guidance for Industry and FDA Staff: Clinical Trial Considerations: Vertebral Augmentation Devices to Treat Spinal Insufficiency Fractures. 2004. Food and Drug Administration. http://www.fda.gov/cdrh/ode/guidance/1543.html.

Humanitarian Device Exemption (HDE) Regulation; Questions and Answers. In *Final Guidance for Industry*. 2001.

Id. § 814.100.

Jurisdictional Update: Human Demineralized Bone Matrix. 2001. Food and Drug Administration.http://www.fda.gov/oc/combination/bone.html.

The Least Burdensome Provisions of the FDA Modernization Act of 1997: Concept and Principles. In *Final Guidance for FDA and Industry*. 2002. http://www.fda.gov/cdrh/ode/guidance/1332.pdf.

The New 510(k) Paradigm—Alternate Approaches to Demonstrating Substantial Equivalence in Premarket Notifications. In *Final Guidance for Industry*. 2000.

Office of Device Evaluation Annual Report. 2004.

PMA/510(k) Expedited Review—Guidance for Industry and CDRH Staff. 1998. Food and Drug Administration.

P.L. 107-250.

Postapproval Study Penalties. In *The Gray Sheet*. 2005.

Prescription Drug User Fee Act. 2005. Food and Drug Administration. *www.fda.gov/cber/pdufa/billable.htm.*

"Real-Time" Review Program for Premarket Approval Application (PMA) Supplements. 1997. Food and Drug Administration. http://www.fda.gov/cdrh/ode/realtim2.html.

Regulation of Combination Products: FDA Employee Perspectives. 2002. Food and Drug Administration. http://www.fda.gov/oc/*ombudsman/ rcpemployee.pdf.*

Summary of Safety and Probable Benefit. 2004. Food and Drug Administration. *http://www.fda.gov/cdrh/pdf2/H020008b.pdf.*

Transcript of Meeting of the Orthopedic and Rehabilitation Devices Advisory Panel. 2003. http://www.fda.gov/ohrms/dockets/ac/03/transcripts/4011T1.htm.

Transfer of Therapeutic Biological Products to the Center for Drug Evaluation and Research. 2003. Food and Drug Administration. http://www.fda.gov/oc/combination/transfer.html.

Vfinance. 2004. www.vfinance.com.

Chapter *16*

Economics and Reimbursement for Spine Technologies

Jordana Schmier, M.A. and
Michael Halpern, M.D., Ph.D.
Exponent, Inc.
Alexandria, VA

16.1 Introduction to Health Economics and Cost Analyses

16.1.1 Why Do Costs Matter and How Are They Used?

Often new health care products or technologies offer a clear advantage over existing products or therapies. Rarely, however, are these new technologies less expensive than existing therapies; with few exceptions, they are more expensive. When the cost of a new treatment is greater than that of current therapies, it is essential to demonstrate that the incremental (i.e., additional) clinical benefits of the therapy over those of the current standard of care are acceptable relative to the incremental cost of the newer treatment. The field of health economics provides a consistent and reproducible framework for the evaluation of value for money, that is, what an intervention provides in exchange for its cost.

The subfield of pharmacoeconomics, valuing the health outcomes compared to the costs of treatment with pharmaceutical agents, is well developed. However, economic evaluation applied to medical devices is a newer discipline. In the current era of increased health care expenditures coupled with budgetary limitations, new medical device interventions face the same requirement of demonstrating benefit relative to cost in addition to demonstrating safety and efficacy. Furthermore, health care organizations and providers often need to know the costs associated with a particular intervention in order to manage limited resources. Thus, presenting the costs and benefits of technologies for treatment or diagnosis of spine conditions has become increasingly important.

16.1.2 Types of Economic Studies

There are several types of health economic studies; the selection of which type of study to use depends on a variety of factors. One type, cost of illness (COI) studies, identifies the total cost of disease across a population. Results from COI studies can reflect costs globally, nationally, regionally, or within a population covered by a given insurance plan. Subsets of COI studies can evaluate specific cost components, such as the cost of hospitalization for a particular condition or the cost associated with administration of a particular intervention. Related to this is cost-feasibility analysis (CFA), which assesses the cost of an intervention to evaluate whether it can be performed within existing budgetary constraints [Levin and McEwan 2001].

Other types of health economic studies compare outcomes between or across interventions. Cost-minimization analysis (CMA) assumes that the outcomes for two interventions are identical, and compares only the costs associated with the interventions. All other types of comparative economic analyses compare both costs and outcomes. Cost-benefit analyses (CBA) compare costs and outcomes in monetary terms (e.g., two dollars saved for every dollar spent on an intervention), while cost-effectiveness analyses (CEA) present outcomes in non-monetary units (e.g., cost per cure, cost per symptom-free day). Cost-utility analyses (CUA), a subtype of CEA, express outcomes in terms of units of patient-perceived value; cost per quality-adjusted life-year (QALY) is the most often used metric.

CBA has been decreasing in popularity in health care analysis, as it is difficult to assign monetary value to outcomes relevant to health studies; for example, there is no consensus on the dollar amount to assign to a year of life [Elixhauser et al. 1998; Gold et al. 1996]. CEA and CUA, however, are not only increasingly used but are now often required by government or reimbursement agencies [Stewart, Schmier, and Luce 1999; Taylor et al. 2004]. Agencies responsible for registration and reimbursement in Europe and Canada, such as the UK's National Institute for Clinical Excellence and the Canadian Coordinating Office for Health Technology Assessment, require pharmacoeconomic evaluations as a component of submission for new drugs alongside safety and efficacy information. In some cases, budget impact models that consider regional patterns of disease prevalence and treatment patterns are required. In the United States, dossiers supporting new products that are submitted to formulary committees often include economic evaluations and pharmacoeconomic models, as per the standard format for dossier submissions developed by the Academy of Managed Care Pharmacy [2005].

The audience to whom an economic evaluation will be presented helps determine the perspective that should be taken in the analysis. The perspective of a third party payer (e.g., a medical insurer or managed care organization) will include only costs to be borne by the paying organization, generally only direct

Table 16.1.

Types of costs and perspectives.

Cost Category	Specific Cost	Included in Which Perspective		
		Third-party Payer	Employer	Societal
Direct medical	Outpatient visits	X	X	X
	Inpatient hospitalizations	X	X	X
	Prescription drugs	X	X	X
	Durable medical equipment	X	X	X
	Nursing/home health care	X	X	X
	Over-the-counter medications			X
Direct non-medical	Transportation costs to/from appointments			X
Indirect	Patient lost productivity/work absenteeism		X	X
	Unpaid caregiver lost productivity/ work absenteeism			X

medical costs. A societal perspective is comprehensive and includes all costs associated with the intervention, including direct non-medical costs (e.g., transportation to and from medical visits) and indirect costs (e.g., decreased productivity, work loss days, caregiver time). Often both perspectives are included, with one presented as the primary analysis and the other as a secondary analysis. Table 16.1 provides an overview of various types of costs and in which perspective(s) they are included.

16.1.3 Analytical Methods for Economic Analysis

There are three principal methods for evaluating the cost-effectiveness (i.e., costs and outcomes) of an intervention: prospective studies, database analysis, and modeling. Often, these methods are used in combination to provide more complete information on cost-effectiveness.

Prospective evaluation of cost-effectiveness can be performed in two settings. First, the costs and benefits of a therapy can be evaluated as part of a clinical trial. As trials collect detailed safety and efficacy information, "piggy-backing" the collection of additional cost data is often feasible. However, clinical trial treatment patterns often do not reflect "real world" practice. For example, there may be more physician visits or laboratory testing required by the protocol than a typical patient would experience or a particular outcome or condition might be detected earlier through more intense follow-up. Further, patients partici-pating in trials may not be representative of the general patient population. These limitations do not indicate that cost-effectiveness analyses should not be performed using data from clinical trials, but that the limitations associated with trial-collected data need to be considered in such analyses. Cost-effectiveness can also be evaluated in prospective "naturalistic" studies. Such studies, generally performed after a drug or device has been approved, may randomize patients to different treatment arms but then follow the patients through their normal course of therapy with no other interventions or restric-tions. While such studies can provide detailed cost-effectiveness information, the time and cost of performing this type of study is often prohibitive. Retro-spective data sources may also be used for these types of analyses, although medical chart reviews are constrained by the type of information regularly recorded, which may not be sufficient for analyses.

Databases used for cost-effectiveness analyses can include medical claims from public or private insurance providers, or databases from registries, health surveys, or other naturalistic prospective studies. Each data source has advan-tages and disadvantages. Claims databases generally include broad and fairly complete information on medical resources used by the enrolled populations, at least on the resources that are covered by the insurance provider. Large claims databases often permit detailed subgroup analyses, such as analyses by comorbidities and specific types of procedures. However, claims databases are essentially designed for billing and administrative purposes and generally do not contain clinical findings (e.g., laboratory test results). Characteristics such as severity of disease, and even disease diagnosis, must be estimated based on resource use and associated diagnostic and procedure codes and often cannot be verified. Registries and health care surveys can avoid these limitations by collecting more complete information on patients' health status and clinical findings. However, such data are often based on patient self-report, which may not be fully accurate. The population included in a database must also be considered. For example, using a national database enhances generaliz-ability of the findings. Databases from particular populations (e.g., from patients receiving treatment at Veterans Affairs medical centers) are less gen-eralizable, but provide greater details on costs and outcomes applicable to specific groups.

In a number of countries, cost of illness studies can be conducted using fairly complete national insurance databases. In the United States, the distributed nature of the health care system makes it more challenging to assemble national costs. However, data on many types of conditions can be derived from nation-ally representative databases managed by the National Center for Health Sta-tistics. These data can be used to determine prevalence or incidence of disease, patient-reported use of health care resources, and mortality associated with a condition. Medicare data, which include inpatient, outpatient, laboratory, durable medical equipment, home health, and nursing home claims, can be used to estimate direct medical care costs (excluding, until recently, self-admin-istered medications) associated with conditions that are more common among the elderly. For example, the use of Medicare data for evaluating the medical costs attributable to nontrauma vertebral fractures is appropriate, as this older population experiences a much higher frequency of vertebral fractures than do those too young for Medicare.

Modeling is the other primary technique used for health economic analyses. Models can be developed using a variety of software packages and can range from simple spreadsheet calculations to very complex simulations with sophisticated graphic and computational capabilities. An important use of models is to assist in evaluating costs and outcomes when not all of the factors relevant to a medical treatment decision are known, that is, decision making under uncertainty. By including assumptions regarding uncertainties, models permit the evaluation of scenarios for which complete data are not available. Assumptions can be included regarding any input parameter to a model: the effectiveness of the intervention, the cost of the intervention, the time horizon over which benefits will accrue, etc. The robustness of models to assumptions (i.e., how much the modeled results change with changes in the assumptions) is evaluated in sensitivity analyses. In this manner, models can be used not only to estimate outcomes, but also to determine the key factors influencing outcomes and to detect thresholds at which certain outcomes will be achieved. For example, models can be developed and used early in a product (drug or device) development life cycle to determine the minimum effectiveness and/or safety needed for the product to be considered cost-effective compared to available competitors. Models that adhere to best practice guidelines for economic evaluation [Halpern et al. 1998] can be valuable tools despite their hypothetical nature; as George Box's words have been paraphrased, "all models are wrong; some of them are useful" [1979].

16.1.4 Keys to Interpreting Health Economic Models

The quality of a health economic study and its findings are dependent on the structure of the model, the appropriateness and reasonableness of the assumptions, and the analytical methods. Details on developing and interpreting models can be found in Halpern et al. [1998]. We provide an overview of issues relevant to economic modeling below.

The structure and duration of the model should be appropriate for answering the question and must reflect the complexity of the clinical situation. For example, a patient experiencing a vertebral fracture may be more likely to experience a second fracture in an adjacent vertebra. A model designed to follow long-term outcomes in this patient population would need to recognize previous experience in order to accurately project subsequent outcomes. A model looking at the infection rate for hip arthroplasty might only follow patients for three months after surgery and ignore whether patients had infections during any previous surgeries (unless prior infection was considered a risk factor for subsequent infections).

No matter how well supported, the validity of model assumptions should always be evaluated in sensitivity analyses. These analyses change the model's input parameters in order to reflect the variance (i.e., lack of certainty) in available parameter estimates. The inputs to the model should reflect anticipated use of the intervention, that is, the population and the setting should reflect real-world expected use. If possible, studies of real-world use rather than clinical trial outcomes should be used. To be more generalizable, costs should be derived from standardized sources rather than from individual hospitals or practices. Utilities (i.e., patient preferences for different health states) used in a cost-utility model should ideally be generated by patients rather than proxies (e.g., medical personnel or caregivers). If the model results change dramatically in response to reasonable changes in one or more input parameters, the model's findings are deemed sensitive to uncertainty and must be regarded cautiously. Every model report should include some overview of the sensitivity analyses performed and the findings of those analyses.

16.1.5 Issues Relevant for Evaluation of Spine Technologies

There are several issues that are important to remember when reviewing cost-effectiveness of medical devices in general. First, the costs may be distributed differently than drug therapies, and the time horizon of the analysis must consider this. For example, drug costs are likely to be fairly consistent over time; especially for patients with chronic conditions who have an established treatment regimen, medication costs will show little variability over the period of study. However, for medical devices, there may be initial high costs associated with a procedure (e.g., implantation) and with the device itself, while maintenance costs may be substantially lower than drug therapy. When comparing therapies with different cost structures, such as drugs versus medical devices, it is important to consider the duration of time over which the patient is expected to benefit. Further, to accurately evaluate both costs and benefits, it is also necessary to apply appropriate discounting (i.e., take into account time preferences, in that individuals generally prefer money and health more in the present than in the future). Health economic analyses use standard methods for incorporating time preferences.

A related question is whether health benefits of different potential therapies occur at the same rate. Medical devices can provide benefits very quickly; for example, in the case of kyphoplasty or vertebroplasty, pain relief and return to usual activities may take place very quickly compared to other treatment options. Thus, in comparing the costs and benefits of alternative therapies, the timing of benefits must be considered.

Another issue relevant to the economics of spine interventions is complete collection of all relevant costs. While many treatments for acute medical conditions may involve only limited categories of costs (e.g., drugs and outpatient visits), spine interventions may also involve costs for diagnostic and surgical procedures, rehabilitation, home health care, care in skilled nursing facilities, etc. For younger patients, the opportunity cost of a longer absence from work can also be important. The perspective of the analysis will determine, in part, the costs to be included. For example, there are likely to be substantial differences in the types of durable medical equipment (e.g., assist devices in the home) that are covered by insurers (either private or government). For a surgical intervention, the reimbursement by an insurer is an economic benefit from the perspective of a hospital while it is a cost in a societal perspective. From a hospital's perspective, additional operating room time may be considered a cost, while it does not affect the costs of an insurer who pays a capitated rate. Thus, careful consideration must be applied to the full range of costs and benefits that are likely to be relevant to different audiences.

16.2 What Do We Know About the Economics of Spine Technologies?

Multiple studies have been published evaluating the costs or cost-effectiveness of pharmacologic treatments for osteoporosis prevention or for rheumatic conditions affecting the spine, such as ankylosing spondylitis. A number of studies have also evaluated the cost-effectiveness of different imaging or rehabilitation strategies for individuals with spinal injuries. However, few studies have specifically evaluated the costs and benefits of surgical procedures and/or medical devices in treating spine conditions. Further, the methods used in published papers are often not thoroughly reported. Table 16.2 provides a summary of published cost analyses examining spine procedures. We exclude studies that evaluate drugs for osteoporosis, rheumatoid arthritis, or related conditions; radiology studies; studies of rehabilitative or preventive interventions; studies of neurological procedures involving the spinal cord or spinal nerves; and studies evaluating specific components of surgery (e.g., anesthesia or blood transfusion). Review of these studies can help identify gaps in the available information regarding spine procedures as well as challenges in applying economic methods to this clinical area. Recent tutorials on methods for economic evaluation in spinal conditions, such as those by Korthals-de Bos and colleagues [2004] and Bozic et al. [2003], summarize some of the key elements in performing these analyses.

16.2.1 Cost of Illness

To our knowledge, there are no studies that assess the cost of illness for spine conditions overall. The available studies either capture broad groups of conditions that include spine conditions (e.g., lower back pain), or focus on subgroups of spine conditions (e.g., vertebral compression fractures). The total cost of medical care for vertebral fractures in the United States has been estimated at $1.61 billion annually using Medicare data [Schmier et al. 2005]. Hospital costs associated with vertebral fractures have been assessed. In the EU, hospital costs for vertebral fractures have been estimated at €377 million annually [Finnern and Sykes 2003], while in the United States, annual hospital costs were estimated at $506 million [Burge et al. 2002].

Table 16.2.
Costs and cost-effectiveness of procedural interventions.

Citation	Study Design	Patient Population	Intervention	Outcomes / Findings
Ackerman et al., 2002	Cost analysis	Patient population from 2 prospective, randomized clinical trials	Bone morphogenetic protein vs. autogenous iliac crest bone graft for single-level anterior lumbar fusion	BMP appears to be cost neutral, based on offsets and reduced need for several medical services/costs associated with its use.
Angevine et al., 2005	Cost-effectiveness analysis: Decision-analysis and Markov models with 5 years of follow-up. Outcome measure is cost per QALY	Patients undergoing treatment for anterior one-level cervical spondylosis	Anterior cervical discectomy with fusion (ACDF) with autograft vs. ADCF with allograft vs ACDF with allograft and plating (ACDFP)	ACDF with allograft was $496/QALY compared to ACDF with autograft. ACDFP was $32,560/QALY compared to ACDF with allograft.
Burge et al., 2002	Cost of illness	Patients receiving inpatient care for vertebral fractures	Not applicable	In 1997, mean charges for hospital admissions for vertebral fractures in U.S. women were $9,532, with a mean length of stay of 6.2 days. More than 40% of admissions were discharged to long-term care facilities. Charges increased with age. Total annual charges for all vertebral fracture care were $506 million.
Castro et al., 2000	Cost analysis using site-specific hospital costs	Patients undergoing multi-level ACDF with ICBG and plating	Anterior cervical discectomy and fusion (ACDF) using titanium surgical mesh, local autologous bone graft, and anterior plate instrumentation (Cases, n = 27) vs. ACDF using autologous ICBG and anterior plate instrumentation (Controls, n = 27)	Cases had significantly shorter operating time (132 vs. 180 minutes) and significantly shorter hospital stays (1.7 vs. 2.9 days) than controls. Operative cost favored the controls (not significant) and total hospitalization costs favored the cases ($6,739 vs. $7,736, not significant). There may be improvements in long-term outcomes that could further offset the increased costs of the titanium surgical mesh.

Finnern and Sykes, 2003	Cost of illness	Patients receiving hospital-based treatment for vertebral fracture	Not applicable	Different practice patterns were evident, with hospital stays ranging from less than one day to more than 20. Total annual cost of vertebral fractures in the EU was estimated at €377 million.
Fritzell et al., 2004	Cost-effectiveness analysis using retrospective data. Outcome measures included societal total costs (direct and indirect), health care costs, ICER based on patient-rated pain, Oswestry disability index, and return to work	Patients with chronic low back pain for 2 years or more	Random assignment to one of three surgical procedures or conservative management	Incremental cost-effectiveness for one unit of improvement was SEK 2,600, for one unit of function 11,300, and for return to work 4,100. Meaningfulness of a unit of any outcome is unknown.
Hitchon et al., 1998	Cost-minimization analysis	Patients with thoracolumbar burst fractures	Operative treatment (n = 36) vs. non-operative recumbency (n = 32)	Surgery was approximately twice the cost of recumbency. Treatment selection should be based on clinical and radiological criteria.
Javid, 1995	Cost analysis	Consecutive patients with single-level lumbar disc disease	Chymopapain chemonucleolysis (n = 100) vs. lumbar laminectomy (n = 100)	Average savings associated with chemonucleolysis was $5,365 per patient. At six months, effectiveness was similar for both treatments, suggesting that chemonucleolysis may be cost-effective compared to laminectomy.
Karpinnen et al., 2001	Cost-effectiveness (data from subgroup of randomized controlled trial) Outcome measure is cost per responder	Patients with unilateral sciatica	Periradicular infiltration with methylprednisolone-bupivacaine (n = 80) vs. saline (n = 80)	For symptomatic lesions L3-L5, steroid treatment was significantly less costly to achieve one pain-free patient ($12,666 less than saline per responder) while it was significantly more costly for extrusions ($4,445 more than saline per responder). Costs and cost-effectiveness were compared by MRI classification and disc level.

Continued

Table 16.2. *Continued*

Citation	Study Design	Patient Population	Intervention	Outcomes / Findings
Katz et al., 1997	Cost analysis using site-specific hospital costs	Patients undergoing laminectomy for lumbar spinal stenosis	Laminectomy alone (n = 194) or with instrumented (n = 41) or noninstrumented (n = 37) arthrodesis	Hospital costs (total, surgical, and blood bank) were significantly lower for laminectomy alone. Length of stay was significantly lower for laminectomy alone. Outcomes (pain, satisfaction) were best for noninstrumented arthrodesis at 6 and 24 months.
Kuntz et al., 2000	Cost-effectiveness: Decision analysis model with 10-year duration. Outcome measure is cost per QALY	Patients with degenerative lumbar spondylolithesis and spinal stenosis	Laminectomy with noninstrumented fusion versus laminectomy without fusion versus no fusion	Compared to no fusion, noninstrumented fusion was $56,500/QALY. Compared to no fusion, instrumented fusion was over $3 million/QALY. Results were highly dependent on the success rate and the patient valuation of utilities.
Malter et al., 1996	Cost-effectiveness analysis. Outcome measure is cost per QALY	Patients with herniated disc	Lumbar discectomy (n = 372) vs. nonsurgical treatment (n = 1,803)	At 10 years after diagnosis, surgery was cost-effective ($33,900/QALY) when costs and outcomes were discounted at 5%.
McLaughlin et al., 1997	Cost effectiveness analysis using site-specific hospital charges. Outcome measures are $/day for return to normal activities, $/day for return to work	Patients with radiculopathy or degenerative disease	Anterior cervical discectomy and fusion with (n = 39) or without (n = 25) rigid internal fixation	Total charges were significantly higher for the plated patients. Return to light activities was similar across groups. Return to unrestricted activities was significantly faster for the plated patients. Incremental cost-effectiveness was $213/day for return to normal activities and $31/day for return to work.

Polly et al., 2003	Cost analysis: Decision analysis model with 2-year duration	Patients undergoing single-level anterior lumbar fusion	Bone morphogenetic protein (BMP) vs. autogenous iliac crest bone graft (AICBG)	Increased BMP costs associated with the index hospitalization were offset over 2 years by savings due to increased costs for AICBG associated with iliac crest harvesting, operating room time, autograft extenders/harvesters, and inpatient stay. Over 2 years, BMP was $9 less expensive.
Ramirez and Javid, 1985	Cost analysis	Consecutive patients with single-level lumbar disc disease being treated at a university hospital	Chymopapain chemonucleolysis (n = 40) vs. lumbar laminectomy (n = 40)	Average cost per patient: $4,163 for chemonucleolysis vs. $6,124 for laminectomy. After weighting costs for re-operation, chemonucleolysis resulted in an average cost per patient $1,808 less than laminectomy.
Rivero-Arias et al., 2005	Cost-effectiveness analysis. Outcome measure is cost (to National Health Service) per QALY (assessed using EuroQol) 24-month time frame	UK patients age 18–55 with chronic low back pain of at least one year's duration who were candidates for spinal fusion surgery	Random assignment to surgery (n = 176) or rehabilitation (n = 173)	ICER: £48,588 per QALY (2002–2003 £) Sensitivity analyses evaluated cost per QALY if all procedures were least or most costly or if it were assumed that patients needed to undergo both therapies over time; surgery generally remained cost-effective.
Shvartzman et al., 1992	Cost analysis	Patients with herniated lumbar intervertebral disc not responding to an initial trial of conservative therapy	Surgical treatment (n = 25) vs. continued conservative therapy (n = 30)	There was no significant difference in effectiveness or costs by treatment. Only direct costs were included in the study; patients who had continued conservative treatment missed significantly more work and may have incurred higher indirect costs.

Continued

Table 16.2. *Continued*

Citation	Study Design	Patient Population	Intervention	Outcomes / Findings
Slotman & Stein, 1996	Cost analysis using site-specific hospital charges	Patients with herniated disks unresponsive to conservative treatment	Laminectomy (n = 23) vs. laparoscopic L5–S1 discectomy (LLD) (n = 22)	Inpatient charges were significantly lower for LLD patients. LLD patients also had significantly shorter stays, less rehabilitation, and quicker return to normal activity. No ICER presented.
Stevenson et al., 1995	Cost analysis	Patients undergoing treatment for contained lumbar herniation in a randomized clinical trial	Automated percutaneous lumbar discectomy (APLD) vs. microdiscectomy	Costs were similar in both groups, but APLD was less effective, suggesting that microdiscectomy is the more cost-effective option.
Tunturi et al., 1979	Cost-benefit analysis	Patients previously failing conservative treatment	Posterior fusion of the lumbosacral spine (n = 133)	Benefits of one lumbosacral fusion equaled $16,075, reflecting a cost-benefit ratio of 1:2.9. Costs included direct medical (hospital) costs, transportation to the hospital, and postoperative work output efficiency.
Whitecloud et al., 2001	Cost analysis	Patients undergoing anterior column reconstruction	Transforaminal interbody fusion (TFIL) (n = 40) vs. anterior-posterior interbody fusion of lumbar spine (n = 40)	TFIL patients had significantly lower hospital costs. No clinical outcomes were reported.

Abbreviations: QALY = quality-adjusted life year; ICER = incremental cost-effectiveness ratio.

16.2.2 Cost-minimization and Cost Analysis

Cost-minimization studies generally fall into two categories. Either researchers have formally decided to conduct a cost-minimization study or they have conducted one by default. In the former case, researchers have recognized that outcomes are likely to be almost identical between treatment groups and they realize that the only difference is cost, thus justifying the cost-minimization approach. In the latter case, they may have designed cost-effectiveness studies that were not fully implemented. Many of the studies identified in the literature as cost-effectiveness are misnamed. Although they present costs and may, in some cases, provide some clinical outcome information, without presenting the cost per outcome achieved, the studies are not true evaluations of cost-effectiveness. A disadvantage of cost-minimization studies is that they may lack external validity, as costs are often based on a single site, and the lack of effectiveness measure makes it difficult to compare results to other interventions or studies.

Bone morphogenetic protein (BMP) was compared to autogenous iliac crest bone graft for single-level anterior lumbar fusion based on data from two randomized clinical trials [Ackerman et al. 2002]. Preliminary analyses suggest that the increased cost of BMP was likely to be offset by reduced costs associated with side effects and a higher failure rate with autogenous iliac crest bone graft. The study also evaluated the increase in fusion success rate that would be necessary to justify various price points for bone morphogenetic protein. For example, considering the costs of the fusion only, BMP would have to increase the fusion success rate by 17.0% in order to justify a cost of $3,000, while if BMP cost $7,000, it would have to increase the fusion success rate by 39.7% to justify its cost. Despite not providing a cost-effectiveness ratio, this threshold analysis is a useful tool for assessing BMP under uncertainty.

Several other studies have also estimated costs and outcomes but do not present cost-effectiveness ratios. Katz and colleagues evaluated laminectomy alone or with instrumented or noninstrumented arthrodesis [1997]. The study found that laminectomy with instrumented arthrodesis did not appear to be cost-effective compared to the alternatives; all costs were lower for laminectomy alone and outcomes were best for noninstrumented arthrodesis. Another study comparing chemonucleolysis to laminectomy found that there were cost savings associated with chemonucleolysis and while laminectomy patients tended to have better outcomes at 6 weeks, by six months, outcomes were similar, suggesting that chemonucleolysis is cost-effective [Javid 1995]. A previous study had found a smaller but still notable cost savings associated with chemonucleolysis [Ramirez and Javid 1985]. Slotman and Stein found that laparoscopic L5-S1 discectomy (LLD) was cost saving compared to laminectomy, as there were lower charges, less rehabilitation, and quicker return to normal activity with LLD [Slotman and Stein 1996]. Hitchon and colleagues suggest that patients' clinical and radiographic characteristics may determine whether surgical or nonsurgical treatment is a more cost-appropriate option for patients with thoraco lumbar junction burst fractures [1998].

Castro et al. found Anterior Cervical Discectomy and Fusion (ACDF) using titanium surgical mesh to be similar in cost and outcomes to using iliac crest bone graft [Castro et al. 2000]. Stevenson et al. found that microdiscectomy appeared to have similar costs but better outcomes than automated percutaneous lumbar discectomy and may be more cost-effective [Stevenson, McCabe, and Findlay 1995]. Patients undergoing transforaminal interbody fusion may have lower costs than those undergoing anterior-posterior interbody fusion of the lumbar spine, but no information on outcomes accompanied a cost analysis [Whitecloud, Roesch, and Ricciardi 2001]. Compared to conservative treatment, surgical treatment for patients with a herniated lumbar intervertebral disc resulted in similar costs and outcomes, when only direct costs were considered [Shvartzman et al. 1992]. Since patients receiving conservative treatment had more lost workdays, if indirect costs would have been considered, it is likely that surgical treatment would have been less costly.

16.2.3 Cost-benefit

Although generally out of favor, there are studies that have addressed the economic impact of spinal technologies using cost-benefit methods. For example, the cost of one lumbo-sacral fusion was found to be $16,075, taking into account hospital costs, transportation to/from hospital, and postoperative work output [Tunturi et al. 1979]. The cost-benefit ratio for fusion was 1 to 2.9; that is, for every dollar spent on fusion, 2.9 dollars were saved in subsequent costs that would have occurred had the fusion not been performed. Given the difficulties and uncertainties of CBA, it is unlikely that newer technologies will be evaluated using this method.

16.2.4 Cost-effectiveness and Cost-utility

Spinal surgeries are good examples of interventions in which a cost-effectiveness analysis is a particularly useful tool for evaluating costs relative to outcomes. The particular outcomes to be used in CEA of spinal interventions require attention. Many spinal injuries cause some amount of morbidity but are not life threatening; therefore, the cost per year of life saved is not an appropriate outcome measure. Similarly, while certain spine injuries do result in increased mortality [Lau et al. 2005], data are not currently available indicating that different interventions have differential impacts on mortality. In these cases, the effectiveness measure between two interventions could be "treatment success," defined as patient satisfaction, relief from symptoms, and/or return to work. Other outcome metrics could be functional status, quality of life, disability, or pain control. There are multiple scales available for assessing these outcomes in spinal injuries, many of which are available in the North American Spine Society's Compendium of Outcome Instruments [Gatchel 2001]. In cost-utility analysis, a subset of CEA, the outcome measure is generally quality-adjusted life years (QALYs). QALYs are calculated using utilities, measures of patient preference for a given health condition rated on a scale from 0 to 1.0 where 0 represents death and 1.0 represents perfect health. Utilities are used to calculate quality-adjusted life years (QALYs) by weighting time spent in a particular health state by the rating provided for that health state, and the resulting ratio metric is expressed as the cost per QALY. Utility values at initiation into a clinical trial for treatment of low back pain through 24 months' of follow-up ranged from approximately 0.35 to 0.55 in a recent study [Rivero-Arias 2005]. Although there is no consensus on the cost per QALY that is a threshold for cost-effectiveness, studies using this common metric of cost per QALY can usually be easily compared with each other.

Several studies have compared surgical vs. conventional treatments. For example, Fritzell et al. compared the cost-effectiveness of lumbar fusion to non-surgical treatment for chronic low back pain [2004]. The study estimated two-year costs for 284 Swedish patients who had experienced chronic low back pain for two years prior to being randomized to lumbar fusion or usual care. Costs are presented for two perspectives, that of the health care sector and societal. Several different measures were used as outcomes, that is, the denominator in the cost-effectiveness ratio: patient-reported global improvement, patient-rated back pain, an index of disability, and time to return to work. They present the incremental cost of lumbar fusion compared to nonsurgical treatment for an additional unit in each of these outcome measures. Fusion was more costly but also resulted in better outcomes. However, because these are study-specific outcomes, it is not possible to compare these findings directly with other studies.

Malter and Weinstein compared the cost-effectiveness of lumbar discectomy compared to nonsurgical treatment among patients with a herniated disc [1996]. This study looked at outcomes 10 years after diagnosis and discounted both costs and outcomes at 5%. Surgery was found to be cost-effective, at $33,900 per QALY. Rivero-Arias and colleagues also looked at the cost per QALY of surgery vs. nonsurgical treatment among UK patients [2005]. This study took the perspective of the UK National Health Service and used clinical outcomes data from a randomized clinical trial. The study used a mix of methods to identify costs. Some costs were standard while others were developed by costing individual resources (e.g., the cost of surgery was based on the cost of all the components of surgery rather than using a single standard cost). Costs and utilities were discounted at 3.5% per year and costs are presented in £2002–2003. In these analyses, surgery was more costly and did not provide sufficiently better outcomes to justify the incremental cost. The analyses generally indicated that the cost-utility for surgery compared to nonsurgical treatment was more than £30,000 per QALY, the de facto threshold in the UK. Sensitivity analyses suggest that a number of factors could affect this conclusion, including the costs incurred after two years and the proportion of rehabilitation patients who later incur surgery.

Laminectomy has also been evaluated using cost-utility analysis. Kuntz and colleagues evaluated the cost-effectiveness of laminectomy vs. laminectomy with concomitant lumbar fusion [2000]. In the base case, the addition of fusion to laminectomy results in $56,500 per QALY compared to laminectomy without fusion. Sensitivity analysis revealed that the results were highly dependent on the proportion of patients experiencing symptom relief (and thus having higher utility ratings, higher QALYs, and a lower cost per QALY).

McLaughlin and colleagues highlighted indirect costs in their cost-effectiveness analysis of ACDF with and without rigid internal fixation [McLaughlin, Purighalla, and Pizzi 1997]. Although their study used hospital-specific costs and may not be generalized, the outcome measures are worth noting: cost-effectiveness was assessed as the cost per day until return to normal activities and cost per day until return to work. Total charges were higher for plated patients, but at a cost of $31/day until return to work, it may be considered the cost-effective option. Angevine et al. also compared types of ACDF: with autograft, allograft, and allograft with plating [2005]. This analysis used decision analysis techniques to follow patients for five years after surgery. ACDF with allograft was cost-effective compared to ACDF with autograft, at a cost of $496/QALY. ACDF with allograft and plating was compared to ACDF with allograft but without plating and was also cost-effective, at a cost of $32,500/QALY. The model was robust and results remained similar in sensitivity analyses.

Cost-effectiveness of periradicular infiltration with steroid was compared to saline in a study of patients with unilateral sciatica [Karpinnen et al. 2001]. The outcome used in this study was the cost per responder, i.e., a pain-free patient. For patients with symptomatic lesions at L3-L5, steroid treatment was less costly ($12,666 less per responder) than saline; however among patients with extrusions, steroid treatment was more expensive ($4,445 more per responder) than saline. This finding reinforces the point that clinical and radiographic characteristics should be considered in determining the most appropriate treatment for patients.

16.2.5 Reimbursement

Approval by the Food and Drug Administration does not imply that a product will be covered by Medicare or Medicaid or that private insurers will decide to reimburse for it. The process of obtaining coverage through the Centers for Medicare and Medicaid Services (CMS) is currently not predicated on cost-effectiveness but rather only safety and efficacy. Suitable codes for reimbursement must be obtained, and ensuring that reimbursement rates are appropriate involves balancing the costs and benefits of new technologies with the corresponding measures for current standards of care. Private coverage does tend to consider costs and cost-effectiveness in determining whether to cover interventions. There is a strong precedent of requiring cost-effectiveness studies for pharmacological agents for registration and reimbursement in Europe and for reimbursement in the United States; it is often considered the "fourth hurdle" after quality, safety, and efficacy [Taylor et al. 2004].

16.3 Conclusions

Economic evaluations of spine technologies are not as common, and in general not as sophisticated, as evaluations for pharmacological therapies. However, an increasing number of rigorous cost analyses are being conducted on spine technologies to answer a growing demand for product registration, insurance coverage, and demonstration of the advantages for new technologies that are more expensive than existing treatments.

There are several important points to consider in evaluating spine technologies. First, studies have identified substantial costs associated with vertebral fractures in the United States and EU. Additional research needs to be conducted into the cost of other related conditions, to justify the costs associated with preventive and therapeutic technologies. Even a small decrease in costs resulting from use of new technologies becomes noteworthy when considering spinal conditions with large numbers of cases overall. Especially when a large insurer, such as Medicare or a national insurance program, is responsible for these costs, small decreases in per patient costs can have a substantial impact on the overall budget.

Second, the duration of the study can have an important impact on costs. Studies that include only acute hospitalization costs may answer questions for which hospitals want answers, but several studies have documented increased hospitalization costs that were in turn offset over time by reductions in chronic care costs. Study duration must be appropriate to the condition and to the technologies being used in order for findings to reflect real differences between treatments and to address the information needs of the health care provider or insurer.

Third, the inclusion of indirect costs, such as lost productivity, is likely to be relevant for spine conditions. Particularly for patients who are younger and likely to be working, differences in anticipated lost work (absenteeism and/or decreased productivity) must be an important part of the decision-making process. Back pain is second only to headache pain in terms of its impact on work absence in the United States [Stewart et al. 2003] and one of the top 10 most costly conditions to employers [Goetzel et al. 2003]. Ekman and colleagues found that indirect costs were responsible for 85% of total costs associated with chronic low back pain [2005]. Workplace effects of other spine conditions should also be considered.

Recent studies of spine technologies have addressed cost comparisons using appropriate methods. As the field continues to grow, it can benefit from ongoing discussions and advances in methodology. Careful attention to existing guidelines for economic and outcomes evaluations will be important to select appropriate methods to capture the specific impacts of spinal technologies and other medical devices. Results from studies using appropriate methods will be crucial in supporting further adoption of cost-effective therapies.

16.4 References

Ackerman, S. J., M. S. Mafilios, and D. W. Polly, Jr. (2002). "Economic Evaluation of Bone Morphogenetic Protein Versus Autogenous Iliac Crest Bone Graft in Single-level Anterior Lumbar Fusion: An Evidence-based Modeling Approach," *Spine* 27:S94–S99.

Academy of Managed Care Pharmacy (2005). *AMCP Format for Formulary Submissions (Version 2.1).* Alexandria: Academy of Managed Care Pharmacy.

Angevine, P. D., J. G. Zivin, and P. C. McCormick (2005). "Cost-effectiveness of Single-level Anterior Cervical Discectomy and Fusion for Cervical Spondylosis," *Spine* 30:1989–1997.

Box, G. (1979). "Some Problems of Statistics and Everyday Life," *Journal of the American Statistical Association* 74:1–4.

Bozic, K. J., A. G. Rosenberg, R. S. Huckman, and J. H. Herndon (2003). "Economic Evaluation in Orthopaedics," *J Bone Joint Surg Am* 85A:129–142.

Burge, R., E. Puleo, S. Gehlbach, et al. (2002). "Inpatient Hospital and Post-acute Care for Vertebral Fractures in Women,". *Value Health* 5:301–311.

Castro, F. P., Jr, R. T. Holt, M. Majd, and T. S. Whitecloud, 3rd (2000). "A cost Analysis of Two Anterior Cervical Fusion Procedures," *J Spinal Disord* 13:511–514.

Ekman, M., S. Jonhagen, E. Hunsche, and L. Jonsson (2005). "Burden of Illness of Chronic Low Back Pain in Sweden: A Cross-sectional, Retrospective Study in Primary Care Setting," *Spine* 30:1777–1785.

Elixhauser, A., M. Halpern, J. Schmier, and B. R. Luce (1998). "Health Care CBA and CEA from 1991 to 1996: An Updated Bibliography," *Med Care* 36:MS1–9, MS18–147.

Finnern, H. W., and D. P. Sykes (2003). "The Hospital Cost of Vertebral Fractures in the EU: Estimates Using National Datasets," *Osteoporos Int* 14:429–436.

Fritzell, P., O. Hagg, D. Jonsson, and A. Nordwall (2004). "Cost-effectiveness of Lumbar Fusion and Nonsurgical Treatment for Chronic Low Back Pain in the Swedish Lumbar Spine Study: A Multicenter, Randomized, Controlled Trial from the Swedish Lumbar Spine Study Group," *Spine* 29:421–434; discussion Z423.

Gatchel, R. J., Ed. (2001). *Compendium of Outcome Instruments for Assessment and Research of Spinal Disorders.* La Grange, IL: North American Spine Society.

Goetzel, R. Z., K. Hawkins, R. J. Ozminkowski, and S. Wang (2003). "The Health and Productivity Cost Burden of the "Top 10" Physical and Mental Health Conditions Affecting Six Large U.S. Employers in 1999," *J Occup Environ Med* 45:5–14.

Gold, M. R., J. E. Siegel, L. B. Russel, and M. C. Weinstein, Eds. (1996). *Cost-effectiveness in Health and Medicine.* New York: Oxford University Press.

Halpern, M. T., B. R. Luce, R. E. Brown, and B. Geneste (1998). "Health and Economic Outcomes Modeling Practices: A Suggested Framework," *Value in Health* 1:131–147.

Hitchon, P. W., J. C. Torner, S. F. Haddad, and K. A. Follett (1998). "Management Options in Thoracolumbar Burst Fractures," *Surg Neurol* 49:619–626; discussion 617–626.

Javid, M. J. (1995). "Chemonucleolysis Versus Laminectomy. A Cohort Comparison of Effectiveness and Charges," *Spine* 20:2016–2022.

Katz, J. N., S. J. Lipson, R. A. Lew, et al. (1997). "Lumbar Laminectomy Alone or with Instrumented or Noninstrumented Arthrodesis in Degenerative Lumbar Spinal Stenosis. Patient Selection, Costs, and Surgical Outcomes," *Spine* 22:1123–1131.

Korthals-de Bos, I., M. van Tulder, H. van Dieten, and L. Bouter (2004). "Economic Evaluations and Randomized Trials in Spinal Disorders: Principles and Methods," *Spine* 29:442–448.

Kuntz, K. M., R. K. Snider, J. N. Weinstein, et al. (2000). "Cost-effectiveness of Fusion with and Without Instrumentation for Patients with Degenerative Spondylolisthesis and Spinal Stenosis," *Spine* 25:1132–1139.

Lau, E., S. Kurtz, J. Schmier, et al. (2005). Mortality Following Diagnosis of Vertebral Compression Fracture (VCF) in the Medicare Population. North American Spine Society 20th Annual Meeting. Philadelphia, PA.

Levin, H. M., and P. J. McEwan (2001). *Cost-effectiveness Analysis: Methods and Applications* (2nd ed). Thousand Oaks, CA: Sage Publications.

Malter, A. D., and J. Weinstein (1996). "Cost-effectiveness of Lumbar Discectomy," *Spine* 21:69S–74S.

McLaughlin, M. R., V. Purighalla, and F. J. Pizzi (1997). "Cost advantages of Two-level Anterior Cervical Fusion with Rigid Internal Fixation for Radiculopathy and Degenerative disease," *Surg Neurol* 48:560–565.

Polly, D. W., Jr., S. J. Ackerman, C. I. Shaffrey, et al. (2003). "A Cost Analysis of Bone Morphogenetic Protein Versus Autogenous Iliac Crest Bone Graft in Single-level Anterior Lumbar Fusion," *Orthopedics* 26:1027–1037.

Ramirez, L. F., and M. J. Javid (1985). "Cost Effectiveness of Chemonucleolysis Versus Laminectomy in the Treatment of Herniated Nucleus Pulposus," *Spine* 10:363–367.

Rivero-Arias, O., H. Campbell, A. Gray, et al. (2005). "Surgical Stabilisation of the Spine Compared with a Programme of Intensive Rehabilitation for the Management of Patients with Chronic Low Back Pain: Cost Utility Analysis Based on a Randomised Controlled Trial," *BMJ* 330:1239.

Schmier, J., M. Halpern, S. Kurtz, et al. (2005). Medical Care Costs Associated with Vertebral Fractures Among Medicare Beneficiaries, 1997 to 2001. North American Spine Society 20th Annual Meeting. Philadelphia, PA.

Shvartzman, L., E. Weingarten, H. Sherry, et al. (1992). "Cost-effectiveness Analysis of Extended Conservative Therapy Versus Surgical Intervention in the Management of Herniated Lumbar Intervertebral Disc," *Spine* 17:176–182.

Stevenson, R. C., C. J. McCabe, and A. M. Findlay (1995). "An Economic Evaluation of a Clinical Trial to Compare Automated Percutaneous Lumbar Discectomy with Microdiscectomy in the Treatment of Contained Lumbar Disc Herniation," *Spine* 20:739–742.

Stewart, A., J. K. Schmier, and B. R. Luce (1999). "Economics and Cost-effectiveness in Evaluating the Value of Cardiovascular Therapies. A Survey of Standards and Guidelines for Cost-effectiveness Analysis in Health care," *Am Heart J* 137:S53–61.

Stewart, W. F., J. A. Ricci, E. Chee, D. Morganstein, and R. Lipton (2003). "Lost Productive Time and Cost Due to Common Pain Conditions in the US Workforce," *JAMA* 290(18):2443–2454.

Taylor, R. S., M. F. Drummomd, G. Salkeld, and S. Sullivan (2004). "Inclusion of Cost Effectiveness in Licensing Requirements of New Drugs: The Fourth Hurdle," *BMJ* 329:972–975.

Tunturi, T., P. Niemela, J. Laurinkari, et al. (1979). "Cost-benefit Analysis of Posterior Fusion of the Lumbosacral Spine," *Acta Orthop Scand* 50:427–432.

Whitecloud, T. S., 3rd, W. W. Roesch, and J. E. Ricciardi (2001). "Transforaminal Interbody Fusion Versus Anterior-posterior Interbody Fusion of the Lumbar Spine: A Financial Analysis," *J Spinal Disord* 14:100–103.

Index

Printed and bound by CPI Group (UK) Ltd, Croydon, CR0 4YY

03/10/2024

01040312-0005